500

of the most important
HEALTH TIPS
YOU'LL EVER NEED

An A–Z of alternative health hints
to help over 250 conditions

Hazel Courteney

Consultant Editor
Dr Karen Vieira

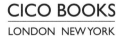

CICO BOOKS
LONDON NEW YORK

Published in 2011 by CICO Books
an imprint of Ryland Peters and Small
519 Broadway, 5th Floor
New York NY 10012
www.cicobooks.com

10 9 8 7 6 5 4 3 2 1

A CIP catalog record for this book is available from the Library of Congress.

ISBN: 978 1 907030 76 5

Printed in the US

Consultant editor: Dr Karen Vieira
Jacket design: Jerry Goldie Graphic Design
Design: Jerry Goldie Graphic Design

PUBLISHERS' NOTE:
Always consult a doctor before undertaking any of the advice, exercise plans, or
supplements suggested in this book. While every attempt has been made to
ensure the medical information in this book is entirely safe, correct, and up to
date at the time of publication, the Publishers accept no responsibility for
consequences of the advice given herein. If in any doubt as to the nature of
your condition, consult a qualified medical practitioner.

The Publishers also accept no responsibility for changes in prices, supplier
arrangements, and locations mentioned herein.

Hazel Courteney is an award-winning, respected health and metaphysical writer and speaker based in the UK. In 1997 she was voted Health Journalist of the Year for her column in *The Sunday Times*. This is her fourth health book. Hazel has also written three highly acclaimed spiritual metaphysical books. For more information on Hazel's work, log on to her website at www.hazelcourteney.com

Other books by Hazel Courteney:
500 of the Most Important Ways to Stay Younger Longer
Divine Intervention
The Evidence for the Sixth Sense
Countdown to Coherence
Mind and Mood Foods
Body and Beauty Foods

Stephen Langley MSc, ND, DipHom, DBM, DipAc, DCH, OMD is a registered naturopath, homeopath, acupuncturist, doctor of Chinese medicine, and medical herbalist. He lectures in naturopathic medicine at the College of Naturopathic Medicine (CNM) in London, Bristol, Manchester, Dublin, Galway and Belfast, as well as running a busy health practice in London and lecturing globally. Stephen has studied holistic medicine in China, India, America, Australia, Tibet, and Japan. He can be reached via the Hale Clinic in London at 011-44-20-7631-0156.

Gareth Zeal BSc is a nutritionist and health writer with 25 years' experience. He runs a busy health practice in North Yorkshire and regularly lectures around the UK. You can reach him via his office at 011-44-1287-280733.

Author's note

Throughout the book, we have in many instances suggested specific amounts of nutrients. This is to ensure that sufficient amounts of the nutrient are taken to benefit a specific condition. In places where no specific amounts are suggested, take the supplements daily, according to the instructions on the label or from your healthcare professional.

We have mentioned books that we have found useful, but whatever you are suffering from, believe me, there is a specialist book on it. Remember, you will fail only if you give up.

This book is not intended as a substitute for conventional medical counseling. Never stop taking prescription medication without first consulting with your doctor. Make sure you always inform your doctor of any supplements or herbs you are taking in case they are contraindicated with your drugs.

During the last 25 years I have read hundreds of books and many phrases and facts have remained in my mind. Wherever possible, I have acknowledged the source of these phrases and facts, and to those whose names I have forgotten, my apologies for any unintentional oversights.

I also want to clarify that I personally am not paid in **any** way whatsoever to mention specific companies, nutrients or products. I mention supplements that have good research behind them or those recommended by highly qualified professionals that will help heal or prevent various conditions.

For the latest update on FDA rulings regarding which supplements may or may not be available in the future, see pages 9–10.

Acknowledgments

Revising and greatly updating this latest edition has been an intensive seven-month labor of love. Several wonderful people have contributed to make this book truly special. To my co-authors, Stephen Langley and Gareth Zeal—thanks for spending several days each with me to keep me up to date on the latest health news and research. And Steve, thanks for reading the proofs; your patience and integrity have been much appreciated.

Thanks also to nutritional physician Dr Shamin Daya from the Wholistic Medical Centre in London. Also to my dear friend Bob Jacobs, naturopath, homeopath and nutritional scientist at the Society of Complementary Medicine in London, for your specialist help with the Breast Cancer, Cancer, Menopause, Osteoporosis, and Thyroid sections. Thank you both for your time, advice, and sharing your cutting-edge knowledge.

My gratitude also goes to bio-electromagnetics scientist Dr Roger Coghill for his help on Electrical Pollution, Jet Lag, and Insomnia.

This section would not be complete without also sending a big hug to my ex-PA, Lindsay Ross-Jarrett, who checked hundreds of contact details.

Finally, thanks as always to my wonderful husband Stuart—who has the patience of a saint.

DEDICATION

This book is dedicated to Sue Croft who for more than
thirty years has devoted her life, often without reward, to
ensuring our freedom to purchase higher-dose vitamins,
minerals and herbs is retained.
Thank you Sue for always being so positive, professional,
cheerful, and helpful. You are a very special lady.

INTRODUCTION

WHY THERE IS STILL AN URGENT NEED FOR THIS BOOK

Einstein's definition of insanity was "To keep doing the same thing over and over again—and expect different results." He was right.

If I told you that 85% of your health problems, including chronic degenerative diseases associated with ageing, could be prevented, cured or greatly alleviated by simply changing your diet and taking the right supplements, would you believe me? Yet it's true.

For example, the World Cancer Research Fund and the American Institute for Cancer Research have stated that as many as 38% of cases of breast cancer in the United States could be avoided by following a healthier lifestyle, drinking less alcohol, maintaining a sensible weight by eating more healthily, and exercising regularly. Published studies carried out at the School of Medicine in Puerto Rico by Professor Jaime Matta have found definitive evidence that women who take long-term multi-vitamins and mineral supplements reduce their risk for developing breast cancer by almost 30%. Another study from the Institute of Brain Chemistry and Human Nutrition at London's Metropolitan University found that women who take multi-vitamins and minerals, including vitamin D, folic acid, B vitamins, antioxidants and iron, give birth to bigger and generally healthier babies.

With more than 500,000 positive research papers regarding diet and supplements, plus freely available health information through the Internet and media, you would think that our overall health would be improving—yet sadly, in many cases the opposite is happening. Without a doubt some people are living longer, but not necessarily healthier, lives. Most people may be aware of what constitutes a healthy diet, yet they continue to prefer junk foods and lifestyles, without taking responsibility, or caring about the long-term consequences of their actions. We are still talking about being healthy, yet the statistics demonstrate that we are becoming one of the "sickest" nations on earth.

The United States spent more than $2.3 trillion on health care in 2008—equating to approximately $7,681 per resident and 16.2% of the nation's Gross Domestic Product (GDP). However, despite this sizable investment, the US consistently ranks as the worst healthcare system among developed nations, especially with regards to infant mortality rate, healthy life expectancy and obesity, diabetes, hypertension and heart attack rate.

Cardiovascular disease remains the largest killer in the West. It kills more than 800,000 people annually in the US alone and cost $475.3 billion in 2009. One in every three people will develop cancer at some point in their lives; 50 years ago, this was 1 in 27.

Obesity is reaching epidemic proportions, and if it continues at this rate it will cost the US healthcare system $344 billion by 2018. Since 1980, the number of children in the US who are obese has tripled. Now one in every five children in the US is obese. Furthermore, more than 72 million men and women in the US—approximately one-third of the population—are obese. With many adults and children ingesting as many as 40 teaspoons of refined sugars daily, from refined cereals, pre-packaged meals, cereals and fizzy drinks, is it any wonder we are piling on the pounds?

Such habits have triggered an explosion of type II (late-onset) diabetes, which affects around 23.6 million people in the US and 246 million globally. And "late-onset" diabetes, which 25 years ago was unheard of in anyone under 50, is now affecting children as young as 15.

All the above, plus an ever-escalating increase in people suffering from age-related conditions such as late-onset dementia, are creating an enormous burden on the US healthcare system.

The continuing tragedy is that virtually all these conditions are, in the majority of cases, totally preventable.
Thanks to First Lady Michelle Obama's high-profile anti-obesity campaign, *Let's Move*, thousands of adults and children are becoming more aware of what constitutes a healthy diet. Many supermarkets and food manufacturers are also gradually eliminating hydrogenated trans-fats, which raise LDL, the "bad" cholesterol, thus contributing to heart disease, strokes, obesity, dementia and cancers. Sodium-based salts and refined sugars are also coming under fire as public awareness grows of their negative effects on health.

However, we still have some way to go: the number of Americans drinking alcohol has hit a 25-year high, as has the incidence of binge drinking.

Even though smoking has thankfully been banned from public places in many states, nearly 25 million people in the US still smoke. And four out of five smokers tend to take up this dreadful habit before the age of 18.

Human nature is perverse: we may know what's healthy, but too many of us are still not acting on the information available! Why? Because most of us tend to think that it's never going to happen to us … until it does.

How much better it would be if we could take not only a lot more responsibility for our own health, but also learn more about our bodies, with the aim of stopping them from becoming sick in the first place. Unfortunately, too many people still hand total responsibility for their health to their overworked doctor. Most doctors are caring, hard-working people, but unless they have a specific interest in how diet and supplements can prevent or heal many conditions, they are often lacking this type of information. During their four years' training at medical school, very few receive even a day's training in how diet, lifestyle and taking the right supplements can greatly improve and prevent many illnesses. Most of their courses are still sponsored by drugs companies, which is why prescribing a pill for our illnesses remains their usual response. But this practice rarely addresses the root cause of the condition.

Almost everyone is looking for a single magic bullet to help alleviate their health problems. Most of us are in a hurry and yet happy to react to misleading and often incorrect or misquoted health information that appears in the media with alarming regularity. But help is at hand. Certified organic food sales continue to grow and, contrary to media reports, organic fruit and vegetables have been proven to contain more vitamins and minerals than their non-organic counterparts.

The more we eat organic, the less hormone-disrupting chemicals we swallow. As an example, a non-organic lettuce may have been sprayed 11 or more times during its brief growing cycle and the average apple is sprayed 18 times with a cocktail of chemicals.

In addition, in 2000 I also wrote about how the millions of cell phones in use were linked with depression and various cancers. By 2010 more than 285 million cell phones had been connected in the US—many for use by children—even though governments around the world have issued warnings that children ages 12 and under should not use mobile phones. If you add the cumulative negative effects of mobile phones, microwaves, computers and all electrical equipment that pulse us with harmful electromagnetic radiation to the effects of a negative diet and lifestyle, you soon realize that all these factors combine to trigger the tidal wave of illnesses we are experiencing today. Our bodies were never designed to eat so much junk and ingest so many chemicals, and they are telling us that they have simply had enough. **We** have caused most of the problems we face today—but the good news is that we can change or reverse many of them.

The development of MRSA and C. *difficile* have been triggered by our overuse of antibiotics, but many doctors don't know that manuka honey as well as herbs such as pau d'arco, beta glucans and essential oils of oregano and thyme are known to help destroy MRSA and other superbugs. They are also unlikely to know that a leaky gut is often the root cause of many other conditions, including eczema, and most autoimmune problems such as lupus, which are now on the rise.

With so many diseases on the increase, and with various bacteria mutating into deadlier strains faster than doctors can kill them, the time has come to discover new ways to protect ourselves.

For this reason I and my co-authors, Stephen Langley and Gareth Zeal, have **completely** revised and updated this book to give you access to the latest developments in the alternative health field. We have included several new headings, including adrenal exhaustion, a multi-factorial and misunderstood problem, which has now, thanks to our high-octane 24/7 lifestyles, reached epidemic proportions.

Also included in this edition is atherosclerosis (hardening of the arteries), which contributes to high blood pressure, heart disease, strokes and erectile dysfunction, plus conditions such as lupus, since these types of conditions are on the rise.

Throughout this book I and my colleagues have given numerous, often little-known but well-researched solutions to many health problems, plus a host of proven remedies, nutrients and ideas to improve your health on a daily basis. We also offer alternative answers to many common symptoms that even your doctor may not recognize, to help you become your own health detective. Remember, the body is perfectly capable of healing itself when and if it is given the right tools for the job.

May our work give you good health—today and all days.

Hazel Courteney

IS OUR RIGHT TO TAKE SUPPLEMENTS UNDER THREAT?

Sue Croft, a director of Consumers for Health Choice (CHC), continues to spend her life lobbying European regulators to help us retain our freedom to choose higher-dose supplements. She says: "As things stand (summer 2010), we (Europeans) are still set to lose our right to buy high-dose specialist nutrients—even a one-gram tablet of Vitamin C is under threat.

"The dose levels of vitamins and minerals they will allow us to buy in the UK and Europe will be set by the 31 December 2010. Also, most of the people in the Member States of the EU are not used to taking higher-dose nutrients, and unfortunately, the majority view that wants low dosages could prevail. For instance, the current RDI (Recommended Daily Intake) for vitamin C, needed for more than 40 functions in the body, is 60mg, but this is only just sufficient to prevent scurvy and deficiency diseases and even a goat can manufacture 4 grams daily. Yet this is the dose that is mostly available in Europe—and those countries with the largest number of votes, France and Germany, want to keep it that way."

If the EU gets its way, this decision could have far-reaching consequences for the use of vitamin and minerals around the world, even here in the US. Even though there are thousands of published and verified scientific studies showing that appropriate higher dosages are both safe and beneficial, Europe sadly considers this a price worth paying. But will we?

"The emerging signs remain positive."

In February 2010, Senator John McCain introduced a new bill called The Dietary Supplement Safety Act (DSSA) which, if passed, would have repealed key sections of the Dietary Supplement Health and Education Act (DSHEA). The DSHEA is currently what classifies supplements as "foods" rather than "drugs" by the FDA and offers supplements some minimal protections against being arbitrarily banned.

This bill would have allowed the FDA to create a list of "accepted" supplement ingredients and required supplement manufacturers to report all adverse events, including non-serious ones, to the FDA. However, in March 2010, Senator McCain withdrew his support of the bill. He is now working with Senator Orrin Hatch, a vocal supporter of dietary supplements, to create a revised bill that would increase transparency and safety within the supplement industry without adding the intensive regulatory intervention found in the original legislation.

Still, the government's unwavering belief in the FDA's ability to protect Americans from harm is fundamentally flawed. Just look at how they police pharmaceuticals.

All medications must first be granted a product license before the makers are allowed to make specific beneficial claims. These can cost millions of dollars that vitamin companies simply don't have, and there is no guarantee that even licensed pharmaceuticals are safe. Vioxx, the arthritis drug, was granted a medicinal license and has been taken by 20 million people. Unfortunately, many are now dead and others have brought massive lawsuits against the makers of this drug. Negative side effects from statins and Tamiflu are also emerging on a large scale.

According to the American Association of Poison Control Centers, in 2008 1,066 deaths were caused by pharmaceutical drugs; however, there were no deaths reported from dietary supplements. Yet these are exactly the products that Congress feels it needs to "more effectively regulate."

It is easy to see how the US could easily head down the road that the EU has already paved. For example, if bodies such as the EU have their way, supplements such as vitamin B6, which can cause tingling if taken in high doses of over 250mg, could be banned because they have a minor reversible effect in some people. This is ridiculous when you consider that more than 770,000 Americans are injured or die in hospitals each year because of adverse reactions to their prescription medications.

Like Sue, I feel very strongly about this subject. I hope you will write to your senator or state representative to tell them about the health benefits you have experienced thanks to taking supplements and to persuade the government to keep the legal protections for high-dose nutrients and other supplements intact.

For the latest news regarding this unwelcome legislation, log on to the Natural Products Association website: www.npainfo.org

WHY YOU NEED NUTRITIONAL SUPPLEMENTS

How many times have you heard people say: "If I eat a healthy balanced diet, I don't need to take vitamins and minerals." "Expensive pee!" others exclaim.

In a perfect unpolluted world, if we all could eat plenty of fresh, locally grown fruits, vegetables and grains from nutrient-rich soils, then of course we should not need extra vitamins and minerals. But since we don't live on a desert island with a pure water supply, fresh fruits and vegetables and little stress, we need to give our bodies some extra protection.

The government's campaign encouraging everyone to eat more fruit and vegetables (approximately 1.5 to 2.5 cups a day) has fallen mainly on deaf ears. One of my co-authors, nutritionist Gareth Zeal, is often asked: "Does ketchup count as a vegetable?" And, I'm afraid to say the answer is still an emphatic NO!

A few people have changed, but the fact remains that as little as 5% of the Western population eats a truly healthy, balanced diet. The majority talks about healthy eating but, in reality, continues to eat far too much pre-packaged, refined junk foods that are often packed with salt, sugar, additives and saturated fats. A few people still do not comprehend that the human body is literally made of food molecules, so your body is largely made up from what you have eaten during the last year.

Also, many commercial growers—especially from overseas—continue to harvest their fruit and vegetables long before they are ripe. Research in Spain and at Oregon State University have found that when, for example, cherries are picked before being ripe, the vitamin C content is halved. When blackberries were picked early, the green ones contained 74mg of anthocyanins (the blue pigment that is great for your eyes and immune system) compared with 317mg in the naturally ripened fruits. Add to this the fact that most fresh produce is flown halfway around the world and is then stored for long periods, which itself hugely depletes nutrient levels. The message is obvious: as much as possible, buy more fresh, ripe, locally grown foods.

To survive, the human body needs 50 factors; these are 13 vitamins, 21 minerals, 9 amino acids, 2 essential fatty acids, plus carbohydrate, fiber, air, water and light. As our bodies cannot manufacture most of these substances, we must take them in from external sources—through our diet and by taking the right supplements. If the body becomes deficient in nutrients, negative symptoms will eventually result.

We can all have treats and really enjoy them, but we must stop living on them. Many times I have watched people fill their shopping carts with white bread, pre-packaged meals, cakes, chocolate bars and carbonated drinks. Almost all this refined, pre-packaged and processed food contains virtually no vitamins, essential fats, minerals or fiber. We are bombarded with food advertisements claiming that products are "packed with added vitamins." Have you ever asked yourself why the manufacturers need to add vitamins if the food is supposed to be nutritious in the first place?

White flour and mass-produced oils are the same. Canned foods are sterilized at high temperatures to kill any bacteria. How many nutrients do you think are left after these processes?

Without doubt, I advocate organic farming—and the more farmers who switch to organic methods, the fewer pesticides and herbicides (known to deplete even more nutrients from our food) will be in our food, water and air. And organic food has been proven to contain more nutrients than non-organic produce. Also, the use of fewer chemicals means less acid rain, less pollution and less sickness. Natural mineral levels in soil in many countries, including the US, are dropping, and if vital nutrients such as selenium, known to reduce the incidence of cancer and heart disease, are not in our soil, they are never going to make it into our fruits and vegetables.

Our eating habits have changed drastically during recent years. As little as 50 years ago, it was routine for the family to sit and eat home-cooked meals with freshly picked vegetables and fruits from a local farm or garden. Today, this tradition seems to have all but disappeared, and some children are not eating even one piece of fresh fruit a week. This is shocking. The longer fresh food is stored and cooked, the more nutrients are lost. If you leave an orange in a fridge for more than three days, up to 50% of the vitamin C content disappears. And, because the modern diet is less than perfect, we need to come to a compromise—which is why I take nutritional supplements and recommend specific nutrients in this book.

Unfortunately, some people still compare vitamins, minerals and essential fats in capsule forms, to prescription drugs—but remember that essential nutrients are essential to life.

On the drugs front, the trend to take statins to lower cholesterol is growing exponentially and people believe that once taking statins, they can eat all manner of high-fat food without risk. Yet statins are known to weaken all muscles, including the heart muscle, and they greatly inhibit natural production of Co-enzyme Q10, a vitamin-like substance needed by the body to protect the heart and produce energy. Statins also deplete the mineral selenium from the body, which is vital for heart health, cancer prevention, healthy sperm and for removing toxic metals such as mercury from the body. Statins are also linked to memory loss, muscle pain and nerve damage. But LDL cholesterol levels can also be controlled by taking supplements such as lecithin granules, garlic, B-group vitamins, vitamin C and pine bark extract known as pycnogenol, among others.

Many governments around the world suggest minimum amounts of nutrients, called RDIs (Recommended Daily Intakes) or DRIs (Dietary Reference Intakes). In the US there are DRIs for 29 nutrients and yet there are 45 essential nutrients required for health. Confusion is rife, as recommended intakes vary from country to country, so whom do we believe? Initially, the idea of RDIs was to prevent obvious signs of deficiency, such as scurvy (vitamin-C deficiency) in soldiers in the trenches in 1941. However, they do not in any way represent the quantities of nutrients we require for optimum health today. Nor do they represent the levels of vitamins and minerals we need to protect our bodies from the pollutants and toxins in our modern environment. What is more, RDIs take no account of individual requirements, such as age, gender or the health status of the person. For example, the current DRI for vitamin C is 90mg for adult men and 75mg for adult women in the US—but to ingest this amount from your diet, you would need to eat more than eight apples, three kiwi fruits or two oranges.

Currently there is no DRI for vitamin D3, a deficiency of which is now linked to 17 types of cancer, as well as to heart disease, diabetes, depression, osteoporosis and more. A growing body of research from highly accredited medical centers now states that this vitamin should be termed essential to life and every one of us needs to take an absolute minimum of 800IU of vitamin D3 daily.

But there is hope. A few years ago, I met a man aged 73 who had been refused heart surgery in the UK because his arteries were so blocked. He was deemed a lost cause; totally breathless, he could not even walk across the room. A nutritional physician friend took him on. First, she completely changed his diet, then gave him supplements proven to thin blood naturally, lower cholesterol levels and to help clear some of the plaque that had built up in his arteries. Under medical supervision, he was also taught yoga. After several months he slowly but surely regained his health. Today he climbs Alpine slopes as a hobby. It's never too late to change. And as Western doctors are now seeing plaques in the arteries of children as young as 10, change is imperative.

We all need to start eating food that is as unprocessed and unrefined as possible. Natural, locally grown, organic food, without pesticides and additives, plus taking the right supplements, is the way forward. There are now more than half a million clinical research papers showing that, taken in the right amounts, nutritional supplements can—and do—work.

IMPORTANT HINTS TO NOTE BEFORE TAKING SUPPLEMENTS

If you are taking any prescription drugs, you **must** advise your doctor of any supplements or herbs you wish to take, in case of contraindications. For example, the drug Warfarin thins the blood, but full-spectrum vitamin E and the herb ginkgo biloba do too. Anyone with HIV, or who is taking immuno-suppresive drugs or the contraceptive pill, should avoid St John's wort, which can reduce the effects of the medication. If you decide to begin taking supplements you must check with your doctor so that you can have regular blood tests. Then, in time and with your doctor's permission, hopefully you can reduce your intake of drugs for conditions such as high blood pressure, high cholesterol and type II diabetes.

- It is important to note that vitamins, minerals and essential fatty acids are nutrients essential to life. However, herbs are powerful medicines. Many prescription drugs are based on herbs. Herbs themselves are not essential to life, but, (like good food) when taken in the appropriate amounts and for the appropriate time, have proven to be of great benefit for many conditions. For instance, rosemary has been shown to protect against a host of cancers. Generally, take herbs for no more than three months at a time, have a month or so without them and then, if you feel the need, begin taking them again. Generally, look for whole herbal preparations in powder form, rather than herbal extracts that have been standardized for one particular "active" ingredient. "Whole herb" preparations can also be safer. For help with any herbs suggested in this book, call a qualified herbalist or health professional, or contact Wholistic Botanicals at 1-800-453-1406 Website: www.drchristophers.com

- Supplements taken regularly in the long term almost always produce beneficial effects, but don't expect miracles in a week. Supplements are not magic bullets, but stimulate the body's natural healing processes, giving long-term health benefits. Generally speaking, supplementation with nutrients produces improvements in health more slowly than prescription medication, which normally just suppresses symptoms. If you start a course of vitamins, minerals or any supplements, take them regularly for at least two months in order to see the benefits. Any changes in your health may be very subtle.

- Some supplements currently on the market have less than optimum quantities of beneficial ingredients. In general, you get what you pay for. Some low-priced supplements contain relatively small amounts of nutrients or forms of nutrients. The better quality and usually more expensive supplements generally provide better value for money in the long term.

- Most vitamins have a good shelf life, but cease to be effective if you keep them for too long. Be aware of sell-by dates and always keep your vitamins in a cool, **dry** place; never expose them to direct sunlight.

- If you find that vitamin C irritates your gut, take it with food or try Esther C, or vitamin C in an ascorbate form. Vitamin C is more effective when taken in repeated small doses throughout the day with food.

- Unless otherwise stated on the label, take supplements with food, because this ensures better absorption. Generally, amino acids such as glutamine are best taken on an empty stomach—check instructions.

- Avoid taking supplements with hot drinks such as tea and coffee, or with alcohol, as these can block the absorption of certain nutrients.
- Some people have reactions to certain supplements, but this is quite rare. This is usually caused not by the nutrients themselves but by a reaction to one or more of the other ingredients contained in the supplement. In general, better-quality supplements containing hypoallergenic ingredients are less likely to cause adverse reactions. If you suffer a negative reaction to any supplement or herb, stop taking it immediately. For example, most glucosamine supplements tend to be derived from crushed crab shells—so, if you are highly sensitive to shellfish, ask for the vegetarian version derived from corn, which is available from health shops.
- Products derived from bees, in extremely rare cases, may cause a reaction in anyone who suffers a severe sensitivity to bee stings. Obviously, if you know this is a problem avoid products related to bees! In the case of bee propolis this would also apply to tree resins, including pycnogenol, which is obtained from tree bark.
- The supplements suggested in this book can be taken by anyone over the age of 16, unless otherwise stated. For children's dosages, seek professional guidance.
- Probiotics (friendly bacteria) should also contain bifidus strain bacteria. Probiotic preparations in general keep better in glass bottles and should be kept either in a fridge or a freezer. There are various probiotics available that do not need to be kept refrigerated and can survive stomach acid—but in general these are best taken immediately after food, unless otherwise directed.
- Natural-source, full-spectrum vitamin E is better absorbed and retained by the body than synthetic forms.
- If you are pregnant, or planning a pregnancy, do not take any supplement containing more than 3000IU of vitamin A per day. Most manufacturers state whether supplements are unsuitable to be taken during pregnancy. Pregnant women should consume no more than one portion of liver a week, as liver is high in Vitamin A—and too much vitamin A is linked to fetal damage. One portion of liver may contain 30,000 to 40,000IU of vitamin A. However, as vitamin A is vital for a healthy immune function, eye health, healthy lungs and bowels, a healthy once-a-day safe level would be 7500IU. To overdose on vitamin A you would need to take something like 85,000IU a day. **However, taking a natural-source carotene complex daily is safe, as carotenes will convert naturally in the body to Vitamin A.**
- Do not take separate iron supplements if you are over 50, unless you have been diagnosed with a medical condition that requires extra supplementation, as iron accumulates in the body, and too high a level is linked with heart disease and strokes—especially in men. **Never leave iron tablets near children.**
- Keep all supplements away from young children. Any substance taken in excess can cause harm—even water. Follow the manufacturer's instructions unless your health professional advises otherwise.
- If you have any problem taking pills and cannot find liquid formulas at your health store, use an inexpensive tablet crusher. They are sold in most drug stores like Walgreens, CVS and Rite Aid, plus online at Amazon.com.
- The supplements we suggest should, in most instances, be taken until the condition is alleviated.
- If you are in any doubt about the amount of supplements you or your children should be taking, always consult a qualified health practitioner.

HOW TO USE THIS BOOK AND KEY TO CODES

Throughout this book we have suggested numerous formulas—and given the names of the companies that make them. All their details are here if you choose to contact them. If we have not mentioned a specific company, store or brand name, then the listed supplements should be readily available from good health food stores worldwide.

No one is more aware than myself of the thousands of alternative supplements now available. In this book we have suggested many specific brands, which we have used, and/or come to trust over many years. If we tried to mention every brand by name, this book would not be an easy-to-read book of hints, but a lengthy encyclopedia. Our choices of specific brands in **no way** infers that they are better or more beneficial than others on the market. If you have specific brands that you know and trust, check with your own suppliers or health store who, I am sure, will stock similar supplements to those recommended. It is well worth noting that virtually every reputable supplement company has its own in-house qualified nutritionists who are happy to help you. Don't be afraid to call them. Most of these suppliers are happy to post orders anywhere worldwide.

BMH
Blessed Maine Herbs
Website: www.blessedmaineherbs.com

GL
Garden of Life
5500 Village Blvd. Suite 202
West Palm Beach, FL 33407
Tel: 1-866-465-0051
Website: www.gardenoflife.com

GNC
GNC
Tel: 1-877-GNC-4700
Website: www.gnc.com

GP
Greens Plus
Orange Peel Enterprises, Inc.
2183 Ponce De Leon Cir.
Vero Beach, FL 32960
Tel: 1-800-643-1210
E-mail: info@greensplus.com
Website: www.greensplus.com

JF
Jarrow Formulas
Tel: 1-310-204-6936
Questions: info@jarrow.com
Sales: sales@jarrow.com
Website: www.jarrow.com

LEF
The Life Extension Foundation
1100 West Commercial Boulevard,
Fort Lauderdale, FL 33309
Order by phone: 1-800-544-4440
Customer Care: 1-800-678-8989
Health Advisors: 1-800-226-2370
Website: www.lef.org

NHC
Natural Healthy Concepts
1620 Appleton Road
Menasha, WI 54952
Tel: 1-866-505-7501
Website: www.naturalhealthyconcepts.com

NOW
NOW Foods
395 S. Glen Ellyn Road,
Bloomingdale, IL 60108
Tel: 1-888-669-3663
Website: www.nowfoods.com

NP
Nature's Plus
Tel: 1-800-645-9500
Website: www.naturesplus.com

OHB
Organic Health and Beauty
23801 Calabasas Rd. Suite 1003A
Calabasas, CA 91302
Tel: 1-800-430-3501
Website: www.organichealthandbeauty.com

OP
The Organic Pharmacy
396 Kings Road, London SW10 OLN, UK
Tel: 011-44-20-7351-2232
E-mail: info@theorganicpharmacy.com
Website: www.theorganicpharmacy.com

PN
Pharma Nord (UK) Ltd
Telford Court, Morpeth, Northumberland
   NE61 2DB, UK
Tel: 011-44-1670-534900
Fax: 011-44-1670-534903
E-mail: info@multivits.co.uk
Website: www.multivits.co.uk

SVHC
Solgar Vitamin and Herb Company
500 Willow Tree Road,
Leonia, New Jersey 07605
Tel: 1-201-944-2311
Website: www.solgar.com

SR
Saffron Rouge
3971 Lakeview Corporate Dr.
Edwardsville, IL 62025
Tel: 1-866-322-3227
Website: www.saffronrouge.com

TFB
Terra Firma Botanicals
PO Box 5680
Eugene, OR 97405
Tel: 1-800-837-3476
Website: www.terrafirmabotanicals.com

VC
Vitacost
130 Lexington Parkway, Lexington, NC 27295
Tel: 1-800-381-0759
Website: www.vitacost.com

VS
The Vitamin Shoppe
2101 91st Street, North Bergen, NJ 07047
Tel: 1-866-293-3367
Website: www.vitaminshoppe.com

A

ABSORPTION

(see also Celiac Disease, Colitis, Crohn's Disease, Indigestion, Irritable Bowel Syndrome (IBS), Leaky Gut, Low Stomach Acid, and Stress)

Many people presume that the nutrients within every item of food they swallow are automatically absorbed into their system, yet there are numerous health conditions, including IBS mentioned above, that greatly affect absorption within the gut. These can trigger deficiencies in most nutrients vital for health. There is also a vital intermediate stage: you swallow food and, if it is chewed thoroughly, a form of amylase (an enzyme in your saliva) begins breaking down your food. As we age, our levels of amylase fall, causing more absorption problems. Amylase is 30 times more abundant in the average 25-year-old than in the average 80-year-old.

The chewing process also alerts the stomach that food is on its way, which triggers stomach-acid production, ready to begin the digestion process. Chewing is the first and very important stage of digestion, and most carbohydrates are partially digested in the mouth if chewed properly, as your stomach does not have any teeth! With aging and problems such as gastritis, stomach-acid production is also reduced. Without these natural digestive aids, the absorption of nutrients through our gut walls and into the bloodstream is greatly diminished. Therefore, vital nutrients needed for tissue repair and cellular regeneration can sometimes pass through the body and out the other end undigested, thus contributing to conditions such as eczema, autoimmune conditions such as lupus, fibromyalgia, and rheumatoid arthritis.

Absorption mostly takes place in the small intestine, but as we age, enzymes produced by the pancreas (which helps to further break down sugars, proteins and fats) are also reduced. As the pace of modern life is increasing, more and more people are suffering varying degrees of absorption problems. Dr Shamin Daya says: "The most likely cause today for malabsorption is a leaky gut, a state in which the small intestine becomes inflamed, affecting its ability to absorb nutrients."

Stress also has a negative effect on the digestive process as it reduces absorption by shutting down enzyme production.

Symptoms of malabsorption include hair loss, low energy levels, chronic fatigue, weight loss or gain, poor bone density, dry and wrinkled skin, and dry hair and nails. Naturopath Steve Langley says, "Almost all disease is linked to a deficiency of nutrients and/or toxicity within the body; therefore, if you get your digestive system in good working order, a huge amount of health problems could be avoided."

Foods to Avoid

■ Avoid too much chewing gum, because it triggers production of stomach acid when no food may actually be following.

■ Reduce your intake of red meats and heavy, rich meals. Concentrated proteins and fats, such as red meat and cheese, are harder to digest as they require more work as well as oxygen to break them down completely. We need to maintain a high oxygen level in our tissues to keep our bodies healthy. And all junk foods reduce oxygen levels and accelerate loss of enzyme reserves in the body.

- Avoid croissants, burgers, fried foods, excessive high-sugar foods and full-fat dairy produce. The more unnatural your diet, the more the body has to produce enzymes to digest your food, and over time negative symptoms can arise.
- Cooked cheese is really hard on your digestive system.
- Modern refined wheat and related products are often hard to digest as we lack the necessary enzymes.
- Avoid drinking too much fluid with meals as this dilutes the stomach acid—the very substance you need for digesting your meal.

Friendly Foods
- Bitter foods such as watercress, spinach or oak leaf lettuce taken in small amounts at the start of a meal will stimulate digestion.
- Aloe vera also qualifies as a bitter food and stimulates digestion as well as soothing the gut.
- Raw, steamed or lightly cooked foods retain more enzymes, which aid digestion.
- Papaya is rich in the enzyme papain, which aids in the breakdown of foods in the stomach and small intestine. It is best eaten before a main meal.
- Pineapple is rich in the enzyme bromelain, which again aids digestion. Eat a small amount before main meals or even as a dessert, as pineapple aids digestion of proteins.
- Generally, increase your intake of fresh raw foods. Eat a salad at least once daily during the summer. Light stir-fries and steamed vegetables are also fine.
- If you have a problem with wheat, try millet, buckwheat, barley, amaranth or quinoa-based breads, which are available in most supermarkets and health stores.

- Try rice, corn, buckwheat or millet-based pastas, which are also easier to digest.
- If you have a problem with cow's milk, try rice, almond, oat or goat's milk, which are gentler on the stomach.
- A glass of red wine can help to stimulate stomach-acid production.

Useful Remedies
- Take a digestive enzyme capsule with all main meals. These are available from health stores.
- You can also take a hydrochloric acid (HCl) with pepsin capsule with main meals, but only if you have been diagnosed as suffering from low stomach acid (see *Low Stomach Acid*). Do not use if you suffer from ulcers or inflammatory bowel problems.
- Bitter herbs such as gentian, in tincture form, can be taken 15 minutes before each meal to stimulate production of stomach acid and digestive enzymes.
- A teaspoon of apple cider vinegar (preferably organic) in a little water taken before main meals can also help increase stomach-acid production.
- I have found Life Extension's Agave Digestive Immune Support, which contains prebiotics, is excellent for staying regular and aiding good gut health. Take one scoop daily with or before breakfast. **LEF**

Helpful Hints
- Try not to eat late at night, as this places an extra burden on the digestive system.
- Chew food thoroughly, and as much as possible eat sitting down in a relaxed frame of mind. Not always easy, but this simple act really aids digestion.
- Avoid eating for about an hour after vigorous exercise.
- Don't attempt to eat a large meal if you are under stress. Keep them small and light.
- If your digestive system is acting up or you have symptoms of an irritable bowel, such as bloating, wind, constipation and/or diarrhea, then eat soups (without bread), brown rice, vegetables, or grilled fish—in other words "easy-to-digest" foods—for a day or so. Also, you could try "food combining." Basically, this means separating concentrated proteins, such as meat, fish, eggs, and cheese, from concentrated carbohydrates, such as potatoes,

rice, bread, and pasta. So if, for example, you are eating fish, eat it with vegetables rather than potatoes. And if you have pasta, then also eat this with vegetables but not with meat or fish. Eat fruit in between meals or 15–20 minutes before a meal, rather than after a main meal. Fruit likes a quick passage through the gut and if it gets "stuck" behind a main meal, gas and bloating can result. This is especially true of melon. Some nutritionists now state that food combining is old fashioned, but naturopath Stephen Langley says: "There is no doubt that anyone with digestion and absorption problems would find, let's say, pasta and meat together pretty hard to digest. I have seen thousands of patients who have been helped by this method of eating—especially those who want to lose weight." For this reason eat melon on its own as a starter. And don't combine it with other fruits since melon has an even quicker transit time than other fruits, which again can trigger fermentation and bloating in the gut.

ACID–ALKALINE BALANCE

(see also Arthritis, Indigestion, and Low Stomach Acid)

Practically every major degenerative disease, including some cancers, is triggered by an over-acid system. When the pH of your blood is out of balance, your skin and hair become dull, the nervous system is affected and you may suffer insomnia, arthritis, rheumatism, aching joints, skin conditions, candida, fungal infections, muscle pain, and gout, which are all common symptoms of an over-acid system.

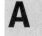

Nutritionists and health professionals have long understood the importance of maintaining a healthy acid–alkaline balance. For good health the body needs to maintain a certain acid–alkaline balance and keeping this balance is one of the crucial keys to remaining healthy and also slowing the aging process. Every cell functions more efficiently when it is predominantly alkaline.

In general, the body needs to be around 70% alkaline and 30% acid. But in the West, the average person is 80% acid and 20% alkaline, which is why we are suffering so many acid conditions such as arthritis. Many people confuse the term acid-forming with the term acidic, but they are entirely different. Everything we swallow, once metabolized within the body, breaks down into either an alkaline or acid mineral-based ash or residue. Whether a substance is alkaline or acid is determined by its pH (potential Hydrogen). Stomach acid can be as low as pH 1.5, which is very acid, whereas saliva after eating could be as high as pH 8, which is very alkaline. Your blood has a pH that is slightly alkaline—between 7.35 and 7.45—and this level needs to be maintained at all costs. If the blood becomes too acid and our buffering systems are not adequate (a common problem), then the body withdraws alkalizing minerals from anywhere it can find them; beginning with the hair, skin and nails and then moving on through the body until it begins drawing minerals from the bones, which in time contributes to conditions such as osteoporosis.

Unfortunately, most modern lifestyles and diets are almost all acid forming, and if the body remains in an acid state for too long, this acidity triggers degenerative diseases. A high acid-forming diet also has a negative effect on tooth enamel—pre-packaged, concentrated fruit juices are particularly at fault. Acid-forming foods deplete calcium from the body, while alkaline foods increase the body's ability to absorb calcium from the diet.

Emotions also greatly affect this balance: stress and anger trigger more acidity within the body, whereas feelings of being in control and in love, as well as breathing deeply through the nose, re-alkalize the system. Basically, harmony alkalizes and disharmony acidifies.

Foods to Avoid

- It's important to realize that just because a food is acid forming it is not necessarily unhealthy. Proteins are acid forming, but they are also essential for good health. Therefore, if you tend to eat two meat-based meals per day, reduce it to one. Make the other a fish-based meal, or eat pulses such as soy, aduki, butter beans, haricot beans or chickpeas (also in hummus).
- Basically, all animal products and egg yolks are acid forming. Duck, venison, grouse and pheasant, lamb, beef, and pork are all acid forming. Fish, turkey, and chicken are also acid forming, but do not contain such high levels of uric acid as red meat.
- Milk and yogurt are alkaline before digestion but become acid forming once digested. This is why milk products are calming to an over-acid esophagus if you suffer from an acid-type reflux after food. But, in the long term, this would exacerbate arthritic-type conditions. It's just a case of getting a balance.
- All nuts are acid forming, except almonds, fresh coconut, and chestnuts.
- All grains, with the exception of millet, buckwheat, amaranth, and quinoa, are also acid forming. Whole grains are a healthy food and remember: these foods are not to be eliminated *per se*, you just need to be aware of what is acid forming.
- All refined sugars found in cakes, cookies, pre-packaged desserts, whipped toppings, and so on are acid forming. Milk chocolate is a truly acid-forming treat; it's high in oxalic acid, which is linked to kidney stones—so don't overdo it!
- Wine, beer, liquor, coffee, tea, carbonated drinks, and sweetened fruit juices are all **highly** acid forming.

- All drugs, prescription and social (such as cannabis), are also acidic.
- Cranberries, plums, prunes, and rhubarb are highly acid forming. But again I reiterate, these foods are healthy—in fact, prunes (dried plums) are very anti-aging. Everything in moderation.
- Mass-produced malt vinegar, a waste product of the brewing industry, is also acid forming in the body.

Friendly Foods

- Honey, agave and brown-rice syrup are alkalizing. But don't overdo these foods, as they are still sugar! If you eat too much of them, the sugar converts to fat and lives on your hips. Again, just find a balance.
- All vegetables are alkaline, but the best are wheat grass, alfalfa, kelp, seaweed, parsley, watercress, cabbage, celery, broccoli, carrots, endives, and celery. All green foods are high in chlorophyll, which is rich in magnesium—a major alkalizing mineral.
- Cabbage, kale, broccoli, spring greens, green beans, and asparagus are all great alkaline foods. Spinach contains oxalic acid, but it breaks down into an alkaline residue.
- All fruits are healthy, and you should eat them freely, but be aware that cranberries, plums, prunes, and rhubarb are highly acid forming and to a lesser degree so are blueberries, blackberries, raspberries, and strawberries.
- The most alkalizing fruits are cantaloupe melons (and all melons), papaya, dates (especially dried dates), mangoes, lemons, limes, and figs. In case you are wondering, it's the alkaline mineral content and not the sugar content that determines whether a food is acid- or alkaline-forming in the body.
- Pineapple, cherries, kiwi and tomatoes contain acids, but they make an alkaline ash within the body after they are digested. People who suffer indigestion immediately after a meal, and may have an over-acid stomach, often say these types of foods make their problem worse. This is because they are acid on contact and until digested. However, they make an alkaline residue once they reach the small intestine. This is why apple cider vinegar or lemon juice,

with a little honey and warm water, help to re-alkalize the body and reduce symptoms of arthritis and inflammatory conditions. Take one teaspoon of each twice daily.

- Use a little organic sea salt, which is rich in alkalizing minerals.
- Drink more green and white tea with a little added raw agave syrup (a natural extract derived from cactus that will not raise blood sugar and is all right for diabetics).
- Apple cider vinegar, preferably organic, has an alkalizing effect within the body. It also helps increase stomach-acid production, as it is acid on contact but alkalizing after digestion.
- If you are a chocoholic, then ask at your health store for a raw chocolate bar. Dark, pure chocolate is usually sugar free and is not as acid forming.

Useful Remedies

- Ask at your health store for powdered organic formulas that contain wheat grass, spirulina, chlorella, alfalfa, broccoli, and green foods, and take them daily.
- I take Green pH powder, made by Metabolics (www.metabolics.com)—one small level teaspoon daily in water, preferably taken 30 minutes before a meal or in between meals. It is a mixture of green beans, garden peas, pea leaf, dry apple cider, watercress, broccoli, and nettle leaf. It doesn't taste great, but it is an easy and quick way to alkalize your body. *Other* companies make comparable products: **JF, VC, VS**
- Dr Shamin Daya suggests that taking a quarter of a teaspoon of baking soda in half a cup of lukewarm water twice a day between meals is an easy way to keep the body alkaline.
- Take a multi-mineral formula that contains approximately 600mg of calcium, 300–500mg of magnesium, 25mg of zinc and 90mg of potassium in a colloidal or chelated form, which are more easily absorbed. These minerals are alkalizing.

Helpful Hints

- Stress, anger and smoking contribute to an over-acid system.
- Breathing deeply and regularly helps to re-alkalize the body. This is because when you breathe more oxygen into the body, it has an alkaline effect. When we are under stress, we tend to shallow-breathe, which leaves more carbon dioxide, and therefore more acidity, in our tissues.
- Do not brush your teeth immediately after eating or drinking high acid-forming foods and drinks, as you can lose more tooth enamel. Simply drink a little water and swish it around the mouth to help neutralize the acids.
- Meditation also re-alkalizes the body.
- Life Ionizers supply alkalizing water filters for your home. Their number is 1-888-688-8889 or visit www.lifeionizers.com
- Otherwise try Kangen Water—a water system that attaches to your kitchen faucet and ionizes and greatly alkalizes water. It's used in Japanese hospitals with highly beneficial health results. For full details visit www.kagenwaterusa.com
- When you first wake up, the body is very high in acid, so having fruit for breakfast will help to re-alkalize the system. This is a great diet for summer breakfasts, but in winter you need to keep warmer so fruit won't do the job. During these months, try eating oatmeal sweetened with a freshly grated apple or any chopped fruit instead. Breakfast is also a great time to drink freshly made juices. But too much orange juice can overstimulate production of stomach acid, so go for diluted apple or pear juice as an alternative. Apple, carrot, or celery juice with a little added fresh root ginger are also highly alkalizing.

ACID STOMACH

(see also Indigestion and Low Stomach Acid)

Many people complain about having an acid stomach, often mistakenly presuming that they produce too much stomach acid—hydrochloric acid, which is known as HCl. In fact, sufferers from acid stomach regularly produce inappropriate amounts (too much or too little) stomach acid at the wrong times; this can occur through overindulgence in caffeine, alcohol, or sugar, or as a reaction to stress. And, as the average person eats approximately 50+ tons of food in their lifetime, which requires nearly 80 gallons of digestive juices to break it down, it's no wonder that we are suffering more and more digestive disorders. Typical symptoms are feelings of heartburn, acid reflux, indigestion, bloating, and general discomfort. When you are under prolonged stress or are exhausted, your digestive system is greatly weakened. Never underestimate how long-term, negative stress and chronic exhaustion can affect the body (see also *Stress*).

Foods to Avoid

- Reduce your intake of coffee, sodas, black tea, alcohol, and sugar.
- Pizzas, which are laden with vegetable fat and cheese, are especially hard to digest, as are large, rich meals and red meat.
- Full-fat cheeses and rich, creamy foods.
- Fried and very fatty foods.

- Oily, spicy foods (such as Indian curries), which are usually packed with refined vegetable oils. These types of meals—if high in fat—are hard to digest.
- Concentrated fruit juices, especially orange, lemon and grapefruit, and raw tomato juice, which can make the problem worse. Buy non-concentrates and dilute with water.
- Reduce your intake of wheat-based foods, which can be a problem for people with acid stomach (especially croissants, which are high in butter), white bread and pre-packaged, mass-produced pies and cakes.

Friendly Foods

- A small amount of aloe vera taken just before eating can greatly aid digestion and help prevent an over-acid stomach.
- Eat more whole grains like brown rice, quinoa, kamut, or amaranth, and try lentil-, corn-, buckwheat-, millet- or spelt-based pastas, breads, and cereals. Rice cakes, amaranth, or rye crackers are often easier to digest than wheat. If you adore bread, try small amounts of whole-wheat varieties.
- Include plenty of lightly cooked vegetables and fruits in your diet, which are easier on the digestive system.
- Try making more fruit compotes or lightly grilled fruit kebabs without sugar. Use a little agave syrup or chopped organic dried fruits to sweeten.
- Choose low-fat meats such as venison, turkey, duck, and chicken without the skin, and include plenty of fresh fish in your diet (preferably not fried).
- Replace full-fat cow's milk with organic oat, rice, soy, or goat's milk.
- Experiment with caffeine-free herbal teas, such as fennel and licorice, which reduce acidity. Chamomile, meadowsweet, and fresh mint teas soothe the gut.
- Fresh root ginger is very calming to the gut, as is lightly cooked cabbage or cabbage juice made from raw cabbage. I always use water from cooking cabbage to make gravy.
- Eat more live, low-fat bio yogurts. But if you are intolerant to dairy products from cows, then try sheep's milk or soy-based yogurts. Please note that low-fat bio yogurts (from cows) are usually okay because they are fermented—but if they trigger bloating, avoid them.

Useful Remedies

- De-glycyrrhized licorice helps protect and heal the lining of the esophagus and stomach. Chew 1–2 tablets 20 minutes before a meal. It can also be used as an alternative to antacids after meals. Available from health stores.
- Ask at your local health store or pharmacy for a Peppermint Formula containing ingredients such as peppermint, gentian, fennel, or chamomile, which can be taken after foods.
- Slippery Elm Plus is a supplement containing slippery elm, marsh mallow, and gamma oryzanol, which all help to soothe the stomach lining.
- Aloe-containing juice makes a particularly good digestive aid juice that greatly soothes the stomach lining. Look for one containing any mix of aloe vera, papaya, peppermint oil, chamomile, and slippery elm.

Helpful Hints

- Chew all foods thoroughly and avoid drinking too much liquid with meals as this dilutes the stomach acid, which you need for digestion. However, a small glass of red wine aids digestion.
- Eat little and often, avoiding large, heavy meals. The larger the meal, the greater the burden on your digestive system. Small meals are especially important if you are stressed, as stress increases stomach acid at inappropriate times.
- Take time out to eat your meals calmly—do not eat on the run. Avoid large meals if you are feeling upset.
- If you are prone to nervous conditions, join a yoga, meditation, or tai chi class and learn to relax. Get plenty of exercise, but no strenuous exercise immediately after eating. Walking for 10–15 minutes after a meal greatly aids digestion.
- Drink peppermint, fennel, chamomile, or licorice teas after a meal.
- Food combining helps relieve an acid stomach: this means separating proteins and starches to aid digestion. Basically, if you are eating a protein such as meat or fish, eat this with salad or vegetables but not potatoes, pasta, or bread; conversely, when you eat bread, pasta, or potatoes, eat them with vegetables or salad, not protein. Many people become reliant on antacids to control their symptoms, even though making a few simple changes to their diet and eating patterns can produce very significant relief in most cases. Antacids can harm the body if used excessively, and many contain aluminum, which has been implicated in Alzheimer's disease.

A

ACNE

(see also Liver Problems and Rosacea)

Many young people, including teenagers, are notorious for eating a poor, nutrient-deficient diet—and ingesting far too many carbonated drinks and too much alcohol, which will exacerbate this problem. Sugar and fat are without a doubt the biggest offenders. Many adolescents experience acne due to the massive increase in hormone production at that age, which often leads to overproduction of sebum, or naturally produced oils in the skin that cause blockages in the skin's sebaceous glands. For adults, acne often results from internal toxicity, which can be caused by many factors. Constipation, candida (a yeast fungal overgrowth; see *Candida*), or food intolerances can all trigger this problem. Pre-menstrual women can also experience acne. The key factor in controling and preventing acne is to look after your liver and ensure that toxins can be eliminated. Once the system becomes overloaded, it begins dumping toxins into the skin—hence constipation and poor skin often go hand in hand.

Foods to Avoid

- Refined snacks, soda-like drinks (many of which contain as many as 8 teaspoons of sugar), croissants, cakes, candy, and so on. These types of foods have to be greatly reduced if the acne is to be healed.
- Most mass-produced, pre-packaged meals, cakes, cookies, and pies, which are high in sugar, salt and saturated fats, because they place a great strain on the liver.
- Full-fat cheeses, pizzas, chocolates and dairy products, fried foods, and greasy burger-type foods.
- In some cases the acne can be triggered by a sensitivity to foods such as cow's milk.

Friendly Foods

- Eat more beets, kale, celeriac (celery root), and artichokes, which help to cleanse the liver.
- A glass of beet juice every day for a few weeks is especially useful for teenagers, because it helps to control the overproduction of hormones.
- Chickpeas, soy, black-eyed, haricot, and cannellini beans, as well as pulses, help the body excrete excess hormones.
- Japanese and Thai foods, such as miso and tempeh, help to regulate hormones.
- Include more fresh vegetables and fruits such as figs into your diet—this is especially true for teenagers, who tend to eat a very poor diet. We can all do this for a certain time, but symptoms will appear once the body becomes very toxic.
- Drink 6–8 glasses of water daily.
- Add a tablespoonful of linseeds (flax seeds) and sunflower seeds to high-fiber, low-sugar breakfast cereal.

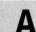

A

- Snack on unsulfured dried apricots and dates as well as raw, unsalted nuts and seeds.
- Avocados are rich in vitamin E, which nourishes the skin.
- Fish—especially sardines, mackerel, salmon—are rich in essential fats, which regulate hormones. White fish, cod, plaice, halibut, sea bass, and so on are rich in zinc and selenium, which are also needed for healthy skin.
- See also *General Health Hints*.

Useful Remedies

- If you take nothing else, take a good-quality multi-vitamin/mineral, containing at least 15mg of zinc and 1mg of copper.
- Zinc has been shown to be as successful as taking certain antibiotics for this condition; if you are not taking a multi-vitamin, take 30mg of zinc up to three times daily for 6 weeks, then reduce to 60mg daily. For every 15mg of zinc, you should also take 1mg of copper to maintain a healthy balance within the body.
- With acne, hormones are often an important factor. Female Reproductive Formula contains herbs that should help, including blessed thistle, squaw vine, cramp bark, and raspberry leaf. These are available as a liquid or capsules.
  Visit www.herbsfirst.com/descriptionsformulas/FemaleReproductiveFormula.htm for more information.
- To help support the liver, try a formula based on barberry, wild yam and dandelion. Take this for 3 months.
- The Organic Pharmacy Clearskin Tincture formula, which contains saw palmetto, red clover, agnus castus, calendula, echinacea, and dandelion, is a very useful formula for balancing testosterone levels in women. Take 15 drops twice daily in liquids. **OP**
- Vitamin A is essential for healthy skin; if you are **not** pregnant or planning a pregnancy, take up to 10,000IU daily for 2 months and then switch to a high-strength, natural-source beta-carotene complex that will convert into Vitamin A within the body. **LEF, NOW, SVHC**

- 200–400IU of natural-source, full-spectrum vitamin E per day reduces the tendency for scarring and helps maintain healthy skin.
- Essential fats are also important because saturated, trans- and hydrogenated fats displace EFAs in the body. Therefore, take 1–3g of omega-3 fish oil daily.

Helpful Hints

- *Rosa Mosqueta*, a Latin American plant-based oil, can be used topically to heal scars, but don't use on active acne. Use once the acne is no longer active. Available from good health stores and pharmacies.
- Taking liquid hyaluronic acid (a natural component of skin) daily in water helps to heal any scarring on the skin.
- Tea tree oil is highly antiseptic. Add a few drops to bath water or use cream, soap or lotion on the affected areas. As teenage boys seem to hate washing, get them to use a tea tree shower gel daily.
- Kali Brom 6c is a homeopathic remedy that helps if the acne is on the face, chest and shoulders. Homeopathic Silica 6c is also useful twice daily. This may trigger symptoms to increase for a short time as toxins are released, but this will balance out after a couple of weeks.
- Exercise encourages the free flow of sebum and detoxification of the body through sweating.
- Many readers have benefited from taking aloe vera juice internally as well as using the gel externally.
- A thorough detox is useful for clearing acne (see *Liver*).
- The Sher System is a skin regime especially formulated for problem skin. Contact The Sher System, 30 New Bond Street, London, W1S 2RN. Tel: 011-44-1784-227805, Monday to Friday from 3:30am–11:30am Eastern. Website: www.sher.co.uk Next-day delivery is available for the US if your order is placed before 10am Eastern.

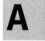

ADDISON'S DISEASE

(see Adrenal Exhaustion)

ADHD—attention deficit hyperactivity disorder

(see Hyperactivity)

ADRENAL EXHAUSTION

(see also Exhaustion, Low Blood Pressure, Low Blood Sugar, ME, and Stress)

Thanks to our fast-paced, 24/7 open-all-hours lifestyle, adrenal problems, which are **hugely** multi-factorial, have reached epidemic proportions. Because symptoms vary greatly, this condition often goes undiagnosed for months or even years, and doctors urgently need to understand and diagnose this condition, which can, if left untreated, become extremely serious.

Naturopath Steve Langley says: "It can happen at any age, but this problem is becoming more and more common in younger people, especially women. Many patients initially report having problems getting up in the morning, but say they get a 'second wind' later in the evening. Other symptoms are cravings for sugar, carbohydrate, stimulants, and salt, tired much of the time, dark circles around the eyes and frequent urination, often at night.

"Mood swings are common, or feeling dizzy or faint, which is linked to low blood sugar.

In some cases, if the person remains under constant stress, then high blood pressure can arise and medical attention needs to be sought. Feeling angry or short tempered can also be common symptoms. If these symptoms are not dealt with, a sense of humor failure can occur, tears can spring up for no good reason, and general malaise and depression set in. The person knows something is wrong, but presumes he or she is just tired and keeps pushing themselves.

"Doctors often prescribe anti-depressants that simply mask symptoms, and if the low blood sugar is left untreated and the person continues to eat sugar in order to function, then eventually they can collapse."

At such a point the person may experience panic attacks. The thyroid can malfunction—becoming either under- or overactive. If the adrenals become totally exhausted, Addison's disease can occur, which thankfully is pretty rare.

Many people are now suffering from burnt-out adrenals, yet clinically they do not have Addison's, which is a serious medical condition that requires long-term, life-long, corticosteroid treatment. Obviously, the secret is to recognize symptoms at an early stage and deal with them.

Your adrenal glands are two small glands, no bigger than large grapes that sit on top of each kidney like tiny pyramids. They produce the hormones adrenaline, cortisol, and DHEA among others. In everyday life, if we become stressed our age-old "fight or flight" mode kicks in and the adrenals start pumping the stress hormones on a signal from the pituitary gland (in the brain). Basically, cortisol signals your liver to "dump" stored sugar into your bloodstream to fuel your muscles and your brain. The problem with this drip-feeding of sugar over a period of time is that it encourages insulin resistance, a common problem these days. (See *Insulin Resistance*.)

Years ago, this "fight or flight" release of stress hormones would save lives, as, once this mode kicked in, our ancestors' blood would start to thicken in case they were injured and give them the energy to run away from any life-threatening situations. Fortunately, most of us today are not being chased by a wild animal—so instead of running away, which would disperse the stress hormones naturally, our response is to head for another caffeine or sugar fix.

The major problem today is that long-term "fight or flight" reactions caused by stress imbalance these stress hormones which, if not dealt with adequately, can become toxic to every system in the body. High and low levels of cortisol can affect brain function. Too much cortisol can deplete calcium and other vital minerals from your bones, which in the long term can trigger osteoporosis. It also depletes vital oxygen from your blood and every organ—which is then under stress. If this continues, you may blow a fuse, be it a "gut fuse," triggering ulcers, or worse, a "heart fuse," triggering a heart attack and so on.

An imbalance of stress hormones can trigger a cascade of "acid" reactions throughout your body. And if this situation continues over time then the adrenals become tired, producing ever less cortisol and therefore lower blood sugar. Depending on the person, this could eventually lead to a complete cessation of cortisol production, thus triggering Addison's disease.

Also, as the immune system is hugely disrupted, a majority of people with adrenal problems are suffering from candida and a leaky gut. See under *Candida* and *Leaky Gut*. Therefore, it's no surprise that many people suffering with adrenal exhaustion are often diagnosed with chronic fatigue syndrome (CFS).

Foods to Avoid

- White flour, sugar, caffeine, and alcohol all need to be avoided.
- See diet under *Insulin Resistance*.
- **It's crucial for the person to totally avoid sugar in any form**—and caffeine drinks such as coffee, sodas, Red Bull, and so on.
- In the initial stages, foods high in potassium also need to be avoided, such as figs, dates, grapes, oranges, raisins, bananas, sultanas, and mango. This is because your body will retain potassium and excrete sodium, and your blood pressure will go down.

Friendly Foods

- Protein is important since it balances blood sugar for longer and because the body requires more protein when it is under stress. Always eat breakfast. Make sure you eat some protein with your breakfast, which could include fish, eggs, quinoa, lean meats, or a good-quality protein powder.
- Oatmeal and whole-wheat bread (unless you are intolerant to wheat/yeast) will also help balance blood sugar levels.
- Use amaranth or rye crisp breads spread with hummus-like spreads.
- Eat more lentils, brown rice, barley, and chickpeas, and experiment with wheat-free breads and rice, lentil, or corn pastas.
- Fresh fish, chicken, lean meats, cooked tofu, tempeh, natto, eggs, goat's cheese, mozzarella, feta cheese would be fine.
- Vegetables such as cauliflower, broccoli, kale, spring greens, bok choi, cabbage, sprouts, etc. are all good.

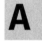

- Once symptoms are more under control sweeter foods such as sweet potatoes, papaya, carrots, and apples should be fine. In fact, sweet potatoes are very useful in controling blood-sugar problems.
- Foods high in natural sodium will help replace lost sodium—samphire grass, kelp, celery, spinach, beets, and any seaweeds would be great (available at health food stores).
- Use Himalayan crystal salt or a nori seaweed shake.
- Licorice supports adrenal function but tends to be high in sugar (and sometimes wheat), which will make adrenal exhaustion worse. It is usually given to Addison's sufferers but would have to be a sugar-free version.
- If your symptoms are not acute, then you can use small amounts of raw organic agave syrup or xylitol sugar (a fruit fiber), which have a lower impact on blood-sugar levels and are available from health stores. **VC** A number of xylitol-based sweeteners are also available for purchase on www.amazon.com.
- Green tea contains L-theanine, which helps you to stay calm. Buy organic de-caffeinated green teas.

Useful Remedies

- Magnesium citrate—as magnesium is nature's tranquillizer, and anyone who is stressed is low in this vital mineral. Take 600mg as a minimum during the day and take 200mg before you go to bed
- Vitamin C plus bioflavonoids—around 2–3g per day, spread out with each meal.
- A high-dose vitamin B complex, 100mg of each—plus 500mg of pantothenic acid (B5) daily, as you cannot make cortisol without B5.
- Good stress formulas contain licorice root, gotu kola, ashwagandha, Siberian ginseng, and shatavari—all of which nourish the adrenals and aid healing. **JF, VC**
  NB: Cannot be taken by anyone suffering from high blood pressure.
- Take Cortico-Zyme, which contains a complex of B vitamins, magnesium, and nutrients to

support the adrenals. Take two with breakfast and then two with lunch. They can be taken by anyone. **NHC**

■ Cortisol Manager tablets contain ashwagandha, phosphatdlyserine, and L-theanine (an extract of green tea). These are excellent for reducing cortisol production and calming you down. If you are a Type A person who rushes around all day, and you are stressed and need to "slow down," then try taking one of these tablets when the adrenaline starts "pumping" and take one or two before bed. I have found they are great at reducing "fight or flight"-type symptoms and they really help me get a good night's sleep. However, if you are at the point of total and utter exhaustion, then your body may not be producing sufficient cortisol, in which case there would be no benefit in taking this formula. Available from www.amazon.com and Natural Healthy Concepts (www.naturalhealthyconcepts.com).

Helpful Hints

■ By now you will have realized that you need help. A saliva test via your doctor or healthcare professional will show your DHEA and cortisol levels. You may also require blood tests for thyroid function. See under *Thyroid*. Once you know how severe or otherwise the problem is, then you can start to heal yourself.

■ With the help of a healthcare professional, you may need DHEA supplementation.

■ If you are at the stage of fainting because of low blood sugar/adrenal exhaustion, then avoid exercise.

■ If you are simply a highly stressed person who produces the "flight or flight" response quickly, then get more exercise to help naturally disperse toxic (in the long term if not dispersed) stress hormones and watch your diet. Also take the Cortisol Manager as directed.

■ Learn to meditate, which helps reduce the stress response.

■ Take deep breaths more often.

■ Eat every 4 hours; the worst thing you can do is miss a meal. Some people with severe blood sugar problems may need to eat every 2–3 hours.

■ Sleep in past 8:00 in the morning. Cortisol production peaks at 8am. The more you can rest and eat sensibly, the faster you will heal. It may take three months to recover from total burn-out.

■ Go to sleep before 11pm.

■ Try to rest at some point during the day. Even a 15-minute nap will help.

■ Read *The Low GL Diet Bible* by Patrick Holford (Piatkus), which is a godsend for anyone with this problem.

AGING

By 2050, 1.5 billion people—that's one in five of us—will be over 65, and more than 5 million people will be over 100. Within 10 years, for the first time in human history, there will be more of us over 65 than children under five—and people aged over 80 are the fastest-growing portion of the total population in many countries.

Governments worry about the health-cost burden of our aging population, and yet, if you begin taking more responsibility for your health from today by eating sensibly, reducing stress and exercising more, then you could live a healthy, productive life until at least 100. In fact, the average child born today can expect to live to 104.

Japan, where the average life expectancy is 82, has some of the longest-living residents. Sweden, France, and Italy all have life expectancies of around 80, and in the US it's 78.4.

As we age, biological changes take place throughout our bodies. Our heart muscle becomes thinner, the capacity of our kidneys reduces, and all of our organs go through some physiological change. However, these changes are not necessarily associated with illness or disease. And none of these changes causes ill health or disease on its own. The process of aging is the breakdown of key biological functions of our mind and body and is directly related to our environment, diet, lifestyle, and outlook on life.

The single most common result of the aging process and the leading cause of death worldwide is cardiovascular disease. Dr Michael Colgan, a renowned nutritional research scientist in the US, says that if people could eat more of the right foods and change their lifestyles, then 98% of cardiovascular disease cases and 80% of cancers would be preventable. He also states that late-onset diabetes, which is reaching epidemic proportions in Western countries, is a direct consequence of over-consumption of sugar, plus stress and overuse of stimulants. It is both avoidable and manageable by good nutrition (see also *Diabetes*).

And if you eat the right foods and take the right supplements and hormones, then a 60-year-old can have the Biological Aging Markers—such as blood pressure, cholesterol count, lean body mass, bone density, skin thickness, and so on—of a 40-year-old.

So, what causes the deterioration of our body that we call aging?

It is now accepted that the aging process and virtually all disease development is the result of free radical damage to the cells in one form or another. This is why antioxidants such as natural-source carotenes (vitamin A), vitamins C and E, plus minerals such as selenium hold one of the major keys to slowing down the aging process. Free radicals are produced by our bodies when oxygen is used to create energy, as well as during everyday processes such as breathing and eating. There is much misinformation concerning the billions of free radicals that are produced every day, though. While it is true that they can wreak havoc on the body's cells, they are also vital to life. They help neutralize viruses and bacteria and help kill cancer cells, so there are benefits for a certain amount of free radicals (also known as oxidants) in the body. But over time, as the body begins to accumulate excess free radicals in the absence of sufficient antioxidants, the system becomes overwhelmed by these unstable molecules, and they are then able to break down our DNA, trigger deterioration in our blood vessels and brain, and cause damage to virtually every cell of our body. You can reduce free-radical accumulation by cutting down on burned or smoked foods, exposure to air pollution and pesticides, overuse of cellular phones, excessive sunbathing, additives and stress, and by taking more potent antioxidants, which are listed below.

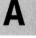

Inflammation is another major contributor to aging. Degenerative diseases that are associated with inflammation in the tissues are arteriosclerosis, Alzheimer's, Parkinson's, diabetes, arthritis, chronic fatigue, cancer, and allergies. Sources of inflammation are chronic low-level infections, toxicity from ingesting too many foods containing additives, a deficiency in essential nutrients, foods to which we have an intolerance, and exposure to heavy metals such as mercury and aluminum.

Physical activity is crucial for helping to slow down the aging process, but severe exertion generates large amounts of free radicals and inflammation in the body. This may explain why people who spend a lot of time at the gym do not always survive longer than those who don't, and why some marathon runners and aerobics instructors age more quickly. As always, we need everything in a balance; this is the secret to slowing down the aging process.

Also, how often do you hear people say, "It's all in my genes"? And if their parents died young, many people presume they have inherited a likelihood to do the same. Yes, our genes do play a huge part in determining how well or otherwise we age, but if our genes stay healthy then our bodies stay healthy. So, if you live a healthy lifestyle you can change which genes are expressed. In other words, if your parents and grandparents died of heart attacks you may well have a predisposition for heart problems at some point. But if you live a different lifestyle and eat healthier foods, you can change the chemistry within the body and tip the scales in your favor. Genes can be repaired and changed; they adjust to our environment and state of mind. Generally people who live to a ripe old age are positive, adaptable, and hard working; they eat breakfast and consume plenty of freshly, locally grown fruits and vegetables.

Jeanne Calment, a French lady, lived to 122. She gave up smoking at the age of 120 in 1995, saying that "it had become a habit" and died two years later. She was one in six billion, which shows that there are always exceptions to every rule.

Don't underestimate the extent to which your thoughts and stress levels can affect both your general health and the rate at which you age. If you repeatedly say, "It's to be expected at my age," don't be surprised if you age faster.

In my twenties and thirties, I was obsessed with aging and spent too much time rushing around having the latest anti-aging therapies instead of simply enjoying being young. Learn to enjoy the moment; know that you can only do your best, and have some fun.

Foods to Avoid

- Sugar triggers an inflammatory response in the body, which contributes to hardening of the arteries, which in turn contributes to heart disease and strokes. Sugar also ages the skin through the process of cross-linking as much as smoking or regular sunbathing. And if you don't utilize sugar during exercise, it converts to fat in the body. Therefore, cut down on foods with a high sugar content, such as refined carbohydrates—breads, cakes, cookies, pastries, and pasta—as well as on sweets and concentrated fruit juice. A diet with a carbohydrate intake of more than 40% can cause insulin resistance and trigger late-onset diabetes (see *Diabetes* and *Insulin Resistance*). Also, the body has a limited capacity to store carbohydrates in the liver and muscles and will turn excess carbohydrate into fat tissue.
- Artificial sweeteners including aspartame (Nutrasweet and Equal), saccharin, and sucralose (Splenda) are synthetic forms of sugar that the body does not utilize well.
- Fried foods and all refined foods containing hydrogenated/trans-fats (see *Fats You Need To Eat*).
- Artificial preservatives and chemicals, including MSG.
- Some municipal tap water is known to contain many chemicals, hormones, antibiotic residues and, in some areas, fluoride—which can accumulate in the body and cause many health problems. As a result, make sure you have (and use) a good water filter and make sure it is serviced regularly. You can also use Kangen Water—a water system that attaches to your kitchen faucet and ionizes and alkalizes tap water. It's used in Japanese hospitals with highly beneficial health results. For full details visit www.kangenwaterusa.com. Otherwise I drink Fiji or Volvic bottled waters.
- Cut down on stimulants such as caffeine and sodas and reduce alcohol consumption. Drinking alcohol to excess is **extremely** aging.
- Reduce your intake of full-fat dairy products.
- Avoid shellfish, which tend to feed in polluted coastal waters.
- Steer clear of non-organic, preserved, smoked, and cured meats (deli-type meats and bacon), as the chemicals used are carcinogenic.
- Avoid canned, microwaved, and pre-packaged foods.
- Avoid industrially produced battery eggs and chickens.
- Cut down on non-organic red meats.

- Cut down on sodium-based table salts. Use mineral-rich sea salts in moderation. I use Himalayan Crystal Salt, which is rich in organic-source minerals. Available from good health stores, www.amazon.com and Natural Health International, Inc., 524 Second Street, San Francisco, CA 94107; Tel: 1-888-668-3661, Monday–Friday, 9am–5pm PDT; email: general@naturalhi.com; website: www.himalayancrystalsalt.com/

Friendly Foods

- Fresh fish, especially salmon, mackerel, and sardines, is rich in fatty acids. These days I avoid tuna, which usually has a high mercury content. White fish is rich in zinc and selenium, which are vital for healthy brain functioning.
- Linseeds (flax seeds) help protect the breasts and prostate and are a good source of Omega 3. I soak a tablespoon of golden linseeds overnight in cold water, then drain them and use over cereals or in fruit blends for breakfast for additional fiber.
- Cook with good-quality olive or coconut oil.
- Begin adding non-GM lecithin granules to cereals and fruit blends. Lecithin is rich in phosphatidyl serine and choline so it provides great nourishment for your brain; it also helps elevate "good" cholesterol and metabolize fats.
- Consume pomegranate—either the fruit or juice—every day because it has been shown to help prevent atherosclerosis from developing, which is a major trigger for heart disease and strokes. This fruit is also highly protective against certain cancers—especially prostate and breast cancer.
- Papaya and blueberries are "super" fruits that help prevent cancer. Papaya also aids in digestion (as does pineapple).
- All fresh fruits, fresh vegetables, salads, nuts, and oatmeal will help reduce inflammation in the body. Eat locally grown fresh foods as much as possible.
- Sip clean water throughout the day; try to drink 6–8 glasses daily.
- Eat organic foods as much as you can since they are known to contain lower levels of potentially dangerous pesticides and chemicals. Also, organic vegetables contain more nutrients than non-organic ones.
- A good anti-aging diet should be composed of 50% vegetables (non-starchy, such as sweet potatoes), 20% protein (meat, cheese, fish, etc.), 20% fruits, and 10% grains (brown rice, quinoa, lentils, buckwheat, millet, or spelt). The vegetables should be raw or lightly cooked to preserve their nutrient content. The protein should include vegetable proteins such as organic soybeans, haricot beans, aduki beans, and so on, as well as some low-fat animal protein. Fruits should be uncooked and whole as opposed to juiced. However, blended fruits remain high in nutrients that are easier for the body to absorb and utilize. The grains are best as whole grains, such as brown rice, rather than flour-based foods.
- Eat more thyme, basil, and rosemary, which have powerful antioxidant properties. Rosemary is highly anti-cancerous.
- Eat more cilantro, which helps remove toxic metal residues from the body.
- Prunes are highly anti-aging as they are rich in antioxidants—but they are also acid forming. Everything in moderation.
- Eat more curries rich in curcumin, which is derived from turmeric—a highly anti-aging spice (see below).

Anti-aging Nutrients

- There are currently dozens of anti-aging formulas and nutrients. But as a base line, always take a daily good-quality multi-vitamin/mineral plus an antioxidant formula that is suitable for your age and gender. Always include an extra gram of vitamin C (at the very least) to help slow the aging process.

■ Below are listed some of the most anti-aging nutrients currently known:

- **VITAMIN C** has more than 40 functions within the body and is essential for immune function, skin repair, eye and joint health, and so on. I take 2–3g per day, at a minimum, with food. Best taken in divided doses for optimum benefit.

- **CURCUMIN** Much research has been done on genes and aging. When studying the long-lived people on the island of Okinawa, Dr Giovanni Scapagnini from The Institute of Neurological Disorders at Bethesda and his team discovered that because the locals eat plenty of curries containing curcumin (turmeric), their Vita Genes—which means genes of life—are "switched on." These people also eat modestly, exercise regularly, hardly drink alcohol, do not smoke, and keep stress at bay with regular spiritual practices such as meditation. If you take 400mg curcumin, with 400mg bromelain and 10–20mg pipperine, this will help increase the "Okinawan effect," A good formula is Super Curcumin by Life Extension. **LEF** Curcumin is also highly anti-inflammatory, and as most diseases of aging are linked to inflammation and oxidation (of cells, tissues, and organs), eating and/or taking curcumin is a great idea. It also helps support liver function.

- **OMEGA-3 ESSENTIAL FATS** More than 2,000 scientific studies have demonstrated the wide range of problems associated with omega-3 fatty acid deficiencies. Unless you eat copious amounts of oily fish, then it's likely that you are part of the 60% of people whom researchers believe are deficient in omega-3 fats. Essential fats keep the skin hydrated and supple and are essential for hormone production, weight loss, and controlling blood pressure. The brain cannot function properly without essential fatty acids. Fish oils are high in EPA and DHA—omega-3 fats that are not generally found in vegetable or nut sources and are vital for the brain and nervous system. The best sources are sardines, wild or organically farmed salmon, mullet, trout, and mackerel. Excellent non-fish sources of omega-3 fats include flax seeds (linseeds), walnuts, hemp and pumpkin seeds, and to a lesser extent soybeans. For a lot more information about including these seeds and unrefined oils in your diet, see *Fats You Need To Eat*. I personally take 3g of pure omega-3 fish oils a day.

- **OMEGA-6 ESSENTIAL FATS** are found in sunflower seeds, sesame seeds, pumpkin seeds, linseeds (flax seeds) and their unrefined oils, as well as evening primrose oil. Most people have plenty of omega-6 EFAs in their diet from vegetable spreads and oils.

- **ALPHA-LIPOIC ACID (ALA)** is an important antioxidant that has the unique ability to pass into the brain where it helps recycle other antioxidants, such as vitamins C and E and glutathione, a vital brain nutrient. ALA also removes heavy metals such as aluminum, mercury, and lead from the brain, which helps protect against Alzheimer's, Parkinson's and senile dementia. Because it is both water and fat soluble, it is easily absorbed in the gut. ALA also helps prevent and treat some of the complications of diabetes. Take 200mg daily with food.

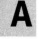

- **CARNOSINE** is a naturally occurring antioxidant made by the body; however, these levels fall as we age. High concentrations of carnosine are present in long-lived cells, such as nerve tissues, and people who live longer have higher levels of this nutrient. Carnosine has been shown to help reverse age-related damage, especially in the skin. It also blocks the production of amyloid, a substance found in the brains of Alzheimer's patients. Other emerging benefits are its apparent anti-cancer effects, the removal of toxic metals from the body, and its immune-boosting potential. Carnosine is found in lean red meat and chicken. For optimum anti-aging results, take 50–100mg daily. Take on an empty stomach in between meals.

- **CO-ENZYME Q10 (CoQ10)** is an essential, vitamin-like substance that is manufactured in the liver. As we age production slows down. CoQ10 facilitates and regulates the oxidation of fats and sugars into energy. CoQ10 also has profound anti-aging effects on the brain and helps protect the heart. Parkinson's patients tend to be low in CoQ10. Supplementation with CoQ10 has been shown to inhibit cancer-cell growth and protect breast tissue, successfully manage allergies, boost energy levels, protect individuals from gum disease, and act as an antioxidant. If you want to stay younger longer, take 100mg daily. If you are taking statin drugs to lower your LDL cholesterol levels, it is important to replenish CoQ10, which is greatly depleted by statin treatment (see *Cholesterol*).

- **COLLAGEN** is a vital component of healthy joints, skin, hair, nails, cartilage, ligaments. and tendons, which also improves bone strength. It is the most widely distributed protein in the body, and we lose about 1.5% annually after the age of 30. I take collagen powder daily in a glass of water or diluted juice 30 minutes before a main meal to help replenish this vital protein. I recommend Super Strength Collagen Drink from Higher Nature, which can be ordered online at www.auravita.com and shipped worldwide.

- **VITAMIN D3** There is now a large body of evidence that shows a lack of Vitamin D, which is synthesized on your skin when it is exposed to sunlight, plays a part in strokes, high blood pressure, diabetes, osteoarthritis, osteoporosis, depression, muscle wasting, and numerous cancers, including colon and breast cancers. For anti-aging, I take 1000IU of Vitamin D3 daily. Thousands of lives could be saved annually if we all did the same.

- **HYALURONIC ACID** (HA) After the age of 40, if you want to help keep your skin and joints more supple, you should begin taking liquid hyaluronic acid in water every day. HA is a naturally occurring protein in the body and is what makes young skin look plump and supple. Unfortunately, as we age, levels of HA in the body decline, resulting in wrinkles and joint problems. HA is used in thousands of beauty salons as an injectable to plump up lines and wrinkles; however, it can also be taken internally in a liquid formula. Taking 1ml daily in water on an empty stomach is very effective. For more details ask at your health store or consult an alternative healthcare professional.

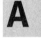

■ Keep your body more alkaline: virtually all chronic diseases associated with aging thrive in an over-acid environment. Take a teaspoon of any organic Green Powder daily. I use Green pH made by Metabolics (www.metabolics.com), which is a mixture of green beans, garden peas, pea leaf, dry apple cider, watercress, broccoli, and nettle leaf, and take one small level teaspoon daily in water. It doesn't taste great, but it is a quick and easy way to alkalize your body. This particular product is only available in the UK, but other companies make comparable products: **JF, VC, VS**

■ After the age of 40, if you tend to eat in a hurry or have a fast-paced lifestyle, you should also take a digestive enzyme with your main meals. There is no point taking all these great nutrients if you are suffering assimilation problems. (See *Low Stomach Acid* and *Leaky Gut*.)

■ As we age, the pineal gland in our brain produces less melatonin, which means we sleep less and sometimes have more problems getting to sleep. Melatonin is one of the most efficient anti- oxidants known to science and helps protect DNA; therefore, it helps keep you younger longer. Bio-electromagnetic research scientist Roger Coghill says, "If you take melatonin supplements that you can buy online and in the States, most synthetic tablets contain thousands of times the natural dose that your pineal gland normally produces." Therefore Roger has developed a supplement called Asphalia, which contains natural melatonin extracted from certain grasses and mimics the normal dose made by your pineal gland to induce sleep at night, rather than the larger doses, which are found in mass-produced tablets. Take 1 to 2 capsules 30 minutes before bed. Roger's exclusive distributor in the US is Diva Marketing, Don't Disturb Me!, 2612 Sleepy Hollow, Pearland, TX 77581; Tel: 1-713-221-1873 or 1-866-692-8037; website: www.dontdisturbmesite.com

NB: This supplement should not be taken by pregnant women in their third trimester, severe asthmatics, or children under one year.

Helpful Hints

- People who are adaptable and have a positive outlook on life tend to live the longest.
- Never underestimate just how much your thoughts and stress levels can affect not only your health but also the speed at which you age. If you keep saying over and over again that "it's to be expected at my age," do not be surprised if you become sicker and age faster (see *Stress*).
- Learn to say yes to what you want in your life and no to what you don't.
- Have fun—laugh a lot. No one ever had engraved on their tombstone: "I wish I had spent more time at the office." Find a balance.
- Stop worrying—as Dale Carnegie once said, "85% of things you worry about never happen," so stop worrying about the things you cannot change. Instead, concentrate on what you can change. And if you really want to change things in your own life and environment, then take the steps necessary to begin the changes that you require. Be willing to act positively for the good of all rather than just talking about it.
- Stop smoking. Every cigarette you smoke can take 15 minutes off your life. Smoking ages your skin and depletes vital nutrients such as vitamin C, which are needed for healthy skin and bones, energy production, and an active immune system.
- Exercise regularly—but not to excess.
- Being overweight can shorten your life by up to 10 years (see *Weight Problems*). so maintain a healthy body weight.

A

- Supplementing the hormone DHEA (see *Menopause*) can help reduce inflammation and aging in the body. Don't take extra hormones unless you need them. Never self-medicate with hormones—have a blood or saliva test. Many doctors administer these tests and there are also home test kits available online.
- Learn to meditate (see *Meditation*), for it has many proven anti-aging benefits. Regular meditation helps you cope more effectively with stress by reducing levels of the highly toxic stress hormones adrenalin and cortisol. It also slows the aging process.
- Reduce your exposure to cellular phones and excessive electrical equipment.
- Reduce exposure to pesticides, herbicides, and toxic chemicals. Consume organic foods and drinks as much as possible.
- Too much sun will age your skin, but we do need some sunshine to produce vitamin D, which helps to keep bones healthy. Sunshine makes you feel good-everything in moderation. Wear a PABA-free organic UVA/UVB sunscreen to protect the skin.
- Try using Real Sunlight lamps by Zadro, available from Target or Amazon. The harmful frequencies of UVA and UVB have been filtered out, making this sunlight safe. These lamps naturally increase levels of vitamin D3, improve collagen production, and boost immune system function.
- Don't overeat. Generally in the West, we tend to eat 40% more food than the body needs. Having said that, there are some people on calorie-restricted diets (proven to slow aging) living on 1,200 calories a day, but some of them look awful! And food is meant to be a pleasure. We can all enjoy treats and not feel guilty, but we must stop living on treats.
- Get sufficient sleep—it's the easiest way to look younger longer.
- A useful website for anti-aging research is the Life Extension Foundation at www.lef.org. They sell a wide variety of supplements, and you can also order hormones such as DHEA and melatonin. However, please check to make sure you need them first.
- Dr Nick Delgardo is a member of the American Academy of Anti-aging and his website, www.growyoungandslim.com, is well worth a look.

- Always use a body lotion after bathing. There are many fabulous organic vitamin creams that are now widely available from health stores. Anne McDevitt offers a great range of organic, biodynamic and glycolic acid creams, which help remove dead skin cells. For details log onto www.annemcdevitt.ie or email: sales@annemcdevitt.com
- The Life Extension Foundation offers numerous creams and serums based on Vitamin C, white tea, pomegranate, etc., which have demonstrated anti-aging properties. **LEF**

AGE SPOTS
(see also Liver Problems and Sunburn)

If you look at young skin, it's almost always clear with an even tone, but age spots can begin to appear from your early 40s and onwards. However, if you look at the buttocks of an average 60-year-old woman, the skin will still look young and blemish free. The best ways to reduce and avoid age spots are to have less exposure to the sun, look after your liver and ingest more antioxidants. Melanocytes are your melanin- or color-producing cells, and over time, thanks to exposure to the sun, these fatty pigments or lipids begin to "clump" together, causing age spots (also known as liver spots) or uneven pigmentation of varying sizes and shapes. And while age spots can appear all over the body, they most commonly appear on the backs of the hands, the face, the forearms, and eventually anywhere that is exposed regularly to the sun.

Foods to Avoid

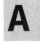

- Fried and barbecued foods, saturated fats found in full-fat dairy products, cakes and fatty meats.
- Alcohol and too many fats, which place a strain on your liver.
- Mass-produced refined foods and meals, which are often packed with hydrogenated and trans-fats, plus sugar, which all age the skin (see *Fats You Need To Eat*).
- Reduce non-organic foods, which are often high in additives and pesticides.

Friendly Foods

- To help avoid age spots it is important that the body is eliminating unwanted fatty deposits properly. Lecithin granules, available from all health stores, help emulsify and break down fats. Take 1 tablespoon daily over cereals, fruits and yogurts. Lecithin is also found in soy products and eggs.
- Eat more antioxidant-rich foods, organic fruit and vegetables, especially red, orange or dark-green fruits and vegetables, such as pomegranates, papaya, blueberries, carrots, apricots, watercress, pumpkin, broccoli, spring greens, bok choy, red peppers, red and purple berries, and tomatoes.
- Use tahini or olive oil instead of hydrogenated margarines and spreads.

Useful Remedies

- Antioxidants help mop up or neutralize the free-radical reactions that are triggered by sunbathing. Therefore, take a high-strength antioxidant formula that includes 200IU of full-spectrum Vitamin E, vitamin C, zinc, and selenium as a base.
- Beta-carotene helps encourage melanin production; make sure it's a natural-source carotene complex that contains all of the carotenoids. **LEF, NOW, SVHC**
- Potassium chloride is important for removing congestion and fatty deposits in tissues. You should take 50mg potassium chloride per tablet three times a day. **VC**
- Take at least 1g of vitamin C daily.
- Essential fatty acids, known as EFAs, help reduce the sun's negative effects. If taken regularly

they help keep your skin looking younger for longer (see *Fats You Need To Eat*). Take 2g of pure omega-3 fish oils daily.

- Pycnogenol, a pine bark extract, has been shown to help maintain elasticity of the skin. Take 80mg daily. **PN, NOW, GNC**

Helpful Hints

- Apply a sunscreen with at least 15 SPF on the backs of your hands and on your face, and take more care in the sun; you really will reap the benefits in later life.
- If you have young children, keep in mind that a huge amount of skin damage can be done before a child reaches 16. If children are allowed to burn, they are more likely to suffer skin cancers later in life. Some sun is healthy, but all things in moderation. Time and again, I see young children and teenagers on beaches in the midday sun with red, blistered skin and no hat! (See *Sunburn*.)
- The secret is not to let the skin burn and turn red. We all know the sensible precautions—to cover up between 11am and 3pm and to always wear a hat in hot midday sun—but a huge majority of us are simply not doing it. Start protecting the skin from an early age. If you do want to tan, do it slowly—don't burn.
- Ask at your health store for an antioxidant-rich cream. There are now dozens of creams containing grape-seed extract, vitamins C and E and so on. Use this daily on any age spots you may already have.
- Cigarettes age your skin. Stop smoking.

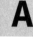

- As we age cell turnover within the skin slows down; therefore, use glycolic acid derived from sugar cane to gently eliminate dead skin cells and skin discolorations. These creams are fairly successful if used now and again, especially when combined with kojic acid. If you use these creams, then always use an SPF antioxidant cream in tandem. To see a range of products, log on to www.annemcdevitt.ie or email sales@annemcdevitt.com
- Modern lasers are highly successful at removing age spots, but make sure you see a dermatologist or doctor who has experience with this work. I had mine done at The Skin Clinic, 144 Harley Street, London W1G 7LD by Dr Thomas Bozek. Tel: 011-44-20-7224-0988. Most dermatology clinics in the US also provide this treatment; visit the American Academy of Dermatology's website (www.aad.org) to find a clinic near you.

ALCOHOL

(see also Liver Problems)

Alcohol is responsible for approximately 79,000 deaths annually in the US, and 504 people die every week from liver disease—making alcohol the third leading cause of preventable death in the US.

Thanks to the incidence of binge drinking, especially among the young, specialists are now seeing more and more young people in their twenties with the liver problems usually seen in people over 50. In fact, approximately 28% of high school students and more than half of college students binge drink.

Every time you drink alcohol, it acts as a diuretic and causes dehydration. It also upsets blood sugar levels, adrenal function, irritates the gut, and causes the body to excrete vital minerals and vitamins, especially the B-group vitamins, which help keep your nervous system, hormone production, hair, and nails in good shape. The more you drink, the more effect it has on your behavior.

Moderate consumption of alcohol, meaning no more than one drink per day for women and no more than two drinks per day for men, has been shown to be slightly protective against heart disease. One drink is equal to 12oz of beer, 8oz of malt liquor, 5oz of wine, or a shot of 80-proof distilled spirits or liquor (gin, rum, vodka, whiskey, etc.) However, the heart-protective effects are most often associated with drinking red wine.

So, while a glass of aged or organic red wine is fine, it's important to remember that the nutrient content of alcohol is very low and that while you may be protecting their heart you are also elevating your risk of hormonal cancers, particularly breast cancer. Alcohol places an enormous strain on the liver, as it reduces its ability to detoxify the body. Over-consumption of alcohol can lead to fatigue and dehydration, as well as disruptive sleep patterns, and can deplete many vital nutrients from the body. In extreme cases of bingeing, the bladder can burst.

Pregnant women risk fetal abnormalities if they consume alcohol during pregnancy, and it should be avoided if you are trying to become pregnant. During pregnancy, give it up. Think of your future. When you are young, you think that "it will never happen to me"—but believe me, it can and does.

Foods to Avoid
- Avoid eating fresh or canned grapefruit juice if you are drinking alcohol as this will increase the toxicity of the alcohol.
- Saturated fats place a great strain on the liver. Avoid fatty, heavy, rich meals—especially sausages, cheese (especially melted cheese as in pizzas), rich pâtés, burgers, and so on.
- Never ply anyone who is drunk with coffee, as this will further dehydrate the body, which can increase the concentration of alcohol in their system. (See *General Health Hints*.)

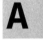

Friendly Foods
- Eat plenty of fresh fruits and vegetables, especially broccoli, artichokes, cauliflower, beets, celeriac (celery root), celery, fennel, and radicchio to help to detoxify the liver.
- Eat plenty of soluble fibers such as linseeds (soaked flax seeds), oat bran, and low-sugar cereals such as muesli or oatmeal.
- Drink at least 6–8 glasses of water daily.
- Use unrefined olive, walnut or sunflower oils for salad dressings.
- See also *General Health Hints*.

Useful Remedies
- The herb milk thistle (silymarin) has been proven to help detoxify and regenerate the liver. Take 500mg of the whole-herb supplement twice a day with meals for one month. During this time you will need to cut down on your alcohol intake to give your liver time to repair. **VC**
- Take a couple of capfuls of organic pure aloe vera juice daily before foods, as aloe supports the liver and acts as a mild anti- inflammatory.
- If you are an occasional drinker, take one high-strength milk thistle capsule before and after drinking.
- Taking 500mg of the amino acid methionine twice a day away from food helps the liver recover. It's a great liver detoxifier.
- Take a good-quality multi-vitamin/mineral for your age and gender daily. **NP, SVHC, JF**
- To avoid hangovers, take 2g of evening primrose oil, 1g of vitamin C, a B-complex supplement, plus 500mg of milk thistle with a full glass of water before going out. Repeat this dosage the next morning as soon as you wake up.
- Chinese kudzu extract contains diadzin, which has been known to be beneficial for treating alcoholism. Not only does kudzu extract help reduce the craving for alcohol, but it also acts as a muscle relaxant, which helps to overcome some of the withdrawal symptoms. Take 10–20 drops of the tincture or 2 tablets before you take a drink. **VC**

Helpful Hints

- Do not give a person coffee to sober them up as coffee is a diuretic, which means it depletes fluid from the body and makes the alcohol content in the blood even more concentrated.
- For every alcoholic drink, make sure you have a non-alcoholic one in between. Generally drink more water, as alcohol severely dehydrates the body. Avoid alcohol when flying, because the pressurized cabins cause considerable dehydration.
- If you have a hangover, you need to raise your blood sugar quite quickly upon waking. Eat a banana or blend various fresh fruits such as figs, papaya, dates and/or raisins with low-fat, live yogurt (or rice milk) and drink immediately, or drink some diluted fruit juice.
- Drink 3 glasses of water slowly as soon as you wake up to rehydrate the body.
- Take one Homeopathic Nux Vomica 30c before bed and another upon waking to help reduce a hangover. This really helps. **VS,VC**
- Bingeing on alcohol is **extremely dangerous**—it creates too much shock in the liver. Vomiting is an indication that the body has reached a danger level, and you must stop drinking.
- If you must drink, have a couple of drinks daily—but do not drink to excess. Better quality red wine, especially Pinot Noir, seems to confer the most health benefits, owing to antioxidant substances called polyphenols present in the skin of red grapes.
- Dandelion root tea tastes bitter but is excellent for cleansing the liver.
- The liver detoxifies most efficiently between 1 and 3am—but for it to do this you need to be lying down, so burning the midnight oil and beyond puts even greater strain on your liver.
- Remember that it takes 20 minutes for alcohol to have an effect and more than one hour for the body to process each unit. If you are concerned about the amount that you (or a member of your family) are drinking, call the National Council on Alcoholism and Drug Dependence at 1-800-NCA-CALL for advice and information. The line is open 24 hours a day, seven days a week. You can also contact your local crisis hotline for help. Most hotlines will be listed in the front pages of your local phone book.

ALLERGIC RHINITIS

(see also Allergies, Candida, Hay Fever, and Leaky Gut)

The incidence of allergic rhinitis is, without a doubt, on the rise as more and more people suffer toxic overload and food sensitivities. Typical symptoms include a runny nose, sneezing, sinus congestion, plus itchy and watering eyes. These symptoms usually appear immediately after being exposed to any foods or external pollutants, such as traffic fumes. Unlike hay fever, allergic rhinitis tends to affect people all year round, although symptoms can be worse at certain times of year when pollen counts are high. In some individuals it is triggered by a food intolerance, the most common being a sensitivity to cow's milk and wheat-containing products. This will need to be addressed for the problem to be resolved. You can take all kinds of herbs and supplements to try to relieve the problem (or worse yet—antihistamines), but this will not address the root cause of the condition. For example, when I eat a high-sugar food, my nose starts running within seconds, which is a shame as I have a sweet tooth! But this demonstrates how immediate any effect can be. This condition can also be linked to candida and/or leaky gut syndrome. See *Candida* and *Leaky Gut*.

Foods to Avoid

- Avoid sugar and high mucus-forming foods, such as full-fat dairy products, cheese and chocolate, as much as possible. Soy milk and foods can also cause this problem for many people.
- Reduce white flour and pasta, orange juice, tomatoes and any other foods to which you may have an intolerance. Keep a food diary and note when symptoms are worse.
- Wheat and dairy products from cows are known to be triggers for this condition, but it could just as easily be bananas or tomatoes.
- Wine and dried fruits, which contain sulfites, can also trigger this condition in some people.

Friendly Foods

- Eat more curries because they are rich in turmeric, which helps calm the inflammatory response.
- Include plenty of garlic, onions, horseradish, root ginger, and freshly squeezed fruit and vegetable juices (but not carton juice) in your diet.
- Fresh pineapple contains bromelain, which reduces inflammation. But don't drink the juice; it is high in sugar.
- If you have an intolerance to wheat, try rye, rice or amaranth crackers and oat cakes. Ask at your health store for wheat-free bread and pasta.
- Dairy alternatives include organic rice, soy, goat's, almond or oat milk. Soy milk does, however, trigger excess mucus in some people.

Useful Remedies

- If symptoms are acute, take up to 5g of vitamin C in an ascorbate form per day with meals spread throughout the day, plus 500mg to 2g of pantothenic acid (vitamin B5).
- Take a bioflavonoid complex—500mg to 2g daily when acute.
- Take 500mg of bromelain, an enzyme from pineapple that helps break down mucus and reduce the allergic response, thereby reducing the discomfort.
- Nettle tincture or tea three times a day helps alleviate symptoms.
- Quercetin, another flavonoid, helps reduce the allergic response. Take 400mg three times a day while the symptoms are acute.
- Beta Glucans 1–3, 1–6, which are derived from yeast cell walls, are proven to strengthen the body's innate immune system (the immune system you were born with), making it more resistant to pathogens from food and the air. Take 250–500 mg daily. **VC**

Helpful Hints

- Keep a food diary and note when your symptoms become worse. You should also note if certain toothpastes trigger the problem or even a walk near a main road can make symptoms worse.
- During an acute attack, a homeopathic nasal spray called Euphorbium Spray is extremely effective. It helps relieve a runny nose, congestion, and headaches. **VC**
- Dust and other airborne allergens can be reduced in your immediate environment with an ionizer.
- Try New Era tissue salt Nat Mur for alleviating allergic rhinitis.
- I recommend that you try taking the Neil Med Sinus Rinse every day. It's incredibly easy to use and really helps reduce allergic reactions linked to the sinuses as well as the incidence of sinus infections. Find details via www.neilmed.com It is also available from most health stores.

ALLERGIES

(see also Leaky Gut and Liver Problems)

Allergy problems, such as asthma, eczema, and rhinitis, are responsible for more than 17 million outpatient doctor's visits a year, and at least 50 million people in the US alone are thought to have either an allergy or a sensitivity to various substances. Allergies are now the fifth most common chronic disease for all age groups and the third most common among children.

Allergies or sensitivities to various foods or substances can cause coughing, itchy skin, skin rashes, joint problems, fibromyalgia, autoimmune conditions such as lupus, wheezing, runny nose, sneezing, watery eyes, chronic sore throats, and so on. Many doctors still state that food intolerances are "all in the mind," but ask anyone who suffers chronic bloating after eating wheat or a razor-sore throat within an hour of eating chocolate if they are imagining their symptoms, which of course they aren't.

The severest form of allergy triggers anaphylactic shock, a potentially life-threatening condition that needs immediate medical attention. People with severe allergies usually carry an injectable form of adrenaline, which would need to be injected immediately if that person were exposed to a specific allergen such as peanuts or a bee sting.

Allergies or sensitivities from external sources such as pesticides, food additives, paints, pollution, perfumes, animal hairs, grass, plant and tree pollens are also widespread. More than 1 billion tons of pesticide products are used on crops in the US every year, and there are more than 13,000 pesticide products registered for use in California alone. Think about this: if you eat a non-organic apple, it may have been sprayed up to 18 times before you eat it, and an average person ingests up to a gallon of pesticides each year. Therefore it's no wonder that we are suffering a variety of reactions. Allergies and sensitivities are the body's way of saying it has had enough and cannot cope with more toxins. This is why symptoms appear when the system becomes overloaded with toxins and/or stress.

Also, many people only partially digest food proteins, which can sometimes break through the gut wall. The body treats these particles as it would an infection and attacks them as an enemy, which if left untreated can cause a myriad of allergic-type symptoms and eventually contribute to the development of an autoimmune disease or severe gut problems. The secret to controlling allergies and sensitivities is to reduce your exposure to all pollutants.

Foods to Avoid
- Eggs, dairy products from cows, wheat, oranges, tomatoes, corn, and soy are all very common allergens.
- All food additives found in mass-produced foods and monosodium glutamate (MSG).
- Caffeine, peanuts, chocolate, beef, yeast, and shellfish.

Friendly Foods
- This is a possible minefield until you know which foods are your problem, but generally eat more brown rice, pears, lamb, cabbage, lentils, papaya, leeks, green peas, aduki beans, and sweet potatoes, which are usually well tolerated. Amaranth crackers, buckwheat or quinoa are also low-allergen foods.
- Include more flaxseeds (linseeds are best soaked overnight in cold water), sunflower seeds and organic sunflower and olive oil in your diet. These foods are a good starting point because very few people react to them.
- It's worth noting that the foods you tend to crave and eat the most are usually the ones that are causing the most problems. Wheat and cow's milk are the most common.
- Papaya is rich in digestive enzymes.

- Live goat's or sheep's yogurt contain friendly bacteria and are more easily digested than cow's milk.
- Raw cabbage juice is high in L-glutamine, which is known to help to heal a leaky gut. Try making fresh juices daily that include a little chopped raw cabbage, a tiny piece of root ginger, carrots, apples, and a tablespoon of aloe vera juice. Drink immediately after blending while all the enzymes and nutrients are still active.
- Drink small amounts of licorice tea to help heal the gut and reduce stress. Nettle tea will help reduce the allergic response.
- Fennel tea will aid digestion if taken after meals, especially if gas and bloating are a problem.

Useful Remedies

- Histazyme, a complex containing calcium, vitamin C, zinc, bromelain, silica, vitamin A, and manganese, acts as a natural antihistamine. BioCare (www.biocare.co.uk) offers international shipping. D-Hist is another natural supplement that works similarly and is available on Amazon.com.
- HEP 194 contains various herbs, the enzyme lipase, the amino acid methionine, and B-vitamins, which all help to support the liver. BioCare (www.biocare.co.uk) offers international shipping.
- Beta Glucans 1–3, 1–6, which are derived from yeast cell walls, are proven to strengthen the body's innate immune system, making it more resistant to pathogens from food and the air. Take 250–500mg daily. It can also be taken by children and reduces the likelihood of food intolerances triggered by a weakened innate immune system. Dr Paul Clayton is a medical pharmacologist based in the UK and US. His website (www.healthdefence.com) is well worth a look. Glucosan, developed by Dr Clayton, is shipped to the US by Nutri Centre (www.nutricentre.com). Other brands of beta glucan are available from Vitacost (www.vitacost.com).

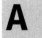

- Betaine hydrochloride—stomach acid—is often lacking in people suffering from allergies and is available from most health stores. You should take one capsule just as you begin eating your main meal but not if you have active stomach ulcers. In this case, try a digestive enzyme tablet (without HCl) that is available at your local health store.
- The amino acid L-glutamine can help heal a leaky gut. Mix 1 teaspoon in a little diluted fruit juice or water (but not orange juice) and take it 30–45 minutes before main meals twice a day until symptoms ease.
- A good-quality daily multi-vitamin/mineral.
- Once you have identified your intolerance, you can reduce your supplement intake to just the multi-vitamin/mineral and the HCl or digestive enzyme every day.
- A common homeopathic remedy for runny eyes and nose is Allium 6c, or if there is swelling Apis 6c, taken three times daily.
- There is now good evidence showing that taking healthy bacteria (probiotics) regularly will reduce the amount of "allergens" from food that can pass through the gut wall. Take one capsule daily after food. For details, ask at your health store or speak to a certified nutritionist.
- H Metabolism tablets by Metabolics (www.metabolics.com) help reduce high histamine levels in the body triggered by the allergy. Take two capsules, three times daily if symptoms are acute. International shipping is available.
- Finnish researchers found that when expectant mothers are given prebiotics (nutrients extracted from the agave plant, which support the growth of healthy bacteria in the gut and enhance immune function) during their final weeks of pregnancy, their babies were far less likely to suffer from respiratory infections or to develop conditions such as asthma. For details about Agave Digestive Immune Support, visit www.lef.org

Helpful Hints

- It is important to have an allergy test to find your worst offenders. One of the best I have found is available from the YorkTest Laboratories, which is located in the UK but can also be utilized overseas; visit www.yorktest.com for more details. Another one is a FACT test from Genova Diagnostics, which looks for any inflammatory markers that indicate the body is reacting to certain substances. Tel: 1-800-522-4762 or visit the website: www.genovadiagnostics.com

- Another excellent method is known as the Bio Meridian Test for food intolerance and leaky gut, in which the practitioner measures via electrodes your reactions to a huge list of foods and substances. For practitioners of the test, visit www.biomeridian.com or call 1-888-224-2337 toll free.

- To receive free allergy alert notices from The Food Allergy & Anaphylaxis Network, register your e-mail address at www.foodallergy.org

- It is vital to chew food more thoroughly.

- Avoid large meals, which overload the digestive system and liver and can trigger an allergic response.

- Many toothpastes, shampoos, soaps, detergents, perfumes, body lotions, and sunscreens contain a myriad of chemicals, so buy products in their most natural and unadulterated state. For anyone who suffers dermatitis or skin allergies, Weleda (www.beautorium.com) makes organic skin, hair and body creams and toothpastes.

- USANA Health Services also makes a natural toothpaste. Visit www.makessense.usana.com to order.

- To test if you have a food sensitivity, first take your resting pulse rate. Then for at least 14 days completely avoid the food you want to test—for example, wheat. Then try eating the food you have avoided on its own—for example, a plate of pasta or plain brown toast. Take your pulse at 15, 30, and 60 minutes after eating the specific food. If your pulse has increased by more than 10 beats a minute, it is likely that you have a sensitivity to the test food. Or have a blood test such as The York Test—details above.

- Many allergic and chemically sensitive people can benefit enormously by switching from tap water to mineral or filtered water. Tests in the US found that 98% of environmentally ill patients improved by eliminating tap water. For details call Pure Water Systems toll free at 1-866-444-9926 or visit www.purewatersystems.com

- Use Kangen Water—a water system that attaches to your kitchen faucet and ionizes and alkalizes water. It's used in Japanese hospitals with highly beneficial health results. For full details visit www.kangenwaterusa.com

- Dr Jean Monro, who has worked at the Breakspear Hospital in Hertfordshire in the UK for 25 years, says: "Before the industrial revolution, conditions such as hay fever did not exist. But since then we have done a great job of polluting our atmosphere and thus our bodies. We now know that an accumulation of a variety of pollutants, such as paint sprays or pesticides (there are hundreds of others), acts as the initial trigger; these chemicals became the sensitizers—and in most cases the membranes within the nose and throat begin to react and become inflamed. Then the body treats the next thing that comes along, such as grass pollens, as a threatening foreign invader, which increases any inflammation and induces allergic-type symptoms. But it's the chemicals that sensitize the body in the first place. Chemicals can have a local affect such as on the skin—and then this effect is communicated to the rest of the body by neural (nerve) pathways and a sensitivity is born.

    "The neural pathway is extremely important because it is the body's sense of awareness, which firstly triggers the dendritic cells, which then send a message to the autonomic nervous system that controls pulse, breathing, and temperature. And if someone suffering a severe reaction to, say, peanuts reacts, even if that peanut happens to be in someone's pocket across the room, we now know that this instantaneous effect is triggered not only by particles of the peanuts but also by the frequencies emitted by the peanut, which have an instant effect. It's important for people to realize that not only do we all emit our own unique signature range of frequencies, but so does everything around us, from asbestos to our foods. And if you have a specific substance/food or whatever emitting a frequency that is incompatible with your own, then symptoms will eventually show up.

"After 20 years' research, we have developed new vaccines based on frequencies that can help to neutralize any reaction to substances found to trigger a response, and these vaccines are proving very effective. This is the medicine of the future. Also, the more that people stay away from synthetic chemicals and reduce the body's toxic overload, the less allergies and sensitivities will occur."

This is fascinating research and for anyone who wants more details about allergy and environmental medicine, log on to www.breakspearmedical.com.

ALOPECIA *(see Hair Loss)*

ALZHEIMER'S DISEASE (AD) *(see also Memory)*

Alzheimer's disease (AD) affects around 5.3 million people to varying degrees in the US and was first described and documented between 1900 and 1906 by the German neurologist Alois Alzheimer—hence its name. The term "dementia" is used to describe the symptoms that present themselves when the brain is affected by specific diseases. Dementia affects one in every 14 people over the age of 65, and as we are an aging population these figures are expected to rise.

More than a third of people over the age of 70 say they suffer from some form of memory loss. The good news is that most of us have similar problems, but only about one in every seven Americans over the age of 70 actually has Alzheimer's disease.

AD is a progressive, degenerative disease that attacks the brain, triggering symptoms such as memory loss (especially short-term), confusion, agitation, and frequently forgetting names, places, appointments, and recent events. Mood swings can become common as well as a gradual withdrawing from everyday life, especially as a person's confidence and his or her ability to communicate is affected. It is the loss of memory of how to do everyday tasks that tends to make a familiar life almost impossible.

In the early stages, AD sufferers have symptoms of absent-mindedness and an inability to learn new things. Judgment and intellectual and social functioning begin to go awry. Later there is loss of logic and memory and poor co-ordination. Speech deteriorates and symptoms of paranoia may appear. In the final stages the AD sufferers completely lose touch with their surroundings and become unresponsive. Needless to say, this is very traumatic, not only for the sufferer but also for their family. *The tragedy is that AD, in most cases, is a preventable disease and can even be reversed to some degree.*

There is no doubt that genes play a part. Researchers have found that those with a variation in the gene MTHFD1L may be twice as likely to develop Alzheimer's—but, by changing our lifestyle and diet, we can, in the majority of cases, change which genes are expressed and load the dice more in favor of good health—even in later life.

One of the most common theories regarding what causes AD is metal toxicity, most likely with aluminum and mercury. A 1980 study of 647 Canadian gold miners who had routinely inhaled aluminum since the 1940s (a common practice thought to prevent silica poisoning), found that all of the miners tested in the "impaired" range for cognitive function, suggesting a clear link between aluminum and memory loss. But while aluminum is certainly harmful to the brain, there are other key factors that can lead to degeneration.

Researchers have found a significant imbalance of metals in AD patients, especially mercury, which has mainly been deposited in areas of the brain related to memory. Mercury is known to cause the type of damage to nerves that is characteristic of AD, and researchers have found that early-onset AD patients have the highest mercury levels of all (see *Mercury Fillings*).

Another factor is homocysteine, a toxic compound produced during the metabolism of proteins. Increased homocysteine levels are a strong, independent risk factor for the development of dementia. At the University of Gothenburg in Sweden, a lengthy study of 1500 women that concluded in November 2009 found that AD was more than twice as common among women with the highest levels of homocysteine. The higher the homocysteine level, the greater the damage to the brain. Homocysteine is readily recycled or broken down within the body by vitamins B6, B12 and folic acid. Therefore, by taking a B-complex supplement daily (or many companies now make Homocysteine support formulas), homocysteine levels can be kept in check. There is also a home test kit from York Test that you can send to the YorkTest Laboratories in the UK to give you your homocysteine level. For details visit www.yorktest.com

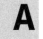

Alzheimer's is also characterized by the buildup of amyloid plaques and, as beta amyloid is an inflammatory protein, inflammation is now considered to be an underlying cause of AD. The amyloid plaques build up outside nerve cells (neurons) and eventually destroy or damage the neurons—thus impairing brain function.

Cortisol, the stress hormone, can also cause great damage to the brain, causing the connections between brain cells to shrivel up, which contributes to AD. There are good supplements to help control cortisol production. See *Stress*.

Free radicals and an excessive intake of refined, processed foods that are low in antioxidant vitamins such as A, C and E are also contributing factors. Basically, the more pollutants and refined foods we are exposed to, the more vital minerals and vitamins are excreted from the body, causing brain function to deteriorate. Eating the right foods, taking supplements that nourish the brain and exercising more increases circulation to the brain, often improving memory. (See also *Electrical Pollution* and *Memory*.)

Foods to Avoid

- Avoid refined grains in products such as white bread, rice, and pasta. These grains have had most of their nutrients, including B vitamins, removed during the refining process. Also remember that elevated homocysteine levels can be controlled by taking more B-complex vitamins such as B6, B12 and folate.
- Avoid foods containing traces of aluminum such as commercial chocolate, desserts, baking powder, processed cheeses, chewing gum, and pickles.
- Eliminate any foods that contain the food additives aspartame (an artificial sweetener) or monosodium glutamate (MSG), which are suspected neurotoxins.
- Avoid ready-made pies, cakes and pre-packaged meals that are not only cooked in aluminum containers but are also packed with saturated fat, sugar and salt.
- Reduce your intake of saturated fats found in fatty meats and full-fat dairy products.
- Reduce your intake of caffeine, sugar, and alcohol, which can all deplete vital nutrients and

interfere with brain function. Sugar is particularly deadly for brain function and contributes to beta-amyloid deposits, which are one of the main problems for AD patients. President Ronald Reagan ate jelly beans by the bag every day and developed AD.

Friendly Foods

- A Japanese study found that AD patients did not eat fish, rarely ate green/yellow vegetables, ate a lot of meat, and and tended to be lacking in vitamin C, carotenes, and omega-3 essential fats. Also a high intake of animal fats and high cholesterol levels can increase the risk of dementia in later life.
- AD patients are often deficient in the vital brain nutrient acetylcholine, which is manufactured by the body and found in oats, soa beans, eggs, cabbage, and cauliflower.
- Sprinkle a tablespoon of soy lecithin granules over breakfast cereals, into yogurt, or over fresh fruit. Lecithin is rich in acetylcholine, but make sure the brand you choose contains at least 30% of this nutrient. Other foods containing this vital brain nutrient are egg yolks and fish, especially sardines.
- Essential fats are vital for proper brain functioning. They also reduce inflammation within the brain (and body), which helps as brain inflammation and poor circulation is also linked to AD. Lack of omega-3 fish oils has now been demonstrated to be a factor in Alzheimer's and dementia. Eat more oily fish, especially organic farmed salmon, mackerel and sardines. Use organic flax or sunflower oil for your salad dressings, and avoid heating these oils.
- Eat more avocado and sprinkle wheat germ over breakfast cereals, fruit dishes, and salads as they are rich in vitamin E.
- Sweet potatoes are high in natural-source carotenes and will help nourish your brain.
- Include organic farmed salmon, herrings, and mackerel in your diet because they are rich in omega-3 essential fats. Include plenty of organic linseeds (flax seeds), sunflower and pumpkin seeds, which are also rich in healthy fats. Sprinkle them into breakfast cereals or eat them toasted or raw with salads and vegetables. Any way you prepare them, these seeds are delicious—and healthy (see also *Fats You Need To Eat*).
- Include antioxidant-rich foods such as berries (especially blueberries and blackberries), pomegranates, and prunes, as well as dark green leafy vegetables. Add plenty of other brightly colored fruits and vegetables to your diet, too. (See *General Health Hints*.)
- Garden sage has been found to prolong and improve memory functioning, owing to its powerful anti-inflammatory and antioxidant effects. Sage also inhibits the enzyme that breaks down acetylcholine. Use plenty of fresh sage over cooked foods or make sage teas. **Avoid sage if you are pregnant as it stimulates the uterus.**
- Use plenty of fresh cilantro in salads or sprinkle it over cooked dishes since cilantro helps remove toxic metals from the body.
- Eat plenty of pomegranate, as it helps keep arteries healthier and blood flowing.
- Blueberries are rich in potent brain-protecting antioxidants.
- Use nori seaweed flakes instead of salt; they also help eliminate heavy metals from the body.
- Adding cayenne pepper to meals aids circulation.
- Eat more fresh root ginger and fresh rosemary for their anti- inflammatory properties.

Useful Remedies

- Take a multi-vitamin/mineral/essential fats/antioxidant formula for your age and gender every day that also contains the brain nutrients mentioned above.
- Magnesium (300mg daily) and potassium phosphate (75mg daily) are important for nerve connections in the brain.
- Silica helps eliminate aluminum from the body. Take 75mg per day. Fiji mineral water is especially pure and rich in silica.

- Taking 600IU of natural-source, full-spectrum vitamin E and 1g of vitamin C three times a day with meals has been shown to slow the progress of Alzheimer's and to help prevent the onset of dementia. Placebo-controlled studies have shown that full-spectrum natural-source vitamin E is more effective than drugs at reducing the symptoms of Alzheimer's.
- Ginkgo biloba is an herb taken from leaves of what the Chinese call the memory tree. Try 120–240mg daily to help increase circulation to the brain and protect neurons. In rare cases ginkgo can cause a rash, which means you would need to stop taking it. **Do not take this herb if you are taking Warfarin or Aspirin stronger than 75mg daily.**
- B-vitamins are destroyed by stress and alcohol but are needed for the formation of acetylcholine and for the manufacture of other neurotransmitters within the brain and nervous system. Therefore, it is important to take a high-strength B-complex daily, especially if you are stressed.
- Curcumin, a substance found in the spice turmeric (widely used in curries), may be part of the reason AD is uncommon in India compared with Western countries. Studies in India found a less than 1% incidence of AD in people over 65. Curcumin reduces degenerative, inflammatory responses to amyloid. Try one or two standardized curcumin extract capsules daily with food.
- Lipoic acid is a vital brain nutrient that can help reduce heavy metals in the brain and body. Because it is fat soluble, it also protects nerve cells from damage. Take 200mg twice daily for prevention.

- Take HM Chelate by Pure Encapsulations Inc, a chlorella-based formula that also contains selenium, zinc, vitamin C, coriander, N-acetyl-cysteine, and lipoic acid—all of which help to pull heavy metals from the body. Take three to six capsules daily well away from food. Available in the US from webvitamins.com and PlanetRx.com
- Take 2g of omega-3 fish oils daily plus one GLA. They are vital for brain function and also highly anti-inflammatory.
- The herb aswagandha has been found to help protect areas of the brain that are needed for memory function. It also helps modulate cortisol production.
- Cognitex from The Life Extension Foundation contains phosphatidycholine, phosphatidylserine, vinpocetine, grape seed extract, wild blueberry, ashwagandha, ginger, and rosemary—all great nutrients to help keep your brain healthy. **LEF**
- More than 15 years of research by Dr Hirokazu Kawagishi of Shizoka University in Japan have demonstrated that pure extract of the Lion's Mane Mushroom has a remarkable ability to increase nerve growth factor (NGF) in the brain, which in turn helps make more neurons. Take it daily for at least 3 months, as nerves do not grow overnight! **VC, VS**

Helpful Hints

- As a general prevention, ask your doctor to measure your C-reactive protein levels to determine the amount of inflammation that is in your body. Inflammation in the arteries triggers a host of problems; therefore, if you have inflammation take steps to reduce it, as it can save your life in the long term. Markers of inflammation are redness, swelling, heat or/and pain.
- Avoid stress. Stress stimulates the adrenal glands to produce a hormone called cortisol, which can **greatly** damage your brain. Learn to relax. Take walks regularly or try yoga, tai chi, massage, or meditation. (See *Stress* for more supplements that can reduce cortisol production.)
- Stop smoking. Research indicates that smokers are twice as likely to develop dementia later in life. Avoid drugs such as cannabis and ecstasy, which are associated with memory loss if used in the long term.

- Have your hormone levels checked, as lack of hormones such as estrogen, progesterone, DHEA, and testosterone are known to affect the brain. Never self-medicate with hormones.
- Regular exercise has helped many sufferers restore some functions, especially memory. Learn ballroom dancing, which is great exercise and good for the brain! Walk daily to increase circulation and get more much-needed oxygen to your brain.
- If you have mercury fillings, you are advised to have them removed. It is imperative this is done by a dentist who specializes in this procedure, as increased mercury poisoning can result if the proper precautions are not taken to protect you during the filling removal (see *Mercury Fillings*).
- Because of the link between aluminum and AD, avoid aluminum cooking utensils and pans, as well as food stored in aluminum containers. Do not allow food to be in direct contact with aluminum foil, and don't heat foods wrapped in foil. Use stainless steel or glass cookware. Some antiperspirants contain aluminum so use natural deodorants such as those produced by TCCD International (www.naturallyfreshdeodorantcrystal.com)
- Simple antacids are often based on aluminum salts and should also be avoided. Aluminum is also found in toothpastes, some cosmetics, processed cheeses, baking powder, buffered aspirin, and table salts, where it is used as a pouring agent. If our mineral levels are low, then the body tends to absorb more aluminum so this is another reason to include a good multi-mineral in your everyday health regimen.
- Chelation therapy helps remove deadly metal toxins from the body. There are a number of clinics around the US. To find one near you, search the directory on www.worldwidehealthcenter.net
- Use it or lose it. Keep the brain healthy with simple exercises like doing crosswords, and force your brain to work by counting down from 500 each day in multiples of various numbers, such as 500 minus 7 = 493, minus 7 = 486 and so on. Try writing and using the opposite hand to the one you normally use regularly. Extend your arms out at shoulder level, rotate one hand clockwise and the other counterclockwise, and then change over to give your brain a workout. Buy a dictionary and learn to use and spell at least one new word every day. Learn sudoku, as it stimulates the brain.
- Eat organic foods as much as possible and drink filtered or bottled water. Many pesticides are now linked to neurological problems, and these chemicals, along with aluminum, are finding their way into our drinking water, so use a good water filter that removes all of these residues. Contact Pure Water Systems toll free at 1-866-444-9926 or visit www.purewatersystems.com
- Use Kangen Water—a water system that attaches to your kitchen faucet and ionizes and alkalizes water. It's used in Japanese hospitals with highly beneficial health results. For full details visit www.kangenwaterusa.com
- Avoid over-exposure to cellular phones and computers. Certain studies have shown that exposure to electromagnetic radiation significantly increases the risk of AD or makes it rapidly worse. So working with or near computers, visual display units (VDUs) and similar equipment may harm your brain. Evidence of how cellular phones affect the brain is also continuing to mount (see *Electrical Pollution*).
- Maintaining circulation to the brain is essential, because poor blood supply to the brain will starve it of oxygen and other nutrients. This is why regular exercise is important.
- Certain prescription drugs, including statins, are known to cause side effects that appear similar to symptoms of senile dementia. Anyone who feels that they may have the onset of dementia should immediately consult a qualified doctor who is also a nutritionist. (See *Useful Information*.)
- For more help visit: www.alz.org

A

- Read *The Alzheimer's Prevention Plan*, a very useful book by Patrick Holford (Piatkus), or *The Better Brain Book* by David Perlmutter and Carol Colman (Riverhead Trade).

ANEMIA

Anemia tends to come in two forms—pernicious anemia and iron deficiency. If you have pernicious anemia, it is because your body lacks an intrinsic factor it needs to absorb vitamin B12, which is essential for the production of red blood cells. In the past it was always thought that B12 injections were necessary; however, research has now shown that 1mg (1000mcg) a day of B12 taken orally can rectify this deficiency. A number of disorders can create B12 malabsorption, including gastritis, Crohn's disease and celiac disease. Smoking also inhibits absorption of iron.

If you have been diagnosed as suffering from anemia, the normal procedure is to take a large amount of iron, but it is very important to make sure that the co-factors, which are vitamin B12, folic acid, and vitamin C, are taken at the same time to optimize absorption.

Iron deficiency can be brought about by a number of factors, such as losing more blood than the body can replace naturally, which is common among women who suffer very heavy periods and should always be investigated by a doctor or a gynecologist. An underactive thyroid is also linked to low iron levels (see *Thyroid*).

Over-consumption of tea and coffee can somewhat inhibit iron absorption from your food. Many people take an iron supplement when they are feeling tired, but it is always worthwhile having blood levels of iron checked before you begin supplementing iron, which can accumulate in the body. Too much iron in older people, especially men, is linked to heart disease. Therefore anyone over 50 should not take iron supplements unless they have a medical condition that requires iron.

Common symptoms of low iron levels are fatigue, headaches, increased heart rate, shortness of breath, bleeding gums, confusion, feeling faint, and pale skin. If you are found to have low iron levels, it's important that your doctor finds the root cause of your anemia. Orthodox cancer treatments such as chemotherapy and radiation are known to induce anemia in some patients. Alcoholics also are often found to be low in folic acid and B12. Lack of testosterone in older men can also trigger anemia. Generally, vegetarians eat less iron than non-vegetarians and are considered to be more at risk for low iron levels. However, in Israel researchers found that blood iron levels were actually higher in vegetarians, which is probably owing to their high consumption of fruit and vegetables. Vegetarians who do not eat sufficient fruit and vegetables can be low in iron. Vegans most definitely would need to take 50–100mcg of B12 supplements daily.

Foods to Avoid
- Excessive amounts of black tea and coffee, which can reduce absorption of iron from food. It's the tannins in the tea that reduce absorption of iron from the diet.
- Excessive intake of high-fiber foods will have a similar effect, but they are needed for good bowel health, so if you need iron supplements, take them in between eating high-fiber foods.

Friendly Foods
- Liver and most meats are rich in iron—especially lean steak and venison. Chicken, pheasant, partridge, grouse, pigeon, kidneys, hare, and cockles are also good sources.
- Wheat bran, whole-wheat flour and wheat germ contain good amounts of iron, and most breakfast cereals contain added iron.

- Dried fruits such as apricots, raisins, and prunes are also a good source of iron. As dried fruits are high in sugar, soak them for a few minutes in warm water to reduce the sugar content. Drain before serving. Buy dried fruits with no added sulfites.
- Almonds, cocoa, curry powder, and raw parsley contain moderate amounts of iron.
- Leafy green vegetables such as watercress; sprouted foods such as alfalfa, broccoli, spinach, pea sprouts, kale and cabbage; and organic tomatoes are also rich in iron.
- Blackstrap molasses is rich in iron, as is brewer's yeast.
- Prune juice is rich in iron.

Useful Remedies

- Take 1g of vitamin C daily with food, plus 400mcg of folic acid and 1mg (1000mcg) of B12 daily, as these help increase iron absorption.
- B-vitamins work together within the body; take a B-complex with the above.
- If you are very anemic then you can also take iron ascorbate, 15–45mg for one week every month, as it is an easily absorbed form of iron. **Avoid iron sulfate, which may damage mucous membranes in the digestive tract and can cause constipation. Always keep iron supplements away from children.**
- Vitamin A and iron together are more effective than taking iron on its own. Take 5000IU. But if you are pregnant then only 3000IU of vitamin A can be taken daily and only while symptoms last.
- Trace minerals such as zinc, copper, and selenium are also needed to aid increased utilization of iron, so also take a multi-mineral daily.

Helpful Hints

- When taking an iron supplement it is generally best to take it with a small glass of pure fruit juice, which seems to aid absorption owing to the vitamin-C content in fruit juice.
- Iron is so vital for health that we store it in our bodies, but if taken in excessive amounts, it can become toxic and is known to cause constipation in some cases. The exception to this is women who suffer from heavy periods and are feeling exhausted. Pregnant women can benefit from liquid formulas such as Floradix or Spatone, which are available online and from health stores.
- Many scientists now state that no one over 50 should take a separate iron supplement unless they have a medical condition that requires it, as high levels of iron are linked to an increased risk of heart disease, especially in men. If large amounts of iron are recommended because of anemia, then it is best to see a qualified nutritionist who can re-balance your diet and supplements (see *Useful Information*).
- As we age our stomach-acid levels fall, which means that nutrients are often poorly absorbed from the foods we eat. Taking a digestive enzyme with meals improves absorption.
- There is a genetic disorder called hemochromatosis, which affects 1 in every 200 women, in which iron and large amounts of vitamin C should not be taken. A simple blood test can detect this condition.

A

ANGINA

(see also Atherosclerosis, Cholesterol, Circulation, Heart Disease, and High Blood Pressure)

Angina affects about one in every 50 people, and in the US there are an estimated 7 million people suffering from this condition. Around 400,000 people go to their doctor with a new case of angina each year. Angina is often experienced as a pain in the chest, most frequently after exertion such as running up a flight of stairs, but in extreme cases it can occur after getting out of a chair. Stress over long periods thickens the blood (see under *Stress*). Angina, meanwhile, is brought on by an inadequate supply of oxygen via the blood to the heart muscle. Over many years arteries begin laying down sticky deposits, which harden and eventually cause a narrowing within the blood vessels. See under *Atherosclerosis* for prevention and self help for hardening of the arteries.

Typical symptoms include pain in the center of the chest, which sometimes spreads to the neck/jaw area and down the left arm. The pain can be accompanied by breathlessness, feeling faint, sweating and/or nausea. If you have any of these symptoms, please seek medical attention immediately as they can be signs of a heart attack. Cocaine use increases oxidation within the heart, and it damages the heart in a very short time—people who use such drugs are potentially inviting heart disease.

If you are diagnosed as suffering from angina, it's time to make lifestyle changes. For example, if you smoke and are overweight but are willing to change your diet, start exercising and quit smoking, you can reduce your risk of a heart attack or stroke by 400%.

Foods to Avoid

- Cut down on alcohol, which in the long term depletes the body of B-vitamins. When you ingest alcohol, levels of homocysteine (see under *High Blood Pressure* and *Alzheimer's Disease*), a toxic amino acid linked to heart disease, are raised. Beer contains folate and vitamin B6—so try an occasional beer instead of spirits and wines.
- Reduce your intake of animal fats, including full-fat dairy produce, pre-packaged cakes, sausages, and milk chocolates.

- Avoid sodium-based salt – use magnesium- or potassium-based sea salts such as Solo Salt available from health stores. Or buy some powdered kelp, which is rich in iodine and minerals, to use as a salt substitute.
- Reduce your intake of refined sugars found in cakes, cookies, sodas, and desserts, which are converted into hard fats inside the body if they are not used up during exercise, contributing to hardening of the arteries.
- Avoid all foods containing hydrogenated or trans-fats and fried foods. Avoid mass-produced, highly refined cooking oils at all costs. You can see rows of them in plastic bottles at every supermarket and they are usually bright yellow. (See *Fats You Need To Eat*.)

Friendly Foods

- Pomegranate has been shown to help reverse atherosclerosis (hardening of the arteries) by up to 25% within a year if taken daily. You can either drink the juice or eat the fresh fruit.
- Oily fish such as salmon, tuna, or mackerel are rich in omega-3 fats, which help thin the blood naturally, as do onions and garlic.
- Cocoa, found in pure dark chocolate, is rich in flavonoids, which help improve endothelial (smooth muscle) function and blood flow. This does not mean that you should be eating lots of dark chocolate, though. Still, one or two squares a day of organic dark chocolate are good for you. Milk chocolate does not have the same benefits as it is higher in fat and sugar and lower in cocoa.
- Use a little extra-virgin olive oil, pumpkin seed oil, linseed oil or walnut oil in salad dressings.
- Eat an avocado a week. They are rich in vitamin E.
- Include plenty of fresh root ginger in your diet, which improves circulation.
- To help lower LDL cholesterol, often a contributing factor of angina, eat plenty of soluble fiber either from fruit, vegetables, oats, or flax seeds (also known as linseeds). See all dietary advice under *Cholesterol*.
- Dried beans such as haricot, kidney, chickpeas, and soybeans as well as whole grains such as

brown rice, buckwheat, quinoa, millet, and barley are all rich in fiber and can help to control cholesterol.

- Margarines such as Benecol are somewhat healthier, or use an olive oil-based spread.
- Use non-dairy, organic rice, oat or soy milks, or try low-fat goat's milk.
- If you can follow a vegan diet with the addition of fish (preferably oily), this would be the ideal solution.
- Sprinkle 1 tablespoon of high-potency lecithin granules over cereals and salads to help lower LDL cholesterol levels.

Useful Remedies

- There are several formulas that offer pomegranate, blueberry, and cocoa in one capsule available from the Life Extension Foundation. I recommend Endothelial Defense with full-spectrum pomegranate. Take two capsules daily. **LEF**
- Taking 1–3g of the amino acid L-carnitine daily helps improve heart function and reduces symptoms associated with angina.
- Taking 100mg twice daily of Co-enzyme Q10 has helped angina patients manage more exercise with fewer symptoms. **JF, VC**
- Taking 400–500IU of natural-source, full-spectrum vitamin E per day for at least 1 or 2 years thins the blood naturally.
- Fish oils supply EPA and DHA—essential fats that thin the blood naturally. Take 3g daily to help reduce chest pain.
- High doses of vitamin C and the amino acid lysine work together to help reverse atherosclerosis. Many companies now make these in a duo formula. To be effective you would need to take 4–5g of vitamin C spread throughout the day with food along with 3g of lysine daily in between meals.
- Magnesium helps regulate the heartbeat. Begin on 200mg daily and increase to 400mg.
- Include a good-quality multi-vitamin/mineral in this regimen.
- As many heart conditions are linked to stress, take a good B-complex daily in order to support your nerves.
- See supplements under *Atherosclerosis*.

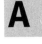

Helpful Hints

- Smoking tends to constrict arterial blood flow, so give it up.
- Remember that negative stress in the long term thickens the blood and constricts arterial flow. (See under *Stress*.)
- If you are overweight, then it is wise to lose weight. Rather than going on a strict diet, this is best achieved by eating healthily. See *General Health Hints* and *Weight Problems*.
- With your doctor's permission, embark on a program of gentle exercise. Start by walking or swimming for 15 minutes a day, gradually building up to 30 minutes, and then an hour. Tai chi and qigong are excellent forms of gentle exercise.
- Intravenous antioxidant therapy (chelation) helps clear blocked arteries and is well worth a try with your doctor's permission. There are numerous doctors and clinics in America that perform this therapy. To find a chelation provider visit www.drcranton.com/chelation/find.htm

ANTIBIOTICS *(see also Candida, Immune Function, MRSA, and Thrush)*

Doctors and public alike are now becoming aware of the dangers of over-consumption of antibiotics. Nevertheless approximately 150 million prescriptions are still written annually in the US, of which the CDC estimates one-third are unnecessary. Because of the overuse of antibiotics, bacteria are mutating and many are becoming resistant to increasing numbers of antibiotics, which has in turn triggered an increase in MRSA, *C. difficile*, and *Acinetobacter*, mainly in hospitals.

Some people still resort to the use of antibiotics whether they really need them or not. Many doctors report that patients continue to demand antibiotics for colds and flu—which are caused by viruses and therefore are not susceptible to antibiotic treatment. It is only if you contract a secondary infection such as bronchitis, which is bacterial, that antibiotics may be valid.

In the long term, antibiotics suppress our immune system and kill the friendly bacteria in the gut, which have an essential role to play in gut and general health. Eventually this can reduce absorption of nutrients from your food (see also *Absorption* and *Leaky Gut*). Therefore, whenever you take an antibiotic, you need a probiotic. Antibiotics mean anti-life and probiotics the opposite—pro-life. Probiotics are supplements containing friendly bacteria called acidophilus or bifidus that can restore a healthy balance of bacteria in our gut.

Antibiotics often allow fungal infections such as candida to flourish and also can trigger athlete's foot (see under *Athlete's Foot*).

Foods to Avoid

- If you have taken antibiotics for one month, avoid foods such as alcohol, sugar, and too much sweet fruit (especially bananas, grapes, dates, mangoes, apples, melons, and kiwi), which ferment easily within the gut. Fermentation tends to lead to an overgrowth of unfriendly bacteria, which can trigger conditions such as thrush and candida.
- Avoid moldy cheeses, which also cause fermentation in the gut.
- Avoid yeast-based breads and foods.

Friendly Foods
- Fruits that don't ferment are okay to eat in moderation; these include berries such as blueberries, blackberries, and raspberries, as well as cherries and tropical fruits such as papaya. Eat fruit 30 minutes before a main meal or in between meals to avoid more fermentation.
- Pineapple contains the enzyme bromelain, which increases the effectiveness of many antibiotics. It also acts as a digestive aid; therefore, eat a couple of fresh pineapple chunks before meals.
- Eat plenty of sugar-free, live, low-fat yogurt that contains acidophilus and bifidus. Read labels as many so-called "live" yogurts are extremely high in sugar, including those that claim to lower LDL cholesterol.
- Artichokes and beets contain inulin, a substance that encourages the growth of friendly bacteria.
- Garlic encourages the growth of friendly bacteria, kills bad bacteria, and helps fight off infections.
- Yeast-free breads and the occasional biscuit are fine, but no butter and jam, please!

Useful Remedies
- Acidophilus and bifidus are healthy bacteria. After completing a round of antibiotics, take two capsules daily after food for four weeks. Keep these sensitive, live, healthy bacteria in the fridge. BioCare also makes Replete powder, which can be dissolved in water and will help the gut to rebalance quickly. You can also buy enteric-coated probiotics that do not need to be refrigerated.
- Prebiotics—nutrients derived from the agave plant—have been shown to increase the natural

production of beneficial bacteria in the gut and enhance immune function. I put one scoop of Agave Digestive Immune Support daily on my morning fruit/nut breakfast blend. **LEF**

- Take a B-complex vitamin that includes 0.5–5mg of biotin daily. Biotin is greatly depleted by antibiotics. Lack of biotin affects your skin, hair, and nails.
- Goldenseal tincture (1ml) or capsules taken twice a day for up to 2 weeks, or grapefruit seed extract, act like natural antibiotics and can also be taken to prevent infections in the first place.
- Olive leaf extract is an anti-bacterial, anti-viral, and anti-parasitic plant extract that helps dissolve the coating of bacteria and prevent viral replication. Take up to 4 tablets daily.
- Beta Glucans 1–3, 1–6, which are derived from yeast cell walls, are proven to strengthen the body's innate immune system, making it more resistant to pathogens from food and the air. Take 250–500mg daily. It works by having one type of yeast kill an altogether more pathogenic type of yeast—the candida.
- Vitamin D3 helps antibiotics work more efficiently, and has anti-bacterial properties in its own right. Take 800IU daily.
- Bee propolis is a natural antibiotic used by bees to sterilize their hives. Many therapists and doctors find that two propolis capsules taken every day with at least 1g of vitamin C can lead to a general improvement in health and enhanced resistance to infections.
- An herbal formula containing echinacea, myrrh, odorless garlic, and other ingredients called Futurebiotics Garlic Echinacea Goldenseal can be taken to help to boost the immune system. Supplement with 3–6 tablets daily. **VC**

Helpful Hints

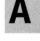

- Some plastic, mass-produced chopping boards—advertised as being anti-bacterial—are helping to make people even more resistant to antibiotics; therefore, use natural wood chopping boards and simply wash thoroughly in warm, soapy water.
- A little dirt never hurt anyone, and our obsession with bleaching and using anti-bacterial cleansers is not only damaging the environment but is also weakening our immune systems in the long term.
- If you feel low when taking antibiotics, rather than waiting until you have finished the course, start taking the acidophilus as soon as you begin to feel below par (with your doctor's permission). Also take a high-strength, B-complex vitamin.
- A naturopath or nutritionist can help you restore your immune system (see *Useful Information* at back of this book).

APHRODISIACS—male and female   *(see Libido Problems)*

ARTHRITIS—OSTEO AND RHEUMATOID

(see also Acid–Alkaline Balance, Gout, and Lupus)

There are more than 200 types of arthritis, and nearly one in every five adults in the US suffers from some form of arthritis. Sadly, around 285,000 children in the US suffer from juvenile arthritis. By the age of 65 as many as 75% of the Western population are arthritic, and women seem to suffer with arthritis far more than men. Arthritis and other rheumatic conditions are one of the most prevalent chronic health conditions, and cost the US $127.8 billion ($80.8 billion in medical care expenses and $47.0 billion in lost earnings) in 2003.

Osteoarthritis

Over time, the cartilage that cushions and surrounds the joints breaks down and the bones can become thickened and distorted, which restricts joint movement. In most cases it affects the load-bearing joints—hips, knees, spine, and hands. There is a popular misconception that exercise makes you more prone to developing osteoarthritis. In reality, exercise helps to keep your bones healthier and joints more supple.

Primary osteoarthritis develops when our natural cartilage repair process can no longer keep pace with the degenerative wear and tear we suffer with age. Secondary arthritis is usually triggered by a trauma, such as a broken joint or a fall, or any underlying joint disease. Arthritis has now reached epidemic proportions in the West.

Weight-bearing exercise such as walking, weight lifting, and so on help prevent bone loss (see *Osteoporosis*). Yoga keeps you supple, but if you play contact sports such as football, soccer, or hockey, then the joints are more likely to be damaged.

The majority of people who suffer from osteoarthritis eat too many acid-forming foods (see *Acid–Alkaline Balance*). Basically, proteins such as meat and dairy produced by cows, plus refined carbohydrates such as white bread and pizzas are acid forming; whereas fresh vegetables and most fruits plus millet are alkalizing. If we could all eat less acid-forming foods, many illnesses could be eradicated.

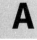

People who develop osteoarthritis are frequently told that they should avoid the nightshade family, which includes tomatoes, potatoes, peppers, and eggplant. Out of these, tomatoes seem to be the worst offender as they contain an alkaloid that can trigger inflammation in the joints. However, any foods a person is sensitive to would need to be avoided as well. It has been shown that 60–70% of people who avoid these foods for at least 6 months or more see benefits. Being overweight places more stress on joints, which will add to the problem in later life. In cultures such as Okinawa, near Japan, where people eat a mainly wholefood, wholegrain, or vegetarian diet, arthritis is virtually unknown.

Foods to Avoid
- Reduce your intake of coffee, alcohol, soda, and pre-packaged cakes, pies, pastries, bread, and pastas that are made with refined white flour and white sugar, which are all highly acid forming.
- Avoid known triggers such as tomatoes, potatoes, eggplant, and peppers.
- Gluten, which is contained in wheat, rye, oats and barley, is a problem for many people.
- Oranges and orange juice can make symptoms worse in some individuals.
- Greatly reduce cow's milk, red meat, high-fat cheeses (especially Stilton), fried foods, sausages, and chocolate (which is highly acid forming).
- Avoid all white and malt vinegars, which are highly acid forming.
- For anyone suffering gout-type problems, also eliminate foods containing large amounts of purines, which break down into uric acid in the body. Excess uric acid can trigger severe inflammation in small joints, especially the toes. High-purine foods are red meats, alcohol, lentils, shellfish, anchovies, mackerel, herring, sardines, and organ meats.

Friendly Foods
- Cherries, plums and blackberries are acid forming, but they help to mobilize uric acid out of the joints so it can be excreted in our urine. Cherries and cherry juice are best for gout.
- Pineapple contains bromelain, which is highly anti-inflammatory.
- If you do not suffer from gout then eat fresh oily fish such as mackerel, organic farmed salmon, or sardines three times a week. Mackerel and sardines, along with herring, are high in purines.

- Sweet potatoes, pumpkin, apricots, papaya, and carrots are rich in carotenes and fiber, and the sweet potatoes are a good alternative to ordinary potatoes.
- Grains such as millet, brown rice, amaranth, barley, quinoa, buckwheat and so on are all preferable to refined wheat products. Choose whole-wheat breads, and try pastas made from corn, buckwheat, rice and lentil flours. Try amaranth crisp breads, sugar-free oatcakes, and low-sugar gluten-free muesli or oatmeal.
- Ask for gluten-free variety breads.
- Eat more fresh green vegetables to re-alkalize your system. One of the quickest ways to do this is to buy a juicer and juice raw cabbage, watercress, celery, parsley, and a little root ginger, and drink immediately. You can also make delicious fruit blends (remember we are blending here, not juicing, so you also get the peel which contains all the fiber). My favorite is half a cup of fresh blueberries, a chopped pear, a chopped apple, and a sliced banana, plus a heaped teaspoon of any organic-source, "green"-based powder from your health store (see under *Useful Remedies*), a tablespoon of soaked linseeds (flax seeds) and aloe vera juice, all blended with a cup of organic rice or almond milk. Fabulous!
- Fresh root ginger can be made into a wonderful pain-relieving tea. Add a small cube of fresh root ginger to a mug of boiling water, add half a teaspoon of honey and apple cider vinegar and sip when warm.
- Blackstrap molasses is rich in calcium, potassium, and magnesium, which all help the joints. Try adding a teaspoon of the molasses to a tablespoon of organic apple cider vinegar or a little lemon juice in a cup of warm water, which helps you to absorb more minerals from your diet and helps re-alkalize your system. For those who prefer honey, buy organic, preferably locally produced, and if at all possible unrefined, which contains more natural minerals. If your symptoms are severe, drink this cocktail up to three times a day.

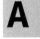

- Use organic, unrefined olive, sunflower, walnut, or sesame oils for your salad dressings.
- Eat at least one tablespoon of linseeds (flax seeds soaked overnight), or sunflower, pumpkin, or sesame seeds daily, as they are rich in essential fats that are vital for healthy joints. Hazelnuts, cashew, almonds, and walnuts are all rich in essential fats to nourish the joints. An easy way to eat more of them is to place 2 tablespoons of each in a blender, grind for 1 minute and store in an airtight jar in the fridge. Sprinkle over breakfast cereal, fruit salads or into low-fat, bio yogurts daily.
- Try herbal teas such as devil's claw and nettle, and use dandelion coffee.
- Add more turmeric and cayenne pepper to your cooking as they help reduce inflammation.

Useful Remedies

- One of the best nutritional supplements known to help this condition is the amino sugar, glucosamine sulfate. A number of studies have found that taking 1500mg daily can substantially reduce pain and improve mobility. Initially, take 1500mg of glucosamine a day until symptoms improve and then lower the dose to 500mg daily. This may take several months. Glucosamine is usually derived from crab shells, so if you have a severe intolerance to shellfish avoid this supplement. But, it is also available in a vegetarian formula derived from corn. The glucosamine combined with MSM, methylsulfonylmethane, a form of sulfur, seems to be even more effective.
- To help re-alkalize my system quickly, I take Green pH made by Metabolics (www.metabolics.com), as one small level teaspoon daily in water provides a mixture of green beans, garden peas, pea leaf, dry apple cider, watercress, broccoli, and nettle leaf. It doesn't taste great, but is a quick and easy way to alkalize your body. Other companies make comparable products: **JF, VC, VS**
- Taking 500mg of niacinamide (no-flush vitamin B3) three times a day is a great alternative to

glucosamine and helps reduce joint pain. Some people reap the benefits in as little as 4 to 5 weeks, but ideally 3 months to a year is a good time scale to take this vitamin. **NB: Be sure to ask for the "no-flush" variety, as common niacin can cause a flushing effect that can be quite shocking if you are unprepared.**

- As all the B-group vitamins work together, add a B-complex to your daily regimen.
- To help reduce pain, take a couple of teaspoons of cod liver oil daily, which also includes pain-relieving vitamin D. Or take three cod liver oil capsules daily. Many fish oils are now high in toxins that have been pumped into the world's oceans, most notably dioxins (deadly chemicals formed during the incineration of plastic) and PCBs (persistent industrial chemicals used in electrical equipment). As a result, many fish oils contain far too many toxins that can adversely affect hormones. Try pure cod liver oil available from most pharmacies and online supplement retailers. Or you can take pure omega-3 fish oils. If the pain is especially bad, you can take up to 3g of fish oil per day.
- 400IU of natural-source, full-spectrum vitamin E daily helps reduce pain.
- Take 1–3g of vitamin C daily in an ascorbate form with meals. It does not irritate the gut and has anti-inflammatory properties. Vitamin C is also vital for healthy synovial fluid that surrounds the joints.
- Ginger, curcumin, and boswellia are herbs with highly anti-inflammatory properties. Take 3–4 tablets a day.
- The formula Ligazyme Plus, made by BioCare, contains vital minerals such as calcium, boron, magnesium, rutin, and silica as well as vitamins A and D and digestive enzymes, which all support connective tissue and encourage healthier bones.
- Include a good-quality antioxidant formula in your regimen, which helps stabilize cartilage membranes.
- Curcumin capsules are really useful for reducing inflammation and increasing circulation. Take 2–3 capsules daily in the middle of main meals.
- Homeopathic Rhus Tox 6x helps relieve stiffness when you first move around. It is especially good for people whose symptoms are worse when it's cold and wet.
- Homeopathic Ruta Graveolens 30c often helps if tendons, the spine, or joints are sore and if they feel worse when it's cold and wet.
- Use liquid hyaluronic acid (HA). HA is a naturally occurring protein found in all bone and cartilage structures in the body. HA provides the cushioning in all joints, and it's the high content of HA in young people that keeps their joints (especially the knees) so supple. As we age, HA levels fall. By taking 1ml daily in water you can help restore some of the elasticity in connective tissue and joints. It is also useful for rheumatoid arthritis.

Rheumatoid arthritis (RA)   *(see also Leaky Gut and Lupus)*

Rheumatoid arthritis is primarily an inflammatory disease of the smaller joints, such as wrists, ankles, fingers, and knees. It is an autoimmune disorder whereby the body's own immune system starts attacking joint tissue and is very much linked to leaky gut syndrome (see this section). RA is also linked to conditions such as lupus. It is a chronic disease and tends to progress with time, but many people find the pain and stiffness comes and goes for varying periods of time. RA affects three times as many women as men, and most often occurs between the ages of 25 and 50. Over-acidity in the body and uric acid deposits in the joints are a contributing factor (see *Acid–Alkaline Balance*).

The pain and stiffness associated with RA are usually worse upon rising and tend to wear off as the day progresses. The joints can become warm, tender, and swollen. Fatigue, low-grade fever, loss of appetite, and vague muscular pain can all accompany RA. Researchers have found that at least one-third of people can completely control their rheumatoid arthritis by eliminating foods that they are intolerant to. The most common culprits are any foods and drinks from cows, plus the nightshade group (see under *Foods to Avoid* under *Osteoarthritis*). Gluten is also a problem for many sufferers of RA. Some people even react to various beans, including kidney, mung, and aduki.

Other triggers are a leaky gut, which is when food molecules pass through the gut wall and trigger an allergic response. Many RA sufferers also have parasites and candida, a yeast fungal overgrowth. There can also be a genetic susceptibility (see *Candida* and *Leaky Gut*).

Heavy exercise may cause RA to progress faster, but gentle exercise such as swimming, tai chi, yoga, stretching, and walking are more helpful. Researchers have found that many rheumatoid arthritis sufferers are deficient in the major antioxidant nutrients; vitamins A, C, and E; and the mineral selenium, but particularly vitamin E. The majority of RA sufferers also appear to have low levels of stomach acid, and supplementing with betaine hydrochloride (stomach acid) can help. (See also *Low Stomach Acid*.) Betaine helps to digest proteins, and most people who have allergies have a problem digesting certain proteins. If you have active stomach ulcers do not take the betaine and use a papaya- or pineapple-based digestive enzyme capsule instead.

RA is virtually unknown in primitive cultures where the diet is mainly alkaline-forming foods and antibiotics and refined foods (which also contribute to RA) are unheard of.

Autoimmune diseases, for the most part, take years to develop—years of eating too many foods that don't agree with your physiology. Stress, lifestyle, and so on all contribute to the condition as well. However, if you change these actions, then over time your body is perfectly capable of healing itself.

Foods to Avoid
- Animal fats eaten to excess tend to aggravate RA. Avoiding all dairy products from cows, meat (especially red meat), sugar, and eggs helps some people.
- Avoid or greatly reduce known triggers such as tomatoes, potatoes, eggplant, peppers, and gluten.
- Oranges and orange juice can be a problem for most people with RA.
- Coffee, chocolate, peanuts, spinach, strawberries, rhubarb, and beets are all high in oxalic acid, which seems to further aggravate RA in some people.
- Greatly reduce your intake of foods and drinks made with refined sugars.
- Avoid wheat and any foods containing gluten, citrus (especially oranges and grapefruit), corn, food additives, colorings, and flavorings. Keep a food diary and note when symptoms are more acute. Eliminate these foods for a week or so and see if this helps.
- Beans such as aduki, mung, and haricot contain lectin, a protein that is hard to digest. If you like these foods, be sure to take a digestive enzyme.

Friendly Foods
- Eat more curries made with curcumin (derived from the spice turmeric), which has powerful anti-inflammatory properties.
- Eat more pineapple—a rich source of bromelain, which has highly anti-inflammatory properties.
- Cherries mobilize uric acid out of the body. Eat them regularly when they are in season or use frozen cherries.
- Eat oily fish such as organic farmed salmon or mackerel at least three times a week or take a

couple of teaspoons of fish oil daily. They contain omega-3 essential fats that reduce uric acid levels. (See also *Fats You Need To Eat*.)

- Use linseed (flax seed) oil plus unrefined olive or hemp seed oil in salad dressings.
- A vegan diet has been shown to help some individuals.
- Root ginger plus the spices turmeric and boswellia have anti-inflammatory properties. These will not alleviate the problem but can substantially reduce the pain and give people more mobility.
- Make a tea using fresh ginger and lemon juice.
- Eat plenty of garlic, and use rice, oat or almond organic milks as alternatives to cow's milk.
- Avocado and raw wheat germ are rich in vitamin E and essential fats.
- Eat lots more green vegetables, especially raw green cabbage, kale, spring greens, watercress, parsley, and endives, or add an organic green food powder based on wheat grass, spirulina, alfalfa, chlorella and green foods that is available from your local health food store to cereals, juices and desserts.
- Under professional guidance juice fasts can greatly reduce symptoms.
- Modest amounts of aloe vera are helpful, as aloe is anti- inflammatory, aids gut health, and improves the production of digestive enzymes.

Useful Remedies

- For those who don't like fresh pineapple, bromelain is available as a supplement. Take one capsule—500mg—of bromelain on an empty stomach to increase its effectiveness.

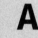

- The herbs curcumin and boswellia are also available in tablet and capsule formulas. Take 1200–1600mg of either one.
- Evening primrose oil can help, but you would need very high amounts. People take EPO for the GLA (gamma linolenic acid) content because GLA is highly anti-inflammatory. However, GLA is also available as a supplement. Take 1–4g daily.
- Take 1–3g of vitamin C daily, spread throughout the day with meals, plus 400–800IU of natural-source, full-spectrum vitamin E.
- A multi-mineral containing 30mg of zinc, 100–150mcg of selenium plus traces of copper is known to help reduce pain.
- EPA-DHA pure fish oil, 1–4g daily, can help.
- Many sufferers of RA benefit from taking vitamin B5 pantothenic acid. 500mg can be taken four times a day. Pure Royal Jelly also has a high B5 content.
- As B-vitamins work together, include a B-complex.
- L-glutamine is an amino acid found in cabbage. Taking 500mg three times daily can help heal a leaky gut. Take 30 minutes prior to a meal.
- Sufferers of RA are often lacking healthy bacteria in their guts; therefore, a daily prebiotic powder with breakfast such as Agave Digestive Immune Support from the Life Extension Foundation can help the gut naturally produce more friendly bacteria. **LEF**
- A multi-mineral formula taken daily helps to re-alkalize the body.
- Vitamin K2 has been found to reduce inflammation in RA sufferers and is vital for bone and arterial health (K2 keeps calcium out of the arteries and in the bones.) **If you are taking blood-thinning drugs such as Warfarin, you need to avoid vitamin K.** Otherwise, try 100mcg daily.
- Vitamin D3 is useful for slowing progression of RA, and, has a protective effect against autoimmune conditions. Take 3000IU daily for one month, then stop for a month, then take a maintenance dose of 1000IU daily.
- A fermented wheat germ extract known as AWGE has demonstrated remarkable immune-modulating effects and helps restore balance to over-stimulated immune systems. AWGE has

been shown in numerous trials to reduce the symptoms of autoimmune diseases, including RA. Take one sachet daily in water at least one hour before breakfast. Also available in capsules. Must be kept refrigerated. For more information and details on where to purchase AWGE, visit www.avemarwge.com

- Olive leaf extract has been proven to reduce inflammation, and some people derive great pain relief by taking 500mg three times a day before meals. It is available from all good health stores.

Helpful Hints for All Types of Arthritis

- A short fast under professional guidance almost always alleviates symptoms, as it reduces the toxic load within the body. And once you look after your liver and heal any gut problems, symptoms are greatly reduced.

- If you are overweight this places more strain on the load-bearing joints, so lose weight.

- Hot and cold compresses applied alternately for 20 minutes at a time will help reduce swelling and pain. Cold compresses are especially good if the affected joints feel hot to the touch. Moist hot packs help reduce pain and stiffness.

- Joint cartilage needs plenty of fluid, so drink six glasses of water daily, which also helps eliminate uric acid. Hard water can sometimes exacerbate arthritic-type symptoms because it is packed with minerals in inorganic forms that are hard to absorb. However, fruits and vegetables are able to absorb these inorganic minerals and can convert them to an organic form when aided by sunlight. When minerals are in an organic form, they become more bio-available to us.

- To ingest the 21 minerals that are essential for life, it makes sense to eat far more fresh fruits and vegetables. Unfortunately, thanks to pollution, over-farming, and acid rain, most soils no longer contain sufficient minerals needed for good health. And if the minerals are not in the soil, they are never going to make it into our vegetables (although organic foods generally contain more minerals). This is why we all need to begin taking a daily multi-mineral.

A

- Numerous people have experienced benefits after taking pure aloe vera juice daily for several months.

- Nettle tea taken regularly has helped reduce the pain and swelling associated with arthritis for many people.

- To re-alkalize your system, take a good-quality green powder that contains a mixture of green beans, garden peas, pea leaf, dry apple cider, watercress, broccoli, and nettle leaf. Mix one small level teaspoon daily in water and take it preferably 30 minutes before a meal or in between meals. It doesn't taste great, but is a quick and easy way to alkalize your body. JF, VC, VS

- Use Alkabath salts, which are more powerful than Epsom salts, to help eliminate toxins from the joints. They are available online, usually from the UK, but can be shipped worldwide. See also *Acid–Alkaline Balance*.

- Use Kangen Water—a water system that attaches to your kitchen faucet and ionizes and alkalizes water. It's used in Japanese hospitals with highly beneficial health results. For full details visit www.kangenwaterusa.com

- Topically applied oil of wintergreen can help ease pain and inflammation.

- Homeopathic Apis 30c helps RA when there is swelling and rheumatic pains that are worse for heat.

- If your RA is in the small joints, ask at your homeopathic pharmacy for Actea Spicata-3c. When taken three times daily between meals, it helps reduce the pain.

- The Chinese exercise regimes of tai chi or qigong have helped many sufferers as these exercises are easy to practice, even with severely impaired mobility. RA can be greatly affected by stress, so make sure you stay as calm as possible (see *Stress*).

■ Visit the Arthritis Foundation's website (www.arthritis.org) to learn more about this disease and to get more dietary advice. You can also contact your local office about activities (www.arthritis.org/chaptermap.php)

ASTHMA

(see also Allergies and Leaky Gut)

More than 20 million people in the US now suffer from asthma, 7 million of whom are children, and the problem is escalating. The annual cost to the US is over $18 billion.

Asthma affects the bronchial tubes leading to our lungs, which results in periods of wheezing and shortness of breath. Pollution from traffic fumes, especially diesel, is without a doubt a huge contributing factor. It has been shown that during school vacations the incidence of attacks is reduced as there is less traffic.

Other atmospheric pollutants such as pollen and cigarette smoke can be triggers, as can house dust mite, molds, and pesticides. Stressful situations and chronic exhaustion can also trigger an attack, as can eating foods to which you have a sensitivity (such as sulfur dioxide, used as a preservative in many dried fruits and salt). You can also suffer exercise-induced asthma. There is also a link between parasites and asthma.

People who take acetaminophen (the active ingredient in Tylenol) every day are twice as likely to suffer asthma, and if you take it twice weekly you are 80% more likely to be affected.

Several studies have demonstrated that expectant mothers given pre-biotics, which enhance immune function by encouraging healthy bacteria to be produced in the gut, are less likely to have babies who suffer from asthma. And infants given prebiotics and probiotics suffer far fewer incidences of asthma.

Foods to Avoid

■ There is a strong association between asthma in children and dairy products, especially cow's milk.

■ Any foods to which you have an intolerance will make you more susceptible to attacks. The most common are wheat, mass-produced cereals, nuts, chocolate, or tomatoes. For details of good tests, see *Allergies*.

■ Reduce intake of all meats, eggs and full-fat dairy products from any source (cows, sheep, goats, and soy), which can increase mucus production.

■ A recent study in Taiwan showed that people who eat a lot of meat, especially liver, and high-fat foods were more likely to develop asthma.

■ Avoid sodium-based salt in any foods. Some people can have an attack after eating too many potato chips.

■ Some mass-produced salads, dried fruits, wines, and beers contain sulfur dioxide, which is known to trigger problems in sensitive individuals.

■ Avoid sodium benzoate, which is frequently found in soft drinks, and MSG.

■ Generally avoid all mass-produced, pre-packaged foods.

■ Avoid aspirin.

Friendly Foods

■ If you have a problem with dairy products, then try rice, almond, hemp, quinoa, or oat milks. Be aware that some people react to almonds, so try the other milks first.

■ Green leafy vegetables, fresh fruits, and organic honey are rich in magnesium, which helps the airways to relax. A lack of magnesium has been linked to breathing problems. Brown rice, avocados, spinach, haddock, watercress, oatmeal, baked potatoes, navy beans, lima beans, broccoli, bananas, soybeans, and unrefined nuts are all rich in magnesium.

- Include more lentils, garlic and onions in your diet, which help fight off infections and clear the lungs.
- Because asthma has been linked by nutritional physicians to a "leaky gut," include plenty of fresh ginger in your diet, which is very soothing. Cabbage and aloe vera juice also help heal the gut (see *Leaky Gut*).
- Aim to eat oily fish three times a week because it is rich in vitamin A and can therefore reduce the severity and frequency of attacks. Sweet potatoes, apricots, papaya, watermelon, and pumpkin are also all high in natural-source carotenes, which naturally convert to vitamin A in the body.
- Use extra-virgin, unrefined olive and sunflower oils in salad dressings and include plenty of linseeds (flax seeds), pumpkin, sunflower, and sesame seeds in your diet.
- Cauliflower, apples, papaya, pears, cherries, grapes, pineapple, kale, and green tea are all great foods for the lungs.
- Buy a juicer and make yourself a carrot, ginger, cabbage, radish, apple, and celery mix—drink immediately. Try different mixes daily, which is a great way to get health-giving nutrients into the body.
- Vine-ripened tomatoes are rich in lycopene, which is beneficial for the lungs (and prostate). Cooking in a little olive oil helps release the lycopene.
- Sprinkle turmeric on your meals or add to cooking as this herb has anti-inflammatory properties and supports the immune system.
- After an attack, drink plenty of fluids to help break up mucus so it can be expelled.
- Children who eat more fresh fruits and vegetables are known to suffer fewer attacks.
- Eat more of the edible white membranes found in lemons. They contain limonene, which is great for the lungs.

Useful Remedies

- Do not give large doses of supplements to young children. Always take advice from a nutritionist. See *Useful Information* at back of book.
- Take a good-quality multi-vitamin daily plus a multi-mineral containing 400–800mg of magnesium and 200mcg of selenium. Low levels of selenium leave you more at risk from an attack.
- Take 1g of vitamin C three times a day with meals to help open the airways.
- Take 150mg of vitamin B6 a day, 1,000–2,000mcg of vitamin B12 a day and a B-complex supplement. Asthma medication depletes B vitamins, especially in people who are sensitive to sulfates.
- Take 400–500mg of bromelain, an enzyme extracted from pineapples, once or twice a day to help reduce mucus production and ease breathing.
- Take 60mg a day of a natural-source beta-carotene complex if you suffer exercise-induced asthma.
- The herb ginkgo biloba—120–240mg of a standardized extract or 3–4ml of tincture taken daily has been shown to improve circulation and decrease asthma symptoms.
- US trials have found that people with low levels of Vitamin D suffer more attacks. Take a minimum of 800–1000IU daily.
- Quercetin, a polyphenol compound found in red wine and garlic, acts as an anti-inflammatory and has been found to greatly reduce the incidence of asthma attacks triggered by chemicals. Take 500mg daily with food.
- Specialist Herbal Supplies "Lung Formula" contains bronchial-dilating herbs that help open

the airways. For further information call Specialist Herbal Supplies at 011-44-1273-424333; they will ship internationally.

- Try Respiratory De-Tox formula made from ginger, myrrh, garlic, Echinacea, and lobelia—15 drops a day. This helps expand the airways and keep the respiratory tract clearer. **OP**
- Pine bark extract, known as pycnogenol, has been shown to ease breathing in asthma patients. Take as directed. **PN, NOW, GNC**
- Take a prebiotic and probiotic formula daily.
- Many people who suffer from asthma have a "leaky gut" (see *Leaky Gut*). If you think you have the symptoms, take a digestive enzyme with all main meals.
- As levels of omega-3 essential fats and GLA (gamma-linolenic acid) also tend to be low in asthma sufferers, take 1g of fish oil daily plus 2g of Mega GLA.
- Colostrum, which is found in breast milk, helps support the immune system and aids with healing a leaky gut. It is very helpful for babies and children suffering from asthma. Up until the age of 2, children should take a quarter of a teaspoon twice daily on an empty stomach. Children over the age of 2 should take half a teaspoon twice daily. Colostrum should only be taken for one month.

Helpful Hints
- People who are overweight tend to suffer more breathing and inflammatory problems.
- Steroidal inhalers deplete magnesium from the body, which can make sufferers become ever more dependent on their inhaler; this is why a daily intake of magnesium is absolutely crucial for them.

- Avoid chlorinated pools as exposure to chlorine can constrict the airways.
- Use an ionizer in any room you are going to spend any length of time in, as it can reduce the amount of pollen and dust in the air.
- Use Ultra Breathe, a very handy, inexpensive device that does a great job of exercising the lungs. It costs $26.95 online plus $3.95 for postage and packing. For details call 011-44-870-608-9019, or visit www.ultrabreathe.com/us/uswelcome.htm
- Try to avoid antibiotics during the infant years as they have been linked to an increased risk of developing asthma later in life.
- Acupuncture has proved useful for many sufferers.
- Check for food and environmental allergens—see details of good tests under *Allergies*.
- It is incredible how many people suffer breathing problems simply because they are not using their lungs properly. Most asthmatics benefit from tuition in proper breathing techniques. Every 20 minutes or so, remember to take a deep breath down into your lower-abdomen area. Buteyko is a breathing technique that has been known to help with asthma. For further information, and to find a local practitioner, call the Buteyko Center USA on 845-684-5456 or visit www.buteykocenterusa.com
- Shallow breathing is associated with being stressed. Learn relaxation techniques or consult a hypnotherapist who can teach you how to relax (see *Useful Information*).
- Do gentle exercise such as yoga, tai chi, swimming, or walking. Exercise reduces stress and helps you breathe better, which should help reduce the incidence of asthma attacks.
- Consult a nutritionist (see *Useful Information*).
- Homeopathy has proved especially helpful for children, but be sure to consult a qualified homeopath.
- Have a regular massage using essential oils of chamomile and lavender.
- A company specializing in indoor, air-quality equipment is Bluepoint Environmental (www.bluepointenvironmental.com).
- Stress is a major factor in asthma—so try to stay calm. (See *Stress*.)

- It may be worth consulting a chiropractor or cranial osteopath, as blocked airways may link back to nerve compression in the spine.
- For a further range of asthma information contact the Asthma and Allergy Foundation of America at 1-800-727-8462 or visit their website: www.aafa.org

ATHEROSCLEROSIS (hardening and narrowing of the arteries)

(see also Angina, Cholesterol, Circulation, and Heart Disease)

Atherosclerosis is technically narrowing of the arteries, but most people call it hardening of the arteries. Over the years, LDL cholesterol forms oxidized fatty deposits that adhere to our artery walls and narrow the space blood has to flow through. In addition, high homocysteine levels, a marker for heart disease, cause inflammation of the inner arterial lining. To try and repair this damage, the body produces collagen to form a cap over the damaged tissue, which can then attract calcium deposits; this is why this condition is most commonly referred to as hardening of the arteries.

Atherosclerosis is the leading cause of disability and death in the Western world and is the major trigger for most heart conditions, including angina, coronary heart disease, strokes, circulation and memory problems, and diabetes complications. My father, although thin like me, died of a heart attack at just 50, and his death certificate read atherosclerosis. He had spent a lifetime smoking, eating the wrong foods, and not exercising sufficiently. He was also exposed to considerable amounts of stress.

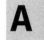

Genetic factors are believed to play a role in hardening of the arteries, but without a doubt, our diet has a huge effect as well. And because of the increase in junk food intake and little exercise, cardiologists are now seeing this condition in teenagers—which is shocking.

Foods To Avoid

- The days of people regularly eating lard as my father did are rare; however, lard has been replaced by hydrogenated and trans-fats found in mass-produced pies, cakes, candies, cheap milk chocolates, ice cream, cookies, sausages, fried foods, and most fast foods.
- Some food manufacturers such as Nabisco and the Campbell Soup Company have removed trans-fats from some of their most popular products. Hopefully others will follow suit.
- Greatly cut down on sodium-based salts, which are found in virtually all pre-packaged meals, pies, pizzas, and so on.
- Avoid cheese in general, but a small of amount of goat's cheese or cottage cheese is fine. You can also ask for low-fat cheeses. Still, think of cheese as an occasional treat.
- Reduce your intake of red meat, but if you have to eat meat try to make it organic and cut the fat off. Venison, turkey, chicken breast, rabbit, guinea fowl, and pheasant are fine in moderation.
- Reduce your intake of all full-fat dairy products. This includes butter.

Friendly Foods

- Pomegranate has been proven during trials in Israel to disrupt the formation of arterial plaque and has also shown some benefit in reducing blood pressure. Practically every supermarket now sells pomegranate seeds ready to eat, and I take at least a tablespoon daily. Otherwise, drink the juice daily. US trials have found that drinking pomegranate juice daily for a year reduces atherosclerosis by as much as 25%.
- Include garlic in your diet as it protects against the oxidation of LDL cholesterol.

- Curcumin (extracted from the spice turmeric and used in curries) lowers LDL.
- Eat more oily fish, especially organic farmed salmon, sardines, and mackerel.
- Pure, dark chocolate is low in fat, dairy products, and sugar and high in flavonoids, which also protect LDL against oxidation and improve blood flow. You can eat two small squares of high-quality dark chocolate a day.
- Eat more fresh root ginger and artichokes.
- Drink more organic green and white tea, which helps lower LDL.
- Red wine contains polyphenols, such as resveratrol and quercetin, which help to protect against one LDL oxidation, of the main triggers of atherosclerosis.
- For a larger list, see *Friendly Foods* under *Heart Disease*.

Useful Remedies

- There are several formulas that contain pure cocoa, concentrated pomegranate, and either blueberry extract or super oxide dismutase, an enzyme known to defend the body against oxidative stress. The Life Extension Foundation makes a good one called Endothelial Defense with full-spectrum pomegranate. Otherwise take a full-spectrum pomegranate formula. **LEF**
- Take a garlic capsule such as Allimax daily. It contains a good level of allicin, the active ingredient in garlic, which helps thin the blood naturally.
- The spice turmeric contains curcumin, which has highly anti- inflammatory properties. Since atherosclerosis is basically inflammation of the arteries, taking this spice daily in a concentrated form with meals can greatly reduce plaque formation. Take around 1g per day in divided doses with food. **LEF**

- Omega-3 essential fats are vital for healthy arteries. Take 2g daily.
- Vitamin C helps protect the artery walls. Take 2–3g daily in divided doses with food.
- Carnitine is an amino acid that helps remove fat that has been deposited in the arteries. Take 500mg three times daily at least 30 minutes or so before eating.
- Full-spectrum, natural-source Vitamin E (400IU daily) protects against oxidation of LDL, as does lipoic acid (200mg daily).
- Take a high-strength B-complex or take Homocysteine Formula by Metabolics (one tablet three times daily).
- If you are taking statins, you need to take the nutrient Co-enzyme Q10 (100mg daily) to protect your heart muscle. Statins reduce production of this essential nutrient and can cause serious side effects.
- Several studies have demonstrated that a lack of vitamin K2 *accelerates* arterial calcification, whereas taking a K2 supplement daily (approximately 100mcg) can help keep excess calcium in the bones and out of your arteries. **NB: Vitamin K cannot be used by people already taking Warfarin.**
- Niacin (vitamin B3) is well known in orthodox medical circles for its ability to reduce arterial plaque and raise levels of the "good" HDL cholesterol, which in turn helps remove cholesterol deposits from artery walls. The downside of niacin is that it triggers a flushing for about 45 minutes after taking it, most especially in women. No-flush Niacin does not have this plaque-reducing effect. For reduction of plaque you would need to take around 500–1000mg of B3 daily for several weeks. I have found that the best way to do this is to begin by taking 500mg of the flavonoid quercetin with breakfast, which greatly reduces the flushing sensations and then taking 100mg of Niacin with lunch and another 100mg with dinner—unless, of course, you are out with someone special and don't want to turn bright red! Be sensible,]and work on increasing the dose so you can take it at times that suit your schedule. Niacin is more effective if taken with 100mcg of chromium daily.

NB: In rare cases, regular intake of niacin can have negative effects on the liver;

therefore, if you have ever suffered from any liver disease do not take niacin. It can also upset a sensitive gut in some people.

Helpful Hints

- Hormones play an important role in this condition. Thyroid, DHEA, progesterone, and testosterone and estrogen levels need to be checked and balanced as required.
- See this section under *Cholesterol, Circulation*, and *Heart Disease*.
- Having an animal that you stroke regularly helps lower cholesterol and blood pressure naturally!
- Have a carotid artery doppler ultrasound to give you and your doctor a good idea of how much plaque you are laying down in your arteries. This test may be covered by your health insurance. Talk to your doctor for more information.
- Several studies have confirmed a link between gum disease and atherosclerosis. Therefore, make sure to have regular dental check-ups and to practice good oral hygiene.

ATHLETE'S FOOT   *(see also Antibiotics and Candida)*

Athlete's foot is caused by a fungal infection of the skin and is characterized by itchy, flaking, and cracked skin, especially between the toes and on the soles of the feet. This problem can be transmitted in public places such as swimming pools, where people walk barefoot in moist atmospheres. To help prevent this condition, wear socks made from natural fibers, such as cotton, silk, or bamboo, which allow the skin to breathe and change your footwear regularly. It is also important that feet are dried properly after bathing or exercise. Persistent athlete's foot is often associated with an overgrowth of candida in the gut (see also *Candida*).

A

Foods to Avoid

- Avoid sugar when symptoms are acute. Sugars ferment and feed yeasts in the body.
- Avoid foods containing yeast such as cheese, wine, yeasty breads, beer, mushrooms, vinegar, and soy sauce.
- Grapes are high in sugar and may have molds on their skin. Blueberries should also be avoided for a short time as they too often have molds on their skin.
- Peanuts should be avoided.

Friendly Foods

- Shitake mushrooms are the exception to the "no-mushroom" rule as they naturally contain beta-glucans, which help reduce fungal infections.
- Eat plenty of garlic and onions, which are anti-bacterial and anti-fungal.
- Live, low-fat yogurt contains acidophlius and bifidus. Eat at least 250g a day.
- The herb pau d'arco is anti-fungal. Take six capsules daily or drink several cups as tea.
- See also diet under *Candida*.

Useful Remedies

- If you have sore open patches, Chiropodist Margaret Dabbs suggests applying salt water to aid healing and then using pure emu oil, which is a good anti-fungal with anti-inflammatory properties to aid healing. For details log on to www.margaretdabbs.co.uk
- Apply some liquid grapefruit seed extract (known as citricidal) externally.
- Black walnut and calendula tincture, applied topically and taken internally twice a day, is effective.
- Try tea tree, manuka, and neem cream. Apply twice daily.
- Pierce a low-odor garlic capsule and sprinkle the powder it contains on the affected area.

- Beta Glucans 1–3, 1–6, although derived from yeast cell walls, are proven to strengthen the body's innate immune system and kill pathogenic yeasts. Pharma Nord makes a version that is free from yeast protein. Take 250–500mg daily. **PN**

Helpful Hints
- Pau d'arco is the bark of a South American tree and boosts immune function as well as helping fight fungal infections. It makes a very pleasant-tasting tea and is easily available in capsules. It can also be added to a foot wash made with tea tree oil.
- Add 5–10 drops of citricidal liquid to a footbath and soak feet twice daily.
- You may not want to try this! Dip an old cloth in fresh urine and wrap it around the affected area. Urine is a natural anti-fungal. Change the "bandage cloth" daily.
- Most sports stores now sell socks made from bamboo, a sustainable material that has anti-bacterial properties.

AUTISM

(see also Allergies and Leaky Gut)

According to the CDC, an average of one in 110 children in the US has an autism spectrum disorder, with four times as many boys affected as girls. And, although more than 80% of parents identify problems with their child by 24 months of age, most children aren't diagnosed until they are 5 or 6. The numerous symptoms of this disorder include an inability to communicate and concentrate, impaired language and learning, disturbed sleep patterns, hyperactivity, abnormal social relationships, rituals, and compulsive behavior.

Because 60% of our brains are made from essential fats (EFAs), some researchers have linked autism to a lack of EFA intake during pregnancy. Low vitamin D levels during pregnancy and in infants are also linked to debilitating brain dysfunction. It also now appears that both genetic and environmental factors contribute to autism.

Meanwhile, ongoing research has linked the increase in autism to toxic overload. This could be from vaccines as I believe that the MMR (measles, mumps, and rubella) vaccine could trigger delayed responses in some cases, which could either be generated by the mercury content of vaccine or the vaccine itself. Other causes are exposure to pesticides, PCBs, and neurotoxic heavy metals such as mercury, lead, and aluminum, plus chemicals in foods such as phenolic compounds and salicylates (see below).

Research also shows that incompletely digested particles of wheat and dairy are found in higher amounts in children with behavioral problems. Problems with digestion, absorption, and elimination are often seen, and most children with autism have a leaky gut. Reduced breakdown of proteins in milk and gluten (wheat, rye, oats, and barley) leads to "neurotoxins" entering the brain and disrupting brain chemistry. Many autistic children have also been given large doses of antibiotics, which in the long term can trigger more gut problems and can initiate intolerances and sensitivities to many foods (see also *Allergies, Candida,* and *Leaky Gut*).

Poor immune function and sluggish liver function (see under *Liver Problems*) can contribute to this condition, as can fungal overgrowth (see *Candida*). I have heard of several cases where autistic children have been referred to psychiatrists, and when given mind-altering drugs the children's symptoms worsened considerably.

Foods to Avoid
- Remove all gluten from the child's diet. This protein is found in most breads, cookies, and cereals. Remember that rye, barley, and oats also contain gluten. Some children suffer from withdrawal-type symptoms and became worse before their parents notice improvements.

- Dairy products from cows should also be avoided.
- Other foods that can potentially cause negative reactions in autistic children include soy-based foods and products, eggs, citrus fruits, chocolate, and peanuts or any other nuts the child is intolerant to. Shellfish have also been found to cause many problems associated with food intolerance/allergy and leaky gut.
- Avoid all pre-packaged, junk-type foods and drinks that are packed with salt, sugar, and animal fats. Keep a food diary and note when symptoms become worse.
- Avoiding additives found in packaged and processed foods is a must, as they may contain compounds that can be toxic to the brain when the body fails to break them down properly.
- For some children, avoiding excitotoxins—chemicals that stimulate the brain—is helpful. Foods rich in salicylates (a form of excitotoxins) are oranges, almonds, apples, apricots, tomatoes, cherries, cranberries, cucumbers, grapes, nectarines, tangerines, peaches, plums, peppers, prunes, and raisins. For a full list visit www.feingold.org **Don't simply remove all of these foods from a child's diet. Have an intolerance test done first and only remove foods to which there is an intolerance. Such foods may be able to be re-introduced at a later date.** One of the easiest is The York Test; for details visit www.yorktest.com or email: customercare@yorktest.com
- To make sure your child does not suffer from nutritional deficiencies when avoiding foods, work with a qualified nutritionist or a nutritional physician (see *Useful Information*).

Friendly Foods

- As much as possible, give your child only organic, whole foods that are free from pesticides and rich in magnesium, vitamin B6, and folic acid, especially green leafy vegetables such as cabbage, watercress, kale, broccoli, string beans, or kidney beans.
- Gluten-free cereals plus carrots, broccoli, baked beans, parsley, spinach, watercress, and sesame seeds are all high in calcium, which will hopefully reduce the incidence of self-injury and have a calming effect. For some good gluten-free recipes log on to www.geniusglutenfree.com
- Most supermarkets and health food stores now offer good gluten-free ranges.
- Essential fats are vital for healthy brain function. Recent research shows that autistic children have lower levels of omega-3 fats in their brains. To increase these levels, give your child oily fish (organic farmed salmon, unsmoked mackerel, or sardines) at least twice a week, and use unrefined, organic pumpkin, sunflower, sesame, flax seeds (linseeds), and walnuts daily if the child does not have a sensitivity to these seeds. Add cold-pressed organic seed oils to cooked foods and use in salad dressings. See also *Fats You Need to Eat*.
- Avocado is rich in monounsaturated healthy fats.
- Papaya, bananas, pears, blueberries, mango, pomegranate, and other fruits should be fine.
- Make sure they eat plenty of fresh fruits and vegetables plus buckwheat-, potato-, or rice-based pastas, fresh fish, lean meats, pulses, brown rice or quinoa.

Useful Remedies

- If you are pregnant, **speak to your doctor** about taking optimum doses of vitamin D, which stimulates proper brain development. Current US guidelines recommend pregnant women take 200–400IU per day, an amount that is far too low. The Canadian Pediatric Society recommends that pregnant women should take 2000IU of vitamin D daily, while recent studies have shown that 4000IU is needed.
- Approximately 9 out of 10 breast-fed babies and less than 37% of formula-fed babies consume the recommended amount of vitamin D. Formula-fed infants need 400IU daily and breast-fed infants can be given 600–800IU of vitamin D daily. Toddlers who do not get regular sun exposure can take 800–1000IU daily.

A

- Magnesium is needed to support nerves and is also known as nature's tranquillizer. Studies have shown that autistic children tend to have low magnesium levels, so give them 6.8mg per pound of body weight daily.
- Supplement vitamin B6 levels with 25–100mg daily for children 2–6 years old. Many children with autism have also been found to be low in folic acid, another of the B-group of vitamins, so try to include a B-complex daily. As children tend not to like tablets, try adding liquid B-vitamins to their food. BioCare makes a liquid formula called Vitasorb B. Nature's Plus also makes great vitamin and mineral products for children.
- Zinc deficiency is also associated with autism, especially in boys; therefore, try adding liquid multi-minerals into fruit desserts as an easy way for your child to ingest sufficient minerals. They will need around 30mg daily. BioCare and Nature's Plus make liquid minerals.
- Many parents have found that including an essential fatty acid formula helps their children tremendously. Try Efamol Efalex capsules or Eskimo Omega-3 fats for kids.
- Dissolve an additive-free vitamin C tablet into water daily to boost immune function; one gram daily taken with meals is sufficient for children who are between the ages of 2 and 6. After the age of 7 the dosage can be increased to 2g daily taken throughout the day with meals.
- A good probiotic taken daily for a month will help build up the good bacteria in the gut and improve digestion. BioCare does a powdered one that can be easily sprinkled onto foods. They contain only the probiotic and either freeze-dried strawberry or banana.

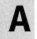

- www.positivehealthshop.com stocks Nutri's low-allergy, cherry-and-banana flavored multi, "Ultra Care for Kids." It has added digestive support and good fats for brain health. Add a scoop to juice and shake, or add to a fruit smoothie.
- Beta Glucans, derived from yeast cells walls, are safe for children to take and improve the function of their innate immune system, which can help reduce the severity of reactions to foods. Dr Paul Clayton, a former scientific advisor to the UK government's committee on the safety of medicines, says: "Thanks to our modern over-sanitized environment and intensive farming methods, which have removed virtually all Beta Glucans from our diet, our ability to resist infections has become compromised." You can break a capsule of the Beta Glucan 1–3, 1–6 daily onto cold foods. Children can safely take 250–500mg daily. Most parents report that when their children are given Beta Glucans regularly, they suffer from fewer infections.
- The Pasteur Institute in Paris studied 250 autistic children and found that their brains synthesized less than half the normal amount of melatonin, the hormone produced in the pineal gland that encourages sleep. When the researchers gave these children tiny doses of melatonin their conditions improved, in some cases radically.
- Scientist Roger Coghill, based in the UK, has developed a supplement called Asphalia, which contains natural melatonin extracted from certain grasses, to maintain melatonin levels. Roger's exclusive distributor in the US is Diva Marketing, Don't Disturb Me!, 2612 Sleepy Hollow, Pearland, TX 77581; Tel: 1-713-221-1873 or 1-866-692-8037; website: www.dontdisturbmesite.com

Helpful Hints

- For a healthy mayonnaise full of healthier fats, add 4 tablespoons of live, sugar-free soy yogurt to 2 tablespoons of cold-pressed linseed oil. Stir in a teaspoon of lecithin granules, which are available in health food stores. Leave to stand for half an hour and then stir again before serving.
- Try to remove all chemicals from a child's environment, including perfumes, chemical cleaning products, and toiletries. Also look out for unnatural flavorings in toothpastes. Jason, Kingfisher, Waleda and USANA Health Services all make safer toothpastes and toiletries.

- Aspirin has salicylate-like qualities so is best avoided by people who are sensitive to salicylates.
- Beware of colorings and flavorings in cheaper vitamin supplements, as even these may cause a reaction.
- Many parents have had some success using homeopathy to minimize vaccine damage. Talk to a certified homeopath about remedies that will suit your child's specific symptoms.
- Dr Ben Feingold researched the link between diet and behavioral problems and created the very successful Feingold diet, which includes avoiding salicylates. Check out his website (www.feingold.org) for lots of helpful information and tips.
- A great book called *New Optimum Nutrition for the Mind* by Patrick Holford (Basic Health Publications), the founder of the Brain Bio Centre, is full of useful information and tips on dealing with autism. Also read *Dietary Interventions in Autism Spectrum Disorders* by Kenneth J. Aitken (Jessica Kingsley).
- For further information and help, contact the Autism Society of America either on their hotline (1-800-328-8476) or visit their website (www.autism-society.org).
- Because each case of autism is so unique, I suggest that you consult a nutritional therapist before embarking on this program. Search for one at www.autismfile.com

AUTOIMMUNE DISEASE

(See Celiac Disease, Crohn's Disease, Lupus, Rheumatoid Arthritis, and Sjogren's Syndrome)

B

BACK PAIN

Every year more than 13 million Americans visit their doctor because of chronic back pain. This condition is the leading cause of disability in the US, leaving 2.4 million people chronically disabled and another 2.4 million temporarily disabled. For years I have suffered chronic back pain after a bad fall onto concrete that resulted in three herniated discs in my spine. If you are a fellow sufferer you have my utmost sympathy. Yet there is so much we can and should do to support ourselves.

As with most health conditions, prevention is better than cure, and as a result, some companies sensibly train their staff how to lift properly. As for treatment, until recently most people thought that bed rest was the most sensible option, but we now know that "right and light" exercise under the supervision of a professional is definitely preferable.

The center of the back can be thought of as a column made up of 33 pieces of bone called vertebrae. The spinal column is strengthened by ligaments, which run the length of the spine, and is supported by muscles, which attach to the vertebrae through tendons. It is important to have back pain diagnosed and, in an ideal world, you should see a chiropractor or an osteopath on a regular basis.

I have seen people with chronic fatigue who have received huge benefits from having their spines and necks manipulated back into place. I have also seen people who have ended up on crutches or even in a wheelchair, when all they needed was a good chiropractor. One lady I knew well was given such strong painkillers after continually complaining of back pain that she ended up wandering the streets suffering from memory loss. Yet when her desperate husband finally paid and took her to a chiropractor, she was able to hugely reduce the painkillers and live a normal life!

Doctors need to refer more patients with back pain to an osteopath, chiropractor, or a cranial osteopath. And if they won't, I suggest you find your nearest practitioner. Many health insurance plans cover chiropractic treatment.

Chronic low-level back or loin pain can also be linked to a kidney infection. Also, the heavier a person tends to be, the more likely they are to experience back pain.

Foods to Avoid
- If you are in pain, it is worth avoiding or reducing foods and drinks containing caffeine, which reduces our ability to make endorphins—the body's natural pain-killing chemicals.
- Reduce your intake of meat and sugar, which will exacerbate any inflammation. (Stress can also exacerbate inflammation.)

Friendly Foods
- Eat oily fish at least twice a week for its anti-inflammatory properties. Anchovies, farmed organic salmon, herring, mackerel, and sardines are all good options.
- Add fresh rosemary to meals to improve circulation and aid healing.
- Ginger, turmeric, and cayenne pepper can improve circulation and have anti-inflammatory properties.
- Adding a teaspoon of turmeric to cooked foods such as soups, stews, curries, and risottos can help reduce pain.
- Cauliflower, sweet potatoes, fresh fruits (especially cherries, berries, and papaya) and green leafy vegetables are all rich in vitamin C, which acts as a mild anti-inflammatory and helps produce the collagen that makes up 90% of our bone matrix.

Useful Remedies
- Collagen is a vital component of healthy joints, cartilage, ligaments, and tendons and improves bone strength. It is the most widely distributed protein in the body, and we lose about 1.5% annually after the age of 30. I take collagen powder once daily in a glass of water or diluted juice 30 minutes before a main meal to support my back. I recommend Super Strength Collagen Drink from Higher Nature, which can be ordered online at www.auravita.com and shipped worldwide.
- Blackcurrant seed oil contains large amounts of gamma-linolenic acid (GLA), which is highly anti-inflammatory. Take 3–4g a day while inflammation is acute plus 2g of omega-3 fish oils.
- While symptoms are acute, take 1500mg of glucosamine plus MSM, an organic form of sulfur, daily. This amino sugar plus MSM will help restore the thick gelatinous nature of the fluids and tissues that surround the joints and vertebrae. Glucosamine plus MSM has been found to be more effective against pain, but this takes time! Once the pain is eased, lower the dose to a maintenance intake of 500mg daily. **If you suffer a severe sensitivity to shellfish do not take this supplement as it is usually made from crushed crab shells.** Instead, look for vegetarian glucosamine, which is derived from corn. For more details visit Health Perception's website: www.health-perception.co.uk
- Taking 3–4 tablets a day of a combination formula containing ginger, curcumin, and boswellia can also help reduce pain and inflammation.
- Calcium and magnesium are known as nature's tranquillizers and help reduce muscle spasm. Take 500–1000mg of calcium and 500–800 mg of magnesium daily; many companies make them in one tablet.
- Take 3g of vitamin C (in an ascorbate form) throughout the day. This vitamin helps produce collagen.

B

- Try Precision Engineered Elite Training Packs, a supplement devised that contains calcium, vitamin C, bromelain, magnesium, rutin, and more, which all help support the skeletal system. Available from Nutrition World (www.nutritionworld.com)
- Cayenne pepper capsules can help reduce inflammation and increase circulation to the affected area. Take 3–4 capsules daily with food. **VC**

Helpful Hints

- Make sure to consult a chiropractor or osteopath as soon as possible after any injury. To help reduce the immediate pain and muscle spasm, wrap some ice cubes or a bag of frozen peas in a towel and place on the painful area for 10 minutes every hour.
- Most cities now have alternative health centers that include chiropractic, acupuncture, and/or physiotherapy. Stop in and see if they can help.
- You can buy from any pharmacy gels that feel cold when applied, and they can help reduce the pain. Creams like Icy Hot or Bengay can also help reduce the muscle spasms.
- Back pain often has its root in poor posture. This is compounded by the fact that we now tend to lead very sedentary lives, which weakens the supporting structures of the spine and makes them much more prone to injury. Many cases of severe back pain are also caused by muscle spasm.
- Work on holding in your core tummy muscles (abs), as this really helps support your lower back.
- If you have a helpful boss and sit at a desk all day, ask for an ergonomic chair. I literally cannot work without mine and find it almost impossible to sit in a normal chair. www.ergodepot.com
- When you are working, take regular breaks, stand up from your desk, walk around, stretch, and roll your shoulders.
- If you have chronic lower back pain, try using a back support seat cushion. I carry mine everywhere—in the car, on planes, in restaurants, etc.—and cannot sit for more than two minutes without it.
- Before agreeing to any surgery, always consult a chiropractor or osteopath for a second opinion (see *Useful Information*). However, always report severe and persistent back pain to your doctor.
- Make sure you have a good bed mattress such as Tempur-Pedic, which supports your spine but is neither too hard nor too soft. Better-quality orthopedic mattresses are expensive but well worth the long-term investment.
- If you are extremely tired and under stress, not only does your immune system begin to suffer but also your body in general. In other words, when you stop supporting your body, it stops supporting you. If this is the case, then you need to take a long, hard look at your lifestyle and get more rest.
- Acupuncture is known to help in many cases and is great for reducing inflammation and pain.
- For general back maintenance, yoga can be very beneficial as it improves flexibility, strengthens the spine, and improves posture, protecting it from injury in the long term.
- Alexander Technique and Pilates teach individuals how to maintain their back and general health through better posture and exercises. With my ongoing chronic back problem, Pilates has been my savior. (See *Useful Information*.)
- Walk more; this helps tighten the abdominal muscles, which in turn supports the back. Treat yourself to a pair of MBT (Masai Barefoot Technology) shoes, which are made using state-of-the-art technology to support the feet. They are used by orthopedic therapists and physiotherapists all over the world. For more details visit www.swissmasai.com
- Swimming is a great exercise because, although the back muscles are worked, they are

B

protected from jarring by the support given by the water. But, obviously, do not swim if your symptoms are acute.

- Use good bath salts such as Epsom salts or Miracle Krystal salts to help reduce muscle spasm. Miracle Krystal salts are more powerful than Epsom salts and help eliminate toxins from the joints and re-alkalize the body.
- Have a weekly aromatherapy massage. The essential oils penetrate into the bloodstream and really help calm the muscle spasms that can leave you doubled over in pain. Roman chamomile, lavender, and eucalyptus oils can all help reduce pain.
- Use a "wheat or lavender bag." These bags are available from most health stores and can also be found in many malls. You heat them in the microwave and apply to painful muscles. Alternate with the ice packs for more relief.

BAD BREATH

(see Halitosis)

BEREAVEMENT

(see also Adrenal Exhaustion, Depression, Immune Function, and Stress)

Losing a loved one at any age can be a devastating blow to your life and wellbeing at every level. Therefore, after a loved one's passing, it is vital for you to express your feelings and let your emotions out. Grief, anger, and guilt have a tremendous impact on the physical body.

Tears shed in trauma contain high levels of stress chemicals, so let them out and don't be afraid to break down. When my mother died in my arms I was inconsolable and, like millions of others, I turned to good mediums who were able to give me specific messages that only the two of us knew.

During the past 17 years, I have written regularly about life after death and have received hundreds of letters from people of all ages who have lost a loved one. Their sense of loss and grief is often overwhelming, but how different might we all feel if we knew that our loved ones live on. During the late nineties I went through a near-death experience with a medical doctor present, and my story is well documented in my book *Divine Intervention* (CICO Books).

These days I write from a totally different perspective as I have an absolute personal "knowing" that we all go on. I, like many scientists, now believe that our unique energy field, which contains all the information about us, simply moves to another frequency level that cannot be seen by our physical eyes. When you turn on your radio or TV you can tune into hundreds of different channels or stations and receive or see huge amounts of information. And just because you cannot see these signals, it doesn't mean they aren't there!

The spirit realms exist on various frequencies, but more sensitive people can hear and see them. I have interviewed and met dozens of people who, by learning to meditate and stilling their minds into a more receptive alpha state, have, after time, heard messages from departed loved ones for themselves. Obviously, some people are better at this than others, but we all have the capability to hear other realms. When some people suddenly begin hearing voices they are labeled as being mentally ill; some are—but others have simply begun hearing the spirit world. It is vital that the medical world begins to recognize this possibility. See also *Spiritual Emergency*. I have listed much of the science in my books *The Evidence for the Sixth Sense* (CICO Books) and *Countdown to Coherence* (Watkins).

Foods to Avoid

- Although during stressful times we tend to crave far more comfort foods, as much as possible keep junk, sugary, pre-packaged meals, which place a strain on your immune system, to a minimum. But then again, at times of extreme stress, the brain burns more sugar. Therefore, if you don't mind putting on a few pounds, enjoy your treats—but don't go overboard.
- Caffeine, alcohol, and sugar place a great strain on your adrenal glands, which further increases feelings of total exhaustion. See *Stress* and *Thyroid*.

Friendly Foods

- At times of extreme emotional stress, it is easy to forget our own health. It is important to eat as healthily as possible, which will not only help your nervous system to cope but also boost your immune system. You help no one by allowing yourself to become ill. Try to eat one meal daily that combines a quality protein such as fish or chicken with fresh vegetables and fruit.
- Make a fruit smoothie. Place one scoop of hemp seed protein or whey protein, half a cup of blueberries, one banana, a spoonful of linseeds that have been soaked overnight in water (or ready-ground Linwood flax seeds), and sunflower seeds, a few raisins (if you like your drinks sweet), and a chopped apple into a blender. Blend with some rice milk, and then drink. This mixture will give you energy and good nutrients. Feel free to experiment by adding any other fruits you love.
- See also *General Health Hints*.

Useful Remedies

- Take homeopathic Ignatia 30c and the Bach Flower Remedy Star of Bethlehem, both of which help reduce feelings of shock and grief.
- Take a high-strength B-complex vitamin supplement daily to support the nerves.
- Take a good-quality multi-vitamin and mineral.
- Kali Phos New Era Tissue Salts are excellent for reducing stress. Take 4 tablets under the tongue in between meals twice daily.
- Try L-theanine and Lemon Balm formula to help keep you calmer. L-theanine is extracted from green tea and helps reduce the production of the stress hormones cortisol and adrenalin. You can also use this at night as a sleep aid. See also under *Stress*.

B

Helpful Hints

- If you have a friend, colleague, or relative who is dealing with the death of a loved one, take the time to prepare an occasional meal for them. Not only will this help support their physical needs, but it will also support their emotional needs by giving them someone to talk to.
- GriefNet.org is an Internet community for people dealing with grief and loss. They have nearly 50 e-mail support groups and two websites.
- The Compassionate Friends is a nationwide organization of bereaved parents offering understanding, support, and encouragement after the death of a child or children. Members of TCF receive regular issues of TCF News and a quarterly newsletter. For further information, contact The Compassionate Friends' helpline (1-877-969-0010) or visit their website (www.compassionatefriends.org).
- To find a medium in your area contact the National Spiritualist Association of Churches, 13 Cottage Row, PO Box 217, Lily Dale NY 14752; Tel: 1-716-595-2000; E-mail: secretary@nsac.org. Or consult the directory posted on their website: www.nsac.org

BLADDER PROBLEMS   *(see Cystitis, Incontinence, and Prostate Problems)*

BLEEDING GUMS
(see also Fluoride)

Bleeding gums can be triggered by over-enthusiastic brushing or by gum disease. They can also indicate a lack of vitamin C, bioflavonoids, or the vitamin-like substance, Co-enzyme Q10 (CoQ10).

Bacteria in the mouth and bleeding gums are also being linked to heart disease, but this could very well be linked back to a lack of CoQ10.

To make sure you are not suffering from anything more serious, go see your dentist and make sure to see a dental hygienist at least twice a year for a proper cleaning. When plaque builds up gum disease, such as gingivitis, can take hold. If left unchecked you can lose your teeth. Believe me, after all the problems I have suffered with my teeth during the last decade, I know your own teeth are very precious and should be taken care of at all costs.

And if you tend to suffer from a constantly dry mouth, you should investigate potential problems such as Sjogren's syndrome (see *Sjogren's Syndrome*), an autoimmune condition that can affect the mouth and gums.

Foods to Avoid
- The plaque-forming bacteria that cause chronic gum disease thrive on sugar. Young children especially should only be allowed small amounts of sodas, candies, and desserts that are high in sugar.

- Keep refined carbohydrates including cookies, cakes, and candies to a minimum. Or make your own cookies using oats, raisins, seeds, and agar or brown rice syrup.
- Avoid all foods and water containing fluoride, which is a by-product of the plant fertilizer industry. Calcium fluoride may have reduced the number of cavities, but sodium fluoride is a poison and, in my opinion, should not be allowed into our drinking water. This is mass medication without consent.

Friendly Foods
- Foods containing plenty of fiber such as leafy green vegetables, brown rice, fresh fruits like apples, papaya, figs, and cherries are all rich in vitamin C, which supports healthy teeth and gums.
- Garden sage makes a great mouthwash for inflamed or bleeding gums, an inflamed tongue, canker sores, or a sore throat. Simply add 1–2 teaspoons of chopped leaves to a cup of boiling water. Once it has cooled, place in a screw-top jar. Use twice daily as a mouthwash. You can also gargle with this mixture while it is still warm. **NB: As sage stimulates the muscles of the uterus, DO NOT use sage during pregnancy.**
- Agave syrup and xylitol can be used as more natural alternatives to refined sugar. A number of xylitol-based sweeteners are also available for purchase on amazon.com and from Vitacost (www.vitacost.com).
- Chew licorice sticks regularly to keep teeth and gums clean and to reduce bacteria in the mouth.
- Drink at least 6–8 glasses of filtered water a day.
- Dilute concentrated fruit juices at a ratio of 1 part juice to 4 parts water.
- Thai foods such as lemon grass, cilantro, and garlic help keep teeth healthy, and the cilantro also helps eliminate heavy metals from the body.

Useful Remedies
- Co-enzyme Q10 is well known to improve gum health. Take 60–100mg a day.
- Take 1–2g of vitamin C with bioflavonoids a day in divided doses with food.
- A good-quality multi-vitamin/mineral for your age and gender.

Helpful Hints
- Do not brush your teeth directly after eating fruit, as you can brush away weakened enamel and cause erosion.
- Mercury from amalgam fillings is also known to cause swollen, bleeding gums (see *Mercury*).
- Eat a piece of fruit after main meals. This increases saliva production, which is alkaline and neutralizes the acid produced by bacteria that is responsible for dental decay. Apples are excellent, but if you eat sweet or highly acid fruits after a meal, such as oranges, then simply rinse your mouth with water immediately afterward.
- Also if you eat very sugary desserts, rinse the mouth with water. Don't brush your teeth for at least an hour.
- Gengigel is a gel and mouthwash that contains hyaluronic acid, a natural substance that plays an important role in gum formation. This gel can also help reduce inflammation. For more details visit www.revital.com International delivery can be arranged or you can order online from a US retailer like www.docsimon.com
- Vitamin C supplements that contain sugar will attack tooth enamel and weaken the lining of the mouth when chewed.
- Use a good electric toothbrush.
- Practice good dental hygiene every day by using floss and a natural tea-tree mouthwash. Clean your teeth and gums daily using a water pick appliance, adding a few drops of tea tree oil and one drop of clove oil, which is an excellent antiseptic, to the warm water. Waterpik Cleaners are available from most large pharmacies (like Walgreens and CVS), as well as from Walmart and Target. Visit www.waterpik.com for more details.
- Toothpaste containing sodium lauryl sulfate (SLS) can thin the lining of the cheeks and may weaken gum tissue. Ask at your health shop or at the pharmacy for toothpastes that are SLS free.
- Avoid toothpastes containing fluoride.
- There are also numerous herbal toothpastes containing everything from Co-enzyme Q10 and vitamin K to support your gums to red clover and herbs known to help ladies through menopause! Find one that suits your needs. USANA Health Services, Pharma Nord, Weleda, and Jason all make healthier toothpastes.

B

BLOATING
(see Candida, Constipation, and Flatulence)

BODY HAIR, EXCESSIVE (Hirsutism)

Many women suffer this problem after going through menopause, although some can be affected when they are much younger. This problem usually begins with extra hairs on the face and sometimes hair begins growing in between the breast area. It is normally caused by an excess of male hormones called androgens, which are produced by the ovaries or the adrenal glands. It is important to consult your doctor if you have unexplained excess body hair, but this condition can often be helped if you can balance your hormones naturally (see *Menopause*). The condition is often related to polycystic ovarian syndrome (see *PCOS*).

Foods to Avoid
- Cut down on alcohol and excess caffeine, which can affect hormone levels—as can stress.
- Reduce animal fats from dairy products and red meat.

- If you cook food in plastic containers, and if you also buy food wrapped in plastic wrap or use plastic wrap at home, then chemicals within the plastic can leach into your food, especially if it is heated in a microwave. The chemicals that are released from the plastic can have an estrogen-building effect within the body, which in turn can trigger a whole host of hormone-related problems.
- If PCOS is a factor, reduce refined sugar to a minimum as this leads to surges of insulin, a chemical needed to balance sugar levels in the body. As far back as 1980, researchers found that an excess of insulin is linked to higher testosterone levels, and higher testosterone levels trigger hair growth.

Friendly Foods

- Include more hormone-regulating foods, such as tempeh, organic tofu, chickpeas, and fennel.
- Eat more beans, lentils, and leafy greens including broccoli, cauliflower, cabbage, artichokes, and beets, all of which help cleanse the liver of toxins and help balance hormones.
- Eat more linseeds (flax seeds should be pre-cracked or soaked overnight in cold water), sunflower, and pumpkin seeds, as well as Brazil nuts, because they are all rich in essential fats, which also help regulate hormones.
- Avocados and oily fish are also rich in essential fats needed to regulate hormones.
- Fill up on fiber, which binds to excess hormones so that they can be easily removed from the body. Oat or rice bran, fruit (especially apples), and whole grains such as brown rice, quinoa, and amaranth would be ideal.

- Fresh root ginger and fish are both rich in zinc, which aids absorption of fatty acids that regulate hormones.
- Make sure you drink plenty of fluids.

Useful Remedies

- The herbs that have proved most useful for reducing excess body hair are dong quai and agnus castus, which help normalize hormonal levels. Take 500mg of either or both daily, but try the agnus castus first. Femarone 40 Plus, available from www.shs100.com, contains blessed thistle, squaw vine, and black cohosh; take 2 capsules three times daily with food for 3 months. (Femarone 40 Plus also comes in drops.) You could also try Female Reproductive Formula available from www.herbsfirst.com/descriptionsformulas/FemaleReproductiveFormula.htm
- Taking 500mg of black cohosh twice a day has been used to successfully inhibit and reverse facial hair growth in women. Many companies now sell all these herbs in one formula—try 500mg twice daily or take 1ml of a tincture.
- Herbs used for the related condition PCOS are licorice, saw palmetto, paeonia, and agnus castus. Take 5ml of each daily.
- Taking 100–150mcg of chromium polynicotinate twice daily helps balance blood sugar and reduce sugar cravings.
- Lipoic acid regulates blood sugar and liver function, which in turn helps regulate hormones. Take 200mg twice daily with food.
- Several companies now make Cruciferous Vegetable Extract Capsules that contain pure extracts of broccoli, watercress, cabbage, etc. Take as directed to help naturally balance hormones. **LEF**

Helpful Hints

- A study of women with excess body hair found that acupuncture reduced both hair density and length as well as significantly reducing their levels of androgens, male sex hormones. See *Useful Information*.
- If you are overweight, this can add to the problem. See *Weight Problems*.

- Women with excessive body hair may be short of the hormone progesterone, which helps balance the male hormones that women also produce in small quantities. Many women don't ovulate regularly (but still have periods), often triggered by stress, excess pollution in the environment, or foods containing herbicides, which have an estrogen-like building effect. Since progesterone is produced only after ovulation or during pregnancy, progesterone deficiency is becoming more common; hairier legs and chins are one sign.
- Natural progesterone, made from yams and sold in a cream, can reduce hairiness when used for some time. It is freely available in the US. You can order natural progesterone creams by calling Pharm West. If you are calling from the US dial 1-310-301-4015. Website: www.pharmwest.com

BODY ODOR

We are all covered in bacteria, and they tend to accumulate in certain parts of the body, such as under the arms and between our legs. Unpleasant body odor is usually associated with poor hygiene habits, but it can also indicate internal toxicity. The skin is a route of elimination that is used by the body when other routes—such as the liver, bowels, and kidneys—are struggling to cope and become overloaded. Also if you eat too much garlic, the smell begins to ooze through your pores. It's very healthy for the person who has eaten it, but not so pleasant for those around you!

B

Foods to Avoid
- Reduce the amount of low-fiber foods you eat such as gelatin, ice cream, white breads and pastas, cakes, cookies, and so on.
- Avoid full-fat dairy products as they trigger mucus production and can exacerbate constipation.
- Any foods that ferment in the gut, such as moldy cheeses or high-sugar fruits like mango, banana, dates, and grapes, can eventually trigger body odor. Eat such fruits in between meals rather than after a meal, as they are more likely to ferment.
- Cut down on sugar and alcohol.
- Red meat and heavy fatty meals such as melted cheeses are hard to digest and slow your digestion and elimination.
- Avoid any foods to which you are intolerant—especially wheat and cow's milk, which trigger constipation in many people. *See Constipation*.

Friendly Foods
- Drink 6–8 glasses of filtered water a day to help flush toxins from the body and reduce constipation.
- Add a tablespoon of soluble fiber to your breakfast cereal. Linseeds (flax seeds need to be soaked overnight in cold water or use ready-cracked linseeds), hemp seeds, and oat or rice bran are all available from health stores.
- Treat yourself to a blender and a juicer. To help cleanse your system blend any selection of fruits you like with a tablespoon of soaked linseeds (flax seeds), two teaspoons of oat or rice bran, plus a teaspoon of a good-quality green food powder or hemp seed protein and a cup of organic rice milk. If you drink this cocktail for brakfast or instead of having an evening meal, it really helps to clear you out! If you add half a teaspoon of powdered essential fats it helps even more. Omega Plex EFA formula is available from BioCare and can be shipped internationally.

- On alternate days, juice any green foods, plus artichoke, celery, apple, raw beets, a little fresh root ginger, and aloe vera juice, which will all help detoxify your system.
- Generally, eat more artichokes, chicory, beets, watercress, alfalfa sprouts, broccoli, cabbage, kale, fennel, leeks, and onions to aid detoxification.
- Adding fresh cilantro to these juices and meals will help keep the bacteria that can cause unpleasant body odor under control.
- Eat more pineapple and papaya, which are rich in digestive enzymes.
- Kelp, almonds, buckwheat, millet, brown rice, and figs are all rich in magnesium, which is often lacking in constipated people.

Useful Remedies
- Healthy bacteria (acidophilus and bifidus) help improve gut functioning. Take two probiotic capsules daily after meals.
- A deficiency of the mineral zinc is related to excess perspiration. Take a multi-vitamin/mineral daily, which usually contains 15mg of zinc, and then take a further 15mg before bed.
- Any organic green food supplement powder that contains chlorella and/or wheat grass is a great way to increase elimination.
- The mineral silica really helps to reduce body odor. Take 75mg daily.

Helpful Hints
- When the bowels are moving frequently, the body doesn't have to try to eliminate toxins through the skin.
- Fresh, live yogurt with acidophilus and bifidus eaten on a regular basis keeps gut flora in good shape.

- Take a shower every day, and change underwear regularly.
- Dry-skin brushing will help break up and remove toxins stored under the skin so that the body can eliminate them. Combine this with an Epsom salt bath to really help flush out toxins that may cause odor. Use 1 cup per 60lbs of body weight and add to a warm bath. Soak for 15–20 minutes and rub your skin all over with a washcloth. Don't rinse off before getting out of the bathtub, just dry off and relax for the evening. Keep some water handy by the tub as a warm bath can make you thirsty.
- Dab milk of magnesia under the arms. Its high pH helps prevent bacteria from proliferating.
- Wear cotton or silk next to the skin, which enables the skin to breathe.
- If persistent, body odor may indicate liver dysfunction, digestive problems, and/or yeast infections, which are probably best investigated by a qualified nutritionist or a doctor who is also a nutritionist (see *Useful Information*).
- Try using a natural, odorless mineral salt deodorant, which prevents bacterial growth without the use of harsh chemicals or aluminum. Just wet the crystal and glide it over the skin. It is also available in a spray. Visit www.naturallyfreshdeodorantcrystal.com for more details.

BOILS
(see also Immune Function and Liver Problems)

Boils are normally triggered by an acute bacterial infection of a hair follicle caused by the bacteria *Staphylococcus aureus*. If you suffer from boils on a regular basis, it's your body's way of telling you that your immune system is very run down, you're most likely consuming a poor diet, and you are full of toxins. Boils are more common in diabetics and AIDS patients and may be accompanied by a slight fever. The secret to controling boils is to keep your liver clean, as once the liver is overloaded, or you become constipated, then toxins are dumped into the skin—your largest organ. See also *Constipation*.

Foods to Avoid

- Any foods and drinks high in sugar, which will lower immune function.
- Reduce your intake of red meats and full-fat dairy products, especially cheese, chocolates, double cream, and so on.
- Avoid all pre-packaged meals and mass-produced cakes, cookies and snacks containing hydrogenated or trans-fats.
- Eliminate mass-produced burgers, fried foods, and oily fast-food meals.

Friendly Foods

- Eat more soluble fibers such as linseeds (flax seeds soaked overnight in water and drained or use the ready-cracked types) or oat or rice bran to encourage faster elimination of toxins from the bowel.
- Use small amounts of xylitol sugar and agave syrup instead of refined sugars, as they have a lower glycemic index. Xylitol also helps reduce constipation.
- Include more garlic and onions, which have antiseptic properties that help cleanse the gut.
- Eat more fresh beets, fennel, celeriac (celery root), and artichokes, which help to cleanse the liver.
- Eat plenty of fiber in the form of lightly steamed vegetables, baked potatoes, brown rice, and fruits with the peel left on when practical. Apples are great for the skin, but make sure they're organic.
- Eat low-fat, live yogurt, which contains the healthy bacteria acidophilus and bifidus.
- Drink at least 6–8 glasses of water a day.
- See General Health Hints.

Useful Remedies

- Zinc is a vital mineral for healing the skin and stimulating the immune system. When symptoms are acute, take 30mg three times daily and then reduce to 30mg daily.
- Take 1g of vitamin C in an ascorbate form three times a day with meals for one month and then reduce to 500mg daily.
- Vitamin A is also great for healing the skin. **If you are not pregnant or planning a pregnancy**, take up to 20,000IU daily for 7 days. Then switch to taking natural-source carotenes daily, which convert naturally to Vitamin A in the body, until the boil has gone.
- Solgar make an excellent carotene complex. Take one daily.
- Place some goldenseal tincture on a cotton swab and apply it directly to the boil. Goldenseal helps to kill off the bacteria Staphylococcus aureus.
- Prebiotic nutrients extracted from the agave plant, chicory, onions, and so on support the growth of healthy bacteria in the gut and enhance immune function. They are extremely useful for reducing constipation. Take one scoop each morning. For details about Agave Digestive Immune Support visit www.lef.org
- Also see the supplements listed under Acid–Alkaline Balance, as an over-acid system can be linked to problems like boils.

Helpful Hints

- Apply a little tea tree oil on a cotton swab to the boil once it has burst.
- Goldenseal can also be used as a poultice. The boils don't normally rupture if you use this herb.
- If you do want the boils to come to a head and possibly rupture, mix about 4 teaspoons of Epsom salts in 1.2 cups of hot water and apply it directly to the boil to enhance draining.
- Try a mixture of homeopathic silica, arnica and belladonna 30, which will help reduce pain and help the boil pop. Once it has popped, clean it with tea tree oil and goldenseal.
- After the boil has come to a head and suppuration has finished, take a mixture of hypericum and calendula 30 twice a day to help it heal.

- Recurrent boils would benefit from a detox.
- Get plenty of exercise, which helps detoxify the skin, and wash as soon as possible after exercise.
- Saunas, particularly infrared, help clear blocked pores and drain toxins from the body.
- Try reading *The Holistic Beauty Book* by Star Khechara (Green Books).

BREAST CANCER *(see also Cancer)*

Although breast cancer remains the most common cancer in women in the US (other than skin cancer)—more than 190,000 new cases were reported last year in the US alone—there are plenty of measures that we can take to help prevent and heal breast cancer. The World Cancer Research Fund now states that as many as 40% of cases could be avoided by following a healthier lifestyle: drinking less alcohol, keeping to a sensible weight, and exercising regularly. Women who are overweight are at a far greater risk of developing estrogen-dependent cancers. In fact, a 2006 British study found that obese women were 60% more likely to develop any type of cancer than normal-weight women. Meanwhile, the incidence of breast cancer in women over 50 has fallen significantly in countries where fewer women take orthodox HRT, which has been shown to increase the risk for breast cancer by over 60%, compared to those who do not use it. Bio Identical Hormone therapy, especially when creams are used, have been shown to be safer. (For more details, see *Menopause*.)

B

A few women are so frightened of contracting breast cancer because their mother, or sometimes their grandmother and other relatives, have died of this disease, that they have their breasts removed as a precaution. My mother died from breast cancer, but I would not undergo such radical surgery unless I actually had cancer. Scientists have now identified that a faulty gene (the NRG1), which is not inherited, is involved in more than 50% of breast cancer cases.

Our inherited genes control the structure and function of our body, but if our genes stay healthy then our body can stay healthy as well. If you live a healthy lifestyle you can mostly change which genes are expressed. In other words, if your parents and grandparents died of heart attacks or cancer you may well have a pre-disposition for heart problems and cancer. But if you live a different lifestyle and eat healthier foods, you can help change the chemistry within the body and stack the odds more in your favor.

Meanwhile, risk factors for breast cancer include orthodox HRT, the contraceptive pill, excessive intake of saturated animal fats, dairy products, alcohol, pesticides, herbicides, and a low intake of protective fruit and vegetables, which are rich in antioxidants. Research from Montreal has also found a link between breast cancer and women who work with synthetic fibers and petroleum products.

Also, many young women overproduce estrogen, and this is one of the reasons they suffer from the symptoms of pre-menstrual syndrome. If you eat a healthy diet, the body excretes these hormones via the liver. However, if the diet is high in saturated animal fats or alcohol, not only is it harder for the body to excrete these estrogens, but it tends to recycle them into an aggressive form, which can begin attacking tissues.

Residues of pesticides and herbicides that are known to trigger various cancers are now in our food chain and drinking water. These toxins are deposited in fatty tissue within the body—so the more you avoid contact with such substances, the more you reduce your chance of contracting cancer.

Foods to Avoid

- Reduce your intake of alcohol to no more than 1–3 drinks a week. See *Alcohol*.
- Animal fats should be kept to sensible levels; eat lean organic meats.
- Reduce your intake of dairy products, especially from cows, sheep and goats, and make sure any dairy product you eat is low fat.
- Pesticides and plastics act like strong estrogens in the body and are known to trigger certain cancers. This is why you need to eat organic food as much as possible. Never re-heat a pre-packaged meal in its plastic container, as the chemicals leach into your food. Transfer them to glass or stainless steel cookware before heating.
- There has been much misinformation in the media about soy that has said it causes hormone activity that is not beneficial to health. While this argument is ongoing, it is generally accepted that fermented soy in the form of miso or tempeh is beneficial. Cooked tofu is fine, but if in doubt avoid unfermented soy products such as soy yogurt or milk. Soy isoflavones act like a weak estrogen, which helps block stronger negative estrogens in our environment so soy isoflavones in capsule or tablet form are fine.
- Avoid fried foods.

Friendly Foods

- As a **preventative** measure eat cooked soybeans, chickpeas, lentils, beans (dried beans are best), and fermented soy products such as tempeh. Japanese and Thai women who do not eat a Western diet have a much lower incidence of breast cancer, and this appears to be due to their regular consumption of fermented soy-based foods, which are rich in phyto-estrogens and isoflavones that contain genistein. Genistein helps inhibit the growth of cancer cells. Eat organic and/or GM-free soy in its traditional form—tofu, miso, soy sauce, and tempeh.
- Broccoli, cabbage, Brussels sprouts, alfalfa sprouts and especially watercress and papaya all contain substances that are protective against breast cancer.
- Raw linseeds (flax seeds soaked overnight in water and drained or use the ready-cracked versions) sprinkled regularly onto meals contain a fiber called lignan, which helps to protect breast tissue.
- Eat more essential fats—see under *Fats You Need to Eat*.
- My favorite way to ingest a lot of nutrients quickly is by juicing. Juice some organic raw carrots, cabbage, apple, fresh root ginger, raw beets, radish, and celery. Also add a teaspoon of any organic green food supplement and some organic-source aloe vera juice.
- The only problem with juicing is that some of the live enzymes and nutrients and almost all of the fiber is left in the juicer, so scrape them out and add them to your juice. It makes the mix thicker, but you receive far more nutrients. For this reason I use my blender quite a lot as then you get the whole fruit, including the peel. A great meal replacement is to blend a banana, an organic apple (remove the seeds), a small box of blueberries, a teaspoon of non-GM soy lecithin granules and some green food powder (I use organic hemp seed powder for its high protein content). I also add some sunflower seeds and soaked linseeds (flax seeds), as well as a cup of low-fat organic rice milk, and then blend the mixture for 30 seconds. It makes the most deliciously healthy and filling shake.
- Replace margarines containing hydrogenated and trans-fats with healthier spreads such as Biona. Or use olive oil or organic coconut oil.
- Many patients with cancer have low levels of the carotenes. Apricots, papaya, sweet potatoes, asparagus, French beans, broccoli, carrots, mustard and cress, red peppers, spinach, watercress, mangoes, parsley, and tomatoes are all rich in carotenes. Fresh, organic carrot juice is a great source, but don't overdo it as your skin may turn orange!
- Pomegranate has been found at City of Hope Hospital in Duarte, California to suppress

B

proliferation of breast cancer cells. Eat this super food or take a pomegranate concentrate capsule daily.

- Take extra fiber daily. It will keep toxic wastes and old hormones from being absorbed from the colon into the bloodstream. The colon must be kept clean and the bowels must be emptied regularly for healing to occur in the body. Add a tablespoon of oat or rice bran (or soaked flax/linseeds) to the fruit blends and drink daily.
- Drink plenty of water to aid elimination.
- Iodine is stored in breast tissue, and low iodine can encourage excess estrogen production and increase the sensitivity of breast tissue to estrogen. Therefore use nori kelp shakes or iodized Celtic sea salt instead of sodium-based salts to naturally increase iodine levels.
- Add more curcumin, which is found in turmeric, to your foods. It is highly anti-cancerous. **NB: If you are undergoing chemotherapy, then check with your doctor before taking large amounts of this spice.**

Drink more organic green or white teas, which have been shown to have anti-cancer properties.

Useful Remedies to Prevent and Heal Breast Cancer

- For prevention, if you don't like soy-based foods, take a one-a-day isoflavone supplement. **VC**
- If you have cancer, you can take 5–7g of vitamin C a day in an ascorbate form with food for a few weeks. In such doses you may experience loose bowels, in which case cut the dose by 500mg at a time until your bowels normalize. For maintenance and cancer prevention, take 2g daily in divided doses with food.

- Vitamin D3 is crucial for preventing cancer of all types. Take a minimum of 1500IU daily for prevention. If you have breast cancer, take 2000–3000IU daily, as this vital vitamin has been shown by scientists at the University of Toronto to prolong survival. A day exposing your skin to sunlight can create 20,000IU of Vitamin D.
- Take a high-strength antioxidant formula that contains vitamins C and E, plus zinc and selenium.
- Natural-source carotenes are vital antioxidants. Take one capsule daily for prevention and two daily if you have breast cancer. Solgar makes an excellent carotene complex.
- **If you have breast cancer,** take 100mg of Co-enzyme Q10 three times daily. This important co-enzyme has been shown to inhibit cancer-cell growth and protect breast tissue. **To aid prevention,** take 100mg daily.
- Beta Glucans 1–3, 1–6 are proven to strengthen the body's innate immune system. Pharma Nord makes a version that is free from yeast protein. Take 250–500mg daily. **PN**
- A good-quality multi-vitamin/mineral.
- Indole-3-carbinol (I3C) is a phytochemical supplement isolated from cruciferous vegetables (broccoli, cauliflower, Brussels sprouts, turnips, kale, green cabbage, mustard, bok choy, and so on) that has been shown to inhibit the growth of estrogen-receptor-positive cells. This supplement has well researched anti-cancer and healing potential. To ingest therapeutic quantities of indole would require eating enormous amounts of raw vegetables, as cooking tends to destroy these phytochemicals. Take one tablet daily or as directed. **VC NB: Pregnant women should not take this supplement, as estrogen is needed for healthy fetus growth.**
- With your doctor's permission start taking the hormone melatonin, the hormone produced in the pineal gland at night that helps induce sleep. A high percentage of women with estrogen-receptor-positive breast cancer have low plasma levels of melatonin. Begin by taking 1mg nightly before bed. This can trigger vivid dreaming in some cases. Your doctor can give you a prescription for melatonin, or it can be bought without a prescription via the Life Extension Foundation. **LEF**

- Bio-electromagnetics scientist Roger Coghill has developed a supplement called Asphalia that contains natural melatonin extracted from certain grasses. Take 1 to 2 capsules 30 minutes before going to bed. Roger's exclusive distributor in the US is Diva Marketing, Don't Disturb Me!, 2612 Sleepy Hollow, Pearland, TX 77581; Tel: 1-713-221-1873 or 1-866-692-8037; website: www.dontdisturbmesite.com
  NB: Should not be taken by severe asthmatics, pregnant women, or children under one.
- For prevention of breast cancer, the methylating B vitamins help switch "bad" estrogens back to "good" estrogens. Either take a high-strength B complex daily or use a Homocysteine Lowering Formula.
- **If you have breast cancer**, AWGE, an extract of wheat germ, has been proven to modulate immune function and improves the effectiveness of conventional treatments if taken daily one hour before food. For details and to view its large body of independent research log on to www.avemarwge.com More information on AWGE is in the *Cancer* section.
- Take three Pomegranate Concentrate capsules daily to help keep breast cancer cells from proliferating. **VC**

Helpful Hints
- Ask your specialist about cryotherapy, a minimally invasive "freezing" therapy that involves destroying cancer cells using a cold gas. Results to date have been very positive.
- If you are going to have chemotherapy, see details of the CTC test under the *Cancer* section, which can help your specialist know which specific chemotherapy suits your unique physiology.
- Examine your breasts once a month. If you find even the slightest hint of anything unusual or any type of lump, see your doctor immediately. Remember, the earlier any problems are detected, the greater your chance of a complete cure. Many lumps are simply benign cysts, so the sooner you see your doctor the better.
- Several studies have linked excessive use of mammogram X-rays to an increased risk of developing breast cancer.
- Antiperspirants often contain chemicals that are absorbed into the body. They also stop you from sweating, which is nature's way of getting rid of many unwanted toxins. The majority of breast cancers occur in the part of the breast closest to the armpit. Use natural tea-tree-based antiperspirants or ones that are free from aluminum such as those available from www.naturallyfreshdeodorantcrystal.com
- Avoid wearing a bra for too much of the day. Women who wore a tight-fitting bra for 14 hours or longer a day were 50% more likely to develop breast cancer. At the very least, find yourself a comfortable, loose-fitting bra that doesn't block lymph drainage.
- Some women who have had their breasts removed find that any remaining lymph glands, especially under the arms, can be really painful. Manual lymph drainage can often relieve the discomfort (see *Useful Information*).
- Keep your stress levels to a minimum (see *Stress*).
- Exercise regularly as much as possible, but not to excess.
- Breast cancer is more common in people who are overweight and obese. Take steps to control your weight (see *Weight Problems*).
- Read Patrick Holford's book, *Say No to Cancer* (Piatkus). If you have specific questions that you would like answered, log on to www.patrickholford.com.
- Read the book by John R Lee, David Zava, and Virginia Hopkins, *What Your Doctor May Not Tell You About Breast Cancer* (Grand Central Publications).
- Another wonderful book is *Your Life in Your Hands: Understanding, Preventing, and Overcoming Breast Cancer* by Jane Plant (Thomas Dunne).

B

- Visit the Office of Cancer Complementary and Alternative Medicine's patient website (www.cancer.gov/cam/health_patients.html) for more information and for advice about selecting a CAM practitioner or paying for CAM treatment.

BREAST PAIN AND TENDERNESS

(see also Breast Cancer and Pre-menstrual Tension)

Tender breasts are a common symptom of pre-menstrual syndrome (PMS, also known as pre-menstrual tension or PMT). During this time prior to menstruation, the breasts can become increasingly swollen and tender. Breast pain is often associated with other symptoms such as fluid retention, abdominal bloating, and an excess of the hormone estrogen. Tender breasts during the first few months of pregnancy are also quite common. But if breasts are tender the whole month or if the discomfort becomes severe, it is important to see a doctor. If you find any lumps of any size or shape in your breasts, seek medical attention immediately. Exercise is one way of reducing PMS symptoms as it encourages lymphatic drainage. On the other hand, wearing a bra for more than 12 hours a day can reduce the body's ability to drain the lymph nodes.

Also, women who take estrogen-only HRT or use estrogen bio-identical hormone creams may find their breasts swell and become tender. If so, you may need to reduce dosage and see your healthcare professional.

B

Foods to Avoid

- Complete avoidance of caffeine can reduce the symptoms of breast pain. Moderate caffeine reduction doesn't always work; it does need to be complete elimination. Remember that caffeine is not just in tea and coffee but also in cola, many energy drinks, chocolate, and some over-the-counter cold remedies.
- Alcohol should be kept to a minimum as it can increase breast pain.
- Sodium-based salt tends to aggravate fluid retention, which can sometimes exacerbate breast tenderness. Ask at your health shop for a magnesium-based sea salt and use it only sparingly. Nori seaweed flakes from health shops can be used instead of salt and are rich in iodine.

Friendly Foods

- Eat plenty of sunflower seeds, sesame seeds, and linseeds (flax seeds preferably soaked overnight in cold water), which all contain essential fatty acids that should help reduce breast tenderness. See *Fats You Need To Eat*.
- Eating organic, fermented soy-based foods such as tempeh, miso, and natto, as well as edamame (fresh green soy beans that you cook like peas) on a regular basis can also reduce the tendency to develop painful breasts and help balance hormone levels.
- Drink herbal teas, such as red clover, and/or dandelion coffee.
- Add kombu or nori seaweed to bean dishes. They contain iodine, which helps reduce mastitis-type pains. Iodine is stored in breast tissue, and low iodine can encourage excess estrogen production and increase the sensitivity of breast tissue to estrogen. You can also use iodized Celtic sea salt instead of sodium-based salts to naturally increase iodine levels. Anyone suffering breast cysts may be lacking in iodine.
- Eat more broccoli, cauliflower, kale, and cabbage, which all help to balance hormones in a natural way.
- Beets, artichokes, and chicory support the liver, which has to metabolize hormones.

Useful Remedies

- Take 400mg of magnesium for its muscle relaxing qualities.
- Take full-spectrum vitamin E, 200–600IU a day, for 3–4 months.
- Take a good-quality B-complex that contains 50mg of vitamin B6 and another 50mg of B6 separately. The dose should total 100mg daily.
- Evening primrose oil is useful for this problem, but you would need around 2–3g daily.
- Taking 500–2000mg of the herb agnus castus a day or 2ml of tincture should help regulate hormone levels more naturally.
- Take a good-quality multi-vitamin/mineral for women.
- For those of you who do not eat enough broccoli, cauliflower, and cabbage, several companies now make Cruciferous Extract capsules, and you can take one or two daily. **VC**

Helpful Hints

- In Chinese medicine breast pain is often caused by liver congestion; see *Liver Problems*.
- Regular exercise (running or walking 1–3 miles a day) can relieve tenderness. Many women find it uncomfortable to run when their breasts are tender, but if you exercise on a regular basis, tenderness should not be as much of an issue for the 7–10 days prior to a period. Wear a sports bra.
- Exercise improves circulation and aids drainage of the lymph system. Mini-trampolines are wonderful, as is any vigorous exercise such as fast walking, swimming, or dancing.
- Lymphatic drainage massage is well known for improving drainage, thereby reducing swelling and pain (see MLD [manual lymphatic drainage] in *Useful Information*).
- Sometimes breast pain is due to an imbalance of estrogen and progesterone, which causes tender breasts and breast cysts—symptoms of a condition known as fibrocystic breast disease. This condition is becoming increasingly common because of the high levels of estrogen pollutants we are exposed to from excess pesticides and herbicides. Using a natural progesterone formula found in creams and capsules may reduce the cysts and tenderness in a few months. You can order natural progesterone from Pharm West (www.pharmwest.com).
- If, after three months, there is no improvement with the above regimen, see a qualified nutritionist who is also a doctor (see *Useful Information*).

BRITTLE NAILS
(see Nail Problems)

BRONCHITIS
(see also Immune Function)

This common problem is triggered when the bronchial tubes—your airways—become infected. Older people with compromised immune systems are more likely to be affected.

Bronchitis can have a viral or bacterial origin, and symptoms normally occur when you have an upper respiratory tract infection. Bronchitis is more common during winter months. If you contract a cold or flu, immune function can become very low indeed—thus allowing any infection to take hold and spread down toward the lungs. For some sensitive individuals, tobacco smoke is enough to set them off, but with other people exposure to pollens and other toxins they inhale can lead to an attack of bronchitis. The effects of prolonged negative stress and/or insufficient sleep can greatly deplete the immune system; and nutrient deficiencies and lack of exercise can also make you more prone to developing bronchitis. This is because at such times you rarely take deep breaths. Having said this, if your immune system is low and you over-exercise, then you can become more susceptible. Do everything in moderation.

Some cases can be managed without the use of antibiotics, but if you find it painful to take a deep breath, have a temperature for more than 48 hours, or can hear a rattle in your chest when you breathe or cough, you absolutely **must** consult a doctor. If the infection reaches your lungs it can develop into pneumonia.

Having suffered bronchitis a couple of times in the past that developed from colds I caught on long plane journeys, I can assure you this condition is no laughing matter. Once you have the weakness, you really need to look after yourself. If my immune system had been in better shape, I would have been better able to fight off these infections. See also *Immune Function*.

From experience, the secret I have found to avoiding bronchitis in the first place is to eliminate all sugar, chocolate, and any "white" foods such as cookies and cakes at the first sign of a sore throat, and by taking the homeopathic remedy Streptococcus 10M. I also use a sinus rinse daily called Neil Med Sinus Rinse (www.neilmed.com); by doing this I can stop infections from developing. In fact, since I started using the sinus rinse daily, I have not suffered a single sinus infection. And no, they don't pay me to say this!

Foods to Avoid

- Greatly reduce your intake of any foods containing sugar, including concentrated fruit juice, because sugar greatly reduces your immune system's ability to fight infections.
- While symptoms are acute, avoid all dairy products from cows and also soy milk. (Rice milk should be okay.) Especially avoid chocolate, cheese, and refined carbohydrates such as cakes, pastries, and cookies, and for some people all other soy products—all of which can create more mucus.
- Avoid any foods and oils containing hydrogenated or trans-fats, as they trigger inflammation in the body and are linked to asthma.
- Reduce fried foods, which can also trigger inflammation in the body.

Friendly Foods

- Eat plenty of fresh fruits and vegetables. When you feel sick, your digestive system can labor under the strain. Therefore, eat fresh vegetable soups, which are an easy way to ingest nutrient-dense foods. Thickening them with sweet potatoes, pumpkin, carrots, and squash—all rich in vitamin A—also helps boost your immune system.
- Barley, brown rice, and miso can be added as well.
- Papaya, mango, pineapple, and apricots are also great lung foods.
- Apples are great for lung health but can be sprayed with many different pesticides. Go organic and eat two apples daily to support your lungs.
- Garlic, leeks and onions are really cleansing and have antiseptic properties.
- Horseradish, which has antibiotic properties, can be used in small amounts to destroy the bacteria in the throat that can cause bronchitis. Take a small amount 10 minutes away from other foods. This also helps clear the sinuses.
- Vine-ripened tomatoes are rich in lycopene, which is great for your lungs. The lycopene is released when the tomatoes are cooked in a little oil.
- Guavas and pink grapefruits are also rich in lycopene.
- Eating fish regularly helps reduce the frequency and severity of bronchial attacks, and if you are undergoing one, the oils in fish can provide a strong anti-inflammatory effect.
- Quercetin—a protective flavonoid—helps defend you from the harmful effects of pollution and smoke. It is found in apples, pears, cherries, grapes, onions, kale, broccoli, garlic, green tea, and red wine.
- Limonene found in the rind and edible white membrane of citrus fruits—oranges, lemons, limes, tangerines, and grapefruit—may help protect the lungs.

- Increasing vitamin B1 (thiamine) is essential for maintaining the health of the lungs. Peas, wholegrain rice, sunflower seeds, and pine nuts are excellent sources.
- Brown rice, avocados, spinach, haddock, oatmeal, baked potatoes, navy beans, lima beans, broccoli, yogurt, bananas, and unsalted nuts are all rich in the mineral magnesium, which is also vital for healthy lungs.
- As zinc has anti-viral properties that fight colds and flu, eat more oysters, pumpkin seeds, fresh root ginger, and unrefined nuts.
- Because you are likely to be running a temperature, drink at least 6–8 glasses of water or fluids daily.
- Make teas with fresh lemon juice, a small piece of root ginger, and a little manuka honey, which has anti-viral properties. Drink lots of herbal teas such as licorice, fenugreek, and elderberry.

Useful Remedies
- Include a high-strength multi-vitamin/mineral suited to your age and gender in your daily regimen.
- Whichever multi you take, make sure it contains 400mg of magnesium, as studies have found that people who take more vitamin C (up to 4–5g with meals in divided doses while symptoms are acute) and magnesium tend to have healthier lungs.
- Bromelain, extracted from pineapples, is extremely effective for bronchial conditions as it improves lung functions and helps loosen up any mucus. While symptoms are acute, take 500mg of bromelain three times daily plus 4–5g of vitamin C in an ascorbate form with meals divided throughout the day.
- N-acetyl cysteine (NAC) helps break up mucus and reduces the bacterial count for people suffering from bronchitis. Take 500mg twice a day 30 minutes before food. Studies have shown that people who take NAC on a regular basis suffer from fewer cases of bronchitis, colds, and flu. NAC also helps support the liver and has been shown to reduce the frequency and duration of attacks of chronic obstructive pulmonary disorder (COPD).
- For 7 days you can also take 25,000IU of vitamin A (if you are pregnant only take 3000IU). After that, for prevention, take 15mg of natural-source carotene daily as it naturally converts in the body to Vitamin A.
- Useful herbs for boosting immune function and reducing bacteria are echinacea, ashwagandha, goldenseal, and elderberry.
- Licorice is anti-inflammatory, anti-viral, and can be very useful for bronchial conditions. Buy whole licorice from health stores.
- Zinc gluconate lozenges really help reduce coughing and sore throat pain.
- Beta Glucans 1–3, 1–6 are proven to strengthen the body's innate immune system (the immune system you are born with). Pharma Nord makes a version that is free from yeast protein. Take 250–500mg daily. **PN**
- Expectorant herbs that help to clear any "gunk" in your lungs are garlic, white horehound and euphorbia. They can be taken either in capsules or as a tincture. **OP, VC**

Helpful Hints
- Inhaling steam is really helpful for opening up the lungs. Add a few drops of olbas oil or any pure eucalyptus oil into a bowl of boiling water. Place a towel over your head and really inhale the steam through your nose. If you do this 4–5 times daily, it helps loosen up your chest.
- If you have a tendency to get bronchitis, take a 3-month program in the fall to boost your lungs and clear out any mucus from the lungs. The herbs in the program include elecampane, golden rod, thyme, and pau d'arco.

- Echinacea taken regularly helps prevent viral bronchitis from progressing into a more dangerous bacterial infection. A good formula is Futurebiotics Garlic Echinacea Goldenseal as it includes astragalus and myrrh, which boost the immune system. **VC**
- If the infection becomes serious and you are prescribed antibiotics, as soon as you finish the course begin taking the healthy bacteria acidophilus and bifidus for at least 6 weeks to replenish healthy bacteria in the gut, which in turn will help immune function. **VC**
- Don't exercise near main roads where pollution levels can be lethally high.
- Learn to exercise your lungs. Professional singers rarely catch a cold because they use their lungs more. Sing along to your radio and give your lungs a workout!
- In general terms, whenever you are suffering from a bronchial infection, you should stay in bed and rest for at least two days. The more you try to struggle on, the slower your recovery will be.
- Use an Ultra Breathe, a very handy, inexpensive device that does a great job of exercising the lungs. It costs $26.95 online plus $3.95 for postage and packing. For details call 011-44-870-608-9019, or visit www.ultrabreathe.com/us/uswelcome.htm

BRUISING

This discoloration of the skin is caused by blood leaking from damaged blood vessels into the tissues of the skin. It is a normal process, but some people bruise excessively, especially older people. Excessive bruising is often due to a deficiency of vitamin C and/or bioflavonoids, the water-soluble pigment in fruits. People who take blood-thinning drugs such as Warfarin are also more likely to bruise easily. If you suffer regular bruising not associated with running into something or some other type of injury, it can indicate a rarer underlying problem such as leukemia. So if you are in *any* doubt, check with your doctor.

Foods to Avoid
- Avoid all highly processed foods such as mass-produced cakes, cookies, and pre-packaged meals, which generally lack any nutrients.
- Don't cook foods for too long as cooking greatly reduces nutrient levels.
- See *General Health Hints*.

Friendly Foods
- Eat plenty of foods high in vitamin C such as kiwi, cherries, peppers, blueberries, blackberries, plums, pineapple, and papaya.
- Include more leafy green vegetables in your diet, especially kale, cabbage, spinach, and bok choy.
- Buckwheat is very high in rutin; therefore, try buckwheat pasta and buckwheat flour in pancakes.
- See also *General Health Hints*.

Useful Remedies
- Take 1–3g of vitamin C in an ascorbate form daily with food spread throughout the day, plus 500–2,000mg of bioflavonoids to help strengthen your capillaries.
- Pycnogenol, a pine bark extract, has been shown to help protect vein walls and reduce the risk of bruising. Take 80mg daily. **PN, NOW, GNC**
- Rutin Complex includes bromelain, a flavonoid extracted from pineapple. It has an anti-inflammatory effect. Take 500mg of bromelain daily until bruising disappears.
- The herb horse chestnut is excellent for bruises. Take 500mg daily until symptoms disappear.

Helpful Hints
- For bruising after a trauma such as surgery, homeopathic arnica is a wonderful remedy. If you have had surgery of any kind, you can take Arnica 30c every 4 hours until the bruising fades. Arnica cream or witch hazel gels used topically are really helpful for reducing the swelling.
- For deeper tissue damage use Ledum 30c three times daily for 4–5 days.
- Comfrey ointment speeds up soft-tissue healing. **OP, VC**
- For sprains and other injuries, use an ice pack to help reduce the immediate swelling. In an emergency, I use a bag of frozen peas wrapped in a towel and place it directly over the swelling for 10 minutes every hour.

BURNS, MINOR

First-degree burns affect the very top layer of the skin. Second-degree burns leave blisters but usually heal without scarring or infection. Third-degree burns are far more serious and affect the full thickness of the skin, leaving it charred or white. These burns need urgent medical attention to reduce the risk of infection and scarring. Also, if you come into contact with acid, solvents, or chemicals that burn the skin, dowse the area with cool, running water as quickly as possible to lessen the damage. If a child drinks any chemical such as bleach that burns the esophagus, do not encourage vomiting, as it will also burn on its way back up. If possible, allow the patient to drink milk and seek immediate medical help.

B

Foods to Avoid
- Avoid too many foods and drinks containing sugar or alcohol, as they will slow the healing process.
- Generally avoid highly processed, refined foods, which contain almost no nutrients.

Friendly Foods
- High-quality protein is vital in the initial stages for tissue healing. Include plenty of organic free-range chicken, fresh fish, beans, and lentils or even a good-quality whey protein powder, such as Solgar's Whey To Go or Hemp Seed Protein Powder, in your diet. These are highly digestible forms of protein that will help speed skin healing. You can also ask for a whey powder that includes extra L-glutamine, an amino acid that will help with tissue healing.
- Unprocessed, preferably organic, nuts and seeds, such as sunflower and pumpkin seeds, are rich in essential fats and zinc, which are vital for healing the skin.
- Wheat germ and wheat germ oil are rich in vitamin E, which aids skin healing and reduces scarring.
- Eat plenty of fresh fruits and vegetables that are high in natural carotenes, such as apricots, sweet potatoes, and spinach, to help heal the skin. Cantaloupe melons, carrots, and green leafy vegetables are good, too. Papaya and pineapple are especially healing.

Useful Remedies
- The herb gotu kola has been used to help heal burns for centuries. You can either take 500mg daily or take 1–2ml of tincture.
- Take natural-source vitamin E, 500IU twice a day, until the wound heals.
- Vitamin C is vital for the production of collagen; take up to 3g daily with food. Buy a formula that also contains bioflavonoids.
- Collagen is the most widely distributed protein in the body and is vital for healthy skin. Therefore, to aid healing take one scoop of marine-extract collagen powder daily 30 minutes before your main meal.

- Also take a good-quality multi-vitamin/mineral supplement that contains 30–60mg of zinc, which aids skin healing and boosts immune function.
- MSM (organic sulfur) encourages wound healing and is anti-inflammatory. Take 1000mg twice daily until the burn heals.
- Pure aloe vera can be applied either topically as a gel or drunk as a liquid (these are two different products). Take daily until healed. **VC**

Helpful Hints
- You can bathe the burn in cold water for up to 30 minutes, if necessary. Dry with a clean sterile dressing and smother with sterile aloe vera gel.
- Try Dr Christopher's Burn Paste. This consists of a mixture of runny honey, preferably manuka, and wheat germ oil (which you buy and mix for yourself), to which you then add comfrey root powder. When you spread the mixture on the skin, it helps to speed up the healing process considerably.
- Take Bach Homeopathic Rescue Remedy every few hours to reduce the feelings of shock.
- Coat the area with a thin layer of manuka honey and cover with a sterile gauze. Honey is a very effective antiseptic, is anti-bacterial, and can also speed the healing process. You buy manuka products from www.manukahoneyusa.com
- In India, fresh potato peelings are placed on burns. The wounds heal more quickly and infection is reduced.
- Papaya pulp has been shown to be effective in sloughing off dead tissue, preventing wound infection. Papaya is rich in enzymes that aid healing.
- Calendula cream helps soothe pain and promote tissue repair.
- Lavender oil helps to aid burn healing.
- Homeopathic Cantharis 6x, taken two or three times daily, will help to reduce the blisters.
- MSM cream (organic sulfur cream), containing vitamins A, E, and B5, aloe vera, and comfrey extract, can be applied topically to aid with the healing of minor burns.

BURSITIS

This condition is also commonly known as tennis elbow or housemaid's knee and is caused by inflammation of the bursa, the sac-like membrane that contains the fluids responsible for lubricating the joints. It is most common in the shoulder, elbow, hip, and knees and can cause severe pain or tenderness, particularly when the person places any weight on that joint. Orthodox medicine offers anti-inflammatory drugs and sometimes cortisone injections. My husband has suffered from tennis elbow, which was triggered by too much weight lifting, and after the injections he found great relief—but within 3–4 months, the pain and tenderness returned and was even worse than before. He has found some relief by resting his elbow completely, and the pain usually recedes when he is under less stress or on vacation.

Foods to Avoid
- Reduce your intake of caffeine, alcohol, and sugar, which can increase inflammation within the body, thus increasing pain.
- Cut down on animal-based foods and junk-type meals, which are very acid forming. See *Acid–Alkaline Balance*.
- Avoid plums, rhubarb, prunes, and orange juice, which are acid forming.

Friendly Foods
- Eat more foods such as kale, watercress, and spring cabbage that re-alkalize the body—the

greener the better. See *Acid–Alkaline Balance*.

- Include plenty of fresh fruits in your diet.
- Millet, quinoa, and buckwheat are alkaline foods. Sprinkle the fine grains over a low-sugar breakfast cereal or use for baking.
- Eat more fresh ginger, oily fish, pineapple, and papaya, which all have anti-inflammatory properties.
- Use turmeric and cayenne pepper in meals as they have anti-inflammatory properties.
- See also *General Health Hints*.

Useful Remedies

- Take 1–3g of vitamin C with bioflavonoids daily in divided doses with meals until symptoms ease.
- Omega-3 fish oils have anti-inflammatory properties. Take 1–3g of fish oils that contain EPA and DHA a day, as these are the key essential omega-3 fatty acids.
- Take 1,000–4,000mcu of the enzyme bromelain, which is extracted from pineapple, for its anti-inflammatory properties.
- Turmeric and Boswellia Complex contains the herbs ginger, boswellia, turmeric, and ashwagandha, which all have anti-inflammatory properties. Take up to four tablets daily. Pukka Herbs (www.pukkaherbs.com) make a good formula; however, they are currently unable to deliver to the US. You can find other similar combinations at your local health store or online.
- Collagen is a vital component of healthy joints, cartilage, ligaments, and tendons. It is the most widely distributed protein in the body, and we lose about 1.5% annually after the age of 30. Take one scoop of collagen powder daily in diluted apple juice 30 minutes before eating. **VC**
- Glucosamine sulfate, an amino sugar with MSM (an organic form of sulfur), helps restore the gelatinous fluids around the joints. Take 1500–2000mg daily, and once symptoms are alleviated reduce to 500mg daily. If you are allergic to shellfish, ask for a vegetarian version, which should available from all health stores.
- 10mg of manganese per day helps to speed up tendon repair and ease pain.
- Liquid hyaluronic acid (HA), taken daily in water on an empty stomach, aids tissue repair. HA is a naturally occurring protein in the body, but as we age our levels fall. For more details ask at your health store or visit www.modernherbals.com

B

Helpful Hints

- Glucosamine gel with horse chestnut extract applied locally can help ease the inflammation.
- Apply a bag of frozen peas wrapped in a dishtowel to ice the painful area for 10 minutes every few hours. This really does help reduce inflammation and pain. You can alternate the cold compress with a warm ginger compress. Simply add a piece of root ginger to boiling water, let it steep for 10 minutes, and then soak a cloth in the mixture before pressing it on the painful area for 10 minutes. Make the compress as warm as possible without burning yourself! Otherwise use a warmed wheat or lavender bag.
- Use an elastic bandage during the day to limit swelling. Elevate the affected area above the level of the heart to encourage fluids to drain out of the injured area.
- Avoid weight training when pain is acute as this will further aggravate the problem.
- Acupuncture works really well for this condition.
- A gentle aromatherapy massage using oils such as Roman chamomile, ginger, marjoram, and geranium can also help relieve pain.
- Check out www.repetitiveusetherapy.com This site gives some great tips plus a list of therapists who specialize in treating this condition.

C

CANCER

(see also Breast Cancer)

One in three people dies of cancer—yet Professor Martin Wiseman, medical and scientific advisor to the World Cancer Research Fund, states that 39% of the 12 major cancers are preventable through better diet, drinking less alcohol, and improving our exercise habits. In the US this means that almost 600,000 cases, out of the more than 1.5 million new cancer diagnoses projected to occur in 2010, could have been prevented.

There are more than 200 types of cancer, each with their own name and treatment. The four most common—breast, lung, colon, and prostate—account for nearly half the deaths due to cancer in the US. Although cancer can strike at any age, the great majority of cancer patients are 60 and over. Yet, whatever your age, there are plenty of things you can do to reduce your risk, or, if you contract cancer, to help yourself heal.

Newer screening methods such as the CTC (Circulating Tumor Cell Test) have been shown to be highly effective in tests by the Department of Internal Medicine at the University Hospital in Essen in Germany. This test helps give your doctors an exact picture of which treatment and type of chemotherapy will be more effective in your unique case. You can send a small blood sample through the mail. More details are available at www.adnagen.com

At University College Hospital in London, a treatment that uses light, known as PDT (photodynamic therapy), is being used to easily kill tumors in a wide variety of cancers and has proven hugely successful. To date, the FDA has only approved the use of PDT to relieve the symptoms of esophageal and early-stage lung cancer, as well as precancerous growths in patients with Barrett esophagus (a condition that can cause esophageal cancer). Many cancer treatment centers around the country offer this type of treatment.

Meanwhile, the earlier any cancer is diagnosed, the more likely the patient is to survive. Thousands of people recover every year, and there is always hope.

It is now known that many cancers are triggered by environmental factors, including excessive free radicals, radiation, viral infections, and chemicals. Diet is another huge factor. Other possible triggers are parasites and fungi. The bacterium *Helicobacter pylori*—the trigger for most stomach ulcers—is also linked to gastric-type cancers.

Free radicals are unstable molecules that are formed within the body during normal metabolic processes or are produced by stress, excessive exercise, pollution, fried food, radiation, and so on. Known risk factors for cancer are diets that are high in saturated fats, sunbathing to excess, exposure to toxic chemicals found in burnt food, petrol fumes, pesticides, preservatives, excessive hormones, multiple nutrient deficiencies, and overexposure to certain electromagnetic fields (see *Electrical Pollution*).

You can inherit a tendency toward developing certain cancers, but you can change gene expression and stack the odds more in your favor by eating a better diet and living a healthier lifestyle. Eating healthily, staying physically active, and maintaining a healthy weight can cut your cancer risk.

Various cancers have been linked to over-consumption of specific foods. For example, people who regularly consume overly processed foods such as hot dogs, smoked and preserved meats, fried foods, bacon, and mass-produced burgers are more likely to develop bowel cancer. Excessive intake of dietary animal-based fats results in higher levels of estrogens, a known risk factor for cancers, especially of the breast and ovaries. Emotions affect our health, too, and tragic stories of people who suffer a major shock in life, such as the loss of a partner through death or divorce, and then develop cancer within a few years, are common. My mother was angry and bitter after my father died at only age 50 from a heart attack. In later life she developed a cancer that killed her, and I firmly believe it was her overall attitude to life, plus her high-sugar diet, that contributed to her contracting cancer. This is why I believe that healing emotional scars, as well as physical ones, is crucial to our long-term health.

There has also been research showing that if you work in an environment with negative people or a boss who tends to be very domineering and controlling, then you are more likely to become ill.

There are always exceptions. Some people eat healthily, exercise, and really take care of themselves but still develop cancer. Others smoke until they are almost 100 and are fine. We all carry within us our own genetic strengths and weaknesses, and if our genetic ability to adapt is overwhelmed by a poor diet, stressful lifestyle, pollution overload, and so on, then naturally occurring genetic errors can accumulate and overpower our body's ability to correct the damage.

The orthodox approaches to cancer treatment mainly rely on surgery, chemotherapy, and radiation therapy. Unfortunately, these approaches place a considerable additional burden on our bodies and often have negative side effects.

However, the picture has begun to improve. Naturopath and nutritional scientist Bob Jacobs, head of the Society for Complementary Medicine in London, says: "Natural extracts such as Avemar (AWGE) [see under *Useful Remedies,* below] have been found to enhance orthodox treatments and patients who, for instance, take Avemar and Tamoxifen together fare better than those who just take the Tamoxifen.

"There are many steps that you can take, if you are to have the best chance of surviving the crisis and going on to enjoy a happy, productive life. Make no mistake, all cancers are a challenge, and surviving and thriving after cancer can mean that healing yourself becomes a full-time occupation. So a holistic strategy should include elements such as detoxification, an optimum diet, nutritional supplements, specific anti-cancer remedies, and mental, emotional, and spiritual healing."

Bob Jacobs adds: "One of the most important things you can do that offers you the best chance of avoiding or beating cancer is to eat a very low animal protein, low sugar, healthier diet—starting NOW."

According to The World Cancer Research Fund (WCRF), eating at least five portions of vegetables and fruits each day could, in itself, reduce cancer rates by 20%. The WCRF asserts that half of all breast cancer cases, three out of four cases of stomach cancer, and three out of four cases of colon cancer could be prevented by dietary measures alone. It must be your choice whether you go the natural route, the conventional route or try a combination of both. There are no guaranteed results, but the more right actions you take, the more positive re-actions you are likely to see.

Foods to Avoid to Help Prevent or Heal Cancer

- All non-organic meat. If you want to eat red meat then have no more than 3–4oz (75–100g) twice weekly. If you have cancer, avoid red meat altogether.
- Eliminate processed meats, sausages, and bacon from your diet.
- Reduce or eliminate all dairy products, especially those made with cow's milk. If you do eat dairy products, make them organic and low fat. Replace cow's milk with organic rice, oat, or almond milks.

- Eliminate white flour, rice, and pasta-based foods.
- Limit your alcohol intake, to say, one glass of organic red wine a day. Eliminate alcohol if you have been diagnosed with cancer.
- Eliminate sugar, coffee, sodium-based salt, and any pre-packaged, canned and mass-produced foods, such as burgers or other fast foods. Especially reduce sugar, as cancer cells feed on sugar.
- Avoid re-heating pre-prepared foods in plastic containers, as the plastics they release into your food can increase your risk for more aggressive hormonal-type cancers.
- When food is fried, burnt or smoked, cancer-causing chemicals are created. Therefore, avoid these types of cooking methods. This is why potato chips, sausages, smoked meats and fish, and barbecued foods should be kept to a minimum.
- Reduce your use of sodium-based table salts. Use an organic sea salt instead and add a little to the food on your plate (see *Anti-cancer Diet*, below). You can also season food with nori flakes, a seaweed that helps eliminate heavy metals such as aluminum and mercury from the body, as these metals are also linked to cancer. **VC**
- You could also use powdered kelp instead of salt.

Friendly Foods to Help Prevent and Heal Cancers

- Eat more pineapple and papaya; they contain the enzymes bromelain and papain. These enzymes help dissolve the protective protein coating that surrounds most cancer cells. Dr Nam Dang at the University of Florida says, "Papaya has a dramatic anti-cancer effect against a broad range of lab-grown tumors, including cancers of the cervix, breast, liver, lung, and pancreas." Eating a small amount of papaya before a meal also aids digestion.
- Fresh mango, which is high in polyphenols, has also been found to kill colon and breast cancer cells in the lab. Eat more mango!
- Eat more organic foods, and if you have cancer, only eat organic. This is because many non-organic foods contain the residues of up to 311 pesticides that are either known carcinogens or hormone-disrupters. They are allowed on food only because the levels are very low—and no negative effect is expected. This might seem reasonable, except we do not know about their cumulative cocktail effect.
- Use more fresh rosemary in foods to reduce the production of HCAs (heterocyclic amines), the cancer-causing compounds created when food is fried, barbecued, etc.
- Eat more rhubarb and strawberries as they are great against cancers—but not if you suffer from kidney stones, as they are high in oxalic acid.
- Most anti-cancer diets recommend juicing, but the pulp of most fruits contains the healthy phospholipids that are essential for healthy tissues. Therefore, chop all of the ingredients and blend, or if you have a juicer, scrape out the pulp and add this to your juice mix; it will be thicker, but healthier. Avoid store-bought fruit juices.
- Eat more garlic and onions.
- For cancer prevention eat soy in its traditional, fermented form, such as tempeh, natto, or miso. Remember that soy is best cooked. Soy contains anti-cancer compounds. A healthy amount is around 2–4oz (50–100g) of fermented soy in total a day. Soy is without doubt beneficial to adults, but it should not be given to small infants and children. Infant soy milk formulas give the infant a daily dose of phyto-estrogens, which helps protect adults against cancer, but the doses may be too high for infants. The obvious first choice is to breast-feed infants for the first year.
- Non-GM soy lecithin granules are also a great food for adults, as lecithin lowers LDL (the bad cholesterol), improves memory, and helps protect against many cancers.
- Eat more organic Brussels sprouts, watercress, cauliflower, cabbage, spring greens, kale,

shitake mushrooms, and garlic, which all help fight cancer. A great quick anti-cancer soup includes mixing two carrots, two heads of broccoli, half a pack of tempeh, a tablespoon of vegetable stock, and some water in the blender. Add almond milk if you want it creamy and spices such as curcumin if you like it hot. Heat and serve.

- Generally, eat more curries or dishes containing curcumin, which can diminish the risk for many cancers, especially gastric and pancreatic cancers.

- Drink plenty of filtered water, which helps to wash out toxins from the kidneys. Try Kangen Water—a water system unit that attaches to your kitchen faucet and ionizes and alkalizes the water. It's used in Japanese hospitals with highly beneficial health results. For full details visit www.kangenwaterusa.com

- You can boil, steam, or bake your foods, but try eating most of your food raw or lightly cooked. Attempt "steam-frying" food using a watered-down soy sauce, plus herbs or spices for taste.

- Non-organic carrots, lettuce, apples, and many other healthy foods are overloaded with pesticides and herbicides that are associated with an increased risk of cancer. Throw away the outer leaves when preparing non-organic vegetables like cabbage or lettuce and always wash these vegetables thoroughly.

- Just one serving of crisp or raw organic cabbage each week can help reduce the risk of colon cancer by as much as 50%. Make more coleslaw: grate raw cabbage, carrot, and apple, and add a few raisins, pumpkin seeds, and a small amount of low-fat mayonnaise.

- Eat at least five pieces of fresh whole fruit a day. Vitamin C, natural beta-carotene, and lycopene are all potent anti-cancer nutrients. Lycopene is a carotenoid found in tomatoes, which has been shown to reduce the risk of many cancers, especially prostate cancer. However, it has also been shown to reduce the risk of cancers in the colon, rectum, pancreas, throat, mouth, breast, and cervix. If you are not allergic to tomatoes, eat 6–10 servings weekly. When the tomatoes are heated in a little olive oil, more lycopene is released. Otherwise, guava or pink grapefruit contain plenty of lycopene.

- All foods that are rich in carotenes help reduce the risk of cancer. These include carrots, apricots, papaya, cantaloupe melons, asparagus, sweet potatoes, pumpkin, parsley, mustard and cress, red peppers, spinach, spring greens, watercress, raw mangoes, French beans, and tomatoes.

- To ingest highly absorbable nutrients quickly, place a selection of your favorite fruits in a blender with a tablespoon of organic green food powder, two teaspoons each of mixed seeds: sunflower, sesame, linseed (one tablespoon flax seeds soaked overnight in a cup of cold water), and pumpkin. Adjust the amount for your personal choice. Then blend with a cup of organic rice or almond milk. If you are undergoing chemotherapy or radiation therapy, add at least a tablespoon of pure whey powder to this mix. Whey is a highly absorbable form of protein containing the amino acid L-glutamine, which helps soothe an irritated gut. As weight loss is often a problem with cancer, whey is a very useful food as long as it is GM-free. Alternatively, you can use organic hemp seed (available at all good health stores), which is a vegetarian protein that's easy for the body to absorb and utilize. This easy shake can be used as a meal replacement. My favorite blend is papaya, blueberries, apple, a slice of pineapple and a banana, plus the seeds and sometimes organic aloe juice with the hemp seed protein. As an easy alternative, I add a pear or strawberries and varying seeds to the blend. It's delicious and highly nutritious.

- Vegetarians seem to develop fewer cancers than non-vegetarians, as animal proteins feed cancer cells. People who live in Thailand and Japan have much lower incidence of most cancers, so adopting a Far Eastern diet with fewer refined foods, less meat and more fish may be a great way to stay healthy.

- Drink more organic green and white tea; it contains powerful antioxidant polyphenols that have been investigated for their cancer-protective effects and found to be even more powerful than vitamins C and E. It is thought that green tea consumption, an average of three cups a day, may be another reason behind the relatively low rate of cancer in Japan. Otherwise try white tea, a variant of green tea from the plant, *Camellia sinensis*.

- Eat whole foods. Anything in its whole form, such as oats, brown rice, barley, quinoa, lentils, almonds or sunflower seeds, is high in the anti-cancer minerals, zinc and selenium. Buy a pack of organic sunflower seeds, pumpkin seeds, sesame seeds, linseeds (flax seeds that have been soaked overnight in water or use ready-cracked linseeds) and, if you do not have a sensitivity to nuts, hazelnuts, Brazil nuts, almonds, and walnuts and grind a tablespoon of each at a time in a blender. Keep the ground nuts and seeds in a jar in the fridge along with the opened packages. Sprinkle daily over fruits, cereals, soups and desserts.

- If you eat bran to keep your bowels regular, avoid wheat bran, which can irritate the gut. Try oat or rice bran instead.

- Minimize alcohol consumption. Alcohol is associated with an increased risk of cancer. Red wine does, however, contain antioxidant nutrients called polyphenols, which are associated with a reduced risk of heart disease. One glass a day is the recommended maximum. Red grape juice contains the same antioxidants without the alcohol content.

- Animal fats are a major contributing factor in cancers; greatly reduce your intake of saturated fats from meat, full-fat dairy products, chocolates, cheeses, sausages, pies, cakes, and so on. Avoid any foods containing hydrogenated or trans-fats. Once you start reading labels you will be appalled at how much saturated fat you are ingesting. Never fry with mass-produced, highly refined oils. Use only organic sunflower, sesame, walnut, or olive oils for salad dressings. Eat more oily fish, which are rich in omega-3 fats, especially sardines, farmed, organic salmon, fresh anchovies, mackerel, herring, and fresh tuna (see *Fats You Need To Eat*).

- Cut down on stimulants such as sugar and caffeine. Sugar has been shown to lower your immune function for up to five hours after consuming it.

- The World Cancer Research Fund offers an online library of healthy recipes. Have a look at www.wcrf-uk.org

- Take 1000IU of vitamin D daily.

Useful Remedies if You Have Any Type of Cancer

- A fermented wheat germ extract known as AWGE, sold in more than ten countries, has demonstrated in numerous studies conducted in the US, Hungary, Israel and Russia remarkably beneficial immune-modulating effects. In more than 100 published research papers based on independent research, this extract has been shown to increase life expectancy without side effects. Most crucially, it reduces the toxic effects of chemotherapy and radiation therapy, while enhancing the effectiveness of orthodox oncology treatments at the same time. AWGE can be taken by anyone diagnosed with solid tumors and malignant hematological diseases, regardless of the stage of the disease. It improves overall health, helps most patients gain weight, and aids recovery from surgery. Take one sachet daily in water at least one hour before breakfast. It must be kept refrigerated. It is also available in capsules, but you would need quite a few; therefore, powder is easier to take once a day. More information and a list of suppliers is available at www.avemarwge.com

- Some cancer specialists fear that vitamins and minerals can prevent orthodox treatments from working. However, numerous studies show that the right nutrients support your immune system and help fight the cancer. A research paper published in the UK stated that even taking a multi-vitamin/mineral can extend a cancer patient's life by two years.

- Take 3 or more grams a day of vitamin C in an ascorbate (non-acidic) form in divided doses with foods. You can increase doses up to bowel tolerance, which would be around 8g daily.
- Take 200mcg of selenium daily, especially if you have any type of skin cancer.
- Find a high-potency multi-vitamin/mineral without iron, as excess iron has been linked to cancer cell growth
- Take 1200mcg of folic acid plus a daily B-complex, which helps to stabilize genes.
- Indole 3 Carbinol (I3C) is a phytochemical isolated from cruciferous vegetables (broccoli, cauliflower, Brussels sprouts, green cabbage) that has been shown to inhibit the growth of estrogen-receptor-positive cells, which are linked to hormonal-type cancers. The Life Extension Foundation makes a Triple Action Cruciferous Vegetable Extract that contains I3C, watercress, and rosemary, plus Apigenin—a powerful plant extract that has been found to block the development of cancer. **LEF**
- If you weigh less than 160 pounds you would only need to take one capsule daily; over this weight you could take two. **NB: Pregnant women should not take this supplement as estrogen is needed for healthy fetus growth. Do not take this supplement if you use antacids.**
- If you have cancer, take 2000IU of Vitamin D3 daily, as a lack of this vital nutrient is now linked to 17 different cancers. In fact, many nutritional physicians now state 4000IU would be preferable. Keep in mind that while spending the day in the sun your body can produce 20,000IU of vitamin D.
- Curcumin helps fight cancer and supports the Phase 2 detoxification pathway of the liver. Take 1–3g daily with food. (See below.)
- Natural-source beta-carotenes, which convert naturally to vitamin A in the body, can boost immune function and are a powerful antioxidant. Take one capsule daily. **PN, SVHC, VC**

C

Supplements to Help Prevent Cancer
- Take a good-quality, high-strength multi-vitamin/mineral every day.
- Additionally, take a good, high-strength antioxidant complex daily that includes natural-source carotenes.
- Curcumin, found in turmeric and used in most curries and Eastern dishes, is a great anti-cancer spice. It enhances immune function and helps inhibit the creation of new blood vessels that occurs as tumors grow. It is especially useful for skin, liver, and colon cancers. It also helps remove toxic metals from the body and helps block pesticide-type pollutants from entering cells. It can be found in capsule form in most health shops. If you are undergoing chemotherapy, make sure that you check with your doctor before taking high dosages of this spice. **LEF**
- 100mg of Co-enzyme Q10 daily helps protect cells from abnormalities.
- Take at least 1g of vitamin C daily, increasing the dose if you're stressed or ill.
- Take 200mcg selenium daily.
- Take 400IU of natural-source, full-spectrum vitamin E daily.
- Take 200mg daily of alpha-lipoic acid, which helps protect the liver and detoxifies heavy metals from the body.
- Vitamin D3 is now known to be a vital anti-cancerous nutrient. For everyday protection, take a minimum of 1000IU daily.
- Calcium and magnesium have been shown to reduce the side effects of chemotherapy. With your specialist's permission, take a duo formula such as Solgar's Cal/Mag twice daily before and during chemotherapy sessions. **SVHC**
- Essential fats help block cancer cell division; take at least 1g of pure omega-3 fish oils daily.

Helpful Hints

- Keeping your body more alkaline improves health and retards cancer. (See *Acid–Alkaline Balance*.)

- With professional help, detox your body. To find a qualified nutritionist, see under *Useful Information* at the back of the book.

- If at all possible, begin taking regular saunas (the best are Far Infra Red Saunas— www.farinfraredsauna.com) as heat helps eliminate toxins from the body. You can buy these for home use. Don't use public saunas if they are busy, as you may pick up other people's toxins. Ask if you can have the sauna on a lower heat (248–284°F or 120–140°C) and then you can stay in for a few minutes longer.

- Minimize your exposure to pollution. Remember, anything that is combusted produces free radicals, so reduce your exposure to car exhaust fumes. Electrical pollutants can also cause problems; only use mobile phones for 10–15 minutes at a time at most. Reduce your exposure to other electrical pollutants, including microwaves, TVs, radios, and so on, and don't sleep with an electric clock by your bed. (See *Electrical Pollution*.)

- Avoid having too many X-rays, most especially CAT Scans which put you at a higher risk (a 1 in 80 chance) for developing cancers. Reduce your number of mammograms, which have been shown to increase the risk of breast cancer.

- Never use chemical pesticides and herbicides in your garden and home. Ask for environmentally friendly natural products. Greatly reduce or eliminate your exposure to non-organic foods, cleaning fluids, garden sprays, and insect sprays.

- If you smoke, give it up and stay away from smoke-filled rooms, as passive smoking has now been shown to trigger cancer.

- I see naturopath, Bob Jacobs, at The Society for Complementary Medicine in London, who uses a dark field microscope that can see details that are not normally found in blood tests. To find a qualified naturopath in your area that does dark field microscopy, visit the American Association of Naturopathic Medicine's website (www.naturopathic.org).

- If you are already undergoing any type of cancer therapy, Dr Rosy Daniel (the former Medical Director of the Bristol Cancer Help Centre) says that nutrition is vital to help bring back up the white blood cell count. She advises patients to eat plenty of organic fresh fruit and vegetables along with whole foods such as brown rice and brown bread. All animal fats should be avoided. She also recommends that cancer patients take a good antioxidant formula, which contains vitamins A, C, and E, plus natural beta-carotene complex, and zinc and selenium. Dr Daniel stresses that fear drains energy levels and advocates any therapy that can reduce anxiety, such as spiritual healing, Reiki, relaxation exercises, visualization, acupuncture, or homeopathy. Dr Daniel has written a wonderful book called *The Bristol Approach to Living with Cancer* (Robinson).

- Contact the Cancer Cure Foundation, a non-profit organization that was established in 1976 to help provide research and information about the alternatives to chemotherapy and radiation therapy. Tel: 1-800-282-2873 or 1-805-498-0185 Monday through Friday, 8am– 5pm PST. E-mail: webmaster@cancure.org. Website: www.cancure.org

- Laugh a lot. Watch films and TV programs that make you laugh, because laughter boosts your immune system. Stay as positive as possible. Without a doubt, the patients with the more positive outlook heal and recover more quickly. This does not mean that you cannot shed tears, as tears release stress chemicals, and you are not meant to be a positive saint all the time! An inspiring book that uses this theme is *Love, Medicine and Healing* by Bernie Siegal (Rider).

- Oxygen therapies are worth looking into. Dr Otto Warburg won a Nobel Prize in Medicine in

1931 for discovering that if the body has sufficient oxygen then cancer cells cannot proliferate. For further information I suggest you read *The Oxygen Prescription* by Nathanial Altman (Healing Arts Press), or *Flood Your Body with Oxygen* by Ed McCabe (Energy Publications).

- At the Hospital Santa Monica in Mexico, Dr Kurt Donsbach has used intravenous hydrogen peroxide for years. For details log on to www.donsbach.com
- In the US some of these therapies are available (as well as high-dose intravenous nutrients such as vitamin C). For further details search online for clinics and practitioners in your area.
- Many associations offer help, counseling, and advice. One is the Cancer Hope Network. This non-profit organization matches cancer patients and/or their family members with a trained volunteer who has been thorough and recovered from a similar cancer situation. For more information, visit their website at www.cancerhopenetwork.org or call 1-800-552-4366 to talk to a support volunteer.
- Read Patrick Holford's *Say No to Cancer* (Piatkus). If you've realized you need to fully educate yourself about cancer and how to avoid it, this book is a great place to start. Or log on to www.patrickholford.com.
- Another useful book is *Anticancer, A New Way of Life* by David Servan-Schreiber (Penguin).

CANDIDA *(see also Allergies, Antibiotics, Leaky Gut, and Thrush)*

Candida albicans is a yeast that is responsible for the condition known as thrush. Common symptoms include itching in the vagina, anus, or penis areas. Doctors estimate that at least 75% of women will experience it at some time during their lives. Although commonly found in the vagina, candida can also occur in the throat, mouth, and gut.

Normally, relatively low levels of candida are present in the gut as they are balanced by large amounts of healthy bacteria, which help keep the yeast in check. Problems arise when the yeast begins to overgrow in the gut. This ultimately triggers a variety of symptoms including bloating, wind, constipation and/or diarrhea, food cravings (especially for sugar and wheat-based foods), headaches, mental confusion, memory problems, impotence, inability to concentrate, spots in front of the eyes, mood swings, skin rashes, persistent coughing, regular bouts of thrush, arthritis-type joint aches, and chronic fatigue. Candida can change its form and irritate, and even burrow through, the gut lining, which increases the risk of food sensitivities and an exacerbation of the symptoms above. If you suffer recurrent bouts of candida, see under *Leaky Gut*.

It is crucial to keep the candida under control by using herbs and supplements and, most importantly, making dietary changes. One of the primary triggers for candida is overuse of antibiotics, plus eating too much refined sugar. Others are long-term use of the contraceptive pill, as well as steroids, chemotherapy, diabetes, HIV, and pregnancy. Many women believe that you cannot have candida if you don't have thrush, but the majority of women with candida do not have thrush. Men are also sufferers. Naturopath Steve Langley says: "Thanks to our over-processed, high-sugar diets and stressful lifestyles, candida imbalances now affect up to 75% of the population, both men and women. It can become a serious condition if left untreated and remains little understood by many doctors." He is right.

During my teens I was given dozens of antibiotics for my acne, thrush, and ear infections. Every time the thrush returned, I would be given more antibiotics, which in the long run made the vicious cycle worse. I strongly advise that anyone testing positive, via stool or saliva tests, for high levels of candida, should consult a doctor who is also a nutritionist (see *Useful Information*).

Foods to Avoid

- Initially, remove all yeast-containing and fermented food from the diet. This includes all breads; aged or moldy cheeses, including Stilton, Brie, Camembert, etc.; alcoholic drinks, especially beer and wine; vinegar and foods containing vinegar (ketchups, pickles, Miracle Whip, baked beans); soy sauce; gravy mixes (many contain brewer's yeast); miso; tempeh, and mushrooms.
- I know it's hard, but try to avoid all white-flour products containing yeast/and or refined sugar for at least two weeks, including crackers, pizza, and pasta.
- Sugar feeds the yeast so avoid sugar in any form for a month; this includes honey, maltose, dextrose or sucrose, and really sweet fruits such as grapes, peaches, kiwi, and melon. Blueberries, blackberries, and strawberries can also harbor molds so avoid these fruits until the candida has been brought under control. I know it will be hard as sugar is highly addictive, but you also need to avoid dried fruits, fruit juices, and canned drinks for this period because they are high in sugar. Artificial sugars such as aspartame should also be eliminated. Sugar is the biggest problem with candida, and we cannot overstate just how much refined sugar needs to be avoided.
- Avoid malted products that can be found in some breakfast cereals, some brown crackers and malted drinks such as Ovaltine, Horlicks, and Milo.
- Avoid peanuts, peanut butter, and pistachio nuts, which tend to harbor molds.
- Avoid cow's milk for one month.
- If you have really severe candida, for the first two weeks also avoid zucchini, carrots, corn, and any of the squash family, as they quickly convert to sugars in the gut.
- Avoid any foods you know you are intolerant to.

Friendly Foods

- Garlic has potent anti-fungal action; raw is best. If you're worried about your breath, chew on some parsley.
- Eat fresh fish and shellfish, chicken, turkey, and other lean meats, as well as eggs, cooked tofu, and pulses.
- Research shows that a candida infection leads to inflammation. To help combat this, eat more oily fish—salmon, mackerel, herring, anchovies and sardines—along with nuts (unsalted and not peanuts) and lots of organic, unrefined seeds, which are also rich in essential fats.
- Include more artichokes, asparagus, eggplant, avocado, broccoli, cabbage, cauliflower, Brussels sprouts, celery, green beans, leeks, lettuce, garlic, onion, parsnips, spinach, tomatoes, and watercress. These types of vegetables encourage healthy bacteria to proliferate.
- Fruits that are okay are apples, pears (not over-ripe), a little pineapple, and cherries. Papaya and pomegranate are okay if not too over-ripe.
- Use organic rice, oat, coconut or almond milk instead of cow's milk.
- Eat live, plain, unsweetened yogurt, which contains the healthy bacteria acidophilus and bifidus. Yogurt is fermented, which means it's easier to digest than milk.
- Brown rice, lentils, corn, millet, buckwheat or rice pasta, oat cakes, soda bread, cookies made with a little butter or organic raw walnut butter are all okay.
- As a wheat substitute, try yeast-free rye bread. It can take some getting used to, but for a month it's acceptable. Most supermarkets and health shops now offer wheat- and/or yeast-free breads.
- Cilantro and thyme are great herbs for helping control this infection, so use liberally in soups and stews.

Useful Remedies

- Prebiotics are certain foods that encourage healthy bacteria in the gut to multiply, thereby enhancing immune function. I have found a great one based on the agave plant called Agave

Digestive Immune Support, which I take every morning in my breakfast shake. You can also just dissolve one scoop of this powder in water. It really helps keep you regular! **LEF**

- Probiotics are the actual healthy bacteria, which help keep the candida under control. Jarro-dophilus EPS, made by Jarrow, will help replenish gut flora; take one daily after food. It is enteric coated, which means it can pass through the stomach lining, and it does not need to be kept refrigerated. **JF**
- Take one yeast-free B-complex supplement.
- Take a multi-vitamin/mineral for your age and gender.
- RidgeCrest Herbals Adrenal Fatigue Fighter, which contains ginseng and pantothenic acid, supports adrenal function. Adrenal function is often exhausted in candida patients. **VC**
- To help cleanse the liver, take one milk thistle capsule and 1g of vitamin C per day. **VC**
- Take a good digestive enzyme with main meals. **VC**
- Use anti-fungals like oil of oregano, which is effective against many yeasts and parasites, plus probiotics. Do not use this combination if you suffer from active stomach ulcers. **VC**
- Take NSI Y-Cleanse, a potent anti-fungal formula that is made specially to help eliminate the fungus. **VC**
- Otherwise, try a formula containing black walnut, pau d'arco, and calendula tincture; take 2–4ml twice a day.
- Glutamine is great for healing and calming an irritated and inflamed gut. Take up to 5g twice a day half an hour before food. **VC**
- I realize I have suggested numerous supplements here, but there is certainly no need to take them all. I am simply giving you plenty of choices!

Helpful Hints

- Follow the yeast/sugar-free diet for 2–4 weeks before you add in any anti-fungal supplements or you may kill off the candida quicker than your body can dispose of it. This can lead to a general feeling of malaise. Should this happen at any time, drink more fluids, up your vitamin C, and reduce your anti-fungals for a day or two.
- If indigestion and bloating are a problem and digestive enzymes do not help, you may still be low in stomach acid. See *Low Stomach Acid*.
- As candida is usually linked to multiple food intolerances (especially to wheat, sugar, and dairy), consider a food intolerance test. Contact Genova Diagnostics. Tel: 1-800-522-4762; website: http://www.genovadiagnostics.com
- A comprehensive stool test and parasitology can also check for evidence of candida (plus other yeasts) in your body, in addition to identifying parasites and monitoring your levels of good bacteria. Check out www.greatplainslaboratory.com for more information.
- Many women who suffer candida are very stressed and exhausted. The best thing you can do to help boost immune function is to go away for at least a week. Get more sleep. Identify and deal with stress (see *Stress*).
- Avoid compost heaps, cut grass, and staying too long in moist, humid atmospheres where molds can thrive.
- Women who wear nylon underwear are twice as likely to suffer from thrush as those who wear cotton underwear.
- Any types of perfumed bubble bath products can aggravate thrush, so are best avoided. A better choice is to add a few drops of tea tree essential oil to your bathwater. It has powerful anti-fungal and antiseptic properties. **NB: Do not apply directly onto areas of delicate skin such as the vagina or penis.**
- For further information visit the UK's National Candida Society website: www.candida-society.org.uk. It is filled with lots of information. Email: info@candida-society.org.

- Recent research indicates that people who have persistent and chronic candida may have intestinal parasites. Herbal combinations containing wormwood, tincture of black walnut hull, and cloves, plus the amino acids ornithine and arginine help eliminate parasites. For details of candida cleansing formulas visit G&G Food Supplies' website (www.gandgvitamins.com) or www.candidasupport.org
- Read Erica White's *Beat Candida Cookbook* (Thorsons), which has more than 250 recipes, many of which are quick and easy to prepare.

CARPAL TUNNEL SYNDROME (CTS)

(see also Sjogren's Syndrome)

Carpal tunnel syndrome (CTS) is caused by the compression of the median nerve that runs under tissues in the wrist. People who use keyboards and other machinery on an everyday basis are the most frequent sufferers. Symptoms range from pain to numbness or tingling in the fingers. CTS is relatively common in pregnancy and more women suffer than men. It is also linked to an underactive thyroid, weight gain, arthritis, and Sjogren's Syndrome. The single most successful supplement for this condition is vitamin B6.

If CTS becomes severe then the protective covering of the median nerve, which is known as the myelin sheath, can be damaged by long-term inflammation, resulting in permanent nerve damage.

Foods to Avoid
- Because this problem is often associated with fluid retention, avoid adding too much sodium-based salt to food. Use a little magnesium-based sea salt for cooking.
- Reduce your intake of salty foods, such as potato chips, pre-packaged meals, soy sauce, and so on.
- Foods containing monosodium glutamate (MSG), which are often found in high amounts in Chinese food and used in many Japanese restaurants, dehydrate the body. MSG depletes vitamin B6 from the body, as does the contraceptive pill.
- In some people, foods such as oranges, tomatoes, and wheat further exacerbate the problem.
- Avoid all foods containing hydrogenated, trans- and animal fats, which increase inflammation.
- Greatly reduce your intake of sugary foods, as sugar also increases inflammation.

Friendly Foods
- Eat foods rich in vitamin B6: liver, cereals, lean meat, green vegetables, unrefined organic nuts (especially walnuts and Brazil nuts), and fresh and dried fruits.
- Eat more brown rice, beans, lentils, pulses, whole-wheat pasta and breads.
- Eat oily fish such as organic-farmed salmon, tuna, mackerel, herrings, anchovies, and sardines, which are rich in omega-3 fats that have anti-inflammatory properties.
- Use organic extra-virgin olive oil for salad dressings and cooking.
- Eat pineapple before meals, which contains bromelain that helps to reduce inflammation.
- Bilberries, cherries, and blueberries are rich in bioflavonoids, which have anti-inflammatory properties.
- Cook with more ginger, turmeric (curcumin), and cayenne, as they are highly anti-inflammatory. Eat more curries.
- Drink at least 6–8 glasses of water a day.
- Drink more organic nettle, green and white tea.

Useful Remedies

- Take 100–400mg of vitamin B6 plus a B-complex daily while symptoms are acute.
- Take 200–600mg of magnesium daily, in divided doses, as it nourishes nerve endings and relaxes muscles.
- Take a multi-vitamin/mineral for your age and gender.
- Take 1–2g of evening primrose oil or 500mg of gamma-linolenic acid (GLA), as GLA is highly anti-inflammatory. **VC**
- Alpha-lipoic acid helps protect against nerve damage; take 150-200mg daily.
- Omega-3 fish oils help protect the myelin sheath that surrounds nerve cells. Take 2g daily.
- The herbs white willow bark and devil's claw are highly anti-inflammatory; take 1–2g daily while symptoms are acute. **NB: If you are allergic to aspirin or taking blood-thinning drugs such as Warfarin, do not take this supplement.**

Helpful Hints

- Glucosamine gel applied topically can help reduce inflammation.
- If you are a regular computer user, try to find an ergonomic keyboard that will be easier to use.
- If symptoms are severe, buy a wrist splint containing magnets, which are available from good pharmacies and health stores.
- Sleeping heavily on your side with your wrists under you can also cause this. If you wake up with numb hands, immediately shake them and give them a massage to restore circulation.
- Acupuncture and daily massages with homeopathic Rhus tox ointment are also helpful.
- Log onto www.repetitiveusetherapy.com, a really useful site that lists therapists who specialize in helping treat this condition.

C

CATARACTS
(see also Eye Problems)

Poor or "foggy" vision affects more than 80% of people aged 75 or over. As we age, the normally clear and transparent lens of the eye oxidizes to become cloudy, which can severely impair vision and changes the way we see colors. Other symptoms include pain in the eyes on exposure to any glaring lights and problems driving at night. Many people who live in the Tropics develop cataracts, and they are a major cause of blindness in developing countries. Cataracts are becoming more common in the West in people who tend to be exposed to too much sun. A poor diet lacking in antioxidant nutrients, smoking, diabetes, and overuse of steroids and other prescription drugs can all cause cataracts. As with so many other conditions, cataracts are much easier to prevent than to cure. Once you have cataracts, the normal approach is laser treatment; however, some individuals claim to have reversed their cataracts with a combination of herbs and nutrients.

Foods to Avoid

- Smoking, fried foods, and sugar speed up the oxidation process and make cataracts more likely to develop.
- Sugar increases cross-linking in the skin and within the blood vessels. The more sugar you eat, the more inflammation you will have in the body.
- Cut down or reduce animal-based fats, and avoid hydrogenated and trans-fats.

Friendly Foods

- Bilberries, cherries, and blueberries are very rich in bioflavonoids, which help protect the eyes. Any blue, red, or orange fruits and vegetables will nourish the eyes.
- Leafy green vegetables, in particular spinach and watercress, contain lutein, which is the

powerful antioxidant found in most green vegetables that has specific properties for protecting the eyes.

- Sweet potatoes and butternut squash have high levels of carotenes, which convert naturally to vitamin A within the body. Other good sources of carotenoids are carrots, green vegetables, mango, papaya, tomatoes, apricots, cantaloupe melons, and pumpkin.
- Include plenty of oily fish in your diet, which is rich in vitamin A.
- All foods high in vitamins C, E, and selenium help support the eyes. These include wheat germ; avocado; green peppers; sprouting seeds such as alfalfa, sunflower, pumpkin, and linseeds; eggs; nuts; lean meats; wholegrain cereals; and fresh fruits, especially cherries and kiwi fruit.

Useful Remedies

- People who take vitamin C on a regular basis over a number of years are at a much lower risk of developing cataracts. The eyes require a high concentration of vitamin C. Take 2g daily in an ascorbate form with food.
- People with low levels of vitamin E are nearly four times more likely to form cataracts, so take 400IU of natural-source full-spectrum vitamin E a day included in a good-quality multi-vitamin/mineral.
- Take 1–2 capsules of Bilberry Eye Formula (www.drchristophersherbs.com) a day. People who consume bilberry on a regular basis have a much lower risk of forming cataracts.
- Ultraviolet light destroys vitamin B2 (riboflavin); therefore, take a B-complex supplement daily.
- Carnosine, an amino acid, greatly reduces cross-linking in the body and brain. Take 100mg a day in between meals.
- Lipoic acid helps prevent cataracts from forming as it helps protect against loss of vitamins C and E. Take 150mg daily with food.

Helpful Hints

- Anyone concerned about developing cataracts should protect their eyes from bright sunlight with sunglasses that have been verified for their UV filtering ability. Wraparound sunglasses are the most effective. If you work outside, wear a hat to protect your eyes. UV filtering contact lenses are also available; ask your optometrist for details.

CATARRH
(see also Allergic Rhinitis, Allergies, and Sinus Problems)

Catarrh, or chronic congestion in the nasal passages and sinuses, can be caused by an inflammatory response to airborne pollutants (from pesticides, paints, insect sprays, chemical-based air fresheners, etc.). This inflammation can then be further aggravated by other substances such as grass pollens, house dust mites, or cat fur. However, in most cases, it is triggered by foods that you eat (or crave and eat) on an everyday basis, such as cow's milk and related products—cheese or chocolate. Wheat-based foods such as croissants are often high in sugar and fats, which can also trigger symptoms in some people.

Many people assume that dairy products cause catarrh, but in reality this is only the case if you have an intolerance to these foods. Catarrh can just as easily be caused by wheat, eggs, citrus fruits, or any foods to which you have an intolerance. It is important to get to the root cause of the problem, so if you are suffering with a lot of catarrh, look at the foods you eat daily. Cut out one food at a time and keep a diary of the results. After a few weeks it is usually easy to spot the culprit (see also *Leaky Gut*).

Catarrh is the body's response to some type of sensitivity, whether it is a food or other substance that does not agree with your physiology.

Foods to Avoid

- Avoid any foods to which you have a sensitivity or intolerance. Typically these might include cow's milk and dairy products, especially full-fat cheeses, yogurts, and chocolate, plus caffeine, citrus fruits and juices, peanuts, wheat, and foods from the nightshade family, which include tomatoes, potatoes, eggplant, and peppers.
- I personally also find that goat's cheese and soy milk or yogurts tend to leave me feeling very "plugged up." Also avoid rich, creamy sauces.
- Avoid foods containing too much refined sugar, which weakens the immune system and makes you more susceptible to food intolerances. Most foods high in sugar are also high in saturated fats.

Friendly Foods

- Garlic, ginger, horseradish, onion, cayenne pepper, pineapple, and pears can all help the body fight off an infection if there is one and loosen up mucus so the body can expel it more easily.
- The herbs thyme, rosemary, and fenugreek make great expectorants, which help relieve congestion. Either use these herbs to make a strong tea or add them to foods.
- Eat plenty of whole grains such as brown rice, quinoa, barley, lentils, plus fruits and fresh vegetables.
- When people go on a cleansing diet, the catarrh almost always disappears. In the initial stages of a detox, the body can produce more mucus for a short time as it cleanses itself.

Useful Remedies

- Try Napiers Sage and Garlic Catarrh Remedy (www.shop.napiers.net).
- Take Mucolixir by Neutrocology. Available online at www.allstarhealth.com
- Take 1g of vitamin C with added bioflavonoids twice daily with meals.
- Sinus and catarrh pills containing a homeopathic mixture of kali bich, pulsatilla, merc sol, thuja, chamomile, and Hydrastis Canadensis 30 can help address infected green or yellow mucus and are suitable and safe for both babies and adults. Cough and Mucus tincture contains elecampane, coltsfoot, pulmonaria, licorice and mullein and helps clear mucus and coughs (even stubborn ones). **OP**
- An excellent nasal spray is Naturade nasal spray with aloe. **VC**
- Quercetin, a flavonoid found in red wine, tea, apples and red grapes, taken in supplement form, helps reduce the inflammatory response. Take 250mg twice daily.

Helpful Hints

- Ask at your health store for a nasal spray to help clear your sinuses.
- Neil Med Sinus Rinse, a saline nasal rinse, has given me huge relief from chronic nasal problems. It is incredibly easy to use. To order call 1-877-477-8633 or visit www.neilmed.com
- Make a soup from vegetable or chicken stock, six onions, a whole bulb of garlic, a small spoonful of honey, 1in (2.5cm) of fresh root ginger, and if you're brave, a bit of cayenne pepper. This will fight off most infections and help clear catarrh.
- Invest in a humidifier/air filter or ionizer to help keep the air free of potential allergens.
- Many people have found that lime flower tea is useful for reducing catarrh.
- If your ears are blocked due to excess mucus, use warm ear candles, which gently remove excess wax and congestion. **VC**

C

CELIAC DISEASE   *(see also Absorption and Leaky Gut)*

Research indicates that 3 million people suffer from this autoimmune condition in the US alone, and it often goes undiagnosed for years. It can happen at any age and sufferers cannot break down a protein called gluten, which is present in wheat, rye, barley, and oats. Some people with celiac disease appear to be able to tolerate small amounts of spelt, a low gluten-type of wheat, but for the majority of sufferers spelt would definitely need to be avoided.

The gluten damages the lining of the small intestine, which can create a leaky gut. This is when food particles "leak" through the gut wall triggering other health conditions. See *Leaky Gut.*

Symptoms include frequent indigestion, abdominal pain, loss of weight, and depression. The stools can be pale, frothy, and foul smelling. It is very important that, if you suffer from any or some of these symptoms over a period of several months, you see a doctor. The longer you suffer from celiac disease, particularly if it goes undiagnosed and untreated, the more likely you are to cause significant damage to your gut lining. This damage greatly reduces the body's ability to absorb adequate levels of nutrients, which can even lead to malnutrition. Celiacs also have a higher risk of osteoporosis, due to mineral malabsorption.

Foods to Avoid

- Any foods containing wheat, rye, oats, barley, and spelt are absolutely crucial to avoid. Quite a few people with celiac disease also have a problem with cow's milk and dairy products or soya foods.
- You will also need to avoid cakes, desserts, and any cereals containing gluten.
- Until the condition is under control, also avoid fatty meats, sausages, pies, and processed-meat products, as they often contain wheat.

Friendly Foods

- Fortunately, these days, there are plenty of gluten-free foods available, and most of them are fairly palatable. Some will be high in sugar so be sure to read labels carefully—sugar converts to fat in the body if not burned up during exercise, and in celiac sufferers, fat can be poorly absorbed. Look out for the gluten-free Enjoy Life Foods, Glutino, KinniKinnick, and Ener-G ranges of products. You can also check out the gluten-free food list at www.glutenfreeinfo.com
- Look for breads, instant foods, and flours made from grain alternatives such as quinoa, amaranth, millet, corn, rice, buckwheat, and lentils.
- You can also try sprouted wheat bread that is free of gluten.
- Dairy alternatives to cow's milk include rice, oat, coconut, quinoa, pea, and almond milk—available from all good health stores.
- Eat plenty of leafy greens, which are rich sources of magnesium and calcium. Cabbage is rich in the amino acid L-glutamine, which helps to heal the gut. Try making fresh vegetable juices that include raw cabbage, a little root ginger, which is very soothing, plus any vegetables that you have on hand. If you cook cabbage in water, save the water and make gravy with it. Or add cabbage to stews and soups.
- Try to eat more fish to provide vitamin D, which is often deficient in celiac sufferers.
- Eat plenty of unrefined organic nuts, seeds, and fish as well as free-range, low-fat meats such as venison, pork, and turkey to keep up zinc intake often deficient in celiacs. Try to use only organic meat.
- Essential fats are needed to heal the gut, so use a little organic sunflower, sesame, olive, or walnut oil for salad dressings.

- Eat an avocado once a week, as they are rich in vitamin E.
- Papaya is very healing for the gut and pineapple breaks down gluten, so if you are gluten sensitive then eat fresh pineapple before meals to aid digestion.

Useful Remedies

- None of the supplements suggested will cure celiac disease; it's just that the vast majority of these nutrients are often deficient in celiac sufferers. Therefore it is very important to increase your intake of these nutrients to prevent deficiency.
- Calcium (500mg daily) and magnesium (250mg daily) are vital minerals, as many celiac sufferers have a low bone density.
- Folic acid (400–800mcg) and vitamin B6 (50–100m)g daily. Include a B-complex as well as the extra daily folic acid and B6.
- Take a high-strength, natural-source carotene complex, which converts naturally into vitamin A in the body—needed for healing.
- Many celiac sufferers are low in vitamin D, a deficiency of which is linked to a host of health problems, including cancers and osteoporosis. Take a minimum 1000IU of D3 a day.
- A high-strength multi-vitamin and mineral (preferably in liquid form) to make up for any other nutritional deficiencies.
- Omega-3 fats are vital: take 2 grams of omega-3 fats daily (see *Fats You Need To Eat*).
- Bromelain helps to break down gluten and is anti-inflammatory.
- If you are gluten sensitive, take 250mg of bromelain before each main meal.
- Take a full-spectrum digestive enzyme to aid absorption. **VC**
- Slippery elm tablets/or aloe vera can help to reduce the irritation. Take one tablet or one capful of the aloe with each meal.

Helpful Hints

- If you have any of the symptoms mentioned, then ask your doctor for a blood test.
- If you are a severe celiac, you will need to avoid utensils that have been in contact with gluten.
- Breast-fed children are much less likely to develop celiac disease than those fed on cow's or soya milk formulas. Formula milks are harder to digest and potentially can cause health problems later on.
- Research from Finland shows that small amounts (50–70 grams) of oat-based products can be tolerated by celiacs without damaging intestinal absorption.
- For further information, visit www.celiac.org

CELLULITE
(see also Circulation)

Nearly nine times as many women as men suffer from cellulite. This is partly due to the different structure of the skin, and the fact that women have more underlying fat cells. Cellulite is mainly due to water retention plus an accumulation of toxins in the body, which have weakened the connective tissue just below the surface of the skin. It is much less common in female athletes who have very low body fat. Cellulite could be greatly avoided if you look after your liver and your lymphatic system.

Foods to Avoid

- High saturated fat foods, such as chocolate, clog up the lymphatic system, which will contribute to more cellulite.
- Refined carbohydrates such as mass-produced cakes, cookies, pies, and pastries.

- Foods with a high salt content, such as canned, pre-packaged and fast foods, also tend to contain a lot of saturated fats. Salt retains more fluid in the tissues, which means you are storing more toxins.
- Also avoid too much coffee and alcohol because they place a strain on the liver, which is already struggling to deal with the toxins from your diet. The more you take care of your liver, the more your skin will improve. (See *Liver Problems*.)

Friendly Foods
- Eat plenty of complex carbohydrates like beans, lentils, fruits, vegetables and brown rice. These foods are fibrous, which aids in the faster elimination of toxins, making fat deposits less likely.
- Make sure you drink plenty of water and add organic seeds like sunflower, pumpkin, and linseeds to fruits, salads and cereals.
- Pectin in apples helps eliminate toxins. Eat an organic apple or two every day.

Useful Remedies
- The herb gotu kola is by far the best researched and most successful remedy for cellulite when taken orally. Try 500mg three times a day for 2–3 months.
- Take a multi-vitamin/mineral daily for your age and gender.
- Horse chestnut cream, gel or lotion applied twice a day reduces some of the swelling and discomfort and helps strengthen the connective tissues, which tend to be damaged when you have cellulite. Available from all good health stores.
- Cellulite tincture contains bladderwrack, alfalfa, horse chestnut, dandelion, and gotu kola to improve microcirculation, elimination, and oxygenation, as well as speeding up the metabolism. **OP**
- A good way to help clean the lymph is with a combination of clivers, blue flag, burdock, and yellow dock. Take one teaspoon of the mix in a glass of water three times daily.

Helpful Hints
- Massage in any form is beneficial, as it increases circulation and lymph drainage. If you are not able to treat yourself to a massage on a weekly basis, invest in a skin brush, which increases circulation and helps eliminate toxins from the body. Skin brushes are available from all health shops and the Body Shop.
- Detox body oil (juniper, rosemary, grapefruit, and fennel) helps detoxify and firm the body by improving microcirculation, oxygenation and elimination. Juniper and fennel are natural diuretics. Use with a skin brush every morning. **OP**
- Begin exercising more to encourage circulation and elimination of toxins. Rebounding on a mini-trampoline and doing yoga are great for reducing cellulite.
- Walk regularly. Stretching aids detoxification from soft tissues.
- If you need to lose weight, do it gradually, as losing weight too quickly can make the appearance of cellulite much worse.

CHILBLAINS   *(see also Circulation and Raynaud's Disease)*

Chilblains are triggered by poor circulation and are characterized by red, inflamed areas that affect the extremities. Chilblains can cause intense itching, swollen toes, and sensitivity to heat and cold. Some unfortunate individuals suffer in both the hands and feet. It is more common in cold weather because the small blood vessels in the skin naturally constrict when it is cold. If you tend to suffer from chilblains every winter, then you need to improve your circulation.

Foods to Avoid
- Avoid anything that worsens circulation. This inevitably means foods that tend to encourage hardening of the arteries such as animal fats, full-fat dairy products, low-fiber foods such as ice cream, gelatin, fatty desserts, chocolates, and cakes. See diet in *Atherosclerosis* and *Circulation*.

Friendly Foods
- Oily fish, cayenne pepper, garlic, onion, ginger, soluble fiber such as linseeds (flax seeds that have been soaked overnight in cold water and drained), plus oat and/or rice bran can all help either improve circulation or reduce levels of LDL (the "bad" cholesterol), which in the long-term will help your circulation. (See *Fats You Need to Eat* and *General Health Hints*.)
- Eat more pineapple, which is a natural blood thinner and acts as an anti-inflammatory.

Useful Remedies
- The herb gotu kola really helps increase circulation to the extremities. Take 500mg twice daily with food.
- Natural-source, full-spectrum vitamin E, 400IU a day, helps thin the blood naturally.
- Take 30–100mg of niacin (vitamin B3) daily to help pump blood into the minor capillaries. **NB: If you are taking niacin for the first time, only take 50mg and then slowly increase to 100mg or more daily, as niacin causes a flushing sensation in the skin. This is simply blood moving into the small capillaries, but it can make you look like a freshly cooked lobster for a while.** As all the B-vitamins work together, also take a B-complex.
- Omega-3 fish oils help reduce stickiness in the blood. Take 1g daily with a main meal.
- Include a multi-vitamin/mineral in this regimen plus 1g of vitamin C with bioflavonoids to help strengthen small capillaries.
- Bromelain, extracted from pineapple, is a natural blood thinner. Take 250mg daily.
- Add a few drops of ginger tincture to water and sip throughout the day. It really helps warm you up.

Helpful Hints
- Smoking restricts circulation, so give it up.
- Have a regular massage or reflexology. Essential oils such as black pepper or rosemary can be rubbed into your feet every morning to improve circulation. Do not use black pepper undiluted.
- Regular exercise, such as walking, rebounding, and skipping, all increase microcirculation.
- I used to suffer chilblains every winter, triggered by having varicose veins removed years ago. After this procedure the surgeon told me that I would still have plenty of veins left, but the legacy has been poor circulation. Obviously, the key would have been for me to have avoided varicose veins in my youth! Keep this in mind and wear bed socks during winter months.
- **Never** wear tight-fitting shoes, especially when it is bitterly cold, as this really aggravates chilblains by restricting circulation to the toes. Invest in fur-lined boots during cold weather.
- Try massaging homeopathic Tamus cream into the chilblains. This cream is made from wild black bryony root and has helped many people.
- Homeopathic Agaricus 3x or 6x can be taken 2–3 times daily. This is a classic homeopathic remedy for chilblains.

CHOLESTEROL, HIGH AND LOW

(see also Heart Disease and Strokes)

Around one in every six American adults has high cholesterol, and the problem is escalating. Every year in the US alone, nearly 2,400 people die every day because of cardiovascular disease, and a high cholesterol count increases your chances of becoming one of these statistics by more than 60%.

Cholesterol is a fatty substance manufactured by the liver and is a vital component of every cell. There are two types of cholesterol: HDL (high density lipoproteins) and LDL (low density lipoproteins). The HDLs are good for us: the easy way to remember this is H is for healthy. The LDLs are generally bad for us: L stands for lethal. Then there are triglycerides, which are another type of fat that is carried in the blood primarily by the LDL, and we generally find high levels of triglycerides associated with high LDL.

A total blood cholesterol level above 240mg/dL is considered high. Interestingly, most people who die of heart disease or stroke have normal or low cholesterol, but having high cholesterol indicates imbalances. A healthy reading should be no more than 200mg/dL. But even within a "healthy" range, it is the specific amounts of HDL and LDL that are the important part. HDL should be less than 40mg/dL for men and less than 50 mg/dL for women. Optimal levels of LDL are less than 100mg/dL, but LDL levels are not qualified as high until they reach 160mg/dL and over.

It appears that the problem lies with the LDL, and specifically whether that LDL oxidizes (like rust) in our blood vessels, causing damage and occlusion. The LDL will oxidize unless we have some form of insurance, such as plenty of "fat-soluble" antioxidants (like vitamin E) to "mop it up."

Ideally, 20–40% of your total cholesterol should be HDL. There is also a type of cholesterol, VLDL (very low density lipoprotein), which is extremely bad for you.

You need cholesterol for healthy cell membrane production and the manufacture of hormones. It is also needed to help in the synthesis of bile acids for the digestion of fats and the production of vitamin D. Low cholesterol levels are linked to depression and in rare cases suicide, which is why fat-free diets are definitely not a good idea. For years we have been told to avoid certain foods, especially eggs, because they contain cholesterol. In fact, blood levels of LDL cholesterol are more affected by eating too much fat and sugar, rather than foods such as eggs that contain cholesterol (see Friendly Foods).

If you do have high cholesterol levels, two of the most important supplements you can take are natural-source, full-spectrum vitamin E, which helps prevent cholesterol from oxidizing, and B-group vitamins such as B12, B6, B3, and folic acid, all of which prevent the elevation of homocysteine levels (see below), which tend to oxidize cholesterol and lead to plaque formation in the arteries. Thanks to eating too much animal fat, many children in the West now have raised cholesterol and arterial plaque by the age of 10. But, while cholesterol levels have been used for many years as a possible way to predict our risk of heart attacks and strokes, that is only part of the story. Medical science is now beginning to re-think the role cholesterol plays in heart disease and strokes.

Homocysteine levels are now also being recognized as an important indicator for heart disease and stroke. Homocysteine is a toxic amino acid produced during the metabolism of proteins, and high levels are associated with an 80% increased risk of heart disease and strokes, even if you have a healthy cholesterol level. The good news is that there is now an easy way to test your own homocysteine levels (see *Helpful Hints*), and you can lower your levels naturally by simply taking more B vitamins (see under *Useful Remedies*). If your homocysteine level is high and you are taking B-vitamins to lower it, retest your levels periodically to see if you are taking sufficient dosages.

High plasma levels of homocysteine damage artery walls, allowing LDL cholesterol (the bad cholesterol) to easily stick to them. This build-up is what triggers the cascade of events that leads to heart disease and strokes. It is also linked to numerous other age-related conditions from Alzheimer's and diabetes to obesity and mental health problems such as schizophrenia.

Places where high levels of saturated fats are consumed (for example, The Netherlands and Finland) have higher elevations of LDL, whereas places such as Japan, where there is a relatively low saturated fat intake, have lower LDL levels. But other factors are important as well. Our cholesterol will naturally tend to rise (as liver function decreases) up until age 65, and high cholesterol will be more common in men younger than 55 years old than in women of the same age. However, after menopause women's cholesterol levels rise, and women over 55 will tend to have higher levels than men.

Around 20% of the body's total cholesterol is obtained from the diet, and the body manufactures the rest. Studies have shown that overweight people produce 20% more cholesterol than people of normal weight for their age, usually triggered by eating too much fat and sugar, stress, and smoking. However, if you have a persistently raised cholesterol level but eat a healthy diet, you may have an under-active thyroid. Also, people with blood type A are more susceptible to high total cholesterol.

Optimum liver function helps you make more good cholesterol; therefore, the more you look after your liver, the more likely you are to have a healthy level (see *Liver Problems*). About one person in 100 has a genetic predisposition to high blood cholesterol levels, but even this can be helped through diet and taking the right supplements.

Statins are being treated as magic bullets to treat high cholesterol, and approximately 24 million Americans take statins regularly. But statins have been found to have considerable negative long-term consequences for some people—including memory loss, loss of libido, muscle pain, and nerve damage (possibly due to damage to the myelin sheath that coats nerve endings).

Statins can mask underlying imbalances such as a fatty liver, and although statins lower LDL and total cholesterol, they only have a modest effect on boosting the artery-cleansing HDL. Statin drugs do not, however, lower the dangerous triglycerides. Also, statins place a strain on all muscles, including the heart muscle, as they lower production of a vitamin-like substance called CoQ10, which is produced naturally in the liver. But as we age production of this vital substance slows, and statins exacerbate the problem further.

Anyone taking statins **must** take a daily CoQ10 supplement. In fact, naturopath Steve Langley says, "The average 70-year-old does not have adequate reserves of CoQ10, and if such a person is then given statins, it could reduce levels to a critical state and trigger heart problems."

Several doctors are now openly linking some of the side effects of statins to lowered levels of CoQ10.

Foods to Avoid
■ Eating too many barbecued or burnt food—especially meat, hard margarines, fried foods, and so on—causes cholesterol to oxidize, which makes it more dangerous because, once oxidized, it begins attaching itself to artery walls. And as we age cholesterol tends to oxidize at a faster rate; therefore, the more antioxidants we eat, the less cholesterol will oxidize, and the more likely you are to remain healthier for longer. Cut down on your intake of animal fats and full-fat dairy products, and eat more essential fats (for a full list, see *Fats You Need To Eat*).

- Read label—and as much as possible, avoid mass-produced foods as well as oils that contain hydrogenated or trans-fats.
- Refined carbohydrates, such as white rice and pastas, processed white breads, cakes etc, can reduce the production of HDLs. White bread eaters usually have higher cholesterol levels than those who eat mainly whole-wheat varieties.
- Sugar, if not burnt for energy during exercise, converts to fat in the body and lives on your hips. In the long run this will help raise LDL cholesterol levels.
- Eggs contain cholesterol, but this is balanced by a high choline content (great for memory), which breaks down the cholesterol. However, some scientists say that if an egg is fried it will cause oxidative damage. Therefore it is the frying that causes the problems, not the eggs themselves. It makes sense then to boil or poach eggs. Buy organic eggs or eggs containing omega-3 fats, which are now available in all major supermarkets.
- Drinking excessive amounts of alcohol and coffee (especially if microwaved) has been shown to raise cholesterol levels.
- Greatly reduce the amount of sodium-based salt you use.

Friendly Foods
- Studies have shown that two glasses of red wine for a man and one for a woman (drunk daily) tend to raise HDL but won't affect LDL levels.
- Generally, you need to increase your fiber intake. Eat more oat or rice bran, rolled oats, wheat germ, and any beans and peas such as soybeans, red kidney beans, lima beans, broad beans, chickpeas, and lentils. Whole grains such as brown rice, whole wheat, barley, rye, millet, and quinoa are great for controlling cholesterol.

- Increase your intake of fresh fruit and vegetables (raw, steamed, roasted or stir fried, not deep fried or boiled). Green vegetables are especially rich in magnesium and potassium, as are cereals (also rich in B-vitamins) honey, kelp, and dried fruits such as dates.
- A couple of raw organic carrots or apples per day can lower cholesterol levels.
- Eat oatmeal for breakfast. Make it with half low-fat milk (or even better rice, almond or oat milk) and half water. Add a chopped apple and a few raisins to sweeten rather than sugar.
- Buckwheat is high in glycine and has been shown to lower cholesterol levels. Buckwheat flour makes great pancakes.
- Fermented soy products, such as natto, miso, and tempeh, can help raise HDLs and lower LDLs.
- Soy lecithin granules are a great way to help lower LDL and control the growth of kidney and gallstones. Sprinkle a tablespoon daily over cereals, into yogurts, and onto fruit salads. Make sure it's a non-GM source.
- Increase your intake of healthier fats found in olive oil, avocados, coconut oil, sunflower, pumpkin, sesame and linseeds (and their unrefined oils), plus walnuts and Brazil nuts (see *Fats You Need To Eat*).
- Oily fish such as salmon, trout, mackerel, anchovies, herring, and sardines contain a fatty acid known as eicosapentaenoic acid (EPA). This helps to make the blood less sticky, so it helps reduce the risk of coronary heart disease. Garlic and onions do the same.
- Look for spreads that are free from hydrogenated and trans-fats such as Promise or Olivio. Or blend a small amount of organic butter with a little olive oil.
- Otherwise use small amounts of walnut, almond or hemp seed butters. Available from most health shops.
- Vegetarians tend to have lower cholesterol levels.
- Use an organic, mineral-based sea salt available from all health stores. I use Himalayan Crystal Salt, which is rich in organic source minerals. Available online and from good health stores.

- Look for eggs that are labeled as containing omega-3 essential fats. These chickens are fed seeds that are rich in essential fats and therefore lay healthier eggs!
- Use dandelion root tea, which helps liver function, and green tea, which lowers cholesterol levels.
- Globe artichoke, celeriac (celery root), kale, and fennel stimulate liver function and cell regeneration. They can also help lower blood cholesterol.
- Eat more live, low-fat, plain yogurt that contains lactobacillus and/or acidophilus. It will help lower blood cholesterol levels by binding fat and cholesterol in the intestines.
- Drink plenty of water, at least 6–8 glasses daily.

Useful Remedies

- If you are taking statins, these drugs block the enzyme that makes cholesterol. This same enzyme also makes CoQ10 (Co-enzyme Q10), a vitamin-like substance, which is needed to protect against heart disease. Therefore, if you are taking statins it is really important that you also take 150mg of CoQ10 per day. Research shows people on statins (such as Lipitor, Crestor, Mevacor and Zocor) have low levels of CoQ10, which can eventually trigger heart problems.
- As a good foundation, take a good-quality multi-vitamin/mineral daily.
- Take 1–2g of fish oil daily.
- Evidence has shown that taking garlic each day could help lower overall blood cholesterol levels and increase the levels of HDL over LDL cholesterol. This is especially true if you are an A or an AB blood type.
- Include a high-strength antioxidant formula that helps prevent cholesterol oxidation.

- Make sure that any multi-vitamin you take includes 400IU of full-spectrum, natural-source vitamin E, which helps protect against oxidation of LDL.
- Alpha-lipoic acid also helps prevent oxidation of LDL; take 200mg daily.
- Folic acid, B12 and B6 all lower homocysteine levels in the blood, thus reducing our risk of heart disease. A good B-complex should contain 400mcg folic acid, 10–20mg B6 and 50–100mcg B12.
- Taking 200mcg per day of the mineral chromium can help elevate HDL levels while reducing cravings for sugary foods.
- The minerals calcium and magnesium are useful for reducing cholesterol. Take 1000mg of calcium and 600mg of magnesium daily.

Helpful Hints

- There is now an easy test to discover your plasma homocysteine levels. Made by YorkTest Laboratories, it is a simple pinprick method that can be done through the mail. For details call York Labs at 011-44-1904-410410 or visit www.yorktest.com
- Exercise is vital for controlling cholesterol. It can raise HDL levels and lower LDL. Try to walk at least 30 minutes every day and do some kind of aerobic exercise three times a week.
- Smoking increases oxidation of LDL.
- Eating smaller meals every 3–4 hours, rather than three big meals a day, can help lower cholesterol.

CHRONIC FATIGUE
(see Exhaustion and ME)

CHRONIC OBSTRUCTIVE PULMONARY DISEASE
(see Bronchitis and Emphysema)

CIRCULATION   *(see also Chilblains, Cholesterol, and Raynaud's Disease)*

Good circulation is fundamental for good health, as all parts of the body require sufficient oxygen and nutrients to function optimally. Good circulation also enables us to eliminate toxins more efficiently, and it's amazing how many conditions are linked to poor circulation. Common symptoms range from cold hands and feet to leg ulcers and varicose veins. Hair loss can be triggered by poor circulation to the head. More serious problems involve restricted circulation to the heart and brain as in strokes.

If you laid out your blood vessels end to end, it is estimated that they would encircle the globe twice over—that's a lot of miles. No wonder we end up with so many circulatory problems. As we age our arteries become thickened (atherosclerosis) or hardened (arteriosclerosis), and many people of all ages are exercising less, so in turn our circulation becomes less efficient.

Numerous conditions associated with aging—leg ulcers, memory loss, atherosclerosis, cold hands and feet—are all linked to poor circulation. Our arteries make up a major part of our blood circulatory system and contain about 15% of our blood supply at any given moment. Healthy arteries have thick, muscular walls, which are necessary for the pressure of the blood moving through them. Your heart weighs just 10–11oz (280–310g) and it is about the size of a clenched fist. The left side of the heart forces blood into the arteries, which carry the bright red, nutrient-rich, oxygenated blood through the body.

The oxygen (from the lungs) and nutrients (absorbed into the arteries via the gut) are taken up by the cells. Then the blood (now a darker, bluish color) is returned to the heart via the veins, and the right chamber of the heart pumps it through the lungs. Veins are more numerous and hold more of the body's blood (about 70%). Their function is to transport blood laden with waste products, and partly depleted of oxygen, back to the heart.

From the lungs the re-oxygenated blood returns, purified, to the left chamber, ready for redistribution, and the whole cycle begins again. Veins are forced to move against gravity much of the time. In order to maintain normal blood pressure, an adequate supply of blood must be returned to the heart from the peripheral vessels. Two main factors are responsible for this "uphill" flow from the legs and abdomen to the heart. Firstly, muscular contractions compress veins, thus squeezing the blood along. When a person stands still for a long time, such as soldiers on sentry duty, the blood pools in the lower limbs due to the force of gravity. In the long term, as the leg valves become weaker, this can trigger varicose veins. This pooling of blood also means that there is insufficient blood returning to the heart to maintain blood pressure, and less blood makes it to the brain. In extreme cases fainting can result, which forces the person into a horizontal position and alleviates the problem.

Secondly, as we get older, especially if we have a sedentary lifestyle, we tend to breathe more shallowly, which has a direct effect on our circulation. Coronary heart disease is almost always due to a condition called atherosclerosis (see under *Atherosclerosis*) where fatty deposits attach themselves to the insides of the arteries. Arteries that were once smooth and elastic become rough, inflexible and narrow (see *High Blood Pressure*). With this narrowing, the volume of blood that the arteries can transport is reduced. Factors that contribute to atherosclerosis are long-term negative stress, cigarette smoking, high cholesterol, a high homocysteine level, a high-fat diet, excessive salt intake, and so on.

Once an area has been damaged, fats from the blood, including cholesterol, accumulate and build up a thick, fatty layer called plaque. This plaque narrows the artery, but clots may detach themselves from the artery wall and enter the bloodstream. If a clot causes an obstruction inside the coronary artery, a heart attack can occur. If it blocks an artery leading to the brain, it can cause a stroke.

This slow build-up of plaque and consequent narrowing of the artery can also lead to a condition called angina, which is very common after age 50. The pain of angina (which can vary considerably) is generally felt when the person is under stress or as more demands are put on the heart muscle during exercise. The pain of a heart attack is a more "crushing" pain in the chest, which can radiate to the jaw or down the left arm (see *Heart Disease*).

Blood pressure tends to increase with age. Normal blood pressure depends on a number of factors, including the elasticity of the arterial walls, amount and consistency of the blood, digestion, smoking, weight, and stress. High blood pressure can cause heart attacks and strokes. An aneurysm can occur when there is a weak spot in an arterial wall that balloons out and releases blood into surrounding tissues, which is why looking after the integrity of your veins and arteries can help keep you healthier at any age.

Foods to Avoid

- Salt hardens your arteries (which need to be elastic) and although it is essential to life, most people consume too much inorganic salt in the form of sodium chloride. Too much salt can result in high blood pressure, because where salt goes water follows! It is found in most canned, pre-packaged, mass-produced foods, burgers, potato chips, laxatives, antacids, and carbonated drinks, especially canned fizzy drinks.
- Reduce animal fats such as red meat, full-fat milk and dairy produce, cheese, and chocolates.
- Pies, pastries, cakes, and foods made with saturated/hydrogenated trans-fats, such as lard and margarines, should be avoided or reduced (see *Fats You Need To Eat*).
- Avoid or greatly reduce your intake of fried foods. Never fry with mass-produced vegetable oils.
- Avoid coffee, caffeine, and other stimulants, which can ultimately lead to a constriction of the blood vessels.
- Avoid excessive alcohol. A glass of red wine with meals, however, can be beneficial.

Friendly Foods

- Try chopping up seaweeds such as kelp and sprinkling them over your food instead of salt. Kelp or nori flakes can be used instead of salt.
- Use organic, mineral-rich sea salt, but only over the food that is in front of you! I use Himalayan Crystal Salt, which is rich in natural minerals. Available from good health stores, some supermarkets, www.Amazon.com and Natural Health International, Inc., 524 Second Street, San Francisco, CA 94107; Tel: 1-888-668-3661, Monday–Friday, 9am–5pm PDT; email: general@naturalhi.com; website: www.himalayancrystalsalt.com
- Vitamin C is vital for healthy circulation because as a major antioxidant it helps protect blood vessels from damage. Foods naturally high in vitamin C include blueberries, sweet potatoes, cherries, guavas, kale leaves, parsley, cantaloupe melon, broccoli, strawberries, and peppers.
- Tomatoes, grapes, and blackberries are high in bioflavonoids.
- Garlic and onions help to thin the blood naturally.
- Wheat germ, avocados, nuts, and seeds are all rich in vitamin E, which also helps to thin the blood naturally.
- Foods rich in rutin help to strengthen the small blood vessels. So eat more buckwheat, the peel of citrus fruits, rose hips, and apple peel.
- Silica-rich foods such as lettuce, celery, millet, oats, and parsnips help to strengthen arterial and vein walls. Fiji mineral water is rich in silica.
- Linseeds (flax seeds soaked overnight in cold water then drained), sunflower and sesame

seeds, and fish oils contain essential polyunsaturated fatty acids, known as omega-3 fatty acids, that have been shown to lower the "bad" LDL fats and thin the blood.

- Try eating at least three portions of fish a week, such as wild organic salmon, mackerel, sardines, or anchovies. Try to avoid tuna as it can be high in mercury.
- Unrefined Brazil nuts, walnuts, hazelnuts, almonds, seeds and their unrefined cold oils, are excellent sources of essential fats. Avocado is also a rich source of mono-unsaturated fats: eat one a week.
- Sprinkle GM-free lecithin granules, which emulsify "bad" fats, over your breakfast cereals, into yoghurts, or over fruit to help lower LDL cholesterol.
- People on high-fiber diets are four times less likely to suffer from circulation problems and heart disease. Soluble fiber (that is, beans, lentils, brown rice) consists of compounds that bind to bile salts and this helps lower cholesterol levels.
- Use oat or rice brans in your diet.

Useful Remedies

- Pycnogenol, a pine bark extract, encourages nitrous oxide production, which in turn relaxes blood vessels and arteries. Take 80mg daily. **PN**
- The herb gotu kola helps increase circulation to the extremities such as feet and hands through its vasodilatory action on peripheral blood vessels. Take 500mg twice daily.
- The herb butcher's broom is high in rutin, a bioflavonoid, which helps to tone the vein walls. It is therefore very beneficial in treating varicose veins. **NB: As butcher's broom is a vasoconstrictor (the opposite to gotu kola), caution should be taken if you suffer from high blood pressure.** Take 500mg twice daily.

- The herb horse chestnut has a similar action on varicose veins as its components help strengthen the small capillaries. Take 500mg daily.
- Use the herbs butcher's broom, horse chestnut, plus B-vitamins and rutin. All the above are usually used for varicose veins, as they strengthen veins, have anti-inflammatory properties, and reduce swelling, thus making venous return to the heart more efficient. Ultra Vein-Gard Leg Therapy Cream, which is available through most US online retailers, contains these ingredients and more.
- Studies have shown that patients suffering from visual and hearing problems linked to poor circulation, such as tinnitus, have demonstrated improvements after taking ginkgo biloba for 3 months. Take 120mg daily in one dose.
- Vitamin C with bioflavonoids helps to strengthen capillaries. Take 2g daily with food—spread throughout the day.
- Vitamin E helps reduce stickiness in the blood; take 200IU daily of full-spectrum, natural-source vitamin E. This is especially true for type A and AB blood types, which tend to be "stickier" than other blood types.
- Niacin (vitamin B3) increases circulation. **NB: Niacin can induce a short-term "flushing" or reddening of the skin, so begin with 30mg and work up to 100mg daily.**
- Ginger helps to warm the body, so make a ginger tea infusion daily and add grated fresh root ginger to stir-fries and fruit salads.

Helpful Hints

- Long-term stress constricts blood vessels and causes the blood to become stickier and will impede circulation. This in turn can trigger heart attacks or strokes, so reduce your stress levels.
- Exercise is a wonderful way to help increase circulation. Just taking a brisk walk every day can be very helpful, as it warms the blood and relaxes the arteries. Skipping, dancing, rebounding, and power walking all help by gently pounding the feet.

- Massage and reflexology are important, especially for people who, for health reasons, cannot exercise much, or for those who lead a more sedentary lifestyle. Aromatherapy massage using essential oils such as rosemary, black pepper, or ginger can be very effective in aiding circulation.
- Skin brushing also aids circulation. Work upward from the feet and hands toward the heart, rubbing briskly; try to do this five times a week in the bath or shower.
- If you smoke, give it up, as it impairs breathing and hence circulation.
- Acupuncture has a long history of treating poor circulation and high blood pressure. The action of the needles promotes better circulation by unblocking stagnation of both qi and blood (see *Useful Information*).

COLDS AND FLU *(see also Antibiotics and Immune Function)*

Colds and flu are caused by viruses, and the secret to avoiding them is to keep your immune system in great shape. See also *Immune Function*. Newer strains such as swine and bird flu, which are potentially a serious threat, are sadly becoming more commonplace, often triggering unnecessary panic. Yet if we could all keep our immune systems functioning optimally, we could avoid becoming sick in the first place.

Flu symptoms are usually far more severe than cold symptoms and include a fever, aching joints, and horrible headaches. With colds there is plenty of congestion, often accompanied by a headache. With worse cases of the flu your joints ache, and all you want is to stay in bed, which is one of the fastest routes to recovery. If you have a temperature, your doctor will likely suggest taking two Tylenol every four to six hours to help bring it down. However, having a temperature is nature's way of killing the invading bugs.

If an infant has a high temperature, you would need for him/her to see a doctor. And if an adult has a high temperature for more than two days, also seek medical attention.

Only if you contract a secondary bacterial infection—meaning if it hurts to breathe and you are wheezing—antibiotics may be necessary; see also *Bronchitis*.

We become more susceptible to colds and flu if we overwork, over-train, or consistently eat a poor diet high in saturated fats and sugars. For example, if you eat a sugar-rich dessert and a bar of chocolate, and are then immediately in contact with someone from a cold or flu, you have doubled your chances of catching it. Also, lack of sleep greatly lowers immune function, as does long-term negative stress.

Foods to Avoid
- Avoid all refined sugars and carbohydrates, such as white bread, cakes, pies, and cookies, as well as high-fat foods, alcohol, and caffeine. All of these can weaken the immune system and make us more susceptible to infection.
- Generally, while you have a cold reduce your intake of mucus-forming foods such as cheese, chocolate, and full-fat dairy products. Mucus will also form as a reaction to any foods to which you have an intolerance; see *Allergies* and *Catarrh*.

Friendly Foods
- It's crucial to keep up your fluid intake—tea and coffee dehydrate the body, so drink plenty of water and herbal teas. Pau d'arco or green tea will help boost immune function. Fluids help the lymphatic system to function efficiently.
- Garlic and onions are great foods, as they are anti-bacterial and have antiseptic properties. A traditional remedy for colds and flu is a soup made with 6 onions, a whole garlic, 1in

(2.5cm) of grated fresh ginger, and some cayenne pepper mixed in a vegetable or chicken stock. You could also add lemongrass to it. For children it is probably preferable to leave out the cayenne pepper, however: although it does make the other herbs more effective, it is often too hot.

- Licorice is a pleasant-tasting food that you can make into tea and eat as confectionery if it is sugar free. It has both anti-viral and anti-bacterial properties and will soothe the throat when it's inflamed (see *Sore Throat*).
- While you have a cold or flu, try to base your diet on fruits, vegetables and brown rice, barley, quinoa, adding in a little fish, chicken, or pulses. Keep your diet clean. See *General Health Hints*.
- Drink plenty of lemon and ginger herbal tea or make your own: finely chop a 1-in (2.5-cm) piece of fresh ginger, stand it in boiling water for 15 minutes with a squeeze of lemon juice and freshly chopped spring onions, strain, and sip.

Useful Remedies
- One of the best remedies I have found is The Wellness Formula, made by Source Naturals Inc. It contains garlic, propolis, elderberry extract, olive leaf extract, vitamin C, astragalus, zinc and grapeseed extract—a perfect combination of nutrients needed to boost immunity, as they are anti-viral and bacterial. At the first sign of a sore throat or feeling that you have something coming, take 1 or 2, three times daily. They are amazing. Available at all good health stores.
- Propolis—from bee hives—has anti-viral and anti-bacterial properties. Taking 1 to 3 grams daily can help reduce the severity of a cold and taken all year round (500mg daily) can help boost immunity.

- Echinacea and golden seal, taken either as tincture or tablets every couple of hours, help fend off a cold or flu. Echinacea has been shown in a number of studies to shorten the length of a cold from 7 days down to 3–4 if taken regularly; generally take 1–4ml of a tincture every 2–3 hours. A great anti-viral formula.
- I tend to take herbs such as echinacea in the winter, when we are more susceptible to colds. It is more effective when taken cyclically. Take for a month, then stop taking for a week. Continue throughout the winter.
- Vitamin C is strongly anti-viral and research has shown that it can shorten the severity and duration of most colds and flu, if taken in sufficient amounts. During the winter, take 1 gram daily, but if you feel a cold coming on, increase your intake to 1 gram, 3 times daily. Take it with meals in an ascorbate form until the cold has gone.
- A huge percentage of people are lacking in vitamin D, known as the sunshine vitamin—and we should all now be taking 1000IU of vitamin D3 daily to keep our immune systems in better shape.
- Take a multi-vitamin and mineral that contains at least 30–60mg of zinc to boost the immune system while fighting an infection.
- If you are suffering from a sore throat, try zinc gluconate lozenges that contain 15–25mg of zinc. Take 1 every 3–4 hours. The zinc lozenges help to kill bacteria in the throat.
- Olive leaf extract acts like nature's antibiotic. I take 2 daily to help keep my immune system in shape when I am feeling run down.
- Sambucol is an extract of the European black elderberry plant, which has potent anti-viral properties. If taken at the onset of a cold or flu, it can help reduce the severity and length of the illness. Available from most health stores and pharmacies.
- Beta Glucans 1–3, 1–6, are proven to strengthen the body's innate immune system and are especially useful for children. Source Naturals makes a version that is free from yeast protein. Take 250–500 mg daily. Can be taken all year round by adults and children (250mg daily) to boost immune functioning.

- N-acetyl cysteine (NAC)) is an amino acid that really helps to boost levels of glutathione, one of the body's most potent antioxidant defenses. In a large study of older adults who took 600mg twice daily 30 minutes before meals for 6 months, only 25% of those taking part experienced any flu-like symptoms. In the placebo group (those who were given a "blank" pill), it was 79%. NAC helps to inhibit virus replication and has shown good results against the H5N1 bird flu virus.

Helpful Hints

- If I start to get a sore throat, I take homeopathic Streptococcus 10M immediately along with the Wellness Formula and my sore throat almost always disappears.
- Homeopathic Aconite 30c can be taken 2 or 3 times daily at the onset of a cold to help stop the cold from developing.
- Oscilliococcinum is a homeopathic preventative for colds and flu symptoms. Take one dose weekly during the cold and flu season as a preventative. Or use it at the onset of a cold or flu to prevent symptoms from developing further. It is sold in most pharmacies and supermarkets.
- Keep warm and avoid changes in the temperature of your surroundings for at least 48 hours until symptoms subside. Rest is essential if you have a temperature.
- Do not struggle into work if you have a really bad cold—all you do is make it last longer and you pass it on to your colleagues.
- Washing your hands regularly, and not shaking hands with anyone who has a cold or flu, are the best ways of avoiding giving your cold or contracting other people's colds and flu, as viruses can easily permeate the soft skin on the palms of the hands. Washing hands is essential for kids, whose hygiene levels are often lacking!
- Use tissues when you sneeze or cough and throw them away immediately. Your germs can spread up to 10 feet around you every time you sneeze.
- Viruses are airborne and spread quickly at large gatherings. Avoid being in stuffy, smoky rooms for too long. Get plenty of exercise and fresh air.
- Use a neti pot daily; it helps remove gunk from the sinuses and reduces bacteria held in the nose and sinuses. Brilliant. Available from most health stores and pharmacies.

COLD SORES

(see also Herpes)

Cold sores are caused by the herpes simplex virus. Once contracted the virus lies dormant in the body and tends to re-activate if you become run down or stressed or after sudden exposure to very hot or cold weather. Some women suffer an attack during menstruation. Others find that if they eat large amounts of nuts or chocolate, containing the amino acid arginine on which the virus thrives, this can also trigger an attack. There have been a number of studies showing that you can reduce the frequency of attacks by taking vitamin C and the amino acid lysine on a regular basis.

Foods to Avoid

- Avoid foods that are very rich in arginine, an amino acid found commonly in chocolate, lentils, beans, and nuts.
- As sugar triggers inflammation and lowers immune function, you should greatly reduce your intake of any sugar. Also avoid refined foods made with white flour, such as cakes, cookies, and desserts, and high saturated-fat foods that are often high in sugar.
- Avoid trans- and hydrogenated fats (see *Fats You Need To Eat*).

- Certain people notice when they eat too much dairy produce from cows they suffer an attack.

Friendly Foods
- Eat good-quality protein, such as lean meats including turkey, chicken, duck (without any skin), lean pork, white fish, salmon, eggs, corn, and soy, all of which are rich in lysine, an amino acid that has been shown to interfere with replication of the virus.
- Plain, live yogurt should be fine and is high in lysine.
- Quinoa is an excellent source of protein.
- Goat's cheese should be fine as it is high in lysine.
- Garlic and onions are highly anti-viral.
- See *General Health Hints*.

Useful Remedies
- At the onset of an attack of this kind, take up to 4 grams of lysine daily. Many companies now make lysine and vitamin C together. At the onset you should also take 4 grams of vitamin C daily with food.
- To help prevent attacks, take 1 gram of vitamin C daily. Take 3 grams of propolis capsules and use the cream topically to help shut down an attack and ease the irritation. Then take 500mg of propolis daily to help prevent further attacks. Propolis is strongly anti-viral—and in studies has been proven to be more effective than some anti-viral drugs. **NB: If you have a severe allergy to bee stings, avoid propolis.**
- Olive leaf extract is another great supplement for cold sores as it is highly anti-viral. At the onset of an attack take 500mg, 3 times daily with food, until symptoms subside.
- If you find that you or your children regularly suffer cold sores you definitely need to include a good-quality multi-vitamin and mineral that contains Vitamin D3 in your regimen. There are now plenty of sugar- and additive-free chewable vitamins for children (Nature's Plus make great ranges for kids), or add liquid vitamins and minerals to their food. **NP, VC**

Helpful Hints
- Make sure you change your toothbrush and face towels regularly as these can harbor the virus.
- Over-exposure to bright sunshine can also encourage replication of the virus.
- Calendula tincture can be dabbed directly onto the sores.
- Homeopathic Rhus Tox 30c helps to eliminate the eruptions. Take as soon as the tingling starts. Take twice daily for 3 days.
- Several people have told me that when they take Bach Rescue Remedy internally and dab it externally onto the cold sores it prevents the cold sores from developing. As Rescue Remedy is also available in a cream, this is certainly worth a try.

COLITIS
(see also Crohn's Disease and Leaky Gut)

Colitis means "inflammation of the colon", and is a chronic, non-specific, inflammatory and ulcerative disease. Most commonly it develops between the ages of 15–40, but it can start at any age.

Symptoms include abdominal pain, tenderness or cramping—particularly in the lower left side. There may be a change in the stools, with episodes of frequent watery bowel movements that usually contain mucus and blood. In severe cases between 5 and 20 motions can be passed daily, causing severe dehydration and/or anemia.

Around two-thirds of sufferers experience intermittent symptoms and for about 5% of people colitis has a rapid onset. This condition tends to start in the rectum and then spreads back up into the bowel.

To make sure you get a correct diagnosis, you need to have stool tests and have an internal examination and a barium enema X-ray. The risk for colon cancer is increased with colitis.

There is an autoimmune component similar to Crohn's and there may be parasites, too much fat in the diet, stress, a leaky gut, food intolerances (mainly to wheat, gluten and dairy produce from cows). Many nutritional physicians now believe that a leaky gut is the root cause for conditions such as colitis—see *Leaky Gut*.

Foods to Avoid
- Any food that is an irritant to the bowel, particularly in the acute stage; this would usually be wheat, gluten, any type of bran, dairy products from cows, including all cheeses.
- Avoid very hot or cold foods, spicy foods, and vinegar.
- Absolutely avoid processed foods, fried foods, and red meats (especially pork).
- In the acute stages also avoid raw fruits and vegetables.
- Avoid refined sugar, which creates inflammation in the body.
- The main intolerances are dairy products, wheat, corn, tomatoes, citrus, potato, and chocolate.

Friendly Foods
- Rice, millet, barley, and quinoa are generally well tolerated.
- Mashed pumpkin, buckwheat, sweet potato, carrots, papaya, mango are all rich in carotenes.
- Chlorophyll heals the bowel—therefore eat more green foods such as watercress, spring greens, cabbage. Green powders such as Greens Plus are useful for these conditions. **GP**
- Eat more home-made soups and stews.
- Alkaline broth can be made with cabbage juice, potato water, and carrots.
- Fresh fish is high in zinc, and zinc aids tissue healing.
- Oily fish are great for their omega-3 content which aids healing.
- Once the healing process has started, then try porridge, oat or rice bran, and generally eat more fiber. Keep a food diary and note when symptoms are worse—also note your emotions.
- If you need sugar use small amounts of organic agave syrup or Xylosweet, which have a low glycemic index. **VC**

Useful remedies
- One of the best gut healers is aloe vera juice. Take before meals three times daily
- Slippery elm bark powder really helps to soothe the gut. Best taken on an empty stomach half an hour before meals.
- Take a natural-source carotene complex, as vitamin A is vital for soft tissue healing.
- Take a multi-vitamin/mineral for your age and gender.
- Licorice root—deglycerinated, sugar free—can help heal the gut.
- Good bacteria are important, especially the Bifido bacteria. Jarro-Dophilus EPS, take one daily with food. **JF**
- You may need DHEA, a hormone usually lacking in these types of conditions. Have a blood test to find out.
- Take vitamin B complex, as folic acid is needed to help reduce the likelihood of colon cancer.
- 2 grams of omega-3 fish oils daily to reduce inflammation.
- Sea buckthorn (an omega-7 essential fat) helps to heal the mucosal lining; try 2 grams daily for a month, then reduce to 1 gram. **VC**

Helpful Hints
- Try Kangen Water—a water system unit that attaches to your kitchen tap and ionizes and alkalizes water. The gut heals more quickly when alkaline. This water is used in many Japanese hospitals with highly beneficial health results. For full details, visit www.kangenwaterusa.com

- As stress is a major factor, deal with stress in your life. Learn to meditate, have counseling.
- Breathe more deeply—learn to let go of the small stuff. It's not worth dying for. See *Adrenal Exhaustion* and *Stress*.
- Try homeopathic Merc cor 6c three times daily if there are hot, bloody stools with mucus and cutting pains in the colon.
- Make sure you get plenty of rest and relaxation, which is the best way to allow the body to heal itself. Be kind to yourself.

CONJUNCTIVITIS
(see also Eye Problems)

Conjunctivitis is an inflammation of the outer surface membrane that lines the eye. This can be triggered by an external allergen, such as perfume or an insect spray, in which case the eyes are usually very red, itchy, and irritated. But if conjunctivitis is caused by bacteria or a virus, this can be accompanied by a yellow or white mucus-type discharge and needs to be treated by a doctor. People who suffer chronic conjunctivitis are often very run down, their immune system is under functioning, and they are usually deficient in vitamins A, C, and D.

Foods to Avoid
- All foods and drinks containing sugar, which reduces the body's ability to fight an infection.
- Reduce your intake of animal fats including cheese and chocolate, plus white-flour-based cakes, breads, and cookies, all of which will weaken the immune system.
- See *General Health Hints*.

Friendly Foods
- Bilberries, blueberries, blackberries, and all blue- and purple-colored fruits are rich in antioxidant nutrients that nourish the eyes.
- Foods rich in vitamin A such as leafy green vegetables, calves' or lambs' liver, cod liver oil, carrots, and fish help encourage healthy eyes.
- Natural carotenes found in tomatoes, sweet potatoes, papaya, apricots, mangoes, spinach and all greens, and raw parsley are all great foods for the eyes.
- Eat more fresh pineapple—rich in the enzyme bromelain, which has anti-inflammatory properties.

Useful Remedies
- Echinacea, eyebright, and bilberry tincture; 1–4ml a day. Available from health shops.
- Bromelain, take 500mg twice daily with food.
- Take a high-strength, full-spectrum carotene complex, which converts naturally to vitamin A in the body. **SVHC**
- Vitamin C (1 gram, 2–3 times per day with meals) and zinc (30–50mg per day) will help strengthen your immune system.
- Take a multi-vitamin/ mineral for your age and gender.
- Omega-3 fish oils help reduce inflammation in the body. Take 1 gram daily.

Helpful Hints
- Do you know that many eye drops are made from urine? Urea is an important component that helps break down mucus deposits and has anti-microbial actions. Bathing the eyes in fresh urine (which is a sterile liquid) on a cotton wool pad can help alleviate most eye problems.
- Conjunctivitis is highly contagious when caused by a viral infection. Be really careful not to use the same handkerchief or tissue to wipe both eyes. Be scrupulous with hygiene and make sure no one else uses your towels, make-up, or pillow.

- Eyebright tincture plus goldenseal tincture: take 2 drops of each and add to an eye bath full of purified or boiled water and use when cool. Use twice daily.
- Dilute homeopathic Euphrasia mother tincture in an egg-cup full of cooled boiled water and use as an eye bath. Alternatively, you can try PrimaVu Herbal Eye Wash with chamomile and eyebright (herbal eye drops also available). **VC**
- Chamomile and calendula herbal teas can be used to make warm compresses to soothe the eye. The heat also helps kill the bacteria that cause the infection.

CONSTIPATION AND BLOATING

(see also Absorption, Candida, and Leaky Gut)

Even though government advisors, health magazines, and doctors all advise us to eat more fiber, we are one of the most constipated nations on earth. In an ideal world we should have a bowel movement after every meal—but most people in the West are lucky if they have one a day. Having clean bowels is one of the best ways to prevent most diseases in later life.

Even if you have a daily bowel movement, you can still be constipated. Over time, we can experience a gradual build-up of matter, which adheres to the walls of the intestines and becomes compacted in certain sections. This build-up is caused by insufficient fiber and too many refined foods, which can eventually inhibit proper assimilation of nutrients from the diet and supplements. It also adds to the weight of the colon, therefore placing more stress on the lower organs such as the uterus and bladder.

Millions of men and women have large, protruding abdomens. This means that all the major organs in that area, such as the liver, heart, and bowels, are surrounded by a layer of deadly fat deposits. They are also likely to be carrying a lot of waste matter. Henry VIII had more than 84 pounds of feces in his bowel after his death and he had a very big abdomen indeed!

When food leaves the small intestine, which is over 20 feet long, it passes into the large intestine or colon where it is gradually compacted into semi-solid feces. The bowel is a term for the large intestine. Most of the absorption of nutrients from our diet and supplements happens in the small intestine.

The large intestine (colon) is primarily involved with the excretion and elimination of foods. The more feces in your bowel, the more toxic your entire system becomes. If you are not eliminating properly, these toxins are re-absorbed into the bloodstream and can be eventually dumped into the skin, resulting in conditions such as acne. People from primitive cultures tend to evacuate twice the amount of feces that their Western counterparts do, due to their higher intake of fiber and raw foods.

Peristalsis is the rhythmic movement of the colon, which helps to move the waste material out of the body. If you tend to eat a poor diet, low in fiber then the muscles in the colon can become lazy, which over time can lead to chronic constipation—and food putrefies in the bowel. Basically carbohydrates (fruit, breads, pasta and so on) ferment if not broken down properly, whereas protein (meat, eggs, cheese, fish) will putrefy. Also if you over-eat, food putrefies in the bowel, triggering symptoms such as bloating, gas, constipation or diarrhea, irritable bowel, poor skin, dull hair, and so on.

Hemorrhoids or piles (similar to varicose veins of the anus) are the result of years of straining to go to the bathroom and straining also contributes to varicose veins in the legs. If ever you experience blood in your feces or any noticeable changes in bowel habits, it is **vital** that you see a doctor immediately.

Foods to Avoid

- Animal products, especially red meats, have a long transit time through the bowel and should only be eaten in moderation.
- Many people do not have the enzyme needed to break down lactose, the sugar in milk, which can also lead to putrefaction in the bowel. This is especially common in Asian, African, and Caribbean people.
- If you tend to be a big dairy fan, try cutting back, as all dairy-based foods are mucus forming, which adds to congestion in the small intestine. However, organic rice, oat, almond, or goat's milk are generally better tolerated.
- Refined sugars found in cakes, cookies, desserts, and highly processed foods ferment in the gut, causing gas and bloating as unhealthy bacteria proliferate. Healthy bacteria, known as probiotics, help break down digested foods and aid in the manufacture of certain B-group vitamins. If these healthy bacteria are missing, your digestion and elimination will be impaired.
- When you mix flour and water it makes a gooey paste; it does the same in the bowel, so cut down on pastries and flour-based foods.
- Many people are sensitive to wheat, so try cutting back and see if the bloating reduces. Keep a food diary and note when symptoms are worse.
- Low-fiber foods such as jello, ice cream, and soft desserts, all white flour products, and refined breakfast cereals contain virtually no fiber and plenty of sugar, which will all "gum up" the works!
- Also avoid foods to which you have an intolerance: for example, cow's milk has been found to be responsible for a lot of infant constipation.
- Cut down on full-fat cheeses and don't eat melted cheese over food—it sets like plastic in the intestine.

Friendly Foods

- Linseeds (flax seeds) are a blend of insoluble and soluble fibers, which bulk the stool, encouraging it to move gently through the bowel. I soak a tablespoon of linseeds every night in cold water and then drain them the next morning and add to a fruit smoothie, which breaks up the linseeds and makes them fibrous. You can buy golden linseeds or ready-cracked flax seeds (which should be kept in the fridge) from all health stores. For a healthy breakfast smoothie recipe, see under *General Health Hints*.
- Bran is an insoluble fiber derived from rice, soya, or oats. The insoluble fiber is needed to stimulate the bowel to work properly. Wheat bran is fine as long as you don't have an intolerance to wheat, otherwise this can actually aggravate the problem.
- Try eating more brown rice (or rice bran) plus beans such as black-eyed, kidney, haricot, butter, and cannelloni beans, which are high in fiber.
- Whole-wheat rye bread, Ryvita-type crisp breads, rough oatcakes, or amaranth crackers can be eaten as an alternative to wheat bread.
- Other high-fiber foods are fresh and dried figs, blackcurrants, ready-to-eat dried apricots and prunes, almonds, hazelnuts, fresh coconut, and all mixed nuts.
- All lightly cooked or raw vegetables and salads will add more fiber to your diet.
- Eat fruit in between meals or before meals.
- Eat more live, low-fat yoghurts, which contain healthy bacteria—a lack of which can exacerbate constipation.
- Drink at least 6–8 glasses of water daily.
- Psyllium husks are a soluble fiber, which add bulk to the stools. Take a tablespoon of psyllium husks in water before breakfast to help keep things moving. Then make sure you drink plenty of water during the day. Water is essential when taking psyllium.

Useful Remedies

- Use 1–2 tsp a day of any good-quality organic green powder, such as New Chapter Superfood Greens, to aid bowel function and alkalize tissues.
- Otherwise use Green Magic Powder—containing Hawaiian spirulina, chlorella, lecithin, barley and wheat grass, kamut, pectin apple fiber, kelp and wheat sprouts, CoQ10, royal jelly, artichoke powder, and lactobacillus acidophilus, it is a great all-round way to ingest good nutrients and healthy bacteria, keep the body more alkaline and help keep you regular. Details on www.naturalways.com or call 1-800-579-8072.
- Acidophilus and bifidus are healthy bacteria, which can be taken after a meal, particularly if constipation has started after antibiotics. Take one daily after food. **JF, VC, VS**
- Prebiotics are plant nutrients that support the growth of your existing good bacteria. They do not overly ferment and really help to keep you regular. I use Agave Digestive Immune Support. One small scoop daily with breakfast. **LEF**
- Another excellent prebiotic is Molkosan drink from Bioforce, proven to help improve bowel transit time (www.bioforceusa.com).
- Vitamin C powder with added calcium and magnesium—1 level tsp 2–3 times a day for a few days with food—can help soften the stool and increase the frequency of bowel movement; magnesium also helps to increase bowel motions, as it is a smooth muscle relaxant.
- One of the best ways I have found to eliminate constipation is to replace one meal a day with a fruit and vegetable blend, while eliminating all flour from any source for at least two days. I put a tablespoon of organic aloe vera juice, a banana, half a cup of blueberries, an organic apple, a slice of papaya and any fruit I have to hand, plus a teaspoon of any good green food mix, a tablespoon of sunflower seeds, and a tablespoon of soaked linseeds (flax seeds) into a blender. To this I add half a cup of organic rice milk and blend. It's delicious and packed with fiber. On alternate days I make a vegetable juice to which I still add the aloe vera juice but not the rice milk.
- The Herbal Cleansing Kit—based on Dr Christopher's (he was a respected naturopath in the US) herbal cascara formula. Visit www.lifebalm.com

Helpful Hints

- Squatting to pass feces helps to encourage elimination, as it is a more natural position for the colon.
- Overuse of laxatives makes the bowel lazy.
- It is very important that you eliminate any underlying causes for your constipation. Visit your doctor and make sure there is nothing more serious going on.
- Do not bear down too much when you have a bowel movement as this places a strain on the vascular system and can, over time, lead to varicose veins and hemorrhoids or piles. Remember, rather than fall asleep after every meal, go for a leisurely walk. This will make you feel less bloated, aid digestion, and encourage healthier bowels.
- In Chinese medicine the best time to walk is between 5am and 7am, which encourages the colon to work more efficiently. I think I'll pass on this one! Walk any time to aid elimination.
- When you feel the need to pass a motion, be sure not to ignore the signal; take the time to read a magazine on the toilet.
- For healthy bowel movements you need about a pint of fluid in between each meal to get waste moving through successfully.
- Stress is a **major** factor, as it slows down the peristalsis movements.
- When you add more fiber to your diet and you're not used to it, it is essential that you drink more water. Adding fiber without more fluid can actually aggravate the problem.

- In the elderly a lack of folic acid has sometimes been found to be the cause of constipation, so supplementing with folic acid in the form of a good-quality multi-vitamin/mineral should be of help.
- For severe constipation, and with your doctor's permission, consider colonic irrigation. If done properly it can be a godsend. For details of practitioners, see *Useful Information*. You can also use a lukewarm water enema at home. Available from most pharmacies.

CONTRACEPTIVE PILL   *(see Infertility and Pill, Contraceptive)*

COUGHS   *(see also Bronchitis and Colds and Flu)*

Coughs are often due to an infection, such as a cold or flu and sometimes asthma. Many people who smoke develop a persistent cough. Sometimes the cough can lead to production of phlegm; if this is yellow or green in color it indicates a bacterial infection, in which case you need to see a doctor. If you have a cough that persists longer than two weeks or produces blood at any stage, it is very important to seek medical attention and have an X-ray. Coughs that produce a lot of catarrh are often helped by mullein and other expectorant herbs. If the cough is dry and tickly, cherry bark is more useful. A persistent cough, especially after eating foods containing wheat, gluten, or sugar may be linked to candida (see *Candida*), a food intolerance, or leaky gut.

Foods to Avoid
- For a few days, eliminate all cow's dairy products—even skimmed milk, low-fat cheeses, and milk chocolate. I find that if I have a cold I also need to avoid soya milk, which can increase mucus production.
- Cakes, cookies, sausage rolls, meat pies, burgers, and so on should all be avoided for at least 14 days in order to give your sinuses and throat time to clear all mucus. Also avoid white bread and pasta.
- Most foods containing sugar tend to be high in fat, and sugar lowers immune functioning.

Friendly Foods
- Manuka honey: 1 tsp before each meal helps coat the throat but also has antiseptic properties. The higher the Umf (5+ to 20+), the stronger its antiseptic properties.
- Drink plenty of water to keep the throat well lubricated.
- Pineapples help loosen up mucus and make breathing easier. Fresh pear juice is also good for easing coughs.
- If the cough is making you feel tight chested and congested, try adding horseradish, cayenne, or ginger to meals.
- Licorice, either as a tea or sucked as a pure (sugar-free) licorice juice stick, can be very soothing.
- Tea made from fresh thyme can ease the cough and has historically been used for whooping cough.
- Eat plenty of fresh vegetables, chicken, fish, pulses, grains, and fresh fruit.
- Drink herbal teas such as lemon and ginger and try organic rice, almond, or oat milk as a dairy substitute.
- Chocolate can give me a sore throat and cough; any food to which you have an intolerance has the potential to affect you in the same way.

- Live, low-fat plain yogurts, (including goat's milk) are usually well tolerated and they help to boost friendly bacteria in the gut.

Useful Remedies

- Comvita propolis elixir is a great remedy for coughs. It contains propolis, tea tree and manuka honey. It is antiseptic, immune boosting, and soothing. From www.comvita.com
- Zinc lozenges. Suck one every 3–4 hours to ease discomfort of sore throats and reduce the tickling of the cough. Ultimate Zinc-C Lozenges from Now contain vitamins A and C, zinc, echinacea, bee propolis, and slippery elm.
- Olive leaf extract acts like a natural antibiotic and has been found especially useful for respiratory problems. Take 3 capsules daily while symptoms last.
- Include a multi-vitamin and mineral in your regimen.
- A quality echinacea product can stop coughs developing further. Take one teaspoon in water 3 times daily until relief is obtained.
- Massaging a little tea tree oil onto your throat externally may help.
- Use a licorice and glycerine herbal syrup called Traditional Medicinals Throat Coat. **VC**

Helpful Hints

- If you begin wheezing after food or when stressed, you may have developed a touch of asthma; see *Asthma*. Consult a doctor.
- If you find you get tight chested after exercise, 2 grams of vitamin C can often be very helpful. But also see a doctor.
- Taken at the first sign of a cough, homeopathic Aconite 6c can help prevent the cough from developing.

- Keep a food diary and note when symptoms are worse. For example, if your nose runs within a few minutes of eating certain foods, especially cow's milk, wheat- and sugar-based foods, then you may be sensitive to those foods. High-sugar fruits such as grapes can be a problem for some people.
- Dilute a few drops of essential oil of sweet marjoram and frankincense in a grapeseed oil base and massage into your chest and back to encourage deeper breathing.
- Take 2 tablespoons of aloe vera juice every day to soothe your throat and boost your immune system.
- Stop smoking.

CRADLE CAP
(see Dermatitis and Eczema)

CRAMPS
(see also Circulation)

Most people will experience cramp at some time or other and it's a painful muscular spasm or contraction, often caused by a poor blood supply to the muscles. It can also be triggered by extreme exercise and certain prescription drugs such as Protelos, the osteoporosis drug.

Unless you live in a very hot country where you are sweating profusely, it is unlikely to be due to a lack of sodium (salt)—that is, dehydration. Chronic depletion of body fluids from diuretics and poor fluid intake predispose seniors to cramps. Cramp is most commonly caused by poor circulation and lack of magnesium, calcium, or potassium. Low levels of calcium and magnesium are common in a normal pregnancy unless these minerals are supplemented to the diet. Magnesium deficiency is very common in the West and cramps are often the first sign of magnesium deficiency.

Foods to Avoid
- Cut down on white-flour-based foods such as white rice, cookies, cakes, pizza, and pasta, and all forms of sugar and coffee.
- Avoid carbonated drinks; they contain phosphoric acid, which increases calcium loss from bone.
- All of these foods deplete magnesium and potassium from the body.

Friendly Foods
- Plenty of fresh fruits and vegetables, especially bananas, raw cauliflower and jacket potatoes, fresh fruit juices, dried apricots and dates, seafood, and all leafy greens, especially watercress, spinach, spring greens, and kale. Avocado, lean steak, mackerel, and beans are all good sources of magnesium and potassium.
- Eating a banana before going to bed helps to reduce cramps, as bananas are rich in potassium and magnesium.
- Snack on almonds, sesame seeds, and Brazil nuts—all rich in minerals.
- Calcium-rich foods are dried skimmed milk, sesame seeds, sardines, muesli, Parmesan cheese, and curry powder.
- Some breads and milks now have added calcium—check the labels and eat wholemeal rather than mass-produced breads.

Useful Remedies
- Black cohosh and cramp bark; 1–2ml as needed. **VC**
- A liquid multi-mineral is easy for the body to absorb and utilize. **VC**
- Take 200mg of magnesium citrate twice daily with food during the day and an extra 200mg at night, which is often lacking in people who suffer cramps. **VC**

Helpful Hints
- If you tend to get cramps at night, try stretching out your calves before going to bed. If you have a friend or a dog you can walk with, take a regular evening walk.
- Exercise regularly, but not to excess, and indulge yourself with a massage on a regular basis. Use geranium, ginger, and cypress oils in your mix of oils.
- Reflexology helps to improve circulation and reduce cramps if undertaken on a regular basis (see *Useful Information*).

CROHN'S DISEASE   *(see also Absorption, Candida, and Leaky Gut)*

Crohn's disease affects an estimated 359,000 people in the US, though the actual number may be much higher. It is an inflammatory disease of the small intestine that can also affect the bowel (large intestine). Sadly, as many as one in every 400 children suffers this condition; this is a 50% increase in the last 10 years. In general, Crohn's disease develops between the ages of 16 and 30, although it can occur at any age.

This condition causes ulcers and scarring to the wall of the intestines and often occurs in patches with healthy tissues in between. Symptoms are similar to those found in ulcerative colitis and tissue samples may need to be taken. It is the scarring that narrows the passages, thus disrupting nutrient absorption and normal bowel function.

Blood in the stool, weight loss, loss of appetite, nausea, severe abdominal pain or cramps after eating (especially on the lower right side of the abdomen), diarrhea, fever, chills, weakness, and anemia are all common symptoms of this disease. It is quite often associated with other inflammatory conditions within the body that affect the joints, eyes, and skin. Malabsorption of nutrients due to inflammation and/or damage of the gut is one of the biggest problems with Crohn's and up to 85% of sufferers are known to have nutrient deficiencies—therefore it's important that you should also read the *Leaky Gut* section. There can also be a genetic link, but Crohn's has been labeled a modern disease, as it is virtually unknown in "primitive" cultures.

Over-consumption of antibiotics and eating meat and milk from herds that have been given antibiotics and hormones are all suggested as possible triggers, as is a possible autoimmune factor, in which the body's own immune system attacks part of the intestines. Children who are breast-fed are less likely to contract Crohn's. Candida is also linked to this disease, as is a leaky gut. See under *Candida* and *Leaky Gut*. Lack of fiber, parasites, stress, and food intolerances have also been implicated in causing this disease.

Fistulas—tubes that form from one part of the body to another—and fissures (cracks) around the anus are a common complication. Crohn's is also linked to osteoporosis, because of poor absorption of nutrients.

Foods to Avoid
- Over-consumption of sugar is strongly linked with the development of Crohn's and some people find that avoidance of sugar slows the rate of progression.
- Tomatoes, raw fruit, and nuts are often problematic for some people.
- Yeast and dairy products are two food groups that many people find difficult to digest and avoidance of them has helped many sufferers.
- Gluten-rich foods such as wheat, rye, barley, and oats are often a problem.
- Avoid and reduce foods associated with inflammation—alcohol, simple sugars, refined white rice, bread, cakes and pastries, and caffeine.
- Foods high in salicylates are a problem for some sufferers, but not all. Tomatoes, eggplants, peppers, zucchini, berries (such as black- and blueberries and strawberries), radish, olives, chicory, oranges, plums, almonds, pineapple, cherries, raspberries, prunes, and guava are high in salicylates. Keep a food diary.
- Aspirin contains salicylates.

Friendly Foods
- Oily fish, which is a rich source of EPA and DHA, two essential fatty acids, have been found to reduce the severity of Crohn's and the frequency of attacks via their anti-inflammatory action. Crohn's sufferers tend to be low in EFAs. Organic-farmed salmon, mackerel, sardines, herrings, and anchovies should be okay.
- It is important to eat unprocessed foods in their fresh state. Fresh organic fruits and vegetables are best.
- Protein is important for the healing and repair of the intestines. Most sufferers can tolerate meat once or twice a week; if this is a problem, lightly steamed or grilled fish and grilled chicken are often easier to digest. Quinoa and cooked tofu are good forms of protein. Eat with plenty of lightly cooked vegetables.
- If raw fruit is a problem, lightly stew or grill fruits, which makes them a little easier to digest. Papaya is very healing.
- Sweet potatoes, cantaloupe melons, carrots, persimmons, pear, mango, marrow, red cabbage, green beans, lentils, lettuce, rhubarb, celery, potatoes, pomegranate, apple, nuts (except almonds), and figs should all be okay to eat.
- A couple of teaspoons of apple cider vinegar in a little warm water sipped throughout the morning helps to correct the pH level within the bowel and aid liver function.
- Drink the water that you cook any cabbage in, as it helps to heal the digestive lining. If you can't face drinking this, at least make your gravy with cabbage water.
- Try wheat- and gluten-free breads such as Genius, available at supermarkets and health stores.

Useful Remedies

- Green powders help to alkalize the body and the chlorophyll is also healing to intestinal walls. Try Greens Plus. **GP**
- As malabsorption is likely to be a problem, liquid vitamins and minerals are a better choice, as they are more easily absorbed. **VC**
- As magnesium and calcium are usually low, make sure that any multiformula contains around 300mg of calcium and 400 mg of magnesium.
- Quercetin is a type of flavonoid known for its anti-inflammatory action. Take 300mg, 1–3 times per day. Solgar's Quercetin Complex is a good one. **SVHC**
- Make sure you take a high-potency B-complex tablet every day, as folic acid and B12 are often lacking in Crohn's patients.
- Glutamine and butyrate are the primary fuels for the repair of the digestive lining, helping repair and healing. Studies show that both are low in Crohn's patients. Take 4–6 x 500mg of glutamine capsules, split throughout the day, before main meals. Or you can take the glutamine powder in water half an hour or more before meals. Whey protein and hemp seed protein are also useful, as they are rich in highly absorbable proteins. **VC**
- Butyric acid can also be taken separately to aid bowel healing. Take as directed.
- Zinc, 30mg a day, to aid tissue healing.
- A high-strength carotene complex, which will convert naturally to Vitamin A in the body, vital for soft tissue healing
- Take 2 grams of omega-3 fats daily.

- Researchers at McGill University in Montreal have linked vitamin D3 deficiency as a contributing factor to Crohn's disease. Take 1000IU of vitamin D3 daily. Due to genetic links, children of people with Crohn's would be wise to take vitamin D3 daily to help switch on the NOD2 gene, which is often defective or deficient in Crohn's sufferers.
- Take digestive enzymes to help absorption of nutrients with meals, after the first few mouthfuls. If you are having a large or rich meal you may need 2 capsules. **VC**
- Make sure you take friendly bacteria daily: acidophilus and bifidus are available at all good health stores and should be taken after meals. These really help to reduce food sensitivities.
- Organic aloe vera really aids healing. Take one eggcupful 3 times daily before meals.
- Curcumin from turmeric has anti-inflammatory properties in the bowel. Take a concentrate capsule with main meals. **VC**
- Omega-7 essential fats extracted from sea buckthorn help heal the mucosal gut lining. Take 2 grams daily initially and then reduce to 1 gram daily for the long term. **VC**

Helpful Hints

- You may need supplementation of the hormone DHEA—have a blood test to check for levels.
- When beginning to use digestive enzymes and other digestive supplements, it is best to do so gradually, so as not to shock the system. For example, if the directions suggest 1 three times per day, build up to this over a week.
- Evidence that food intolerances trigger Crohn's are thin on the ground, but it is widely acknowledged that they may aggravate and irritate the intestines—thus making the condition worse. It may be worth checking for intolerances and avoiding offending foods. ALCAT offers comprehensive food tests (www.alcat.com)
- Smoking has been linked with the development of Crohn's disease.
- Lymph drainage massage and skin brushing help to eliminate toxins from the body.
- Buy foods as fresh as possible—they will be more nutrient rich. Everything will taste better and you'll appreciate the effort in the long run.
- Crohn's disease is greatly exacerbated by stress, therefore any techniques known to reduce

stress, such as yoga, t'ai chi, meditation, massage, or hypnotherapy will help. Spiritual healing has helped many sufferers (see *Healing*).

- Adequate rest is essential for any Crohn's sufferer, and gentle exercise, such as walking and swimming, will also help.
- To re-balance your diet and make sure you are taking the right supplements and herbs in the correct amount for your case, I strongly suggest that you consult a doctor who is also a nutritionist (see *Useful Information*).
- Avoid wearing tight clothing around the waist as this can make you more uncomfortable.
- For further help, contact The Crohn's and Colitis and Crohn's Foundation of America (CCFA), 386 Park Avenue South, 17th Floor, New York, NY 10016. Information Line: 1-800-932-2423. Email: info@ccfa.org. Website: www.ccfa.org The site has helpful information and resources for children and teens with Crohn's.

CYSTITIS
(see also Candida and Thrush)

Cystitis is far more common in women than in men and can also affect children. One-third of all women contract a urinary tract infection such as cystitis before the age of 25. It is caused by a bacterial infection in the bladder and symptoms include a frequent and urgent urge to urinate, plus a burning sensation when passing urine. With cystitis or thrush there can be a whitish/yellow discharge—but this is more common with thrush, which is a yeast overgrowth. Whatever the cause, the entire outer area can swell, which makes sitting extremely uncomfortable indeed.

If lymph nodes in the groin begin to swell (near the bikini line) or if you have pain in the loins, blood in your urine, or a fever, this denotes a kidney infection and you **must** see a doctor. A urine test can confirm which bug is responsible and usually antibiotics are then prescribed. Women who suffer from candida and food intolerances regularly suffer thrush or cystitis (see also *Candida*).

These types of infections are more likely to occur in warm, moist, humid atmospheres. If you are run down, you are more prone to an attack, as your immune system is functioning under par. If you suffer thrush regularly you may be diabetic, in which case a blood test should be taken to eliminate this possibility.

Foods to Avoid
- While symptoms are acute, avoid as much as possible all foods and drinks containing sugar and yeast—especially cheeses, malt vinegar, ketchups, soy sauce, miso, pickled foods, yeast-based breads, mushrooms, and alcohol.
- Avoid sugar in **any** form, including honey, maltose and so on, as all sugars will feed the yeast. For the first week also avoid all cakes, cookies, pizza, or fizzy cola-type drinks and desserts.
- Avoid junk-type burgers and fried foods, which are hard to digest and add to the toxic load.
- Also you will need to avoid high-sugar fruits, such as grapes, melons, and bananas for the first few days.
- Dried fruits are very high in sugar.
- See this section under *Candida*.

Friendly Foods
- Eat plenty of live, low-fat yoghurt that contains the friendly bacteria, acidophilus and bifidus.
- Try cranberry juice without sugar or eat fresh or frozen cranberries. They are rich in hippuric acid, which helps prevent bacteria clinging to the bladder walls. The concentrate in capsules is in this case is more effective.

- Drink plenty of fluids but no sugary drinks.
- As these types of conditions thrive in an acid environment, eat plenty of salads and green vegetables, especially watercress, cabbage, spring greens, kale, and so on, as these are all alkaline.
- Include apples, cherries, pineapples, papaya, and pears for fruits.
- Eat more garlic and onions, which are highly anti-bacterial.
- See also this section under *Candida*.

Useful Remedies

- Nature's Way Cranberry Fruit capsules are made from 100% cranberry fruit solids and are sugar- and preservative-free. One 465mg capsule daily will help to fight and prevent urinary tract infections. **VC**
- Take bromelain, extracted from pineapple, for its anti-inflammatory properties—500mg twice daily.
- A high-strength, natural-source carotene complex, which converts naturally to vitamin A in the body, taken daily helps support immune function.
- To help to re-alkalize your system, which will benefit your immune system and thus reduce incidence for problems such as candida, you should take a green powder—one small level teaspoon daily in water, preferably taken 30 minutes before a meal or in between meals. **VC, VS**
- Vitamin C and flavonoids help to fight the infection. Take up to 4 grams daily with food for the first week and then reduce to 1 gram daily. When you take large doses of vitamin C, make sure it's in an ascorbate form, which is gentle on the stomach.
- Take 2 acidophilis/bifidus capsules daily with food for at least 6 weeks. With Jarro-Dophilus EPS, take one daily with food. **JF**
- Include a high-strength multi-vitamin and mineral in this program.
- Try GSE grapefruit seed extract, which comes in liquid form, and is anti-fungal. Take a few drops in water or juice. **VC**
- Or take an oregano tincture, 4 drops in half a cup of water; it has powerful anti-bacterial and anti-fungal properties (www.amazon.com).

Helpful Hints

- To make your own sodium citrate (which is what chemists sell for this problem), squeeze half a lemon into a glass, add a quarter of a glass of water, and then add a third of a teaspoon of bi-carbonate of soda. This mix will fizz; stir and drink while it is still fizzing. Do this three times daily between meals, starting before breakfast, until the symptoms have gone. If you took this blend every day before breakfast it would help stop the condition re-occurring.
- Urinate as soon as possible after having sexual intercourse to stop transmission of bacteria into the bladder. If symptoms are acute, avoid intercourse for at least one week, as you can pass the bacteria from one partner to another.
- Consuming live yogurt on a daily basis can reduce the incidence of developing cystitis or thrush.
- Drink organic aloe vera juice containing extract of cranberry and cherries three times daily.
- Drink three to four cups of nettle tea daily. Goldenseal tea may also be helpful, as it contains berberine, an alkaloid that inhibits bacteria from adhering to the wall of the bladder.
- Drink plenty of water each day to help flush out unhealthy organisms from the bladder.
- Avoid perfumed soaps and vaginal deodorants at all times.
- Wear cotton underwear. Avoid tightly fitted jeans, especially in hot weather.
- As much as possible when you are at home, wear a skirt and no underwear to keep the vaginal area cool.

- If you have to sit all day, get up and walk around regularly.
- Get plenty of rest.
- Use a pH-balanced soap.
- Douche daily with diluted tea tree oil, crushed garlic, and lavender oil or add a few drops to your bath.
- Acupuncture and homeopathic remedies such as Cantharis 30c will help reduce the burning sensation, while Apis 30c can be taken if stinging is a problem (see *Useful Information*).

DANDRUFF   *(see Scalp Problems)*

DEEP VEIN THROMBOSIS (DVT)   *(see Jet Lag)*

DVT occurs when a blood clot forms within a deep vein, most commonly in the lower leg or the calf area, but in rarer cases it can occur in the thigh or even the arms. DVT can be mistaken for leg cramps or sore muscles, but as DVT is life threatening, urgent medical attention is needed. Symptoms are swelling in the leg affected by the clot, pain and tenderness, and difficulty in placing any weight on the bad leg. The skin may also become red and feel warm to the touch. If you have any of these symptoms seek immediate medical advice, especially after a lengthy flight or if you have been bedridden for any reason. DVT can also occur after lengthy periods of stationary activity such as sitting at a desk or in a car.

Pulmonary embolism is a serious complication of DVT, which happens when a piece of a blood clot travels via the bloodstream to the lungs. This can be fatal if immediate medical intervention is not available. Typical symptoms would be chest pain, breathlessness, potentially coughing up blood, or fainting. Dial 911 immediately.

It's worth noting that people who have Type A or Type AB blood are more prone to clotting disorders.

Foods to Avoid
- See this section under *Circulation*.

Friendly Foods
- Drink plenty of fluids to keep the lymph system functioning.
- Eat light meals when traveling and while in the hospital. (See this section under *Circulation*.)

Useful remedies
- If you are worried about contracting DVT on a long flight, take some high-strength ginkgo biloba and gotu kola (500mg daily) a few days before you leave as well as during your flight. These natural remedies increase circulation. The gotu kola helps increase circulation in the lower limbs, and a positive side effect is sometimes a slight loosening of the bowels!
- Bromelain from pineapples helps thin the blood naturally. Take 500mg three times daily, starting two weeks before you travel. **NB: If you are on Warfarin, check with your doctor before taking this supplement.**
- Natural-source, full-spectrum vitamin E thins the blood and reduces the risk of clotting on

long flights. Take 400IU at least two weeks prior to traveling and during the journey. **NB: If you are taking blood-thinning drugs, check with your doctor.**

- There is also a supplement called Zinopin, which contains pine bark extract (pycnogenol) and ginger. It has the anti-clotting activity of aspirin, only without the negative side effects. Ginger is also useful against travel sickness. Available from www.zinopinusa.com
- Take 2g of omega-3 fish oils daily.
- Take a teaspoon of baking soda in warm water twice daily (away from meals) to re-alkalize your body's fluids. When the body has too much acid, you are more likely to get too much stickiness in the blood. Start taking this remedy a week before your flight and a week after.
- Nattokinase, an extract of Natto, helps break down fibrin in the blood to prevent blood clots. Take in between meals for a few days before, during, and after traveling. For more information about a good Natto product called NKCP, visit www.nkcp.org **NB: If you are taking Warfarin, you should not take this supplement.**

Helpful Hints

- Buy some good support hose or socks. These are now sold at all major airports and pharmacies. A neck pillow can also be useful so you can try to relax and sleep more comfortably.
- Keep walking around the plane as much as you can. Use the aisles to do a few squats and raise your arms up and down; stretch out as much as you can.
- If you are in the hospital or confined to your bed, then with medical supervision, start moving around as much as you can.

- Keep in mind that DVT can also occur after long car trips and in people who sit too long at their desk. To keep blood flowing, and when safe to do so, press both feet firmly into the ground and flex your leg muscles. You can also flex your feet up and down and round and round to get your circulation moving.
- People more at risk for developing pulmonary embolism are those undergoing major surgery, women who are pregnant, people who have been confined to their bed, women taking HRT or the contraceptive pill, or those who are obese and/or suffer from high blood pressure.
- Smoking more than 25 cigarettes a day can increase your risk.
- Walk and move regularly; have a good stretch.
- Massage your lower legs from the feet upwards every hour or so. Go quite deep to "rev" up your circulation.

DEMENTIA
(see Alzheimer's Disease)

DEPRESSION
(see also Adrenal Exhaustion and Stress)

According to the National Institute of Mental Health, one in four American adults suffers from some type of diagnosable mental disorder, and anxiety and depression are the most common. Around 10% of the adult population struggles with depression and its affects on self-esteem, work and home life, and relationships. More women tend to suffer from depression than men. In fact, women have twice the risk of depression as men. Growing numbers of children—around one in five under the age of 18—have a mental health problem, including depression.

There is a world of difference between having a bad day and suffering from full-blown depression. Older people tend to suffer more incidences of depression due to poor nutrition, the loss of a loved one, feelings of no longer being useful, and so on. Persistent mild depression at any age lowers immunity and the ability to fight off disease.

A truly depressed person has an all-pervading feeling of sadness. Other typical symptoms include feeling worthless, inadequate, or incompetent. If you also suffer from loss of interest or pleasure in your job, family life, hobbies or sex, difficulty concentrating or remembering, insomnia, over- or under-eating, unusual irritability, a sense of humor failure, a feeling of being downhearted that just won't go away, frequent unexplained crying spells, or recurrent thoughts of death or suicide, then you may be clinically depressed and should seek help.

Depressed people often isolate themselves by withdrawing from friends and family. However, not all symptoms denote clinical depression. For example, if you are feeling total apathy, like you just don't want to get up in the morning, then such symptoms can most definitely be linked to adrenal exhaustion (see *Adrenal Exhaustion*). Hormonal imbalances, low blood sugar, and poor thyroid function can also trigger depressive-like symptoms (see these specific sections for extra help).

The more junk, pre-packaged, high-saturated fat, sugary-type foods and drinks you ingest, the more likely you are to feel depressed. This is because you are deficient in vital nutrients and essential fats, and your body's demand is exceeding its supply. When violent, hyperactive, and depressed people are given a healthier diet, exercise more, and take the right supplements, their personalities usually alter completely for the better. Sugar and stimulants alter brain chemistry, which alters behavior. This has been proven time and time again, and it's now time for us to take notice and act.

Foods to Avoid
- Avoid or reduce alcohol because it can make depression worse. Alcohol lowers levels of the feel-good hormone serotonin, plus the B-vitamins needed for energy and nerve health in the mind and body.
- If you eat too much refined sugar, your blood sugar levels keep fluctuating, which can greatly affect your mood. (See *Insulin Resistance* and *Diabetes*.)
- Excessive consumption of refined, processed, fatty foods and caffeine can make your depression worse, as they deplete vitamins B (needed for healthy nervous system) and C as well as the mineral chromium (if you do not have sufficient chromium, your blood sugar levels will become unbalanced, triggering mood swings).
- Avoid the sweetener aspartame at all costs. It can have neurological side effects and has been shown to interact negatively with antidepressants. For further information visit www.dorway.com.
- Which foods do you tend to crave and eat the most? I'll bet it's wheat and sugar. If this is the case, be aware that the foods you crave are usually the ones that make your symptoms worse. It takes discipline, but for 7 days avoid these foods and replace with fresh fruits, vegetables, and grains like brown rice and see how much better you feel.
- Lack of iron is also linked to depression, but iron accumulates in the body and is linked to heart disease in those over 50. Your doctor can find out via a blood test if you are deficient.

Friendly Foods
- The brain is made up of around 60% fats, so eat more of the right kind of fats including oily fish such as farmed organic salmon, mackerel, anchovies, and sardines; linseeds (flax seeds); hemp seeds; soybeans; and wheat germ, which are all rich in omega-3 essential fats.
- Sardines are high in DMAE, a brain stimulant that helps elevate mood. (See below: vitamin B5 encourages the body to produce more DMAE.)

- Walnuts, pecans, Brazil nuts, and hazelnuts, plus sunflower and pumpkin seeds are all rich in omega-6 essential fats.
- Use unrefined nut and seed oils for salad dressings. (See *Fats You Need to Eat*.)
- Make sure you eat breakfast. A good option is to make oatmeal with half rice or almond milk and half water. Sweeten with a little honey and raisins, and add a few blueberries, banana, or chopped apples to sweeten. Even better, sprinkle a few sunflower seeds over the top for EFAs.
- Increase your intake of fresh fruits, vegetables, and whole grains such as brown rice, quinoa, non-wheat pastas, barley, and lentils.
- To help raise serotonin levels, eat more foods containing tryptophan, such as fish, turkey, avocado, cottage cheese, organic meats, beans, lentils, cooked tofu, wheat germ, and bananas.
- Foods containing the amino acids phenylalinine and tyrosine can also help to raise mood and boost motivation; these include low-fat meats, fish, eggs, wheat germ, dairy foods, oats, nuts, avocados, bananas, and chocolate. This is why eating chocolate often makes you feel good. But eat dark chocolate, not milk. If you are a chocoholic, try taking 250–500mg of DLPA (DL-phenylalinine) with 2mg of vitamin B6 and 500mg of vitamin C on an empty stomach before breakfast.
- Spicy foods that contain cayenne pepper produce endorphins that help raise your mood.
- Drink 6–8 glasses of water daily to help remove toxins.

Useful Remedies

- If you are taking prescription drugs for clinical depression, you must check with your doctor before trying these remedies.
- First, begin taking a high-strength multi-vitamin/mineral to give you a good nutrient base plus the B-vitamins, a lack of which can trigger depression and low mood.
- Various B-vitamins play a major role in maintaining proper brain chemistry, and deficiencies of B-vitamins are common in depressed people. Therefore, take a high-strength complex that contains at least 50mg of all the Bs. B2 turns your urine bright yellow—but this is normal!
- As well as the B-complex, also take 250–500mg of B5 (pantothenic acid), which supports your adrenals and increases levels of DMAE in the brain, which raises mood.
- Most people over 65 are deficient in Vitamin D, a lack of which is now linked to 17 different medical conditions. There is no doubt it raises mood, so take 800–1000IU of vitamin D3 daily.
- Take 1g of vitamin C daily with food.
- Omega-3 fats are vital for improving depression and have been shown in many cases to be more effective than antidepressant drugs. If you are not eating oily fish three times a week, then take 2g of omega-3 daily.
- Sprinkle one tablespoon of non-GM soy lecithin granules over cereals and fruit dishes. Lecithin is high in the brain nutrient, phosphatidyl serine.
- 5-Hydroxytryptophan (5-HTP) helps raise serotonin levels in the brain. Extracted from the griffonia plant from Africa, 5-HTP helps balance mood, aids you in falling asleep more easily, reduces aggression, reduces appetite, and creates a more relaxed waking state within 45 minutes. Recommended dose: 50mg up to 300mg per day. For best results, start on a low dosage; take at bedtime along with a small carbohydrate snack such as an oatcake. If you need to, gradually work up to 300mg. If your mood stabilizes, gradually lower the dose until you find how much you need. Taking more than you need will not be helpful in the long run. This supplement is more effective if taken with B-vitamins and 10mg of zinc. Be patient, as it can take a few weeks for the full effects of 5-HTP to work. **VC, NOW**
- In a clinical study, DHEA hormone supplementation was tested on middle-aged and elderly

patients with major depression for four weeks. Depression ratings and memory performance significantly improved. DHEA in other human studies significantly elevated mood in elderly people. Recommended dose: 50mg a day for men and 15–20mg per day for women. **VC, LEF**

- Ginseng is an adrenal tonic that is useful for people who are depressed, as their adrenal glands are usually functioning under par (see *Adrenal Exhaustion*). Take two Panax Red Ginseng capsules, one with breakfast and one with lunch. Not at night. **NB: Do not take ginseng if you are on blood thinners.**

- The herb St John's wort has been proven to help milder forms of depression. In more than 25 double-blind studies of more than 1,500 people, St John's wort demonstrated its effectiveness in improving mood, lessening anxiety, and reducing sleep disorders. St John's wort helps reduce the sadness, stress, and feelings of helplessness that come with depression. Recommended dosage: 900mg daily of 0.3 percent hypericin concentration, 600mg with breakfast and 300mg with lunch. **NB: Do not take St John's wort if you are pregnant or on the contraceptive pill. Also avoid intense sun exposure while using it, since this herb can make the skin more sensitive to sunlight. Do not take St John's wort with 5-HTP and drugs such as Prozac, Zoloft, and Paxil.**

Helpful Hints

- Natural sunlight helps suppress production of the hormone melatonin, which is produced by the pineal gland at night. This is why we tend to feel more depressed and sleepy during the winter months. Melatonin aids sleep and acts as an important antioxidant, but if you are depressed then you need less melatonin. Therefore, get out into the sun as much as you possibly can, especially in the mornings, and if you work in an office without full-spectrum lighting, make sure to use full-spectrum light bulbs at home and where you can at work.

- Try using Real Sunlight lamps, available online from Amazon. The harmful frequencies of UVA and UVB have been filtered out to make this sunlight safe. These lamps were developed in Sweden and are now used in many homes to boost immune function and relieve depression. These lamps naturally increase levels of vitamin D3, boost immune function, and reduce depression.

- Regular exercise is vital in the fight against depression. Exercise and sunlight release endorphins, natural antidepressants, which raise your mood. Regular exercise can also help you sleep better, feel better, look better, and provide you with an enhanced self-image. A German study showed a significant reduction in depression when patients walked for 30 minutes a day, and other studies have shown that regular exercise is as effective as antidepressants and that it can be more effective against relapse than drugs.

- Studies have shown that having control over roles, such as being a parent, grandparent, or provider, can add value to an elderly person's life. Many companies are at last waking up to the fact that people over 65 are more committed, take fewer sick days, and are more experienced workers who tend to be more cost effective than younger people. Take charge of your life!

- Consider seeing a counselor—a problem shared is a problem halved and counseling is often far more successful than taking antidepressants. You can also try talking about your innermost fears with a friend or relative; they may not even realize you are depressed. To find a qualified counselor near you, contact the American Counseling Association, 5999 Stevenson Ave., Alexandria, VA 22304. Tel: 1-800-347-6647. Website: www.counseling.org

- Do volunteer work, as helping others can boost self-esteem.

- Watch videos, DVDs, and films that make you laugh. Laughter produces natural mood-boosting chemicals in the body.

- Be sure to get enough quality sleep, but get up after 8 hours or so.

- Blend pure oils of bergamot, clary sage, geranium, and neroli in a base of almond oil and ask a friend or relative to give you a massage. These aromatherapy oils will help lift your mood.
- For further help, read *New Optimum Nutrition for the Mind* by Patrick Holford (Piatkus), available in most book stores and online at Amazon.
- Mental Health America is the largest and oldest community-based mental health network in the US. They have more than 300 affiliates throughout the country and provide education, prevention, and recovery programs and other services. For more information call 1-800-273-TALK or visit www.mentalhealthamerica.net

DERMATITIS—SEBORRHEIC DERMATITIS (cradle cap)
(see also Eczema and Leaky Gut)

Seborrheic dermatitis is basically a type of eczema (see under *Eczema*) that commonly occurs on children's scalps. This is why it's often called cradle cap. In most infants it tends to clear up in the first year or so. Symptoms are thick scaly tissue on the scalp, in particular, and sometimes around the eyes and ears. The problem is linked to a deficiency in essential fatty acids and one of the B-vitamins, biotin. Eliminating allergens from the diet usually helps clear cradle cap. Fungi are also implicated in this problem because as children's immune systems develop, they are more susceptible to various organisms.

You can also suffer varying degrees of dermatitis in adult years—triggered by exposure to hair colorants, paints, hairsprays, and all manner of chemicals in cosmetic products, household cleaners, and detergents. Non-specific skin rashes can also be linked to liver toxicity (see *Liver Problems*), poor immune function and food intolerances (see *Allergies* and *Leaky Gut*).

Foods to Avoid
- The most common offending foods for causing cradle cap and eczema are cow's milk and products, wheat, and eggs. As with any problem that may be influenced by food intolerances, it is important to identify the problematic foods. (See *Allergies*.)
- Avoid mass-produced, refined, white-flour-based foods and any foods and drinks that are high in sugar.
- Colorings, additives, and preservatives in shampoos, toiletries, toothpastes, and foods (especially sweets and drinks) are well known to trigger reactions, especially in children.

Friendly Foods
- Make your child nutrient-rich fruit blends—chop any fruit you have on hand (such as bananas, papaya, apple, pears, etc.) and place in a blender. Add a couple of teaspoons of sunflower seeds and flax seeds that have been soaked overnight in cold water (flax seeds/linseeds are rich in essential fats). Add a low-fat, live yogurt (try goat's or sheep's yogurt) and blend for 30–40 seconds. This makes a healthy dessert. Children can usually digest dairy products made from goat's and sheep's milk more easily than those from cows.
- Oils such as Udo's Choice, a blend of omega-3 and -6 fats, can be added to food once cooked; a teaspoon a day should be fine. I find that if you cook some sweet potatoes and mash them with a little almond or oat milk and then add the oil as they are cooling, the child cannot taste the oil. Otherwise, add to thick vegetable soups and stews before serving.
- For adults with dermatitis, eat plenty of fruits, vegetables, oily fish, and whole grains such as brown rice, quinoa, and barley. (See this section under *Eczema*.)

Useful Remedies

- Many companies make liquid multi-vitamins and minerals for children, which you can add to cold dishes to make sure your child is not malnourished. Nature's Plus makes an excellent children's range. **NP**
- Alternatively, you can add organic-source green food powders rich in vitamins, minerals, and essential fats to breakfast cereals or desserts.
- Supplement biotin, a B vitamin that is often lacking; take 6mg daily.
- As all the B vitamins work together in the body, if you are breast-feeding or an adult with this condition, also take a B-complex daily. Children would get this in their multi.
- If the child is being breast-fed, it is useful for the mother to take 10mg of biotin—which will in turn be delivered through the milk—or to eat more biotin-rich foods, such as liver and egg yolk.
- Essential fats can be applied directly to the affected areas. It should be applied twice a day for 2–4 weeks. Use either evening primrose or borage oil. You can also take 2000mg of evening primrose oil daily.
- Adults should take a high-strength multi-vitamin/mineral plus an essential-fatty-acid formula daily.
- Colostrum, which is found in breast milk, helps support the immune system and aids in healing leaky guts. It's very helpful for babies and children suffering from eczema. Until the age of 2, take a quarter of a teaspoon twice daily on an empty stomach. Over 2 years—half a teaspoon twice daily. Take this for just one month. **VC**

Helpful Hints

- Buy products in their most natural and unadulterated state, as they are gentler on a child's delicate skin. For anyone who suffers from dermatitis or skin allergies, Weleda makes organic face creams, shampoos, body lotions, deodorants, toothpastes, and even baby care products. Tel: 1-800-241-1030. Email: info@weleda.com Website: usa.weleda.com
- Note that many toothpastes, shampoos, soaps, detergents, perfumes, and so on contain a myriad of chemicals. I have met several dozen hairdressers who suffer from this condition caused by all of the chemicals they are in contact with every day.
- Apply a little manuka honey cream from Living Nature or the Organic Skin Rescue Oil from the Organic Pharmacy. You can also contact an organic pharmacist, who can suggest a specific remedy for your particular symptoms. **OP**
- Use aloe vera gel topically to help calm the itching.

DIABETES—TYPES I AND II

(see also Circulation, Insulin Resistance, and Weight Problems)

Approximately 23.6 million people in the US suffer from diabetes. Only 5–10% have Type I—a life-long condition that requires insulin—meaning that the vast majority of diabetics have Type II, triggered by our ever-escalating rates of obesity and poor diets. Most alarmingly, children as young as eight are now developing late-onset (Type II) diabetes—which 20 years ago would only be seen in people over 50. This is shocking, especially when you consider that around 80% of late-onset diabetes patients will die of cardiovascular disease. Make no mistake: late-onset diabetes can shorten your life, and yet it is totally preventable.

Type I diabetes is caused by the failure of the pancreas to secrete adequate insulin. Type II diabetes, however, is generally characterized by adequate insulin production, but, the body has become resistant to it and simply doesn't respond to the insulin as it should. Type I diabetes is a life-long condition, which usually starts during early childhood. Both types of diabetes involve very high levels of sugar in the blood. The hormone insulin is responsible for lowering blood sugar levels.

Symptoms of Type I and II diabetes are: increased thirst, fatigue, unexplained weight loss, blurred vision, increased urination, especially at night, and regular episodes of thrush. Complications associated with diabetes include peripheral neuropathy such as numbness, tingling, or throbbing in extremities, poor circulation, slow wound healing, and in adults, impotence and eye problems. There is a greater risk for gangrene, heart disease, and blindness.

The cascade of late-onset diabetes is placing a huge burden on the US healthcare system, costing approximately $174 billion in 2007. This situation has been triggered by our over-consumption of refined, sugar-based foods such as cakes, cookies, and sugar-filled carbonated drinks. Therefore, despite high levels of insulin, glucose is not properly transported into the cells and it increases to unacceptable levels in the blood. Your body tries to get rid of excess sugar in the urine, which is why doctors test for diabetes through urine—although a blood test is more accurate.

While diabetes can have a hereditary link, your genes interact with your environment (including your diet) to either improve or worsen your health. We can inherit more from our parents than just their genes; their eating habits are often passed on, too.

If you are diagnosed with diabetes by your doctor via a fasting blood test, you will very likely be offered various courses of action. In mild cases, late-onset diabetes can be kept in check by diet alone. If severe, the diet is accompanied by oral medication or injections to either increase the production of insulin or improve your sensitivity to insulin. Over the years I have interviewed many elderly diabetics and have been appalled that they have not been offered any advice on diet. Most cases of late-onset diabetes can be kept in check by eating a healthier diet!

Foods to Avoid

- See also diet in *Insulin Resistance*.
- Avoid sugar and foods containing sugar, such as carbonated drinks, chocolate, desserts, and sweets, which release their sugars too quickly into the bloodstream. According to the American Heart Association, sugary drinks alone contribute to 130,000 cases of Type II diabetes annually—and these figures are rising fast.
- Avoid refined, mass-produced "white" flour and rice-based foods such as pizza, white rice and pastas, white breads, cakes, and cookies, which are usually high in sugar and saturated fats.
- Honey, maltose, and dextrose are still sugars and can exacerbate the problem.
- Be aware that most foods advertised as being low in fat are often high in sugar.
- Don't drink concentrated store-bought fruit juices. Make fresh juices or dilute low-sugar juices with one part juice to two parts water.
- Reduce saturated fats from animal sources to less than 10% of your daily food intake. Cheese, chocolates, full-fat dairy products, red meats, pies, sausages, and fried foods need to be kept to a minimum.
- Cut out red meats or only eat occasional organic lean steak, turkey, pork, venison, or chicken with the fat removed.
- Reduce your use of sodium-based table salts; look for magnesium- rich sea salts instead. Also, only add a little to the food on your plate. Otherwise, used powdered kelp or nori flakes as a salt substitute. Himalayan Crystal Salt is another healthier alternative. Available from good health stores, www.amazon.com and www.himalayancrystalsalt.com

- Too much iron and copper in the body increases the risk of diabetes and heart disease. Read labels, especially on fortified cereals, and cut right down on red meat. Eat more curcumin (turmeric), which detoxifies the body of these metals.

Friendly Foods

- Eat more unrefined, high-fiber carbohydrates, such as whole-wheat or rye bread, oat cookies, amaranth crackers, brown rice, buckwheat, oats (especially oatmeal), and sweet potatoes, plus low-fat proteins such as beans, pulses, lentils, and barley.
- Eggs, tofu, low-fat meats, fish, hemp seeds, lentils, chickpeas, and all pulses help balance blood sugar.
- Fruits and vegetables are high in antioxidants and soluble fiber; eat them raw as much as possible.
- Fish oils have been shown to improve pre-diabetes and insulin resistance, and help prevent full-blown late-onset diabetes from developing. Therefore, eat more oily and fresh fish, but don't fry it—poaching or grilling are best.
- Eat more unrefined sunflower, pumpkin, sesame and linseeds (flax seeds) and their unrefined oils, which are rich in omega-3 and -6 essential fats.
- Blend these oils half and half with extra-virgin olive oil for salad dressings.
- Vitamin E-rich foods help lower the risk of many conditions associated with diabetes, such as circulation and eye problems. Food sources are soybeans, raw wheat germ, sprouting seeds, avocados, green vegetables, eggs and unrefined and unprocessed nuts, especially almonds and hazelnuts. Look for low-sugar muesli that is rich in nuts and oats, and sprinkle raw wheat germ onto it.
- Eat fresh bilberries, blueberries, blackberries, papaya, spinach, watercress, sweet potatoes, pumpkin and apricots, as these fruits help protect the eyes.
- Use lots of cinnamon in your foods, as it has been shown to help reduce glucose levels in the blood.
- Eat more curries, as curcumin has been shown to reduce the chances of developing diabetes if you are overweight.
- Organic agave syrup and xylitol (found in fruit fiber) are natural sugars that have low glycemic counts and therefore a minimal impact on blood sugar levels. Use small amounts. Available online and from most health stores.

D

Useful Remedies

- A high-strength, multi-vitamin/mineral complex taken every day provides a good foundation of nutrients.
- The mineral chromium (200mcg) is vital for helping control and prevent late-onset diabetes. Scientists in the US found that taking 200mcg of chromium daily helped reduce the incidence of late-onset diabetes by up to 50%. Chromium also helps reduce cravings for sweet foods. And in time, chromium should enable you to reduce your medication, which you would need to discuss with your doctor.
- Lipoic acid and L-carnitine are two potent nutrients that help dramatically lower blood sugar. Take 250 mg of lipoic acid daily and 500mg of L-carnitine twice daily.
- Vitamin C (1g twice daily) can lower glucose response.
- Magnesium, needed to process insulin, is usually lacking in diabetics. Take a multi-mineral daily that contains 300–450mg of magnesium, 20mg of zinc, and a trace amount of copper.
- Take a B-complex, as diabetic patients are usually deficient in B vitamins, which are needed for energy production and nerve health.
- If you don't eat oily fish regularly, take 2g of omega-3 fish oil daily. Make sure it is free from PCBs and dioxins. BioCare and Seven Seas make pure fish oil capsules.

- The hormone DHEA (see *Menopause*) helps lower insulin levels and protects vital organs, particularly the kidneys, against damage due to high blood glucose. Don't take hormones unless tests have shown that you need them.
- Aloe vera juice helps lower blood-sugar levels in non-insulin-dependant diabetes.
- Nettle tea helps lower blood sugar.
- As we age we produce less Co-enzyme Q10, a vital vitamin-like nutrient that protects against heart disease. Take 100mg daily with either breakfast or lunch.
- Researchers at the University of Granada in Spain found that taking olive leaf extract helps stimulate the production and utilization of insulin. Take 500mg twice daily.
- Pine bark extract, known as pycnogenol, has been shown to help protect against diabetic retinopathy. Take 80mg daily. **NOW**
- **NB: Taking supplements can affect blood sugar levels, so any supplement regimen should only be undertaken with the help of a medical doctor and/or a nutritionist.**

Helpful Hints
- If you are overweight you greatly increase your risk for diabetes, especially after age 50. (See *Weight Problems*.)
- Regular exercise is vital, because it reduces the need for insulin, reduces blood cholesterol, and prevents obesity. It doesn't have to be intense exercise, but try to walk for at least 30 minutes daily, as regular walking has been shown to improve insulin sensitivity and glucose management. If you have been a "couch potato" for a long time, just start gently. Walk for 15 minutes a day and then build up over a month to 30 minutes daily and within another month to 45 minutes or even an hour.

- Have regular eye check-ups and see a podiatrist who can keep an eye on your feet, as both can be affected by diabetes.
- Have regular reflexology on your feet, which improves circulation. (See *Useful Information*.)
- For further help contact the American Diabetes Association. Tel: 1-800-342-2383, Monday–Friday, 8:30am–8pm EST. Website: www.diabetes.org
- Try reading *How To Prevent and Treat Diabetes with Natural Medicine* by Dr Michael Murray. You can also take a look at the author's website: www.doctormurray.com

DIARRHEA   *(see also Crohn's Disease, Colitis and Irritable Bowel Syndrome)*

Diarrhea can have several causes including infectious bacteria, food poisoning, food allergy or intolerance, IBS or yeast overgrowth (see also *Candida*). It may also be associated with more serious conditions such as Crohn's disease or ulcerative colitis. If it is a chronic problem, diarrhea is more likely to be associated with a food intolerance or a parasite. Severe diarrhea, especially in babies and children, must be treated quickly, as the body can rapidly become dehydrated, and the person can eventually lose consciousness. Adequate intake of fluids, particularly water, as well as powdered electrolyte drinks should be given hourly to prevent severe dehydration. Babies and children must see a doctor.

Foods to Avoid
- Many people who have a sensitivity to wheat and possibly gluten suffer from chronic diarrhea.
- Certain foods—example, concentrated fruit juices or overripe fruits—can make the situation worse. However, it's important to discover if you have food intolerances and to keep a food diary and note when symptoms are worse.

- Avoid sorbitol, which is used as a sweetening agent.
- Lactose, the sugar in milk, is a common cause of chronic diarrhea.
- If you are a regular coffee drinker, it's worth giving it up for a few days to see if this helps.

Friendly Foods

- Try arrowroot, tapioca, or semolina—made with rice milk—as they are less likely to make the situation worse and provide much-needed nourishment.
- Drink barley water and keep up your fluid intake, or try ginger ale.
- If you cook rice, drink the water it's been cooked in, once it has cooled.
- Although we tend to associate fiber with ensuring adequate bowel movements and frequency, it can also help to control diarrhea, as the fiber will give bulk to the stool. Try eating soluble fibers such as oat or rice bran, linseeds (flax seeds that have been soaked overnight in cold water, then drained), and psyllium husks. Also make sure that you drink plenty of water or electrolyte drinks.
- Drinking 3–4 cups of chamomile, fennel, or black tea a day has been used for centuries as a gentle way of dealing with diarrhea.
- Eating dried bilberries or drinking bilberry juice can also help (but not fresh bilberries, as they can actually aggravate the problem).
- Fresh vegetable soups with a little root ginger or a small portion of poached fish and brown rice are usually well tolerated. Move on to solids only when the symptoms begin to ease, as sometimes diarrhea is your body's digestive system telling you it needs a rest.
- Eat plenty of low-fat, live yogurt to replenish healthy bacteria in the bowel.
- For acute diarrhea, grate an apple, let it go brown, and then eat it. Greenish bananas are also very binding.
- Slippery elm powder can be mashed into a paste with banana and honey. **VS, VC**

Useful Remedies

- While symptoms last, take 10,000IU of vitamin A daily for one week (**but no more than 3000IU if pregnant**), as it helps protect the lining of the gut. Also take 30mg of zinc, as too little zinc has been shown to trigger diarrhea.
- After that, take a good-quality vitamin/mineral to help prevent malnutrition. Liquid formulas are easy to absorb.
- The herb pau d'arco in combination with propolis helps kill many harmful organisms. Take 2–3ml of tincture two or three times a day or 1g in capsule form two to three times a day.
- If you are susceptible to diarrhea when you travel to foreign countries, taking acidophilus for two weeks prior to your trip can help increase the number of healthy bacteria in your gut, which reduces the risk of picking up any nasty stomach bugs. You should also take these for at least a week after suffering from food poisoning to help repopulate your gut with healthy bacteria and eliminate any remaining bad bacteria. Jarro-Dophilus EPS is a good formula. **JF**
- Buy a probiotic supplement with healthy bacteria plus supplements of garlic, oregano oil, clove oil, cinnamon, and rosemary. These can be taken daily with food when you are out of the country to help kill off any invading bacteria. They can be very handy for vacations, but do not take them if you are pregnant.
- Bee propolis, grapefruit seed extract, and olive leaf extract are all natural antibacterials.

Helpful Hints

- Drink water from cooked brown rice or mix 15g of carob powder with some applesauce to make it palatable. Carob has a history of helping alleviate diarrhea.
- Never drink tap water unless you are sure it is safe to do so. Avoid salads and fruit washed in local tap water in places like India, Africa, the Far East, and any country that you think the water may be questionable. Avoid ice cubes made from local tap water, too. You can drink

D

bottled water and soft drinks, but only if they have sealed tops. Only eat foods that have been thoroughly cooked.
- If the diarrhea resembles water coming out of a hose, try homeopathic Podophyllum 30c every few hours for a day. Charcoal tablets are also useful for stopping diarrhea.
- For teething children who have this problem, use homeopathic Chamomila 30c three times daily.
- If you suffer persistent diarrhea, you **must** see a doctor.

DIVERTICULAR DISEASE or DIVERTICULITIS

Diverticulitis is a disease of modern Western civilization, as it rarely occurs in people or cultures that eat a high-fiber diet. Years ago it occurred in older people, usually over 50, but these days, thanks to our over-processed diets and 24/7 lifestyles, younger people in their 20s and 30s are regularly diagnosed with this condition.

D Diverticular disease occurs when the mucous membranes lining the colon form small finger-like pouches, known as diverticula, that protrude out of the intestinal wall. Thirty to forty percent of people over the age of 60 have diverticular disease, and generally these pouches do not cause problems. If, however, they become inflamed and infected, diverticulitis results. It causes extreme pain—primarily in the descending colon, which is situated on the left-hand side of the abdomen. Symptoms include pain, bleeding, diarrhea, and fever. Chronic constipation is the most common underlying cause of this condition. A soft, bulky stool is easy to push along the colon, but a hard, dry stool makes the muscles of the colon work too hard. Also, if we don't evacuate impacted feces, then the muscular walls of the colon lose their integrity, increasing the risk for herniated pockets. Most sufferers have a tendency not to drink enough water or ingest insufficient fiber (see also *Constipation*). Occasionally, a pouch may burst, which requires urgent medical attention.

Foods to Avoid
- Avoid foods that contain seeds, such as tomatoes, grapes, and strawberries, as well as poppy, sesame and pumpkin seeds. Seeds can lodge in the intestinal pockets and cause inflammation and pain.
- Although fiber is necessary for a normal bowel movement, the abrasive fibers in wheat bran or high-fiber breakfast cereals, such as All Bran, can temporarily aggravate the problem.
- For many people wheat found in bread, cakes, cookies, pizza crust, pasta, and so on can have a constipating effect. Try avoiding these foods for 2 weeks to see if it helps.
- Avoid fried or spicy foods.
- Reduce saturated fats such as full-fat milk, cheese, and chocolates, as these can trigger inflammation, are mucus forming, and can make constipation worse.
- Avoid as much as possible white bread and pasta, white rice, cakes, cookies, fast foods, and mass-produced burger-type foods.
- Greatly reduce your intake of red meat, which takes a long time to pass through the bowel, as does cooked cheese. Pizza would be one of the worst foods that you could eat with this condition.
- While symptoms are acute, also avoid all yeast-based foods including bread, cheese, soy sauce, vinegar, and so on.

- Avoid all sweeteners containing fructose, sorbitol, and aspartame.
- Carageenan is a milk protein stabilizer often used in ice cream that causes problems for people with digestive/bowel problems.
- Tea, coffee, soft drinks, and alcohol can dehydrate the bowel.

Friendly Foods

- When the bowel is inflamed, eat soothing foods such as vegetable soups with cabbage, celery, and ginger, plus lightly stewed apples, apricots, prunes, papaya, and oatmeal made with non-dairy light soy, almond or rice milk.
- Mashed pumpkin and sweet potato are rich in carotenes that help heal the gut.
- Once the inflammation is under control, introduce a little steamed or grilled fish and low-fat, organic meat such as skinless poultry.
- Gradually increase your intake of high-fiber foods such as brown rice, gluten- and wheat-free breads and pastas, fresh vegetables, pulses, oat-based cereals, and fruit (especially figs). There are many excellent organic high-fiber mueslis and cereals made from grains such as amaranth, kamut, and quinoa. Remember, it's important to check which foods are making your condition worse before you remove too many foods from your diet. (See under *Allergies*.)
- Live, low-fat yogurt containing acidophilus and bifidus helps maintain the level of bacteria in the bowel and stool, which encourages regular bowel movement.
- Drink at least 8 glasses of water daily to make sure there is adequate fluid in the bowel.
- Use extra-virgin, unrefined olive or sunflower oils for your salad dressings.
- Eat more garlic and onions for their antiseptic qualities.
- Add ginger to foods and juices, which soothes and heals the gut.
- If you cook cabbage, let the cooking water cool and then drink it. It contains cabigin, a nutrient that helps to heal the bowel.

Useful Remedies

- The anti-inflammatory essential oils found in evening primrose oil also promote healing and repair; take 1–2g daily. You could also take 1g of gamma-linolenic acid (GLA) daily. **VC, VS**
- Add half a cup of aloe vera juice to fresh vegetable juices daily to help heal the gut, soothe the mucous membranes, and increase bowel movements.
- Slippery elm is gentle, soothing, and nourishing to the digestive lining. Drink as a tea, chew on the bark, or take 2–3 tablets before meals. Contact Specialist Herbal Supplies, who make pure slippery elm tea, and they can recommend specific herbs for your particular symptoms. **VC, VS**
- Good bacteria (acidophilus/bifidus) can help fight infection while they are active and help reduce constipation. During a flare-up, take two capsules three times per day. To protect for the future, take one capsule twice a day.
- Prebiotics are plant compounds that encourage the growth of healthy bacteria in the bowel. Try Agave Digestive Immune Support. One scoop daily with breakfast really helps keep you regular. **LEF**
- A natural-source carotene complex will aid soft tissue healing. Take 60mg daily.
- Calcium fluoride tissue salts help strengthen the intestinal walls. Take four daily.
- Chlorophyll found in green plants is very healing to gut lining. Take an organic green food complex twice a day in between meals.

Helpful Hints

- Exercise regularly. Gentle walking and swimming help work the stomach muscles and encourage bowel movements.
- Leave time to go to the bathroom. Relax and don't rush.

- Remember to drink plenty of fluids, which helps prevent constipation.
- Anxiety of any kind affects the bowel.
- Stress makes any digestive, gut, or bowel problem worse. Look at your lifestyle and take time out to practice meditation, yoga, or tai chi.
- For more information visit www.digestive.niddk.nih.gov
- Lots of useful fact sheets about diverticular disease can be found at www.corecharity.org.uk

DIZZY SPELLS

(see Adrenal Exhaustion, Low Blood Pressure, Low Blood Sugar, and Vertigo)

EARACHE   *(see also Glue Ear, Ménière's Syndrome, Tinnitus, and Vertigo)*

Most earaches are caused by the build-up of fluid in the middle ear, which can lead to an infection causing pain, fever, or loss of hearing. Children under the age of five are particularly prone to ear infections, usually triggered by a sensitivity to foods such as corn, eggs, peanuts, cow's milk, and wheat. Cow's milk and milk products are without doubt the most likely culprits. Soy milk and products can also trigger mucus in many people. I have vivid memories of when I was a child, screaming with a chronic earache until eventually both my ear drums burst. My poor mother had no idea that it was our diet of cow's milk, creamy desserts, cheese, chocolate treats, and lots of lard and dripping (solidified beef, lamb, and pork fat) sandwiches that caused the problem.

I was prescribed with almost continuous rounds of antibiotics, which undoubtedly contributed to my acne, thrush, and chronic fatigue during my teens. So if you have young children, try as much as possible to avoid antibiotics by changing your child's diet and giving them supplements to boost their immune function.

Cutting down on sugar and saturated fats also helps. Remember, most foods that contain saturated fats also contain sugar, which converts to fat within the body if not used up during exercise. Also note that many yogurts and "low-fat" foods are high in sugar! To make sure your child does not become malnourished, I suggest you consult a qualified nutritionist. (See *Useful Information*.)

If the earache is persistent, many doctors suggest insertion of tubes through minor surgery, but in the majority of cases this procedure can be avoided.

Foods to Avoid
- Avoid any food to which there is a sensitivity, particularly dairy products from cows plus wheat-based foods and eggs. Greek yogurts are very high in fat and should be avoided.
- Generally, while symptoms are acute, avoid mucus-forming foods, such as chocolate, milks, soy (in some people), cheese, and so on, but note that any foods to which you have an intolerance will trigger mucus production.
- Stay away from any sugar as it tends to weaken the immune system and leaves children more susceptible to infections. This includes sodas and desserts, which are often packed with sugar.

- Avoid excessive amounts of fruit juice, as these are often citrus based, which sometimes adds to the problem. Remember that most canned sodas contain up to 10 teaspoons of sugar. Never buy drinks containing aspartame, as they place too much of a strain on the liver, which can further exacerbate the problem.

Friendly Foods

- Once you have identified any problem foods, such as cow's or soy milk (see under *Helpful Hints*), look for alternatives such as oat, rice, or almond milk. I would not recommend soy milk or soy-based foods for any child under the age of 5.
- There are plenty of wheat-free pastas now available based on lentils, buckwheat, quinoa, rice, corn, and vegetables.
- Wheat can be replaced by rye or rice bread; rice, rye, or amaranth crackers; and oatcakes.
- Eat plenty of fruits and vegetables to keep the immune system in good shape, particularly those rich in the carotenoids such as sweet potatoes, pumpkin, papaya, mango, apricots, carrots, watercress, and spinach. Other useful foods for the immune system are cauliflower, broccoli, kale, and Brussels sprouts.

Useful Remedies

- Take an echinacea tincture (one drop per 13lb [6kg] of body weight) three to four times a day for up to 3 weeks at a time.
- To help fight infection and boost immunity, take 1g of vitamin C with food daily. Children generally find it easier if vitamin C powder is dissolved in diluted low-sugar apple juice.
- Beta Glucans, derived from yeast cells walls, are safe for children to take and improve the function of their innate immune system, which can help reduce the severity of food reactions. Dr Paul Clayton, a former scientific advisor to the UK government's committee on the safety of medicines, says: "Thanks to our modern over-sanitized environment and intensive farming methods, which have removed virtually all Beta Glucans from our diet, our ability to resist infections has become compromised." You can break a capsule of the Beta Glucan 1–3, 1–6 into cold foods, and children can safely take 250–500mg daily. Most parents report that when their children are given the Beta Glucans regularly, they suffer fewer infections.
- Children's multi-vitamins/minerals can make sure that children are not deficient in any nutrients, which can impair their immune system. Nature's Plus makes an excellent children's range. **NP**
- As antibiotics destroy healthy bacteria, encourage your children to eat low-fat live yogurts that contain the friendly bacteria acidophilus once a day. Try giving them goat's or sheep's milk yogurts, which are usually better tolerated than those made from cow's milk. If they hate the taste of plain yogurt, add any fresh fruit you have on hand and mix in the blender for a few seconds.
- To sweeten desserts, use a little agave syrup or xylitol—natural sugars that have a low glycemic factor. Available online and from health stores.

Helpful Hints

- If you smoke, it is definitely worth trying to stop or, at the very least, refrain from smoking near your children, as this has been strongly linked to the development of ear infections.
- A warm hot water bottle wrapped in a towel can be placed by the ear. Or you can buy a wheat bag: warm through, then place it near the ears.
- Warm an onion and place the core of the onion just inside the affected ear wrapped in muslin, or squeeze a small amount of onion water into the ear. Onion and garlic are natural decongestants.
- It is important to have an allergy test to identify the foods that affect you the worst. One of the best I have found is available from YorkTest Laboratories in the UK (tel: 011-44-1904-

E

410410; website: www.yorktest.com); Genova Diagnostics do a FACT test that looks for inflammatory markers indicating that the body is reacting to certain substances. Tel: 1-800-522-4762. Website: www.genovadiagnostics.com

■ Another excellent method is the Bio Meridian Test for food intolerance and leaky gut, in which the practitioner measures, via electrodes, your reactions to a large list of foods and substances. For practitioners visit www.biomeridian.com or call 1-888-224-2337 toll free.

■ Taking homeopathic Pulsatilla 30c or Belladonna 30c every 3–4 hours helps if the earache is in the right ear. If it is in the left ear, try Hepar Sulph 30c. If there is a sticky discharge, try Kali Bic 30c.

■ Do not let a child swim under water if their ears become infected.

■ Children who are given pacifiers are more prone to ear infections.

■ Consult an allergy specialist who can test for food intolerances, which can exacerbate and trigger this problem.

■ See a cranial osteopath or chiropractor to check the alignment of the head and neck, as misalignment and poor drainage can cause earaches. (See *Useful Information*.)

■ For irritations in the ears and sinuses, mucus, and catarrh use ear candles, which gently remove excess earwax without pain. These are excellent for children, as they are fun to use and not painful. Available from all good health stores.

■ The NeilMed Sinus Rinse (www.neilmed.com) is easy to use and helps reduce sinus and ear infections.

ECZEMA

(see also Allergies, Asthma, Leaky Gut, Irritable Bowel Syndrome, and Liver Problems)

According to various estimates, anywhere between 10 and 32 million Americans suffer from some type of eczema, including about 1.5 million children. Eczema can be an inherited condition and is also linked to asthma and rhinitis/hay fever.

During flare-ups the skin can become very inflamed, itchy, and may develop into open bleeding sores. Eczema is sometimes triggered by an external irritant, such as perfumes, laundry detergent, shampoos, paint, house dust mites, or cat hairs; but most commonly it is linked to food intolerance (as many as 80% of sufferers show a positive reaction to allergy testing) or a leaky gut. Therefore, please make sure to read the *Leaky Gut* section. It can also be associated with an under-functioning immune system.

Eczema can appear at any age, seemingly from nowhere. It tends to be aggravated by stress, exhaustion, sometimes by heat, and frequently by exercise. Eczema does tend to come and go.

For most people, symptoms worsen when they are under stress, but others notice that the condition is aggravated by certain foods, especially sugar, wheat, orange juice, and cow's milk, or drinking too much tea or coffee. If eczema starts in early childhood, the most likely culprit is cow's milk and dairy products. Either the child has been fed formula milk or the residues are ingested via the mother's breast milk. The most common triggers for eczema in babies are dairy products, eggs, citrus, and wheat. Avoidance of the offending food often resolves the problem.

It is very important to remember that by the time the eczema shows up on the skin it has worked its way through the body, and you really need to address the root cause of the problem. With any skin condition it is a good idea to support the liver, which is the most important cleansing organ for the body. If the liver becomes overloaded with toxins it tends to start dumping them into the skin—so anything you can do to keep your liver functioning more efficiently will, in the long term, help your skin.

Also, drugs such as ibuprofen have been known to trigger an attack in some people, as this drug can contribute to a leaky gut.

Foods to Avoid

■ As much as possible, avoid or greatly reduce your intake of all dairy products from cows, as well as coffee, tea, chocolate, beef, citrus fruits, eggs, wheat, alcohol, tomatoes, and peanuts. This is a long list of foods to avoid, but if you have eczema and do cut them all out, the eczema is virtually guaranteed to improve. Start keeping a food diary and note when symptoms are worse.

■ Sugar greatly affects the immune system, so try to cut down on sugary foods and drinks.

■ It is important to note that even decaffeinated coffee causes problems in people who are sensitive to coffee—it's not just the caffeine. The solvent used to extract the caffeine can affect a number of skin conditions.

■ As much as possible, avoid preservatives, additives, pesticides, food colorings (such as in the bright red glacé cherries on fancy cakes), and refined sugar-based, mass-produced cakes, cookies, and pies. (See also *Allergies*.)

Friendly Foods

■ Wherever possible, go organic and eat plenty of fresh fruits and vegetables.

■ Include plenty of cabbage in your diet. Also drink any water the cabbage has been cooked in because it contains L-glutamine, which helps heal a leaky gut.

■ Beets, artichokes, celeriac (celery root), celery, and radicchio all cleanse the liver.

■ Freshly made vegetable juices with celery, apple, cucumber, carrot, kale and half a cup of aloe vera juice will all help re-alkalize the body and heal the gut. (See *Acid–Alkaline Balance*.)

■ Diluted pear juice is a good alternative to orange juice.

■ If you react to cow's milk, there are plenty of alternatives such as rice, oat and almond milk, all of which have a much lower incidence of reaction.

■ Oily fish can be particularly beneficial, as the essential fatty acids in fish are anti-inflammatory and have been shown to improve eczema conditions. Eat more sardines, organic-farmed salmon, mackerel, anchovies, and herrings.

■ Eat more sunflower seeds, sesame seeds, linseeds (flax seeds), and pumpkin seeds, as well as nuts (with the exception of peanuts). The fatty acids and high levels of zinc and protein in these foods will help nourish the skin and speed up the healing process.

■ Wheat germ and avocados are rich in vitamin E, which also aids skin healing.

■ Use extra-virgin olive oil plus unrefined walnut and sunflower oil in salad dressings.

■ Use non-hydrogenated spreads such as Biona and Vitaquell instead of mass-produced hard fats. (See also *Fats You Need To Eat*.)

■ Orange-colored fruits and vegetables contain beta-carotene, the vegetable source of vitamin A, which is known to be beneficial to skin health. Try squash, pumpkin, red grapes, sweet potatoes, mango, cantaloupe melon, peppers, carrots, and apricots.

Useful Remedies

■ There is now good research showing that people who take healthy bacteria (probiotics) regularly are less likely to suffer from eczema, as healthy bacteria help improve digestion and reduce any immune response. Talk to a qualified nutritionist at your local health store to find which probiotic would suit you best.

■ A good probiotic that I recommend is Jarro-Dophilus EPS (one daily). **JF**

■ Prebiotics are plant compounds that encourage the growth of healthy bacteria in the bowel.

Try Agave Digestive Immune Support. One scoop daily with breakfast really helps keep you regular, which takes the burden off the liver. **LEF**

- Cabbage contains the amino acid L-glutamine, which greatly aids healing of the gut. Take a teaspoon twice daily in water 45 minutes before main meals.
- Colostrum, which is found in breast milk, helps support the immune system and aids healing of a leaky gut. It's very helpful for babies and children suffering from eczema. Until the age of 2, an infant can take a quarter of a teaspoon twice daily on an empty stomach. After that, children should take half a teaspoon twice daily. Only take this for one month. **VC**
- Take 1–4g of evening primrose oil a day. This has been shown to help heal eczema.
- Also take 400IU of full-spectrum, natural-source vitamin E daily. The vitamin E will help prevent scarring and itching.
- The mineral zinc is needed to ensure adequate absorption of fatty acids, and it's invariably deficient in eczema sufferers. It also speeds up skin healing. Take 30mg twice daily for a couple of months, and then reduce to 20mg per day.
- Research shows that selenium levels are low in people with inflammatory conditions such as eczema. Make sure your multi-vitamin provides 200mcg of selenium as it works well with vitamin E.
- Vitamin A is really important for skin healing. For just one week each month (for up to 6 months) take 10,000IU of vitamin A daily to boost levels in the body. **NB: If you are pregnant or planning to become pregnant, then never take more than 3000IU of vitamin A per day.**

- Include a high-strength multi-vitamin/mineral that includes a full spectrum of B vitamins, which help reduce stress, improve digestion, and increase the absorption of fatty acids.
- Nettle works as a mild antihistamine, which can reduce the itching. This tincture can be applied both externally and taken internally. Ideally, do not apply to broken skin, as the small amount of alcohol would sting. For young children use one drop per 13lb (6kg) of body weight. This will ensure you don't give them too much.
- The herb milk thistle has been shown to help regenerate and support liver function. Take 500mg twice daily with meals.
- Omega-7 fats extracted from sea buckthorn berries are highly effective at relieving dry skin. **VC**
- Also take 1g of omega-3 fish oils for their anti-inflammatory properties.

Helpful Hints

- Many people have found that aloe vera juice taken internally, and the gel used topically, are very helpful for eczema.
- Allergenics cream soothes the majority of cases, and some people have said it has actually cleared their eczema up. For details of the cream, visit www.wellbeing-uk.com; they will ship internationally.
- To help relieve the itching, place two cups of any kind of bran or oatmeal in your bath and soak for 20 minutes.
- It is important to have an allergy test to find out the triggers for your eczema. Either try YorkTest Laboratories (tel: 011-44-1904-410410; website: www.yorktest.com) or Genova Diagnostics' FACT test that looks for inflammatory markers indicating that the body is reacting to certain substances (tel: 1-800-522-4762. website: www.genovadiagnostics.com).
- Do something positive to help relieve the stress that may be aggravating your eczema. Try meditation, yoga, tai chi, or some other means of relaxation. If you can, get away and bask in some sunshine and salt water, which usually aids eczema.
- If you have access to, and can afford, reflexology treatment or aromatherapy massage, not only will the oils improve the condition, but they are also incredibly relaxing. A few drops of

essential oils of lavender, Roman chamomile, geranium, rose, and cedar wood, mixed in a good base carrier oil such as calendula, can be applied to the affected areas.

- Exercise is generally beneficial for both reducing stress and improving the condition; however, wear lightweight, cotton, loose-fitting clothing, as if you get too hot and sweaty this may aggravate the condition.
- Relief Cream, made from calendula, manuka honey, aloe vera, and gotu kola, works really well on eczema and psoriasis and is great for babies. For details visit www.planetblueshop.com. Or try Ultra Dry Skin Cream by the Organic Pharmacy. **OP**
- Constipation and having a liver under stress are also associated with eczema because toxins cannot be broken down and removed from the body efficiently. (See also *Constipation* and *Liver Problems*.)
- If sensitivity to certain foods is suspected, then avoid the offending food. (See *Allergies*.)
- Avoid mass-produced soaps and soap powders. Ask at your health store for pH-balanced soaps or natural soaps that contain olive oil or vitamins A and E.
- Chinese herbs have proved helpful in many cases, but you need to see a qualified Chinese herbalist and may need to have your liver function checked before and during treatment. Others report great success through homeopathy. (See *Useful Information*.)
- Reduce your exposure to house dust mites by using a vacuum cleaner with an allergy filter. Also vacuum mattresses once a week.
- Putting blankets, bedspreads, and pillows out in bright sunlight for a few hours a month will help to kill off dust mites.
- For further help, contact the National Eczema Association, 4460 Redwood Highway, Suite 16D, San Rafael, CA 94903. Tel: 1-800-818-7546. E-mail: info@nationaleczema.org. Website: www.nationaleczema.org

E

ELECTRICAL POLLUTION AND ELECTRICAL HEALING

In 2004 there were 180 million cell phone subscribers in the US. By 2010 more than 285 million cell phones have been connected—many for use by children—in spite of the fact that governments around the world, including the UK, France, and Austria, having issued warnings that children under 12 should not use mobile phones and that masts should be situated well away from schools.

There is now a considerable body of evidence from highly accredited sources, including SAGE, the UK's Government Advisory Body, and the Bioinitiative Working Group (scientists from the US, Sweden, Denmark, Austria, and China, who in 2007 released a 650-page report citing more than 2000 studies), linking electromagnetic fields from computers, mobile phones, household electrical goods, satellite receivers, transmitters, TVs, fluorescent light bulbs and dimmer switches, microwaves, and other electronic devices to childhood cancers, depression and suicide, brain tumors, dizziness and headaches, short-term memory loss, Alzheimer's, tinnitus, and extreme fatigue.

Roger Coghill, a bioelectromagnetics research scientist based in Torfaen in Wales and one of the UK's leading authorities on this subject, sits on the SAGE committee that advises the UK Government on how to mitigate EMF exposure. He says: "First, people need to understand that we are electrical beings in a physical shell and electricity can be used to harm or to heal us. Every cell in the human body emits its own unique range of frequencies. These frequencies are as unique to us as our DNA. When functioning properly, our cells or groups of cells, such as our liver or kidneys, emit a harmonic signal (denoting that the organ is healthy), which can clearly be seen on specialist scanners. If we become ill, cells begin emitting a disharmonic set of frequencies, which again can be detected. Every food you eat also emits a specific range of frequencies, as does every nutrient and everything on the planet—even rocks. This is how scientists measure what other planets and stars are made of, by measuring their spectral frequencies. But electrical pollution from external sources, such as WiFi equipment, which is now referred to as 'dirty electricity,' is without doubt a major contributing factor to many illnesses and we need to protect ourselves.

"For instance, a study in Sweden has suggested that a person has a five-times increased risk of brain cancer if they start using a mobile phone in their teens. Israel has banned the placement of cellular antennae on residences, and we now believe that up to 3% of the population are clinically hypersensitive.

"In 1981, a study by a British Doctor, Dr Stephen Perry, was published which clearly demonstrated that significantly more suicides occurred at locations of high magnetic field strength.

"There is now a critical mass of evidence to show that excessive use of mobile phones, and the EMFs that come off various sources, can trigger a variety of cancers, impair immune functioning, and contribute to Alzheimer's disease, heart disease, and other health disorders."

Coghill continues: "The hands-free kits are also linked with health problems and if you use these phones for more than ten minutes at a time you are at a much greater long-term risk of brain tumors. We are living in a sea of artificial frequencies and because animals, especially whales, dolphins, insects, and birds, are more sensitive to these man-made emissions, their sensory abilities are being greatly affected—which is why so many whales are beaching themselves. Humans are also becoming more electro-sensitive, and there are even societies that help people who are either affected by, or whose fields affect, electrical equipment.

"Also if you have subterranean flowing water under your home or office, this often compounds health problems, as the water can create an inharmonious electromagnetic field. Hundreds of years ago, builders would watch carefully where sheep settled at night and would not build in places where sheep refused to sleep. Studies show that rats also avoid areas of high electromagnetic fields. Every time you turn on a light switch or any electrical equipment, your brain's rhythms change immediately. Spending too much time under fluorescent lighting or in front of a computer screen can suppress the brain chemical melatonin, which can have negative effects as diverse as sleep disturbance, depression, and infertility."

Foods to Avoid
- Junk foods have a dull energy field frequency that will eventually trigger negative symptoms if you eat them to excess. It is also important to note that since all foods emit their own frequency; if you eat certain foods, whether they are considered healthy or not, that emit a frequency that is incompatible with your own frequency range, this too can trigger symptoms in sensitive individuals.

Friendly Foods
- Eat foods in as near a natural state as possible. For example, if you look at the energy field of a raw cabbage it has a really bright energy field; once cooked, however, the energy field is greatly reduced. (See *General Health Hints*.)

Useful Remedies
- One of the best ways to help protect yourself is by taking the hormone melatonin. EMF pollution reduces your pineal gland's ability to synthesize melatonin, which is why exposure affects sleep patterns. Radiation creates free radicals in the body, and highly potent

antioxidants that can pass through the blood brain barrier, such as melatonin, help protect you from electrical pollution. Coghill has developed a supplement called Asphalia, which contains natural melatonin extracted from certain grasses to maintain melatonin levels. Roger's exclusive distributor in the US is Diva Marketing, Don't Disturb Me!, 2612 Sleepy Hollow, Pearland, TX 77581; Tel: 1-713-221-1873 or 1-866-692-8037; website: www.dontdisturbmesite.com

Helpful Hints

■ The Bicom Resonance machine developed in Germany picks up on the electromagnetic frequencies emanating from the body. An experienced practitioner can interpret these frequencies and then determine which ones should be amplified back into the patient's energy field to enable the body to heal itself. Cells carry a memory of certain diseases that you thought had left your body long ago. For example, when I was tested with the Bicom my cells showed a positive reading for the memory of glandular fever, which I had suffered during my teens. To counteract this, the therapist inverted the frequency of the Epstein Barr virus (from a tiny vial containing Epstein Barr) back into my body to neutralize any remaining memory. The Bicom is good for helping people eliminate allergies, chronic fatigue, endometriosis, as well as for treating intestinal parasites and eczema. To find a practitioner in your area, visit www.energetic-medicine.net/practitioners

■ Another excellent method similar to the Bicom is Bio Meridian Testing. Via electrodes placed on acupuncture meridian points, the practitioner can measure electric currents being emitted by various organs and musculoskeletal systems, which gives the therapist accurate feedback as to the health of various systems. This method can also determine which supplements and/or drugs agree with your unique physiology and can help determine what foods and substances you are sensitive to. For practitioners, see www.alternativesforhealing.com/cgi_bin/practitioner-biomeridian-testing.php If you are ever in the UK, Dr Shamin Daya at the Wholistic Medical Centre in Harley Street, London, is one of the most experienced practitioners of the Bio Meridian practices I have ever encountered.

■ Electro-crystal healing, invented by bio-physicist Harry Oldfield, works on similar principles. First the patient's energy fields are scanned via a specialist scanner, which enables the therapist to view negative frequency emissions and thus determine which areas of the body are under-functioning. An experienced practitioner then pulses calming or stimulating frequencies through crystals suspended in a saline solution to encourage healing of the affected areas. I have interviewed dozens of people crippled with arthritis and other conditions who have been greatly helped by this type of therapy. Harry has trained hundreds of therapists worldwide. For details of your nearest therapist, log on to www.electrocrystal.com/links.php

■ The basic rule is that moving electric fields—for example, mobile phones or power lines—are harmful, while static magnetic fields, such as the earth on which we all evolved, are beneficial to health.

■ Avoid using a mobile phone inside a car, building, or any enclosed space because the phone is forced to increase its output power, which can affect your health more quickly. Never use a mobile phone for more than 5–7 minutes at a time.

■ Never charge your mobile phone by your bedside.

■ If you are pregnant, do not sleep with an electric blanket on and keep mobile phone use to a minimum.

■ When you put a phone earpiece directly into your ear, Roger says that you risk pulsing radio waves straight into your brain. Roger also advises that you look for sets that have ferrite components, which block radiation from traveling up the wire.

- Keep electrical appliances in the bedroom to a minimum, and turn off all mains switches in the bedroom at night. If you live near an electrical power station, put large copper jugs or ornaments in the windows. Avoid placing "touch lamps" with thyristor dimmers anywhere near your bed. Also turn off computers and TVs at the mains at night, as leaving them on "standby" wastes huge amounts of energy and still creates an electrical field.
- Turn off your Wifi router box at night.
- Avoid sleeping with an electric blanket on. Warm the bed thoroughly before you get into bed, and then switch it off for the night. However, if you are over 60 and have poor circulation and have been specifically told to sleep with it on, for goodness sake don't get too cold!
- Studies show that microwave ovens alter the chemistry of food. Irradiating (x-raying) food could, in the long run, prove very dangerous. If any foods like strawberries are still healthy looking after being in your fridge for a few days, then they have most likely been irradiated.
- DECT (digital enhanced cordless telecommunications) cordless phones give out some of the worst EMF signals that arc across the room. So change to a low-radiation cordless phone. Contact Orchid on www.lowradiation.co.uk or call 011-44-20-8398-9925. Unfortunately they are not available outside of Europe at this time.
- Avoid having too many CT scans and X-rays unless they are deemed essential. One CT scan is equivalent to 400 X-rays.
- You can buy an ELF Meter to tell you the field strengths in your home. Available online from Amazon. Or read Roger's book, *Something in the Air*.
- Have your home dowsed by an expert if you are worried about suffering from electricity overexposure. Contact the American Society of Dowsers (www.dowsers.org) or see their list of experts at asdowsers.hostcentric.com/ds_list/Specialty_List.htm
- For further news on pollution issues, visit: www.pollutionissues.com or www.pollutionissues.co.uk

EMPHYSEMA

(see also under Bronchitis)

The group of conditions that includes emphysema and chronic bronchitis is known as chronic obstructive pulmonary disease (COPD).

Bronchitis means "inflammation of the bronchi," and this inflammation increases mucus production in the airways, causing a sufferer to produce more phlegm as they cough.

Emphysema, on the other hand, is a serious disease that occurs when the air sacs or alveoli (the place where carbon dioxide is exchanged for oxygen (the lungs' main function) lose their elasticity, and the airways narrow. This means that your lungs are not as efficient at getting oxygen into the body, so you need to breathe harder, which triggers shortness of breath.

Any chronic lung condition that causes narrowing of the airways, such as asthma or bronchitis, may contribute to emphysema, but 80% of cases are triggered by smoking. As this condition can take years to develop, it usually manifests in midlife or later. According to the CDC, an estimated 10 million Americans were diagnosed with COPD in 2000, but national health survey data suggests that up to 24 million are affected by this condition.

Other potential triggers for COPD are exposure to coal dust, toxic molds, cotton, flour, wood or grain dusts, welding fumes, and minerals such as cadmium and vanadium. Pollution from industry and our roads definitely plays a part in chronic lung disease.

It's a sad fact that many patients lose up to 70% of their functional lung tissue before they realize that they have a chronic disease; therefore, the earlier a diagnosis can be made, the less damage will be done.

Low levels of protective antioxidants (such as vitamins C and E) and high levels of oxidative stress caused by damaging free radicals from burnt food, pollution, chemicals, and so on, alongside exposure to toxins will only exacerbate onset of this condition.

Symptoms might begin as a chronic cough or bouts of bronchitis, phlegm, or shortness of breath, especially in the winter. However, as the condition progresses the patient will suffer shortness of breath more regularly, until it happens daily.

Other symptoms include skipped breaths, wheezing, insomnia, fatigue, swelling of feet, ankles or legs, irritability and unexplained weight loss. Emphysema patients have an increased risk of contracting pneumonia so keeping the immune system strong is essential. (See *Immune Function*.) Heart disease is another risk, as the heart has to work extra hard to make up for the lungs. The more you can avoid developing infections, the better.

Foods to Avoid

■ Avoid foods that contain hydrogenated and trans-fats, as they can trigger inflammation. They also compete with the healthy fats that help keep the alveoli in the lungs supple so that they can do their job more easily. Also avoid the oils found in many pre-packaged and processed foods. (See *Fats You Need to Eat*.)

■ Steer clear of any foods that you are intolerant to, the most common being wheat and any dairy food/milk from cows.

■ If you find you are making too much phlegm, this is almost always linked to high-fat foods, including full-fat cheese, chocolate, cow's or soy milk, white bread, croissants, and bananas.

■ Avoid fried and barbecued foods, as they have high levels of damaging free radicals.

■ Generally, cut down your intake of red meat. If you choose to eat meat, make it organic and always cut off the fat first.

■ Eggs are hard to digest for some people, and it's well worth being tested to see if they are a problem. (See Genova and YorkTest details under *Allergies*.)

■ Sugary foods and drinks suppress immune function, which leaves you more susceptible to infections. Also, most foods high in sugar are also high in animal fats. And keep in mind that many low-fat foods are high in sugar which, unless burnt during exercise, will be converted to fat within the body.

Friendly Foods

■ People who eat fruit and vegetables on a regular basis seem less likely to develop emphysema; therefore, try to focus on foods which are rich in natural sources of carotenes, which help protect the mucous membranes in the lungs. Eat more apricots, mangoes, green vegetables, pumpkin, parsley, red peppers, spinach, sweet potatoes, watercress, and cantaloupe melon.

■ Vine-ripened tomatoes are rich in the carotene lycopene, which helps support the lungs. Cook in a little olive oil to help release the lycopene. Guava and pink grapefruit also contain a fair amount of lycopene.

■ Go organic whenever possible, as fruit such as apples, which are great for lung health, can otherwise be covered in up to eighteen different pesticides.

■ Quercetins—flavonoids found in apples, pears, cherries, grapes, onion, kale, broccoli, garlic, green tea, and red wine—help protect the lungs from the harmful effect of pollutants and cigarette smoke. Also eat more fresh pineapple.

■ Use organic rice or almond milk as non-dairy alternatives. Some people find low-fat goat's or sheep's milk better.

- Choose low-fat dishes including cottage cheese. You should also replace butter with spreads such as Biona and Olivio or try organic raw walnut, hemp seed or almond butter.
- Use olive oil for salad dressings and eat plenty of brown rice, lentils, barley, oat-based dishes, and wheat-free breakfast cereals. There are also plenty of wheat-free pastas available such as lentil, rice, corn and potato pasta and flour.
- Liver, kidney, butter, and skimmed milk contain retinol, the animal form of vitamin A, which is good for tissue healing. Don't go mad on the butter (see above)—and make it organic.
- Eat more garlic and onions, as these help to fend off infection and clear the lungs.
- Fenugreek or licorice tea can help to soothe the lungs.
- See *General Health Hints*.

Useful Remedies

- People with lung conditions tend to be low in Vitamin A. If you are not pregnant or trying to become pregnant, take 25,000IU of vitamin A daily for one month and then reduce to taking two natural-source carotene complex daily. **SVHC**
- Take 500mg of N-acetyl cysteine (NAC) one to two times a day. This amino acid is one of the best-researched nutrients for emphysema. It helps break up mucus and has been shown to reduce the frequency and duration of attacks of COPD if taken twice daily for at least 6 months. NAC also helps the body produce the powerful antioxidant glutathione in the liver.
- Take 1–2g of vitamin C daily with food in an ascorbate form to help clear mucus and improve respiratory ailments. It works well with NAC (above).
- Take 2g of L-carnitine daily if breathing is made worse by exercise.
- Take a multi-vitamin/mineral containing high-potency lycopene, selenium, zinc, alpha-lipoic acid, and vitamins A, C, and E, which all help support lung tissue.
- Bromelain, extracted from pineapples, is great for helping break up mucus and is anti-inflammatory. Take 500mg twice daily.
- Co-enzyme Q10 is a powerful antioxidant that helps restore energy to damaged lung cells. Take 100mg twice daily with food, but not at night as CoQ10 also increases general energy levels.
- Magnesium helps relax bronchial muscles for easier breathing. Take 200mg three times a day.
- The amino acid taurine can help improve breathlessness. Take 1000mg twice a day before meals.
- Lipoic acid is a very important antioxidant for lungs. Take 200mg daily.

Helpful Hints

- Don't smoke, and if you do smoke, give it up. Avoid smoke-filled rooms and sources of second-hand cigarette smoke.
- Regular exercise before the onset of COPD can help increase lung capacity and strengthen the heart.
- To help break up any thick mucus that may collect in the lungs, drink plenty of fluid.
- Avoid air pollutants such as dust, aerosol sprays, herbicides, pesticides, fumes from fuel and exhausts, smoke from bonfires and barbecues, and dust stirred up by house cleaning.
- Use Ultra Breathe, a very handy, inexpensive device that does a great job of exercising the lungs. It costs $26.95 online plus $3.95 for postage and packing. For details, visit www.ultrabreathe.com/us/uswelcome.htm
- Gentle exercise can help relieve the symptoms of this condition by building lung capacity and cleansing the lungs of stale air. Start slowly and then build up gradually. Choose walking, swimming, or cycling.
- Reflexology has proved successful with some sufferers. Yoga can also be beneficial, as it will teach you relaxation techniques and how to breathe properly. (See *Useful Information*.)
- Aromatherapy has also been of benefit to some sufferers. Fill a basin with boiling water and

add three drops of eucalyptus essential oil. Put your head over the basin with a towel over the top and inhale the steam.

- Be careful about visiting high altitudes as this makes it harder to breathe.
- Using an ionizer in your home may be useful for lowering levels of dust.
- Sing when you can, as this helps increase lung capacity. Take deep breaths regularly. You can increase the efficiency of your lungs a thousand fold by increasing your air intake by 5% on each breath.
- Environmentally friendly cleaning products are kinder to your lungs as they don't contain harsh chemicals that can be inhaled. Try Ecover products—available in health stores and supermarkets.
- The Life Extension Foundation offers a wealth of information for people with emphysema. **LEF**

ENDOMETRIOSIS   *(see also Thyroid, Underactive and Overactive)*

Ten to twenty percent of women of childbearing age in the US suffer from this problem, which most commonly occurs between the ages of 25 and 45. Endometriosis is a condition where tissue that normally lines the womb grows outside the womb. The endometrial tissue can be found in places such as the ovaries, fallopian tubes, pelvis, cervix, colon, appendix, and vagina. In more severe cases, adhesions of endometrial tissue are found on the bladder, kidneys, lungs, or even in the nasal lining. Some doctors believe that endometriosis is an autoimmune disease, as higher rates of rheumatoid arthritis, MS, and lupus are found in women suffering from this condition.

E

The chemical dioxin (from vinyl and plastics and produced during incineration and forest fires) and numerous other toxic chemicals found in our air and water have also been linked to this condition. This is because dioxins can interfere with the metabolism of B vitamins, which are needed for optimum liver function. This, in turn, is essential for breaking down excess estrogen. Also excess pollutants mimic estrogen in the body, triggering hormonal imbalances.

Most nutritional practitioners also believe there is a strong link between endometriosis and candida overgrowth (see *Candida*) because candida treatments greatly alleviate the symptoms of endometriosis. Many of the women suffering from this condition find that their symptoms are definitely worse when they are stressed out or really tired.

The current theory is that, during menstruation, womb tissue flows not only down to the vagina but also up through the fallopian tubes, eventually sticking to other structures. The displaced tissue acts in the same way as it would if it had stayed in the womb and has a monthly bleed. In mild cases the blood is reabsorbed, but in more severe cases cysts can form and irritate the pelvis. It can be very painful, particularly during ovulation, menstruation, and sexual intercourse. Pain can also be triggered by a bowel movement or emptying the bladder. Internal examinations are necessary to diagnose this condition, but sometimes they can make things worse. Nevertheless, they are necessary to rule out anything more serious. Endometriosis is one of the more common causes of infertility.

Foods to Avoid
- Avoid alcohol, saturated animal fats found in red meat and dairy produce, as these can elevate estrogen levels and place a greater workload on the liver, which in turn can increase the pain and inflammation.
- Sugar and sugary foods trigger inflammation in the body, so candies, puddings, cakes, sodas, and pastries are best avoided or greatly reduced.

- Caffeine reduces the body's ability to cope with pain and blocks absorption of some minerals.
- If you suspect candida—symptoms include bloating, constipation and/or diarrhea, thrush, food cravings and chronic fatigue—then avoid sugar, refined carbohydrates, cheese, mushrooms, concentrated fruit juice, and yeasty breads for a couple of weeks to see if this helps. (See *Candida*.)
- As with so many other conditions, if there is a food intolerance it will almost certainly aggravate the problem. Avoid wheat and dairy products from cows for at least one cycle. Keep a food diary and note when symptoms are worse
- Peel all fruit and vegetables if they are not organic, as this is where the pesticides and herbicides that disrupt hormones are more concentrated.
- Reduce your intake of wheat and wheat bran as they contain phytic acid, which binds to essential minerals such as zinc and magnesium that are needed for hormone balance and muscle relaxation.

Friendly Foods
- Eat more foods that are rich in I3C (indole-3-carbinol) and known to eliminate excess hormones from the body, such as broccoli, cauliflower, cabbage, and Brussels sprouts. Another option is to take one Triple Action Cruciferous Vegetable Extract capsule daily. **LEF**
- Fermented soy-based foods such as tempeh, miso, natto, and tofu can control excessive estrogen levels, as do beans, lentils, chickpeas, cauliflower, Brussels sprouts, and broccoli.
- Add sunflower, pumpkin, sesame, and ready-cracked linseeds (or, if whole seeds are used, soaked overnight in cold water and drain) to your breakfast cereal, as they provide essential fatty acids and zinc that are vital for soft tissue healing. Nuts, with the exception of peanuts, are a good source of fatty acids and zinc.
- Eat more oily fish—farmed, organic salmon, trout, mackerel, sardines, and anchovies—along with nuts and seeds for their anti-inflammatory properties.
- Pineapple is rich in bromelain, which has a potent anti-inflammatory affect. Eat before main meals.
- Ginger and turmeric (curcumin) are also anti-inflammatory, and ginger is very soothing within the gut.
- Eat foods high in natural carotenes—spinach, carrots, apricots, pumpkin, watercress, papaya, parsley, mangoes, cantaloupe melons, and sweet potatoes.
- Dark fruits, including blueberries, prunes, cherries, and blackberries, are high in bioflavonoids, which ease inflammation.
- Natural wheat germ and avocados are rich in vitamin E, which is known to help reduce scar tissue associated with endometriosis.
- Eat more magnesium-rich foods—cashew nuts, almonds, broccoli, bananas, and prunes—as these will help reduce cramping.
- Brown rice, millet, and oats contain lots of fiber, which binds to excess estrogen so that it can be removed from the body.
- Dandelion coffee helps support the liver so that it can remove excess hormones more easily.
- Add fresh cilantro and sea vegetables such as nori and kombu to your diet, as they help remove toxic metals from the body.

Useful Remedies
- Gamma-linolenic acid (GLA) is the omega-6 essential fatty acid found in evening primrose and borage seed oil and really helps reduce inflammation. Take 500mg of GLA twice daily or 3g of evening primrose oil daily.
- Omega-3 fish oils (DHA and EPA) are vital for controlling the inflammation associated with endometriosis. Take 3g daily.

- Full-spectrum, natural-source vitamin E helps protect cell membranes. Take 400IU daily
- Take one soy/isoflavone supplement daily if you do not eat fermented soy foods or chickpeas every day. Take 50–100mg daily.
- Include a high-strength multi-vitamin/mineral in your regimen that is suitable for your age.
- Pycnogenol, pine bark extract, helps reduce inflammation, bleeding, pain, and the formation of endometrial tissue. Take 120mg daily.
- Vitamin C is a vital antioxidant when excess estrogen is a problem. Take 2g daily in divided doses with food.
- Beta-carotene, which converts naturally to Vitamin A in the body, is important because it helps protect against the effects of dioxins found in our air, water, and foods. Take 20,000IU daily.
- Most sufferers have low levels of the mineral magnesium. Take 200–600mg daily.
- If your multi-vitamin has a daily total of 30mg of zinc, this is fine. If not, you need an additional zinc supplement (30mg) daily, as most sufferers are deficient, Zinc ensures proper absorption of fatty acids and aids hormone balance.
- A strong B-complex will help absorption of fatty acids and support liver enzymes in the breakdown of excess estrogen. If you have a high-strength multi-vitamin, the Bs should already be included.
- Take 500mg of the amino acid L-methionine, which helps detoxify estrogen from the liver. Take one to three capsules daily 30 minutes before food.

Helpful Hints

- Almost all cases benefit from using natural progesterone cream. **VC, VS** Also see details of natural progesterone bio-identical hormones plus suppliers under *Menopause*. **NB: Do not self- medicate with hormones. Have a blood or saliva test to find out if you need them. Do not take progesterone if you might be pregnant or are breastfeeding**

E

- Anthony Porter, a reflexologist since 1972, went to China and the Far East to teach reflexology during the 1980s and found that their methods combined with his own gave even better results. He has taught his advanced techniques to thousands of reflexologists internationally and says: "With Advanced Reflexology Techniques (ART) we can not only balance various parts of the body (which is what happens with normal reflexology), but we can also feel more subtle changes within the 7000 nerve endings or reflex areas of the feet, and after working on them this has a profound therapeutic affect. Medical research with a leading gynecologist has shown huge success with easing the pain and distress in these types of conditions." To find an ART therapist in your area, visit www.artreflex.com and click on Practitioners in the menu.
- Naturopathy and Chinese medicine have proven beneficial to many sufferers. If you decide to try Chinese herbs, make sure your doctor keeps an eye on your liver function. (See *Useful Information*.)
- Epsom salts added to hot bath water relaxes and soothes; add a drop of lavender oil to relax.
- Avoid heating foods in plastic containers or those covered in plastic wrap. Once heated, these plastics can leach chemicals that act like estrogens, which are "builders" in the body.
- As much as possible, remove chemicals from your home that can have a hormone-disrupting action and use biodegradable products whenever possible. Use Ecover products, available in most supermarkets and health food stores.
- Use a hot water bottle or alternatively a heat pad to help relax cramping muscles.
- Massage your abdomen with gentle strokes using lavender and neroli essential oils, as they both have a calming and antispasmodic effect and will help reduce cramping.
- Acupressure: you may be able to alleviate cramping by applying pressure to Spleen 6, located on the inside of the leg 3–4 in (7.5–10cm) above the center of the ankle bone.

- Always use pure cotton towels that are guaranteed to be free from dioxin. Beware of tampons, as they can exacerbate symptoms.
- Light exercise will help to raise levels of endorphins, which make you feel good and help relieve pain. During the winter, double the benefit by walking in daylight as this can also lift your spirits.
- To reduce tension, drink soothing herbal teas made with herbs such as hops and valerian.
- Read *Women's Encyclopedia of Natural Medicine*, by Dr Tori Hudson (McGraw Hill).
- Further help and information on the subject is available from The Endometriosis Association, 8585 N. 76th Place, Milwaukee, WI 53223. Tel: 1-414-355-2200. Website: www.endometriosisassn.org

EXHAUSTION   *(see also Adrenal Exhaustion, ME, and Stress)*

Being "tired all the time" or "tired and toxic" have become modern-day mantras. If you are a Type A person who lives life in the fast lane and eats in a hurry or if you suffer from bloating and/or constipation or food cravings, especially for carbohydrates such as bread, cakes, and pasta, read the *Adrenal Exhaustion* section before this one, as adrenal problems are now at epidemic levels.

As well as adrenal stress, being tired much of the time can also be linked to toxicity in the body (see *Liver Problems*), long-term stress (see *Stress*), and/or being overweight (see *Weight Problems*). It is also heavily linked to food sensitivities, most especially to wheat and cow's milk. However, the list of possible causes is fairly extensive, and you may also need to have your thyroid checked as chronic exhaustion is also linked to an underactive thyroid.

One of the most common causes of constant tiredness may simply be lack of sleep. And the quality of sleep is very important. When you are under pressure you have more difficulty getting to sleep, and then you have to get up for work feeling almost as tired as you did the night before. There is no right or wrong amount of sleep; we are all unique. Thomas Edison could manage on 4 hours, but I need 8. Everyone knows how much sleep they need to be fully functional the next day, but the average is 7–8 hours. (See under *Insomnia*.)

Obviously, there are varying levels of exhaustion, but if you find you are suffering bouts of palpitations during the day, chronic headaches, have an urgency to keep going to the bathroom, or experience a red flushing in your upper chest and throat area, this is most likely your adrenal glands telling you that your body is exhausted. And if you start crying without cause and begin to suffer a total sense of humor failure, you urgently need to listen and take note of the signals—or worse is to come. Your immune system is lowered, and you are more likely to pick up anything that's going around. Rest is your best option at this point. Know when to walk away. It's not worth dying for—literally.

Foods to Avoid
- Stimulants such as coffee, tea, alcohol, and sugar give a short-term energy boost, but unfortunately this soon wears off, leaving you craving more sugary, refined foods. Therefore, greatly reduce your intake of colas and carbonated drinks, chocolates, cookies, cakes, snacks, croissants, and mass-produced refined foods. Not only do these foods leave us feeling tired, but they also deplete important nutrients such as magnesium, chromium, and the B-vitamins from our bodies, and we become even more exhausted.
- Don't eat heavy protein meals late at night as they take a long time to digest.

Friendly Foods

- Eat more high-energy foods such as alfalfa, aduki bean sprouts, wheat grass, and fresh fruits and vegetables.
- Include more whole grains such as brown rice, oat-based cereals, and millet, which are packed with B-vitamins and therefore help support your nerves.
- Try wheat-free breads like Ener-G, which are delicious.
- Try almond or oat milk instead of cow's milk.
- Eat breakfast every day. Good-quality protein will keep you feeling fuller for longer, reduce cravings, and increase energy. Eggs, fish, lean meats, hemp seed protein powder, and peanut, almond, or walnut butter would all be fine.
- Magnesium and calcium are known as nature's tranquillizers, so eat more green vegetables such as kale, cabbage, and broccoli, as well as almonds, Brazil nuts, sesame seeds, pineapple, papaya, Parmesan cheese, fish, dried apricots, sardines, and skimmed milk. Chocolate is also high in calcium, but the benefits are offset by the caffeine content. Just eat it in moderation; and make it dark and organic.
- At night, eat whole-wheat pastas, baked potatoes (especially sweet potatoes), pumpkin, and oats, which are more calming. Make thick vegetable soups, which are easier on the digestion.
- Turkey, bananas, oats, and avocado are high in tryptophan, which aids natural sleep.
- Generally, control your blood sugar levels by eating small meals regularly instead of bingeing on junk foods. This will help reduce the constant exhaustion. (See *Low Blood Sugar*.)
- Drink herbal teas throughout the day that are free from caffeine. Choose a calming blend such as licorice, yerba mate, or chamomile. Green tea is rich in L-theanine, which is known to induce feelings of calm.
- As your digestive system is bound to be stressed, eat a low-fat, live yogurt with meals.

Useful Remedies

- Take a high-strength B-complex to help calm your nerves and aid digestion. Add 500mg of pantothenic acid (vitamin B5) to help support adrenal function. If you regularly wake up between 3 and 5am, this can be linked to adrenal exhaustion; also if you find you need to urinate regularly but don't have a bladder infection, this can also denote that your adrenals are on the edge. (See also *Adrenal Exhaustion*.)
- Since the digestive system begins malfunctioning when we are really tired, take a digestive enzyme or betaine hydrochloride (stomach acid) with meals to improve the absorption of nutrients. Do not take the betaine if you have active stomach ulcers; instead, take a digestive enzyme capsule (without HCl) with main meals.
- Co-enzyme Q10 is a supplement that is well proven to boost energy levels. The body produces CoQ10 naturally, but as we age or when we are stressed we produce less. And as most people no longer eat organ meats that are rich in Co-enzyme Q10, it is best taken as a supplement (100mg daily with breakfast).
- Calcium and magnesium are often depleted. Take 300mg of calcium with 200mg of magnesium an hour before going to bed. Stress and exhaustion make the body more acid, and these minerals help re-alkalize your system. They are also known as nature's tranquillizers. **SVHC**
- Siberian ginseng is useful as a general tonic that helps support adrenal function. There are plenty of liquid formulas, and this can be taken for a month. Jarrow makes an advanced stress formula containing Siberian ginseng, ashwagandha, and gotu kola along with other ingredients, which helps regulate cortisol levels. **JF**
- L-carnitine is an amino acid that helps to improve energy levels, Take 1g a day before meals for a month.
- Take L-theanine and lemon balm before going to bed. They really do help. **LEF**

E

Helpful Hints

- If you are at rock bottom, a few vitamin pills and a couple of nights' sleep will help, but they are definitely not the long-term solution. You must try to address the root cause of your exhaustion.
- Generally try to take at least one day a week for yourself, making time for exercise or simply some "me time."
- Breathe deeply into your belly every hour. Get up, walk around, and stretch.
- If your exhaustion is linked to personal problems, think about seeing a counselor. Talking problems through gives you a better perspective. (See also *Depression*.)
- Never take work to bed and always finish work at least one hour before going to bed. Otherwise, your mind simply keeps churning your thoughts over and over.
- Gentle exercise like yoga, tai chi, qigong or strolling through nature helps make you feel more positive and re-builds energy levels.
- Find a practitioner who can really sort out your diet, such as a nutritionist or a naturopath. Then make a determined effort to improve your food intake. (See *Useful Information*.)
- If at all practical, treat yourself to three days at a health spa to rejuvenate and rest.

EYE PROBLEMS

(see also Cataracts, Conjunctivitis, Glaucoma, and Macular Degeneration)

Eye problems are highly varied, ranging from simply being tired, to suffering blurred vision, redness, dark circles and so on. I have covered several of the more common problems—but please, if any eye problem becomes chronic, you must see an optometrist, ophthalmologist, or your doctor. Your eyes can become bloodshot if you cough too much, sneeze a lot, or if you have high blood pressure.

Generally, if the whites of your eyes appear yellowish, it means that your liver is somewhat toxic, and you need to clean up your diet. If you suffer "floaters" in your vision, this can denote poor liver function and possibly candida, a yeast/fungal overgrowth. However, if there are large numbers of floaters and you also have a curtain-like darkness coming across your eyes from the outside in, this can indicate a detached retina, and you **must** seek urgent medical attention.

Blepharitis

If red eyes are accompanied by a burning sensation, excessive tearing, itching, sensitivity to light, swollen eyelids, blurred vision, frothy tears, dry eyes, or crusting of the eyelashes on awakening, then blepharitis (inflammation of the eyelid caused by an infection) should be considered. Visit an eye-care specialist to check this out. (See also *Red-rimmed Eyes*.)

Foods to Avoid

- Avoid saturated fats found in red meat and dairy foods, as well as sugar, as these foods create inflammation in the body and can block the essential lubricating fats found in oily fish, nuts, and seeds from doing their job.

Friendly Foods

- Eat plenty of dark-purple fruits like bilberries, blueberries, blackberries and cherries, as they are rich in bioflavonoids, which protect and strengthen the eyes and help reduce the risk of eye damage from other diseases.

- Eat more green vegetables, especially raw spinach, cabbage, kale, and watercress, plus sweet potatoes, pumpkin, papaya, cantaloupe melons, and carrots, which are all rich in carotenes that nourish the eyes.
- Eat more oily fish—salmon, trout, mackerel, tuna, sardines, and anchovies—along with nuts and seeds. These are rich in essential fats, which help to lubricate the eyes from the inside out.
- Immune-boosting foods rich in vitamin C and zinc are essential, as they will help the body fight off any infection. Eat more red and yellow peppers, kiwi fruit, green leafy vegetables, whole grains, nuts, and seeds.
- Green and white teas supply catechins, which reduce oxidative stress in the eyes. Drink them black without milk

Useful remedies

- Higher Nature's Visual Eyes contains a good combination of vitamins and antioxidants. These antioxidants are believed to help protect the retina from free radical damage. Available from www.swallowhealthydiet.com
- If the blepharitis is severe, an eye-care professional may prescribe antibiotics. Healthy bacteria found in the gut need to be taken along with the antibiotics. Take Jarro-Dophilus EPS probiotics as far away from the antibiotics as possible. (See *Antibiotics*.) **JF**
- Bromelain, extracted from pineapples, really helps reduce inflammation. Take 500mg twice daily while symptoms are acute.

Helpful Hints

- Castor oil has traditionally been used as an anti-inflammatory remedy for the treatment of blepharitis. Eyelid inflammation may initially increase after starting this treatment, but with repeated use of it over a week, the inflammation should be reduced. Refresh Endura contains castor oil and is available from most health stores. Use one to two drops a few times a day.
- Gently massage the eyelids with a clean, warm, steamy flannel (change each time) for 5 minutes two to four times daily. Wipe all debris off the lids with a cotton ball soaked in warm, salty water.
- Note that many eye drops are on based on urine (urea). Therefore, if you can stand it, use fresh urine—which is a sterile liquid—and dab it around the eyes.

Dark circles under the eyes

(see also Adrenal Exhaustion, Allergies, Hay Fever, and Thyroid)

The obvious culprit for dark circles is lack of sleep, and if you are chronically short of sleep, then your adrenal glands will become exhausted, making the circles under your eyes even darker. Panda-like "black" eyes are also a common symptom of thyroid problems. (See under *Thyroid*.) Dark circles can be triggered by sensitivities either to products that you are using (creams, hair sprays and so on), or by foods to which you have an intolerance. And if you suffer from hay fever, then rubbing your itchy eyes can make dark circles worse.

If you have truly "black," panda-like eyes, ask your doctor to check for an underactive thyroid or low iron levels. Food intolerances are one of the most common causes of dark circles, and wheat is usually the main culprit. In a few cases it can also be hereditary (see below). Pregnancy and menstruation can cause the skin under the eyes to become paler, which allows underlying veins to show through, thus making the circles look darker. This also can happen with certain medications used to dilate blood vessels. Too much ultraviolet light, from the sun or tanning beds, and smoking can also make dark circles worse, as can water retention caused by kidney problems (in Chinese Medicine the eyes relate to the liver) or PMS (see *Pre-menstrual Syndrome*). If you have a tendency to develop dark circles under your eyes, they are likely to become more noticeable and permanent as you grow older. Excess folds of skin under the eyes will also make dark circles more pronounced. Therefore, it makes sense to first make sure you are getting enough sleep, and if you are, but still suffer from dark circles, try eliminating wheat for seven days. You will be amazed at the difference.

Also, it's important to realize that as we age, some people will develop what is known as periobital volume loss. Consultant ophthalmic surgeon Mr Raman Malhotra, based at Gatwick Park Hospital in the UK, says: "This is a combination of loss of bone volume and soft tissue volume, including fat and thickness of skin under the eyes, which can give rise to the appearance of under-eye dark circles partly due to the concavity that occurs as a result of hollowing. In addition, darkness occurs due to the visibility of the underlying orbicularis eyelid muscle underneath thinner skin."

My mother suffered from this dark hollowing under the eyes and so have I. For years I always looked "tired all the time" until I discovered that Mr Malhotra has developed a method of injecting fillers such as Restylane directly into the hollow, dark, under-eye circles (details at www.ramanmalhotra.com). His injections have completely (unless I'm really exhausted) eradicated this hollow look. Many plastic surgeons offer dermal filler treatments. This treatment is well worth looking into.

Foods to Avoid
- Cut down on alcohol and salt and drink plenty of water to flush toxins out of the body.
- Processed foods, sauce packets and other ketchup-style condiments often contain huge amounts of hidden salt, so are best avoided.
- If you are sleeping well but still have circles after three or four good nights' sleep, then eliminate wheat for a week to see if this helps. If there is no change, then also try eliminating cow's milk. These are the most common triggers.

Friendly Foods
- Drink plenty of water to eliminate toxins and generally eat a clean diet, avoiding too much refined food and sugar. (See *General Health Hints*.)
- Green leafy vegetables, seaweeds, kelp, lentils, and peas are all rich in vitamin K, which has been shown to help reduce bruising and under-eye circles.
- Natural-source carotenes, especially lutein, plus vitamin C are great eye nutrients. Eat more strawberries, kiwi fruit, red, yellow, and green peppers, squash, sweet potatoes, pumpkin, papaya, oily fish, spinach, watercress, mangoes, and green leafy vegetables.

Useful Remedies
- If you are totally exhausted, see *Useful Remedies* under *Adrenal Exhaustion*.
- OcuPower Advanced multi-vitamin from Synergy contains bilberry extract, antioxidants (vitamins A, E, and C, plus selenium), ginkgo biloba, lycopene, and chromium. **VC**

Helpful Hints
- Do not drag or rub the delicate skin under the eyes when using cleansers and make-up.
- Use specific skincare products made especially for the eyes, as regular moisturizers can be too heavy and lead to puffy, dark circles.
- Beware of using concealers as many are too heavy for this delicate area and actually make the problem worse. However, one of best I have found is Jane Iredale's mineral make-up (www.janeiredale.com). See the Where to Buy section of the website for retailers near you.

Detached Retina

This is when the retina separates from its normal position at the back of the eye —much like wallpaper peeling off a wall. This can occur if there is a trauma to the eye (such as being hit by a baseball), as a complication to diabetes, or sometimes during cataract surgery.

If you suddenly begin to experience large numbers of floaters in your vision and if you also have a curtain-like darkness coming across your eyes from the outside in, this can indicate that the retina has, in fact, become detached or developed small holes, in which case you **must** seek urgent medical attention. Otherwise, you risk blindness in that eye.

■ Follow diet as above.

Dry Eyes   *(see also Sjogren's Syndrome)*

Dry eyes can be triggered by being in a dry environment for lengthy periods of time (such as on an aircraft) or working on a computer all day. Contact lens users often complain of dry eyes as well. Chronic dry eyes, though, is a classic symptom of Sjogren's Syndrome. (See under this heading.)

There are two types of dry eyes. The first, and less common, is known as aqueous or tear deficiency (linked to Sjogren's), while the second type, which is more common, is known as evaporative dry eye. Evaporative dry eye occurs as a result of meibomian gland dysfunction. The meibomian glands are oil glands along the eyelid margin that produce oil as a component of tears to prevent evaporation. Treatment includes regular use of artificial tears (available at all pharmacies) and regular use of warm compresses to help maintain good meibomian gland function and healthy oil turnover.

A hormone imbalance can play a significant role in dry eye development related to meibomian gland dysfunction and in particular, androgen deficiency, which can occur post-menopause but also in the perimenopausal period. Certain types of hormone replacement therapy can be androgen suppressing and can therefore exacerbate dry eyes. If a patient is found to be androgen deficient, then switching to a more androgen-friendly hormone replace-ment therapy may be of some help. (See *Hormones associated with the menopause* under *Menopause*.)

■ For foods to avoid and eat more of, see under *Blepharitis*.

Useful Remedies
■ Essential fats are vital for healthy eyes. Take 2g of omega-3 fish oils daily.
■ Flax seed oil has been shown to be of benefit for people with meibomian gland dysfunction. Take 500mg daily. **VC**
■ Omega-7 found in sea buckthorn is particularly useful for reducing dry eyes. Take 2g daily for one month, then reduce to 1g daily. **VC**
■ Natural-source beta-carotene is also crucial for healthy eyes. Take 7–10mg daily. **SVHC**
■ Take a good-quality multi-vitamin/mineral with 15–30mg of zinc.
■ Natural-source, full-spectrum vitamin E helps nourish and protect the eyes. Take 400–500IU daily.
■ Hyaluronic acid (HA) is a naturally occurring protein in the body. HA is what makes young skin look plump and supple. It also helps keep your eyes moist from the inside out. To supplement your HA levels, take 1ml of a liquid formula daily in water on an empty stomach; it takes time to work, but it does help. HA will also help your skin and joints remain supple. **VC**

Itchy eyes
(see also Conjunctivitis and Hay Fever)

Itching of the eyes can be due to an infection such as conjunctivitis, allergies, or hay fever, as well as to exposure to a smoky or polluted atmosphere. As I can attest, dry eyes can also be due to over-exposure to computer screens. Eyes also become irritated on long-distance flights and when they are tired. If you suffer from dry, itchy eyes after a long flight, then use Natural Tears Eye Drops regularly and take more essential fats, which help nourish your eyes from the inside out. (See *Fats You Need to Eat*.)

If the problem is linked to your computer, take regular breaks, get out in the sunshine, and get some rest. Dry, itchy eyes are also a classic symptom of Sjogren's syndrome, an autoimmune condition. (See under that section.)

Foods to Avoid
■ Avoid dehydrating beverages, such as caffeine and alcohol. Just like every other part of the body, the eyes need plenty of fluid intake to keep them in good shape. Drink more water.
■ Processed flour dries out the body; therefore, reduce your intake of flour-based foods.
■ Avoid saturated fats found in red meat and full-fat dairy products, as they create inflammation in the body and can block the essential lubricating fats found in oily fish, nuts, and seeds from doing their job.

Friendly Foods

■ Eat plenty of dark-purple fruits like bilberries, blueberries, blackberries, and cherries, as the bioflavonoids in these fruits not only protect and strengthen the eyes but also help reduce the risk of eye damage from other diseases.
■ Eat more green vegetables, sweet potatoes, pumpkin, and carrots, which are all rich in the carotenes that nourish the eyes.
■ Eat more oily fish. They are rich in essential fats, which helps prevent the eyes from drying out.
■ Eat more unsalted nuts (not peanuts) and seeds, which are high in zinc and selenium.

Useful Remedies
■ Take 25,000IU of vitamin A a day for one month. **NB: You can only take 3000IU of vitamin A per day if you are pregnant or planning to become pregnant.** After one month, take around 10–15mg of natural-source carotenes daily. These convert naturally to vitamin A in the body. Carotenes are safe even in higher doses and are fine to take during pregnancy. SVHC
■ Zinc (30mg a day) is essential for enhancing vitamin A absorption.
■ B-vitamins, in particular vitamin B2, are necessary to prevent dry eyes. Take a strong B-complex daily.
■ Take a high-strength multi-vitamin/mineral and an EFA formula. There is no need to take the extra zinc or B vitamins if you are taking a high-strength multi.

Helpful Hints
■ Euphrasia (eyebright), raspberry, and pau d'arco can be made into an infusion, strained and, when cooled, applied to each eye using an eye bath. Make sure to sterilize the eye baths before use. The infusion has anti-inflammatory, astringent, antiseptic, and anti-catarrhal properties. The powder, capsule, teabag, or liquid form of these herbs can all be purchased online from Amazon sellers or from most health stores.
■ I often find that if I sleep in an air-conditioned room it can make my eyes very sore; similarly in rooms that are too hot. In the winter, I keep a small bowl of water near my heating vents to keep the air in the room moist.

- The homeopathic version of eyebright (euphrasia) can be used for bathing the eyes and is very soothing. Use Euphrasia Mother Tincture about four times a day, using a disposable eye bath. Available online from www.amazon.com.
- Heel Homeopathics makes disposable remedies in single vials. Oculoheel can be used to treat conjunctivitis and dry eyes. You can find this product through most online retailers, including www.amazon.com and www.drugstore.com
- Another way to relieve itchy eyes is to brew a pot of chamomile tea and lay the tea bags, once they've cooled, on your eyelids. Ideally, leave them on for about 15 minutes.
- Don't use anyone else's washcloth or towel just in case the problem is infectious.
- Pinhole glasses help take the strain off the eyes and help your eyes focus properly (pinhole-glasses.com).
- If you suspect allergies are the problem, keep your home free from pet dander and house dust mites and stay inside when there is a lot of pollen is in the air. Air ionizers can help keep the air clean. (See also *Allergies*.)

Macular degeneration   *(see under Macular Degeneration)*

Optic neuritis

This is an inflammation of the optic nerve, which carries information from the seeing part of the eye, the retina, toward the brain. It can cause partial or complete loss of vision, which comes on over a few hours or days and may be accompanied by pain in the eye. Optic neuritis can be one of the symptoms of multiple sclerosis but can also be triggered by sinus problems, severe high blood pressure, post-viral and post-meningitis infections, or more serious problems. Always check your symptoms with your doctor.

Foods to Avoid
- Foods that would aggravate inflammation, including red meat and dairy products (butter, cheese, cream, and milk).
- Try to avoid alcohol and caffeine, which can interfere with blood circulation to the eyes.
- Cut down on sugar in any form, as sugar triggers inflammation in the body. All the usual suspects I'm afraid: cakes, cookies, candies, desserts, and soft drinks.

Friendly Foods
- Pineapple is a rich source of bromelain, an anti-inflammatory enzyme that really helps the eyes.
- Oily fish is rich in essential fats, which are anti-inflammatory. Eat more mackerel, sardines, anchovies, organic salmon, and herrings.
- Spices such as ginger, turmeric, and cayenne are all great for reducing inflammation as well as improving circulation to the eye.
- Bilberries, blueberries, blackberries, and all other blue and orange fruits will help nourish the eyes.
- Resveratrol is an anti-inflammatory compound that helps relieve the pain associated with inflammation. You can find it in red grapes, so enjoy a glass of red grape juice daily or an occasional glass of red wine (preferably organic).
- Sugar-free blueberry, plum, or cherry jams would be fine.

Useful Remedies
- Taking 500mg of bromelain twice a day can reduce inflammation and improve circulation.

- The herb ginkgo biloba helps strengthen the capillaries in the eye and improves circulation; take 120–240mg of standardized extract a day.
- Take 10,000–25,000IU or vitamin A a day for one month. **NB: Only take 3000IU if you are pregnant or planning to become pregnant.** After a month take a natural-source carotene daily, which is safe at any dose. Take 10mg daily. **SVHC**

Puffy eyes

Puffiness and bags under the eyes can denote kidney problems and a build-up of toxins within the body. The condition also signifies that the sodium and potassium levels within the body are out of balance. In this case, take 100mg of potassium daily for a week or so and reduce your intake of sodium-based salts. Puffiness can also be associated with food intolerances and conditions such as hay fever. (See *Hay fever*.) In these instances, drink more water to flush the kidneys, and avoid wheat and dairy products for at least three days. Puffy eyes can also indicate an underactive thyroid; therefore, if the problem continues after making these changes, have a check-up with your doctor.

Foods to Avoid

E

- If underneath the eyes is both puffy and dark, it is very likely that you have food intolerances, so it is important to identify these. The most common intolerances are to dairy products from cows, wheat, citrus fruits, eggs, and nuts. Salt is also a major trigger and definitely exacerbates any water retention, which increases swelling in all parts of the body.
- Mass-produced breakfast cereals often contain more salt than the average bag of potato chips.
- Dairy products from cows, cheese, and cottage cheese are high in sodium.
- Most pre-packaged, refined foods will have additional salt, and a lot of foods that are naturally sweet have salt added as a preservative and to take the edge off the sweetness.
- Look out for hidden sources of salt/sodium such as ketchup, pickles and relishes, olives, and hotdogs. These foods contain sodium benzoate —a preservative—and monosodium glutamate (MSG), which contribute to high levels of sodium.
- Cut down on all foods and drinks that contain caffeine and alcohol, which further dehydrate the body.
- Reduce red meat consumption to lessen the burden on the kidneys.

Friendly Foods

- Water is really important; drink 6–8 glasses a day.
- Eat lots of fruit and green vegetables—especially celery and dark green leafy vegetables. Dried fruits, nuts, sunflower seeds, and seafood are also rich in potassium, which can improve the balance of minerals in the body, particularly if your salt intake is high.
- Eat more artichokes, beets, celeriac, celery, and fennel.
- If you are not a big fan of fruit and vegetables, at least try drinking a couple of glasses of non-concentrate fruit juice or freshly made vegetable juice every day, as they are rich in potassium. Avoid orange juice, which is a common trigger for puffy eyes.

Useful Remedies

- Drink dandelion tea or take a tincture with every meal; total 5ml daily.
- Take a digestive enzyme with all main meals.
- Take a good multi-vitamin/mineral that is suitable for your age and gender
- Take 1g of vitamin C daily in an ascorbate form to encourage lymph drainage. **VC**
- Take 500mg of celery seed extract twice a day to aid drainage. **VC**

Helpful Hints

- One of the most effective ways of getting rid of puffy eyes is to have regular acupuncture, which can help tone up the kidney meridians. This in turn should reduce the swelling. Facial acupuncture is great for reducing eye problems. (See *Useful Information*.)
- Manual lymph drainage (MLD) can also aid this condition. (See *Useful Information*.)
- Dry skin brushing will help break up toxins stored under the skin so the body can eliminate them. Combine skin brushing with an Epsom salt bath to really help flush out toxins. Use one cup per 60 pounds of body weight and add to a warm bath. Soak for 15 to 20 minutes and then rub your skin all over with a flannel. Don't rinse off before getting out of the bath; just dry off and retire for the evening. Keep some drinking water handy by the tub as a warm bath can make you thirsty.
- Make an infusion with chamomile tea bags and, when cool, apply to the eyes.
- Take the homeopathic remedies Apis 6c and Kali Carb 6c, which are excellent for reducing puffy eyes.
- Lymph drainage done mechanically through massage, reflexology, or even bouncing up and down on a rebounder can be quite helpful.
- If you suspect a food intolerance, get this checked out by YorkTest Laboratories. They offer a home test kit called The Food Intolerance Test that is available in the US. The test checks for the most common culprits and gives you the option of going on to a more thorough test should you have a positive result. Visit www.yorktest.com for more information.
- Puffy eyes may be related to an underactive thyroid, so it is worth checking with your doctor and getting a thyroid test.

E

Red-rimmed eyes

Consistently red-rimmed eyes can be a sign of malnutrition or a lack of B-vitamins. It can also be a sign of malabsorption of nutrients within the gut from your diet (see also *Absorption* and *Leaky Gut*) or can be associated with hay fever or hangovers. If symptoms also include a burning sensation, excessive tearing, itching, sensitivity to light, swollen eyelids, blurred vision, frothy tears, dry eyes, or crusting of the eyelashes on awakening, then blepharitis— inflammation of the eye lid—should be considered. Visit an eye care specialist to rule this out. Red-rimmed eyes can also, of course, simply denote extreme tiredness, so get some rest.

Foods to Avoid

- Refined carbohydrates, such as cookies, cakes, white bread, pizza, and pasta, all deplete the B vitamins you need for good eye health.
- Avoid caffeine in foods and drinks, as these tend to over-stimulate the system and deplete B vitamins even further.

Friendly Foods

- See *Friendly Foods* under *Itchy Eyes*.

Useful Remedies

- Take a high-strength B-complex daily.
- Take 1–3ml of dandelion and burdock tincture a day (available from www.zooscape.com). If the red-rimmed eyes are due to a build-up of toxins, these herbs can help eliminate them from the body, as well as improving liver function and digestion.
- Always include a high-strength multi-vitamin/mineral and an essential fats formula in your daily regimen.

Helpful Hints

- Bathe the eyes in cooled chamomile tea bags, which are very soothing, or apply cool slices of cucumber.
- Soak some pads in witch hazel and rose water and then lay them on the eyes for 10 minutes. You could also use a soothing eye balm made from cucumber extract.
- If the condition is linked to blepharitis, then massage the lids with a clean, warm, steamy flannel (change each time) for 60 seconds and wipe all debris off the lids with a cotton ball soaked in warm, salty water. If the blepharitis is severe, an eye care professional may also prescribe antibiotics or steroid eye drops, which need to be followed by a course of healthy bacteria. Take Jarro-Dophilus for a month. **JF**

General Hints for Eye Problems

If the whites of your eyes are dull or yellowish in color, this indicates that your liver is struggling. Eat more green vegetables, fruits, and whole grains, also try drinking dandelion coffee and taking herb milk thistle to help cleanse the liver. Consume less saturated fats, sugar, alcohol, and coffee. (See also *Liver Problems*.)

Pinhole glasses help strengthen weak eye muscles (www.pinhole-glasses.com).

Dr Hauschka's Eye Solace is an organic and environmentally friendly solution that you can simply add to cotton balls or pads, lie back and enjoy. It contains eyebright, anthyllis, and chamomile extracts, which soothe and refresh sore, reddened, overtired eyes. Available from www.amazon.com

For people like me who spend a lot of time reading and working in front of a computer screen, take breaks as often as you can and get out in the fresh air and natural sunlight. While sitting at your desk, you can stretch your eye muscles by looking into the distance.

Get plenty of sleep.

FATIGUE *(see Adrenal Exhaustion, Exhaustion, ME, and Stress)*

FATS YOU NEED TO EAT

For more than 16 years I have been telling people about the health benefits of essential fats—as have many other health writers, doctors, scientists and nutritionists—and at long last the message is finally filtering through. It needs to.

After all, your brain is almost 60% fat, but it needs more of the right type of fats to function effectively. Essential fats (EFAs) are essential to life, hence their name, and, as we cannot manufacture them in our bodies, we must take them in from external sources through our diet. Most people consume approximately 42% of their calories from fat, but unfortunately it's usually the wrong type of fat.

Dr Udo Erasmus, a Canadian-based bio-chemist and world renowned authority on fats and oils, says: "A huge proportion of degenerative health conditions are triggered not only by eating excessive animal fats, but also over-consumption of mass-produced fats and oils. The majority of vegetable oils found in supermarkets have been refined, bleached, and deodorized and then used for frying, which introduces huge amounts of aging free radicals into the body." To compound the negative health effects, a commercial practice called hydrogenation, in which liquid oils are turned into spreadable fats called trans-fatty acids, found in some margarines, mass-produced cakes, cookies, cereal bars, chocolates, potato chips, and so on, are also unhealthy fats.

Some food manufacturers, such as Kraft, have taken the positive step of banning trans- and hydrogenated fats from hundreds of their most popular products. Let's hope more follow.

Erasmus adds to this list sweet and starchy foods—desserts, high-sugar fizzy sodas, filled pastries, chocolates and so on—which tend to be high not only in sugar but also in saturated fats. If it is not utilized during exercise, sugar converts to fat in the body and sits on your hips, thighs, and stomach. But before sugar turns into fat, it triggers cross-linking in the skin, which means you develop wrinkles faster; bacteria thrive on sugar, which will impair your immune system; and sugar increases inflammation in the body, and inflammation can trigger practically every disease from arthritis to Alzheimer's and cancer to Parkinson's.

Having said this, some children, especially young girls, are becoming obsessed with eliminating all fat from their diets. This is dangerous. If the body becomes too low in fat, then chronic depression and a host of skin disorders such as eczema can result. Children (and adults) need fats for vital functions, such as the manufacture of hormones and energy. That said, I would not encourage really overweight children, who do little or no exercise, to eat lots of junk fatty foods; but I would never recommend that normal-weight children give up all fats. We all enjoy treats, but we do need to stop living on them. The body also needs essential fats to encourage weight loss, as EFAs help to burn stored fat.

F

There are two main types of EFAs, omega-3 (alpha-linolenic acid) and omega-6, which comes in two forms, linoleic acid and gamma-linolenic acid (GLA). There is more about GLA under *Useful Supplements*.

The best source of omega-3 is oily fish, which contains EPA and DHA (easily utilized types of omega-3 fats). Eating lots of oily fish is why Eskimos rarely suffered heart disease—until they began eating a Western diet. Linseeds (flax seeds), walnuts, hemp seeds, and pumpkin seeds also contain omega-3 fats, which the body then converts into the useful EPA and DHA forms; in fish oil this has already been done by nature. There are a few people who cannot easily convert the essential fats in seeds and nuts into EPA and DHA, which is known as atopic tendency, and common characteristics of this condition are asthma, eczema, and hay fever.

Therefore if you suffer from these conditions, take fish oils as your first line of defense. Omega-3 fats help transfer oxygen around the body, relax blood vessels, and are vital for hormone production, healthy eyes, gut function, weight loss, reducing inflammation, speeding wound healing, and so on. Unfortunately, most people eat 80% less oily fish now than we did in the 1940s, and 60% of people are deficient in omega-3 EFAs.

The second type of EFAs, omega-6, is found in evening primrose, starflower, blackcurrant, and walnut and sesame oils. Walnuts, Brazil nuts, pecans, almonds, as well as sunflower, pumpkin, and sesame seeds are also rich in omega-6 EFAs. These fats help lower blood pressure, thin the blood and help insulin work, which keeps blood sugar levels in balance and helps reduce the cravings for sweet foods.

Most people ingest plenty of omega-6s from nuts and non-hydrogenated vegetable oils and margarines, but normally from poor-quality sources such as bread, cookies, cakes, etc., which are usually made with vegetable oils.

To absorb **any** essential fatty acids, the minerals zinc and magnesium plus vitamins B3 and B6 are necessary and are often depleted by our over-consumption of omega-6s.

"Undoubtedly," says nutritionist and my co-author Gareth Zeal, "we need to take far more omega-3 plus these co-factors daily, and to address our modern dietary deficiencies, we need to consume twice as much omega-3 as -6."

Another beneficial fat, omega-9, is found in unrefined extra-virgin olive oil, a monounsaturated fat, which is far more stable for cooking (but never heat until it spits and produces smoke). A lesser-known EFA is omega-7, also known as palmitoleic acid. This polyunsaturated fatty acid is found in the sea buckthorn berry. It is useful for dry skin and dry eyes, and for mouth and vaginal dryness. (For more information about omega-7 visit Pharma Nord's Nutrient Information Service's website: www.pharmanord.co.uk)

Polyunsaturated fats (also found in seeds, nuts, and their oils) are healthy in their cold, unrefined form, and they are rich in omega-6 EFAs. So if you use sunflower, walnut, sesame seed or grape seed oils in their unrefined forms in salad dressings they are healthy. However, once the polyunsaturated oils that you find in most cookies, margarines and mass-produced vegetable oils are heated, they become unhealthy.

Many people cook (mostly frying) with oils and margarines labeled "polyunsaturated," believing them to be healthier, but it is not so. If the oils that you buy are mass produced, all the processes I mentioned earlier will have long ago destroyed the majority of any health benefits. Butter is actually better for cooking at low temperatures, as it does not turn rancid like the essential fats. Coconut oil has similar properties. Butter contains vitamin A and butyric acid, which has anti-cancer properties, and a little butter, preferably organic, is okay, if you have sufficient EFAs in the body.

All essential fats need to be kept cool and never heated, as the heat destroys their delicate make-up; this includes all oil-based supplements, which should be kept in the fridge.

Typical symptoms of insufficient EFAs are dry skin and eyes, cracked lips, water retention, increased thirst, physical and mental exhaustion, mood swings, inflammatory conditions such as eczema and arthritis, frequent infections, hay fever, allergies, mental health problems including depression, poor memory and learning difficulties, and cardiovascular disease. Most of these conditions we tend to accept as we age, but if you take sufficient EFAs then you should avoid such symptoms for many more years.

Foods to Avoid
- Reduce your intake of full-fat milk, cheeses, chocolates, potato chips and refined mass-produced cakes and cookies, which are usually high in hydrogenated or trans-fats, and are not good for your health.
- Avoid as much as possible all refined vegetable oils, typically found in margarines, cookies, cakes and, of course, mass-produced vegetable oils.
- If you like red meat, just eat lean organic meat once a week. Hugely reduce or eliminate hamburgers, sausages, and so on. With chicken, turkey, duck, venison, buffalo, quail, or other game, cut off the skin. If you eat bacon, make it a rare treat only: grill and cut off the fat.
- Eliminate or greatly reduce the amount of fried foods you eat.
- Remember that sugar, if not used up during exercise, converts to fat inside the body and that many foods advertised as being low in fat are usually packed with sugar!

Friendly Foods
- Look for non-hydrogenated spreads such as Biona and Olivio or try organic raw walnut, almond, hemp, or pumpkin seed butters. These should be available in your local health store or larger natural/organic supermarkets like Whole Foods.

- You can also buy coconut oil spreads—coconut is unadulterated and helps lower LDL cholesterol.
- If you need to shallow fry, use a little organic olive oil, coconut oil, or butter. Although butter is a saturated fat, it does not turn rancid like vegetable oils when heated. I also use a little butter for baking cakes. For cookies, I use extra-virgin olive oil.
- Nutritionist Gareth Zeal recommends blending extra-virgin olive oil with butter to use as a healthier alternative to hydrogenated and trans-fat-based margarines, also for spreads and making cakes and cookies.
- If you like stir-fries, use a little olive, canola, coconut, or groundnut (peanut) oil. Heat through (but not until "spitting or smoking," which means the oil has become carcinogenic), then add vegetables and so on and stir for a minute. Then add a little water and "steam fry" for a couple more minutes. This helps to reduce the amount of free radicals that are produced when you fry food.
- Oily fish, such as mackerel, organic salmon, trout, sardines, anchovies, and herrings, are all rich in omega-3 fats.
- Soy and kidney beans also contain some omega-3 fats, but try to use only GM-free and organic soybeans.
- Walnuts, pecans, and almonds are all rich in omega-6 fats.
- If you use flax seeds to increase your omega-3 intake, buy them ready-cracked (available from most supermarkets). Keep cracked flax seeds in the fridge. Grind them first before eating. Use a coffee grinder, which breaks them up in seconds, or simply crush them with a mortar and pestle. Otherwise, soak whole linseeds overnight in cold water and drain before eating.
- Seeds,such as sunflower and pumpkin, which are high in omega-6, can be eaten as a snack or sprinkled on soups or salads, and added to meals.
- Hemp seed is readily available and is a good blend of omega-3 and -6 fatty acids. You can also buy excellent organic-source hemp seed protein powders.
- Eat more (but not to excess) monounsaturated fats, such as those found in avocados and olive oil.
- Eat more raw wheat germ and rice bran, rich in vitamin E, which helps you absorb the EFAs more effectively.
- Buy good-quality, unrefined and preferably organic sunflower, walnut, and sesame oils and mix them half and half with olive oil to make delicious salad dressings, or drizzle them over cooked foods (once they are on your plate). Keep them in the fridge to protect the EFAs.
- Once a week I pop a tablespoon each of sunflower, pumpkin, sesame seeds, hazelnuts, hemp seeds, walnuts, almonds, and Brazil nuts into a food processor and pulse for a few seconds. I then place them in a glass jar in the fridge and use them over breakfast cereals, yogurts, desserts, fruit salads, and so on. This is a great way to get more EFAs.

Useful Remedies

- If you are not vegetarian, then take 1–3g of fish oil capsules daily. Many people no longer take fish oils, as they worry about the concentrations of toxins, such as PCBs and dioxins, but many brands of fish oils are guaranteed to be free from toxins. Eskimo 3 stable fish oil capsules are one of the best and can be ordered through online distributors like Vitacost. **VC**
- Gamma-linolenic acid (GLA), is an omega-6 EFA that is found in evening primrose oil, blackcurrant oil, and borage oil. It has anti-inflammatory properties, helps increase your metabolic rate, and reduces symptoms of PMS. Most supplement companies sell GLA, and you can take around 250mg daily.
- If you want pure flax seed)oil try Omega Nutrition (www.omeganutrition.com).
- Udo's Choice Oil is made from organic flax, sunflower, and sesame seeds, plus rice and oat germ oils, in the perfect ratio for good health. Dr Udo Erasmus says we need approximately

1 tablespoon for every 50lbs of body weight, and we need more EFAs in winter than in summer. It is available as an oil, which can be blended with other oils for salad dressings or a little can be drizzled over cooked dishes. It is also available in capsules. These oils are highly unstable, should never be heated and need to be kept in the fridge. Udo's Choice is available from health stores worldwide, or to find your nearest supplier, contact Flora Incorporated, Box 73, 805 Badger Rd, Lynden, WA 98264 or call 1-800-446-2110. Website: www.florahealth.com or e-mail: florainc@worldnet.att.net

- When supplementing with fatty acids, either in capsule or liquid form, it is very important to take a natural-source, full-spectrum vitamin E, at least 100IU a day.
- For anyone who has had his or her gallbladder removed, suffers from Crohn's disease or colitis, or has a sensitive gut or irritable bowel and cannot tolerate too much oil (as the liver has to metabolize all fats and oils), use DriCelle Omega Plex essential fatty acid powder by BioCare. The EFAs have been microencapsulated into water-soluble fiber and then freeze-dried using no oxygen or heat. This powdered formula is therefore stable, which increases absorption dramatically. It bypasses the liver and is 100% absorbed in the intestines.
- Read Dr Udo Erasmus's book, *The Fats That Heal and Fats That Kill* (Alive Books). He has also written *Choosing the Right Fats*, which contains recipes that show you how to integrate healing oils and fats into your daily meals naturally. To find a retail store near you visit www.florahealth.com/flora/home/USA/Stores/_Search.htm

FIBROIDS

A fibroid is a benign tumor made up of muscle and fibrous tissue that grows in the muscular wall of the womb. Fibroids often produce no symptoms at all, but they are known to cause heavy menstrual bleeding and may contribute to infertility. The growth of fibroids seems to be related to a hormone imbalance, especially an excess of the hormone estrogen. If you are on the combined pill or HRT, both of which contain estrogen, you may wish to discuss coming off these drugs with your doctor in order to prevent further growth. If you suffer heavy periods over several months, please have this checked out. With any condition that is linked to hormones you really need to detoxify and support the liver. (See *Liver Problems*.) Basically, fibroids are another symptom of the body holding on to excess toxins.

Foods to Avoid
- Any foods that can trigger elevated estrogen levels or will recycle estrogen into its more aggressive form. These include alcohol, animal fats, such as red meats or any fat on any meat including chicken, cheese, milk (other than fully skimmed), cream, ice cream, butter, and chocolates.
- Most importantly, don't heat ready-made meals in plastic containers as the plastic residues leach into the food, which again has an estrogen affect. Never heat plastic wrap if it's next to food.
- Avoid as much as possible non-organic foods that are often high in pesticides and herbicides, which migrate into fatty tissue and increase estrogen activity in the body.
- Avoid refined soy milks and products.

Friendly Foods
- Chickpeas, broccoli, cabbage, Brussels sprouts, and cauliflower are all beneficial foods, as they encourage excretion of excess hormones.
- Fermented soy-based foods, such as tempeh, miso, and natto, have a regulating effect on estrogen levels and are protective against aggressive estrogens.

- Flaxseeds contain lignan, which also helps balance hormones naturally. I soak a tablespoon of Linusit Gold flaxseeds in a cup of cold water overnight and then use in fruit breakfast blends, in oatmeal, or over cereals.
- Don't overcook your vegetable. Make fresh vegetable juices every day and drink immediately after juicing.
- Eat plenty of foods containing natural carotenes such as cantaloupe melons, apricots, sweet potatoes, parsley, carrots, spring greens, watercress, pumpkin, and spinach. Eat more almonds, cod liver oil, avocados, wheat germ, and hazelnuts, which are all rich in vitamin E.
- Eat more oily fish rich in omega-3 fats.
- Use plenty of rosemary and pineapple, which are anti-inflammatory.

Useful Remedies
- To regulate hormone levels, take 50–100mg of soy isoflavones and add wild yam (1–3ml of tincture or 1–3g of tablets) to help curb excessive bleeding.
- Triple Action Cruciferous Vegetable Extract by the Life Extension Foundation contains broccoli, watercress, and rosemary, which include I3C, a compound known to neutralize harmful estrogens. Take one capsule daily. **LEF**
- You need plenty of essential fats, which play a vital role in hormone production. Take 2–3g of omega-3 fish oils daily.
- Include a high-strength multi-vitamin/mineral for women. **VC, JF**
- Some women stop ovulating at some point between their 35th and 40th birthdays, which means they no longer make progesterone but continue to make estrogen. Talk to your doctor about using a natural bio-identical progesterone cream, which can help reverse fibroids. Contact PharmWest at 1-310-301-4015; e-mail: infodesk@pharmwest.com; website: www.pharmwest.com
- The Life Extension Foundation (www.lef.org) also supplies bio-identical hormones. **NB: Never self-medicate with hormones unless you have had a blood or saliva test showing that you need them.**
- Silica and calcium fluoride tissue salts can help to break down the fibroids. Take four of each one daily.

Helpful Hints
- Once you go through menopause, the fibroids should shrink naturally.

FIBROMYALGIA

(see also Candida, Irritable Bowel Syndrome, and Leaky Gut)

The word "fibromyalgia" is derived from the Latin *fibra*, meaning "fiber," and the Greek word *mys*, meaning "muscle." This syndrome generally affects more women than men and is characterized by aching and stiffness in the large muscle groups, especially in the neck, shoulders, and pelvis. There also may be pain in the chest and ribcage, often combined with stiffness in the morning and sometimes with a feeling of nausea. A low-grade fever and/or anxiety, depression, and sleep problems are also common. Some sufferers experience an irritable bowel and bladder, even when no bladder infection is present. In virtually every case this condition can be greatly alleviated or cured by dietary changes, since fibromyalgia is closely linked to the yeast fungal overgrowth candida and a leaky gut. (See also both of these sections.)

Many people tend to confuse polymyalgia with fibromyalgia; however, Polymyalgia Rheumatica (PMR) is an autoimmune condition more closely linked to rheumatoid arthritis.

PMR involves inflammation of the muscles whereas fibromyalgia is associated with low pain tolerance in the muscles and connective tissue. If you have been diagnosed with PMR, I suggest that you read the *Rheumatoid Arthritis* and *Sjogren's Syndrome* sections.

People who suffer from chronic fatigue, such as ME, also tend to suffer from fibromyalgia. High homocysteine levels (which are a toxic by-product of protein digestion) may also be linked to these types of conditions. (For more information about homocysteine see *High Blood Pressure*.)

Doctors have also noted that several other conditions can trigger fibromyalgia-type symptoms, such as thyroid problems, lupus, and rheumatoid arthritis. Blood tests can confirm if any of these conditions are an underlying cause of your fibromyalgia.

Foods to Avoid
- Any food that you have an intolerance to will make this problem worse. Without a doubt these are usually the foods you tend to eat and crave the most. The most common culprits are wheat, sugar, cow's milk, soy, corn, citrus fruits, and tomatoes.
- Avoid caffeine and alcohol, as they affect hormones in the body that are linked to pain receptors. Caffeinated drinks include soft drinks, hot chocolate, coffee, and so on. Alcohol also acts like a depressant.
- Greatly reduce your intake of sugar, which can trigger inflammation and low blood sugar in the body as well as mood swings.

- Read product labels and make sure to avoid hydrogenated and trans-fats, which are found in most mass-produced pies, sausages, salamis, margarines, cakes, cookies, and so on. (See *General Health Hints* and *Fats You Need To Eat*.)
- See this section under *Candida* and *Leaky Gut*.

Friendly Foods
- Eat more cold-water fish, such as herring, mackerel, and organically farmed salmon and trout, as they are high in omega-3 essential fats, which reduce inflammation. If you are sensitive to fish, include flax and hemp seeds in your diet instead.
- Eat more whole foods (preferably organic). These include fruits and vegetables, especially squash, carrots, pumpkin, papaya, watermelon, watercress, cantaloupe melon, mango, sweet potatoes, cabbage, and kale.
- Grains can be a problem, and flour really dries out the body. Avoid white flour and wheat, which can irritate the gut. Try millet, buckwheat, quinoa, and amaranth grains, which can be found in breads, cookies, pastas, and crackers from any good health food store and a number of supermarkets.
- Eat more brown rice.
- Eat a little fresh pineapple before main meals, as it has anti-inflammatory properties and aids digestion.
- Eat more cabbage. You should also try drinking the water you boiled the cabbage in (once it has cooled), as it contains L-glutamine, an amino acid that really heals your gut.
- Take aloe vera daily. Lakewood Organic makes a great pure aloe juice. (Visit www.lakewoodjuices.com.)
- Use more turmeric (found in curries) as it is highly anti-inflammatory.
- Drink nettle leaf tea.
- Since dehydration is often a problem, drink more water.
- See also *General Health Hints* and the dietary advice listed under *Rheumatoid Arthritis*.
- It is worth pointing out that, although fibromyalgia is not strictly an inflammatory condition, it would be helpful to avoid inflammation-causing foods (such as those listed above) and eat

the anti-inflammatory foods suggested. This will help reduce the overall burden on your pain receptors.

Useful Remedies

- Beta Glucans 1–3, 1–6, derived from yeast cell walls, are proven to strengthen the body's innate immune system (the immune system you were born with). They also can kill pathogenic yeasts such as candida. Adults and children who take Beta Glucans suffer from fewer food intolerances. However, if you make ALL of the necessary dietary changes and eliminate foods that you are sensitive to, your immune system would improve naturally and you would not need the Beta Glucans! Until then, take 250–500mg daily
- Take a multi-vitamin/mineral for your age and gender .
- B-group vitamins, especially B6, B12, and folic acid, are needed to support the nerves, and they also help lower high homocysteine levels. Therefore, if you don't take a multi, make sure to take a high strength B-complex daily.
- Minerals such as magnesium and calcium help relax the muscles and often come as a duo formula. You need to take 600mg of magnesium and 400mg of calcium daily. Of the two, magnesium is the most important. If you buy it in capsule form, ask for magnesium citrate and take your last 200mg before bed. **VC**
- To help absorb the calcium, you also need to take 1000IU of vitamin D3 daily.
- Omega-3 is usually deficient in people with this condition. Take 2–3g daily.
- MSM, a type of organic sulfur, helps reduce pain, inflammation, and muscle spasms. Take 2g daily, spread throughout the day.
- The amino acid L-theanine, which is extracted from green tea, acts like a natural tranquillizer. You can take 100mg three times daily (the last one at bedtime) to help calm the brain and reduce anxiety.
- If you suffer from insomnia, the hormone melatonin may prove very useful. (See this section under *Insomnia*.)
- Take a digestive enzyme with all main meals.
- Taking liquid hyaluronic acid (a natural component of skin, joints, and tendons) daily in water helps keep the joints supple and helps reduce pain. Take one sachet in a full glass of water before breakfast. **VC**
- Healthy bacteria known as probiotics can often help, as sufferers also tend to have leaky guts. (See *Leaky Gut*.)
- Creams containing capsaicin (the natural chemical that makes chili peppers hot) have been shown to be very effective at reducing pain associated with these types of conditions. The cream can be applied topically to the painful areas three or four times a day, but it may take a couple of weeks before the effects are felt. Don't use this cream on broken skin or if you are pregnant or breastfeeding.

F

Helpful Hints

- It is important to have an allergy test to find your worst food offenders. Try the YorkTest Laboratories (www.yorktest.com). Tel: 011-44-1904-410410. The FACT test by Genova Diagnostics is another option. This test looks for inflammatory markers that indicate the body is reacting to certain substances. Tel: 1-800-522-4762. Website: www.genovadiagnostics.com
- Another excellent method is the Bio Meridian Test for food intolerance and leaky gut. During this test the practitioner measures your reactions to a huge list of foods and substances using electrodes. For a list of practitioners, visit www.biomeridian.com
- People who don't get sufficient amounts of sleep tend to suffer from more muscle pain; therefore, getting more sleep is very important for this type of condition.
- Moderate exercise, such as swimming, walking, cycling, and so on, will help.

- Have a regular massage using therapeutic grade oils, such as diluted oil of wintergreen, which has anti-inflammatory properties.
- Regular acupuncture is wonderful for reducing the pain and stiffness associated with this condition.
- Soak in a warm bath with Epsom salts or sea salt to help relax your muscles.

FLATULENCE   *(see also Candida, Constipation, and Irritable Bowel Syndrome)*

Flatulence, wind and bloating is, to say the least, often very embarrassing and sometimes extremely uncomfortable. It can be due to partially digested foods fermenting in the gut and/or to an imbalance of the organisms that reside in the bowel. Because unhealthy bacteria thrive on less healthy foods, particularly sugar, as well as the bi-products of partial digestion, the yeast fungal overgrowth *Candida* is often the root cause of this problem.

It is very important that you chew your food properly, as the digestive process begins in the mouth. Almost 60% of carbohydrate digestion is done in the mouth if foods are properly chewed. The majority of protein digestion is done in the stomach, so it is crucial that we have adequate levels of stomach acids and enzymes to break down these foods. Various factors can weaken our ability to digest foods properly: smoking is notorious, but alcohol, sugary foods, high-fat foods, caffeinated beverages, and prolonged stress can all progressively weaken digestion. Another important factor is food intolerances, most especially to cow's milk, wheat, and, in my case, chocolate, which causes me to bloat!

F

Foods to Avoid
- Beans such as cannellini, kidney, black-eyed, and so on, plus lentils, artichokes, broccoli, Brussels sprouts, soft drinks, and beer are all famous for causing wind. In some people, taking a digestive enzyme with these foods it does help.
- Some people also have problems with cabbage and onions.
- Also avoid any food to which you have an intolerance, the most common being dairy products from cows.
- Cheese, especially melted cheese, is incredibly hard to digest. Avoid pizzas!
- Try to note any foods that make you feel bloated or cause a lot of wind and see if there is a common denominator.
- If you have eaten a large meal, don't eat large amounts of fruit directly after, as the fruit will ferment in the gut as it becomes stuck behind the other food. Because fruit likes a fast passage through the gut, eat fruit before or in between meals. Generally avoid large meals that place a huge strain on your gut and liver.
- I often begin a meal with a few chunks of fresh pineapple or papaya, which aid digestion.

Friendly Foods
- Certain foods help improve digestion, notably fennel, celeriac, radicchio, young green celery, and watercress. They all help to stimulate gastric juices.
- Try wheat-free breads or use amaranth crackers or oatcakes.
- Rice, corn, and lentil pastas are now freely available.
- Drinking peppermint, fennel, or chamomile teas, or a combination of them, after meals can often make digestion easier and make you feel more comfortable. Fennel seems to be the most effective.
- Add a strip of dried kombu seaweed when cooking any bean dishes; this helps predigest the enzymes that cause gas and bloating.

- Include more fresh root ginger in your cooking, which aids digestion.
- Eat more low-fat, live yogurts.
- Try low-fat goat's milk, or almond or oat milk instead of cow's milk.

Useful Remedies
- With breakfast take one scoop of Agave Digestive Immune Support Powder, extracted from the agave plant, as it contains inulins that help you naturally produce more healthy bacteria. It is very useful for helping to keep you regular. **LEF**
- Otherwise, Bioforce makes Molkosan, a prebiotic drink made from concentrated fermented whey and minerals, which has been shown to help improve bowel transit times. For more information contact Bioforce USA on 1-800-641-7555 or visit www.bioforceusa.com
- Taking one capsule of betaine hydrochloride with meals helps improve digestion, which tends to weaken as we get older. If you have active stomach ulcers do not take this remedy; instead, take a digestive enzyme that does not contain hydrochloric acid.
- Taking one to two capsules of a probiotic containing acidophilus and bifidus at the end of a meal will help replace healthy gut flora, which in turn will help manufacture gastric enzymes and keep *Candida* under control, if this is the root cause of the problem.
- Take peppermint oil capsules before meals. But generally once you remove the foods such as wheat that trigger these types of problems, your digestion will work a lot more efficiently.

Helpful Hints
- Try to eat smaller meals, which places less strain on the digestive tract and liver. This really does help.
- Stress can trigger bloating and flatulence.
- Eat far fewer grain-based foods.
- Many people have benefited from following the principle of food combining, separating carbohydrates and proteins.
- Chronic flatulence can also be a symptom of food intolerance, irritable bowel syndrome, candida, or gut infections. If you are concerned, see a qualified nutritionist. (See *Useful Information*.)

FLU
(see Colds and Flu)

FLUID RETENTION
(see Water Retention)

FLUORIDE
(see also Bleeding Gums and Thyroid Problems)

No essential function for fluoride has been proven in humans. Fluoride compounds generally have a toxicity between that of lead and arsenic. Calcium fluoride occurs naturally in most US drinking waters, usually at levels less than 1 part per million (ppm). However, more than 60% of the population with access to a public water supply has fluoridated water, which means that artificial fluoride, such as fluorosilicic acid—a waste product from phosphate fertilizer plants and one of the more toxic fluoride compounds—is added to drinking water by water companies to a concentration of 1 ppm at the request of health authorities. This is not done to make the water safe to drink, but to medicate those who drink it. To put these levels into context, lead and arsenic in drinking water are limited to 25 and 10 ppb, respectively.

This practice is not limited to the US, though. The number of people drinking artificially fluoridated water worldwide is 300 million.

Regardless of fluoride intake, mother's milk is very low in fluoride, at 4–10 ppb. This means a baby who is fed formula that is reconstituted with fluoridated water will ingest up to 250 times more fluoride, compared to a breast-fed baby. In late 2006, the American Dental Association issued advice to dentists on how to address parental concerns. Their advice was that baby formula should be reconstituted with water that has no or a low level of fluoride. Health authorities did not issue this advice directly to parents in any other country that fluoridates.

The problem today is that we get fluoride from so many sources—certain foods, tooth-pastes, mouthwashes, medicines (Prozac is fluoxetine), anesthetics, pesticides, and polluted air. Volcanic dust also contains fluoride. Half of the fluoride ingested is retained in our bodies. Dental fluorosis (mottled teeth), a manifestation of systemic toxicity, is common in areas where the water is fluoridated. The accumulation of fluoride in bone and soft tissue causes many health problems, including irritable bowel syndrome, bone deformities, arthritic pain, and hypothyroidism. However the vast majority of doctors carry out no tests to link these problems to fluoride.

In 2006 a team of Harvard University scientists, led by Dr Elise Bassin, published a study that reported a five-fold increased risk of teenage boys exposed to fluoridated water between the ages of 6 and 8 developing osteosarcoma.

In his analysis of the 2000–2003 National Diet and Nutrition Survey, Dr Peter Mansfield, a York Review Advisory Panel member, found that a quarter of the UK population exceeds the safe intake defined by the Committee on Medical Aspects and Food Policy. In fluoridated areas this rises to two-thirds! Studies in the US show that, on average, adults ingest over 2mg of fluoride daily since two-thirds of American drinking water is fluoridated. There is an ongoing controversy over what levels of fluoride are actually safe to ingest.

Since 1997 the FDA has required a poison label on all toothpastes containing fluoride. In 1999 the Centers for Disease Control (CDC) conceded that the predominant "benefit" of fluoride is topical. This means for the "benefit" perceived by the promoters of fluoride, we do not need to swallow it! In areas with added fluoride, many doctors have noticed an increase in thyroid problems. (See *Thyroid*.) This is because fluoride is a halide (a group of chemicals) that competes with iodide receptor sites in the body and can therefore interfere with proper hormone production.

Foods to Avoid
- Read labels carefully and note that tea, salmon, and sardines are rich in fluorides. As much as possible, avoid non-organic foods that have more than likely been sprayed with pesticides containing fluoride. If you live in a fluoridated area, as much as possible drink bottled, distilled or reverse osmosis de-ionized water. Visit www.freedrinkingwater.com

Friendly Foods
- Eat organic foods that are free from harmful pesticides and herbicides.
- Drink plenty of fluoride-free water in between meals.
- See *General Health Hints*.

Helpful Hints
- If you drink fluoridated tap water, do not use fluoridated toothpastes or mouthwashes.
- To avoid cavities, greatly limit your child's intake of sugary foods and drinks.
- Buy fluoride-free toothpastes, such as Tom's of Maine or Burt's Bees, containing ingredients like aloe vera, Co-enzyme Q10, tea tree oil, silica, and so on, which all promote healthy gums and teeth.

- Young children tend to swallow toothpaste; therefore, make sure it is fluoride free.
- Consider having a fluoride-removing water filter fitted at home. Water Filters.net offers a broad range of water filters. Call them on 1-800-801-7873 or visit www.waterfilters.net
- Ask your doctor to test for levels of fluoride in the body.
- Read *The Fluoride Deception* by Christopher Bryson (Seven Stories Press) and *Fluoridation: Drinking Ourselves to Death* by Barry Groves (Newleaf).
- Support The Fluoride Action Network (www.fluoridealert.org), which is fighting against the fluoridation of US tap water.

FOOD POISONING

(see also Diarrhea, Irritable Bowel Syndrome and Vomiting)

Each year an estimated 76 million Americans, that's one in every four people in the US, suffer from some kind of food poisoning. And this figure is on the low side, as many mild cases go unreported. Approximately 5,000 people die annually from food poisoning, which is mainly caused by various bacteria found in food, mainly meats, reheated foods, and shellfish, home-made ice creams and jams, but can also be caused by viruses, parasites, and toxins in foods such as those in many wild field mushrooms.

The most common and widely known bacteria are salmonella, campylobacter, E-coli, listeria, staphylococcus, shigella, and botulism. The more bacteria that are present in a food, the more likely you are to become ill. These bacteria are hard to detect, as they don't usually affect the taste, appearance, or smell of food. Having said this, if foods such as fish, shellfish, or meat smell extra strong or "high," then to be safe, don't eat them.

Food poisoning is more likely to affect people with lowered resistance to disease, such as the elderly or sick, babies, young children, and pregnant women. Symptoms of food poisoning are nausea, vomiting, diarrhea, abdominal pain, headache, and low-grade fever.

The most serious types of food poisoning are due to bacteria, which can cause poisoning in two different ways. Some bacteria infect the intestines, causing inflammation and problems with the normal absorption of nutrients and water, which triggers diarrhea. Other bacteria produce toxins on the food that are poisonous to the human digestive system. When eaten, these chemicals trigger nausea and vomiting, kidney problems and, in extreme cases, death. Bacteria multiply very fast, especially in warm, moist conditions. The presence or absence of oxygen, salt, and sugar as well as the acidity of the surroundings, are also important factors. In the right conditions, one bacterium can multiply to more than 4 million in just 8 hours.

Bacteria generally like temperatures between 41°F (5°C) and 145°F (63°C) where they can multiply easily. They are killed at temperatures higher than 158°F (70°C). Most bacteria multiply very slowly at temperatures below 41°F (5°C), and some bacteria die at very low temperatures. Unfortunately, many can survive these low temperatures and can start multiplying again if warm conditions return. This is why proper handling and storage of food, plus sensible hygiene precautions, are of utmost importance in preventing food poisoning.

Foods to Avoid

- Beware of eating wild mushrooms unless you are absolutely certain of which types you can eat. Only gather mushrooms that you can positively identify; however, I personally would **never** eat a wild mushroom that had not been identified or picked by an expert, as some varieties are deadly (such as Death Cap and Destroying Angel).

- To help prevent an attack, avoid food that has been reheated more than once, especially rice dishes.
- Avoid eating any foods that have been left standing in warm conditions, such as at picnics and buffets, and foods that you know have been sitting there for a while.
- Avoid food that is not piping hot—especially chicken or any meat dishes.
- Do not eat any food that has come into contact with raw meat or poultry.
- If you are in any country that has poor-quality drinking water, take the following precautions:
  - Drink only bottled water, and avoid salads at all costs, as the salad has likely been washed in local water. The worst case of food poisoning I ever had was in India because I thought, "Oh, raw food is fine." Big mistake! Hot food that has been well cooked is preferable.
  - Similarly, if you are offered bottles of water or other drinks that are not properly sealed, say no thanks.
  - It may sound ridiculous, but if cutlery has been washed in local streams in, say, India, you would be wise to take your own cutlery.
  - Peel fruit.
  - Beware of ice cubes unless they are made with bottled water.
- Do not eat any of the following under-cooked or rare: poultry, burgers, sausages, chicken nuggets, and kebabs. Also avoid uncooked fish, which can be lethal.
- Short episodes of vomiting and small amounts of diarrhea lasting less than 24 hours can usually be cared for at home. When an episode of food poisoning is under way, it is best to rest and starve yourself of solid food for 24 hours as this will also starve the bacteria. But if you are not holding down any fluids, you **must** seek medical help, as dehydration can kill you. This is especially true for young children and babies.

Friendly Foods

- During an attack drink plenty of boiled or bottled water, or sip ginger ale to avoid dehydration.
- Regularly sip an electrolyte drink, such as Pedialyte, or mix up an electrolyte powder like Emergen C. These are available from any pharmacy.
- After 24 hours of avoiding all foods, and when you are successfully tolerating fluids, start eating small amounts of brown rice, soups and dry toast or crackers and see how this goes. Don't try to eat anything heavy for the first couple of days—be kind to your system.
- Try making oatmeal or semolina with almond or oat milks. Don't use cow's milk.
- Mashed pumpkin, sweet potato, and a little grilled fish should be fine.
- Hemp seed protein powders mixed with a banana and a small amount of aloe vera juice and rice milk should be well tolerated and give you some much-needed nutrients.

Useful Remedies

- One or two drops of liquid grapefruit seed extract can be added to water and sipped throughout the day, as it has strong anti-bacterial action.
- Whenever you have had an episode of food poisoning, probiotics—healthy bacteria found in the bowel—are really essential. They help re-populate the bowel and help protect against further growth of the offending bugs. If you are susceptible to diarrhea when you travel overseas, taking acidophilus for two weeks prior to your trip can help increase the number of healthy bacteria in your gut, which reduces the risk of picking up a stomach bug. Jarro-Dophilus EPS is a good broad-spectrum formula. **JF**
- Take healthy bacteria probiotics supplements plus supplements of garlic, oregano oil, clove oil, cinnamon, and rosemary. They can be taken daily with food when you are abroad to help kill off any invading bacteria. They can be very handy for vacations, but do not take them if you are pregnant.

- Homeopathic Arsen Alb is good for reducing stomach cramps; Nux Vomica helps reduce feelings of nausea; and Mag Phos is also great for cramps.
- Once symptoms have begun to settle and nausea and vomiting have ceased, you can try taking the herb goldenseal. It helps increase appetite and reduce nausea and vomiting. It also has strong properties for fighting off bad bacteria, and it has a soothing effect on the mucous membranes in the gut. Solgar's Goldenseal Root Complex provides 500mg. Initially, take one a day with food and then increase to one tablet three times day for two weeks. **SVHC**
- Charcoal capsules or tablets may help in the case of diarrhea. The charcoal will help bind to the toxins that are produced by the bacteria and both can then be excreted through the bowel. These are available at most health food stores and some pharmacies.

Helpful Hints
- Most cases of food poisoning clear up on their own after a few days, but you should visit a doctor if the symptoms of food poisoning last for more than two or three days. Also, if there is a fever and the diarrhea is very watery, or there is blood, pus, or mucus mixed in with the stools, please seek medical help.
- Signs of dehydration are intense thirst, dry lips and tongue, increased heart rate, and weakness.
- Bacteria thrive on dirty, damp cloths. So it's very important to wash kitchen cloths, towels, and sponges regularly. Choose the hottest wash that your washing machine permits to make sure all bacteria are killed.
- Bacteria love to travel and will hitch a ride on anything they can—hands, chopping boards, knives or tongs—and find their way onto foods such as bread or salad. Make sure you thoroughly wash hands and utensils in warm, soapy water after touching raw meat and poultry, going to the bathroom, touching the trashcan, or touching pets.
- Don't forget to dry your hands thoroughly, because if they are wet they will spread bacteria more easily.
- Cook meats thoroughly—especially poultry. If you are serving poultry cold, make sure it's kept really cool; and if re-heating, make sure it's hot all the way through. Chickens need to be roasted at 400°F, or gas mark 6, for 20 minutes per pound, plus an extra 20 minutes.
- Citricidal—grapefruit seed extract—has wonderful anti-bacterial and anti-parasitic actions and has been proven in laboratory tests to be 10 times more effective as a disinfectant than chlorine. Available from health stores.
- If you have cooked food that you aren't going to eat right away, cool it as quickly as possible (ideally within 1–2 hours) and then store it in the fridge. Do not cool it down in the fridge, as this can raise the overall temperature in the fridge, which will enable bacteria on food already stored in there to grow.
- Don't store leftovers for longer than two days.
- Never use cracked raw eggs, although well-cooked eggs are fine for anyone recovering from food poisoning.
- Don't put raw chicken or meat next to cooked food on the grill or barbecue.
- Don't add sauce or marinade to cooked food if it has been used to baste raw chicken or meat.
- Store raw chicken and meat on the bottom shelf of the fridge, where it can't touch or drip onto other foods.
- Use separate tongs and utensils for raw chicken and meat and for cooked chicken and meat.
- Keep raw meat and ready-to-eat food separate in the fridge and also in the kitchen area. This is especially important because foods such as salad, fruit, and bread won't be cooked before you eat them, and any bacteria that get on them won't be killed.

F

FOOT PROBLEMS

All too many of us spend far too long on our feet. A typical person walks about 71,000 miles during their lifetime. Our often-neglected feet contain 26 bones, 56 ligaments, and 38 muscles, so there is an awful lot that can go wrong with them. Wearing shoes that are too high can trigger back problems, and if your shoes are too tight they will restrict circulation, triggering problems such as blisters, corns, and chilblains. One of the best ways to keep your feet pain free is to visit a podiatrist regularly.

Cold feet

Cold feet usually relate to poor circulation (see *Circulation*), but can also be associated with low thyroid function (see *Thyroid*). If your feet are chronically cold, even when the weather is warm, ask your doctor to check you for an under-active thyroid or for Raynaud's disease (see *Raynaud's Disease*).

Regular exercise, massage with essential oil of black pepper (mixed with a base oil), acupuncture, and reflexology can all help alleviate cold feet. Wearing bed socks helps—and keeping a magnet in your shoes encourages better circulation to the feet. For all foods and supplements, see *Circulation* and *Raynaud's Disease*. One very useful herb for cold feet is gotu kola, as it increases circulation in the lower limbs. You can also include more fresh root ginger in your diet or take ginger capsules, as they bring more warmth to the body.

Cracked heels   (see also Thyroid)

Also referred to as fissures, for most people cracked heels just look unsightly, but for others they can become quite painful. Cracked heels are mainly due to excessive callus build-up, as well as very dry thin skin on the outside of the heels. But they can also be due to a thyroid problem, lack of essential fats, prolonged standing, inactive sweat glands, obesity, wearing flip-flops or open-backed shoes, flat feet (see *Fallen Arches*, below), use of excessively hot water, walking abnormally, eczema, and psoriasis. Cold weather greatly dehydrates the whole body and therefore this problem is more likely to occur during the winter months.

Foods to Avoid
- Avoid alcohol and caffeine found in coffee, tea, power drinks, and some painkillers, as these dehydrate the body.
- Reduce saturated fats found in red meat and dairy. Trim all fat from the meat, and grill rather than fry your food. These "bad" fats prevent the good fats from doing their job. (See also *Fats You Need To Eat*.)
- Grains in the form of flour of any type will dehydrate the body if eaten to excess.

Friendly Foods
- Aim to drink plenty of water per day to help rehydrate your body and skin.
- Zinc-rich foods, such as brown rice, lentils, and pumpkin, sunflower, and sesame seeds, as well as almonds, are all rich in minerals and essential fats that nourish your skin from the inside out.
- Use more organic olive, walnut, sesame, and avocado oils in salad dressings or drizzle over cooked foods. Eat avocado twice weekly.
- Generally, eat more oily fish —organic salmon, trout, anchovies, mackerel, and sardines—as they are high in essential fats.

- Magnesium-rich foods are dark green leafy vegetables, cashew nuts, broccoli, bananas, and prunes, while selenium-rich foods are Brazil nuts, oats, and brown rice.

Useful Remedies

- Choose a good all-round multi-vitamin/mineral for your age and gender.
- Break open a vitamin E capsule and apply to the affected area.
- There are dozens of nutrient-dense creams made for the feet that will help keep the area nourished. **VC**
- Take 3g of omega-3 essential fats daily if your skin is dry.

Helpful Hints

- Avoid using thick creams on fissures, which can sit on the skin and make the problem worse. Instead, use a trans-dermal moisturizer that contains Emu Oil, which soaks into the hard skin on the feet more easily.
- Find a really good cream for extra-dry skin. Apply twice daily, especially before going to bed, and then put on a pair of old cotton socks so that the cream can really soak into the dry areas.
- Soak your feet daily in warm, soapy water for 15 minutes and use a good pumice stone or foot scrub on the thick skin on your heels. Then thickly apply a moisturizing cream, sit back, and let it soak in. Avoid open-backed or thin-soled shoes, and buy shoes with a good shock-absorbing sole. Never try to cut back hard skin yourself with a razor blade or a pair of scissors—see a podiatrist. To find a qualified podiatrist in your area, visit the American Podiatric Medical Association's website: www.apma.org

Fallen arches

F

When standing, most people have a gap between the inner side of their foot and the ground they are standing on—this is called the arch. Fallen arches—also known as flat feet—happen when the foot rolls over, so there is little to no gap. Symptoms depend on the severity of the condition, but corns, hard skin under the sole of the foot, and a tender arch area are common; shoes will also tend to wear out more quickly. In severe cases calf, knee, hip, or back pain can be experienced. Fallen arches may be hereditary, but in most cases the condition is caused by abnormal walking, whereby the joints in the foot roll in too much. Fallen arches can also cause plantar faciitis, a painful condition where the tight band of connective tissue in the arch of the foot becomes highly inflamed. A ruptured tendon can also lead to a flat foot, as can cerebral palsy, spina bifida, and muscular dystrophy.

Helpful Hints

- Find a good local health clinic that deals with sports injuries. If they have an in-house podiatrist you can be fitted for individual orthotics—inserts made specifically for your feet. These will give your feet all the support they need. Otherwise, large pharmacies and foot specialists such as Scholl offer a variety of orthotic inserts especially made to support the arches. One of the best inserts I have found is Orthaheel, which is available worldwide. Visit www.orthaheelusa.com
- To find a qualified podiatrist in your area, ask in any large pharmacy or visit the American Podiatric Medical Association's website: www.apma.org
- MBT shoes (Masai Barefoot Technology) are state-of-the-art shoes that support the feet really well. These shoes greatly alleviate many structural problems including back, knee, and joint pain. Visit http://us.mbt.com for more details.

Hot, burning feet

Poor circulation is often the cause of this problem (see *Circulation*). It is also common in people suffering from diabetes, as diabetics frequently have problems with the nerves in their feet because of a deficiency in B vitamins. Alcoholics often suffer from this problem, as they are greatly deficient in B vitamins as well. Other than diabetes, circulation can be affected by eating too many of the wrong types of fats, which tend to clog up the system. Dehydration can compound the problem, because it makes it harder for fluid and nutrients to move around the body. Improving circulation to the feet can often relieve symptoms.

There may also be a link between this condition and trapped nerves in the lower spine; therefore it may be a good idea to consult a chiropractor.

Foods to Avoid
- Avoid saturated animal fats found in red meat and full-fat dairy products, plus the hydrogenated and trans-fats rich in processed foods—especially burger-type foods, cakes, and pastries.
- Reduce or avoid alcohol, as it is dehydrating.

Friendly Foods
- Increase your intake of the essential fats found in oily fish, such as mackerel, sardines, organic-farmed salmon, and anchovies, plus nuts and seeds.
- Blueberries and cherries contain bioflavonoids that help keep the walls of your blood vessels strong so they can carry fluid and nutrients around the body more easily and efficiently.

Useful Remedies
- Take a high-potency B-complex daily—aiming for 50mg of the majority of B-vitamins.
- Look for oil or capsules that contain the correct ratio of the essential oils (twice the amount of omega-3 than omega-6). Take three capsules daily, or buy the oil and drizzle it over cooked vegetables and rice dishes or use it for salad dressings.
- Otherwise take 2–3g of omega-3 fish oils daily.
- The herb gotu kola is very useful for increasing circulation to the feet. Try 1–3g daily with food for a month and see if this helps.

Helpful Hints
- Acupuncture and reflexology are useful for alleviating this condition. (See *Useful Information*.)
- Exercise is great for stimulating the circulation. Take a regular 30-minute walk each day. Any exercise that gently pounds the bottom of the feet will help improve circulation. Try, dancing, skipping, or rebounding.

Numb and tingling feet

It is very important to see your doctor if you have this problem for more than a few days in order to find out if there is anything more serious going on, as numb or tingling feet can be due to peripheral neuropathy, which can denote late-onset diabetes. A blood test is all that's needed to clarify if this is the case. A lack of calcium may also cause this problem. Try taking 1000mg of calcium daily for a couple of weeks. Epidurals can also be associated with this problem. Any spinal misalignment can trigger these types of symptoms as well; see a chiropractor.

If you have numb and tingling feet, take the supplements suggested under *Circulation* and get plenty of exercise such as walking, skipping, or rebounding, which really help bring more blood to the feet.

Consult a chiropractor who can check for trapped nerves and any misalignments that might be triggering this problem. (See *Useful Information*.)

Try reflexology and acupuncture to further improve circulation.

Smelly feet   *(see also Athlete's Foot, Candida, and Body Odor)*

Smelly feet, also known as bromihydrosis, can be highly embarrassing for you and those around you—and in most cases are easily preventable. Initially, wash your feet a couple of times a day in warm water with a little added tea tree oil, and then use natural talcum powder to help keep them drier. Several companies make foot sprays that help kill bacteria on the feet such as Crystal (www.thecrystal.com), which is available from good health stores. Always wear 100% cotton socks and leather shoes, as synthetic fibers lead to increased sweating and it is the bacteria in the sweat that create the unpleasant smell. Change your shoes often: alternating pairs daily would help, as this gives your shoes a chance to breathe. Also, avoid wearing closed shoes without socks. Going without shoes whenever possible is another good idea, as the fresh air will help reduce sweating. Some people find that if they put their shoes in a freezer overnight it helps to kill off the bacteria responsible for the odor. Eat more cilantro, which helps destroy "smelly" bacteria in the body.

Swollen feet and ankles   *(see also Water Retention)*

F

As we age, the ratio of water found inside and outside our cells changes, and we find it harder to properly absorb water into our cells. This extra fluid triggers edema (collection of water in the body's tissues), which with gravity heads south toward our feet! This problem is common in middle-aged and older ladies and can also happen during pregnancy. Again, this is mainly linked to circulation and the body's ability to remove excess fluid (see *Circulation*). Any injury of the feet, ankles, or legs can also contribute to swelling in this area.

Foods to Avoid
- Avoid all foods that are high in salt and sodium, such as preserved meats and fish, potato chips, processed foods, sauce packet, and ketchup-style condiments, which often contain huge amounts of hidden salt. Salt exacerbates any water retention and increases swelling in all parts of the body if you already suffer from fluid retention.
- Check the salt content of breakfast cereals and cereal bars. Look for low-salt/sodium alternatives such as Himalayan Crystal Sea Salt or use nori flakes.
- Look out for hidden sources of salt/sodium. It is found in high quantities in ketchups, pickles, relishes, and olives, as well as in sodium benzoate—a preservative—and monosodium glutamate (MSG). Stop adding salt to your food and cooking or use nori or kelp flakes for their natural salts.
- Avoid burger-type meals that are high in salt and fat; also avoid sausages and mass-produced pies, cakes, and cookies.
- Avoid caffeine in any form (watch out for it hidden in energy drinks and some painkillers), plus tea and alcohol, as these will dehydrate the body.
- Cut back on saturated fats found in red meat and dairy products. These clog up the lymphatic system, which is responsible for removing excess fluid. (See *Fats You Need To Eat*.)
- See also *General Health Hints*.

Friendly Foods
- Eat foods rich in potassium, such as green vegetables, fresh fruit, dried fruits, unsalted nuts (not peanuts), fresh fish, bananas, potatoes, and unsalted sunflower and pumpkin seeds.
- Eat more oily fish and use unrefined walnut, olive, hemp, and sunflower oils for your salad dressings.
- Try a little magnesium-rich Solo Sea Salt. Visit www.soloseasaltusa.com for details on where to find it.
- Otherwise use nori or kelp flakes.

Useful Remedies
- Celery seed extract acts like a diuretic. Take two capsules twice daily until symptoms ease. **VC**
- Also take 1g of vitamin C in an ascorbate form to improve lymph drainage. This should help remove excess fluid.
- Take a silica and sulfur compound such as Eidon Ionic Minerals Liquid for three months to help improve tissue tone. **VC**
- On days when your ankles are very swollen, take 15 drops of dandelion tincture three times a day before meals. Dandelion leaves are a potassium-rich diuretic, which also help cleanse the liver. **VC**
- As a lack of B vitamins is linked to this problem, take a B-complex daily. Look for one that contains 50mg of B6. Otherwise, take a good-quality multi-vitamin/mineral that contains a full spectrum of B vitamins.

Helpful Hints
- Reflexology and acupuncture are usually highly effective for helping to alleviate this condition. (See *Useful Information*.)
- Sit with your feet at hip level for at least 15 minutes every day, moving your feet back and forth to improve circulation.
- Rebounding (jumping on a mini-trampoline), gentle jogging and skipping are especially good for boosting lymphatic drainage. Deep-tissue lymphatic drainage can help if the problem is caused by a stagnant lymph system.
- Dry skin brushing helps to remove excess fluid. Buy a natural (not synthetic), long-handled brush, which shouldn't scratch the skin. Begin by brushing the soles of the feet, as the 7,000 nerve endings there affect the whole body. Next, brush the ankles, calves, and thighs before brushing across your stomach and buttocks. Lastly brush your hands and up your arms. Always brush in the direction of the heart. Follow all this brushing with a warm bath or shower and complete the process with a cool rinse to really invigorate circulation. I find this a great way to wake up every morning, and it really helps my skin stay soft and in good condition.
- Call a homeopathic pharmacy, which can suggest a remedy to suit your particular symptoms.
- If the symptoms persist after following the advice given here for more than six weeks, ask your doctor for a thorough check-up, as occasionally swollen feet and ankles may be a sign of heart, liver, or kidney problems.

FROZEN SHOULDER

This condition is often characterized by pain and limited movement in one, and very rarely both, shoulders. It is triggered by inflammation of the muscles, ligaments, or tendons around the shoulders. Exercise can be very painful, especially if you try to lift your arm higher than the shoulder joint; however, gentle exercises that encourage blood flow and does not overstrain the joint or tendons is often helpful. Frozen shoulder is common between the ages of 40 and 60 and affects about 2% of the US population.

Foods to Avoid

- Avoid any foods and drinks that contain caffeine because it greatly reduces our body's ability to make painkilling endorphins.
- Animal fats from meats, butter, cheese, and milk tend to increase inflammation in the body, as they are acid forming. (See *Acid–Alkaline Balance*.)
- Sugar and alcohol greatly increase inflammation in the body.

Friendly Foods

- Oily fish contain anti-inflammatory essential fatty acids—especially organic-farmed salmon, mackerel, sardines, trout, black cod, or red snapper.
- Cherries are high in bioflavonoids, which are mildly anti-inflammatory. Eat more pineapple for its bromelain content, which is also anti-inflammatory.
- Ginger, turmeric, and cayenne pepper are all spices that, when used liberally, can help to decrease pain.

Useful Remedies

- Look for a ginger, curcumin, and boswellia blend or individually; take up to four tablets a day, which should help reduce the inflammation.
- Magnesium helps relax the muscles. Take 1000mg per day while the symptoms are acute.
- Taking liquid hyaluronic acid (a natural component of skin) daily in water helps to lubricate joints. Take daily before breakfast in a full glass of water. **VC**
- Glucosamine with MSM (a type of sulfur) is very useful for easing discomfort and gradually healing the joint. Take 2g of glucosamine and 1g of MSM. Many brands make a duo formula. **NB: This supplement is usually derived from crab shells. If you have an intolerance to shellfish, take the vegetarian version.**
- Bromelain is highly anti-inflammatory; take 500mg twice a day, as it will also help improve the elasticity of tissues.

Helpful Hints

- Creams or ointments made with cayenne pepper can bring rapid pain relief. **VC**
- Glucosamine gels with capsicum and MSM can also be applied daily.
- Bags of cherry stones or wheat can be either heated or frozen and then applied to the affected area for 10 minutes at a time to ease pain and inflammation.
- Traditionally, frozen shoulder is treated with regular physiotherapy. Find a local sports injury clinic, as they have experts who deal with these types of conditions on a daily basis. Alternatives are chiropractic and osteopathy, which may be covered by your insurance.
- Use your local swimming pool, as gentle movement in warm water loosens the shoulder.
- Acupuncture is highly effective for reducing the acute pain associated with frozen shoulder. Aromatherapy massage with essential oils of eucalyptus, ginger and juniper is also helpful. (See *Useful Information*.)

F

G

GALLBLADDER PROBLEMS

(see also Gallstones and Liver Problems)

Gallbladder and gallstone problems are far more common in women than in men, and many people end up having surgery that could be prevented by making dietary changes. The gallbladder is a small pear-shaped organ (sac) that sits underneath, and is connected to, the liver. The gallbladder's main function is to store bile that is made in the liver. Water is removed from the bile, thereby concentrating it to be stored in the gallbladder. The gallbladder passes bile into the small bowel, where the bile helps break down fat during digestion. If the liver is overloaded, this prevents efficient gallbladder function. The gallbladder can be affected by gallstones, inflammation, and infection. Each of the problems may produce pain on the right side, encasing the center of the abdomen. In some cases the pain can be so severe that the patient feels nauseous and faint. Food intolerances definitely play a part in gallbladder problems, and you can avoid the need for surgery once the diet is balanced.

Foods to Avoid
- Anyone who has a tendency to develop gallbladder problems usually eats too many fatty foods. Eggs and cheese can also cause problems in some people, especially melted cheese, which is very hard to digest.
- High-fat and fried foods put an extra load on the gallbladder and its ability to digest fats.
- Alcohol, coffee, and chocolate place an extra strain on the liver, which can worsen the problem.
- Many people who have gallbladder problems are overweight and tend to love creamy, unhealthy foods. Cut these out, and generally eat less, otherwise you'll end up having your gallbladder removed and then your body will find fats difficult to metabolize, causing you to put on even more weight.
- See also *General Health Hints* and the dietary advice under *Liver Problems*.

Friendly Foods
- People who eat more beans and lentils are less likely to end up with gallbladder or liver problems.
- Foods such as celeriac, artichokes, beets, and celery are all good for liver and gallbladder function.
- Try making fresh vegetable juices daily with celery, artichoke, parsley, raw beets, apples, carrots, and any other green vegetables you have in your fridge. Add this to half a cup of organic aloe vera and drink daily to help detoxify your liver and gallbladder.
- Use small amounts of unrefined extra-virgin olive, walnut, or linseed (flax seed) oil in salad dressings, as they all help diminish the risk of developing problems.
- Drink plenty of fluids.

Useful Remedies
- Milk thistle and dandelion are very effective at maintaining a healthy gallbladder. Milk thistle encourages better liver detoxification, and dandelion stimulates bile flow.
- Sprinkle 1 tablespoon of lecithin granules over breakfast cereals, fruit whips, or yogurts to help emulsify LDL cholesterol within the body.

- Swedish Bitters is a bitter tonic that aids the liver by enhancing the flow of bile. Put a few drops in a little water before main meals.
- See also *Useful Remedies* under *Gallstones*.

Helpful Hints
- To avoid gallbladder problems you generally need to control your LDL cholesterol and stress levels. See also *Cholesterol* and *Stress*.

GALLSTONES

Although 1 in 10 Americans (10%) has gallstones, only about 10% will eventually develop symptoms. Gallstones are four times more common in women, especially after 40. The classic description for a gallstone patient is "fair, female, fat, and forty!"

Many women end up having their gallbladder removed, yet changes in diet could prevent this major surgery in most cases. After surgery it's harder for the body to metabolize any fats, so prevention is definitely preferable.

People who tend to eat high saturated-fat and sugary diets without sufficient fiber, or those who are obese, constantly dieting but rapidly gain weight or suffer from Crohn's disease, are at a higher risk. Multiple pregnancies, the contraceptive pill, and HRT are other factors, as is a high stress level. The gallbladder can become congested with substances such as cholesterol, which causes stagnation. Most gallstones consist of a sediment primarily made up of cholesterol, bilirubin, and bile salts. They tend to develop in individuals with excess cholesterol in their bloodstream or as a result of stagnation of bile flow in the gallbladder.

Small gallstones often produce no symptoms, but if they become large enough to obstruct the bile duct they can cause jaundice, inflammation, intense pain, and vomiting. Symptoms tend to be much worse after high-fat meals or after foods to which the individual has a sensitivity, such as eggs. Constipation can be linked to the risk of gallstones, so it is very important that adequate fiber is eaten to reduce the likelihood of constipation and thus re-absorption of toxins.

Foods to Avoid
- To avoid gallbladder attacks and gallstones, you really have to stick to a low-fat diet by greatly reducing your intake of animal fats from any source.
- Low-fiber foods, such as white bread, cakes, cookies, ice cream, most desserts, and pre-packaged meals, should be avoided as much as possible.
- Foods such as eggs, pork, onions, pickles, spicy foods, peanuts, and citrus fruits are likely triggers.
- Regular coffee drinkers (that's real coffee, not decaffeinated) have a much lower risk of developing gallstones, but if you have a sensitivity to coffee then you need to avoid it.

Friendly Foods
- Drink plenty of water/fluids to prevent bile from becoming too concentrated—around 6–8 glasses a day.
- Small amounts of lean-cut lamb (without the fat), plus brown rice, peas, pears, and broccoli are usually no problem.
- Keep a food diary and eliminate any foods that you react to within an hour of eating them.
- Include more beets, artichokes, chicory, radicchio (Italian chicory), dried beans (adzuki, kidney, pinto, haricot and so on), linseeds (flax seeds soaked overnight in cold water, drained and eaten with any cereals), and oat or rice bran—all of which are high-fiber foods—to reduce constipation.

- Sprinkle a tablespoonful of lecithin granules over a low-sugar, oat-based muesli or cereal, as soy lecithin helps break down the fat in foods.
- Eat more oatmeal.
- Use whole-wheat bread and pasta made from corn, lentil, rice, or potato flour.
- Include fresh fish, a little chicken without the skin, plenty of salads, and fresh fruit in your diet.
- Replace full-fat milks with skimmed and try more herbal teas. Use organic rice, almond, or oat milks.
- Use organic extra-virgin olive, sunflower, and walnut oils for salad dressings. These are all rich in essential fats, which help to dissolve stones.
- Freshly made carrot, beet, and cucumber juices help support better gallbladder function.

Useful Remedies

- Milk thistle and dandelion in combination as tablets or capsules, or dandelion formula are really helpful. Take one or two tablets or 10–20 drops of tincture with every meal.
- As people suffering from gallstones process large amounts of toxins, they are frequently deficient in B vitamins, which are crucial for enzyme production and for helping the liver function. Therefore, take a multi-vitamin/mineral that contains 50mg of each of the B-group vitamins.
- People with gallstones tend to be deficient in vitamins C and E. Take 2g of vitamin C daily with food, which is needed for the conversion of cholesterol to bile acids. Take 200–400IU of full-spectrum, natural-source vitamin E.

- Take betaine hydrochloride (stomach acid)—one capsule with meals—as many people with gallstones have food intolerances and digestive problems. Many practitioners find that gallstone sufferers are deficient in stomach acid. **NB: Don't take this remedy if you have active stomach ulcers; instead, take a digestive enzyme that is free from hydrochoric acid.**
- Shuessler silica and calcium fluoride tissue salts can help to break down and expel the stones. Take four of each daily. Available from www.well.ca
- Please remember to use lecithin granules daily. They are very important to help prevent this condition. Always use granules from a non-GM source.
- L-methionine is an amino acid that greatly aids detoxification of the liver. Take 500mg twice daily an hour before breakfast and dinner. **VC**

Helpful Hints

- As multiple food sensitivities are linked to gallbladder problems, it is well worth your while to consult a qualified nutritionist or naturopath who can sort out your diet. The initial few weeks may be hard, but there are plenty of foods you can eat. (See *Useful Information* for details.)
- It is important to have an allergy test to discover your worst food offenders. Try the YorkTest Laboratories (www.yorktest.com). Another option is the FACT test from Genova Diagnostics, which looks for inflammatory markers indicating that the body is reacting to certain substances. Tel: 1-800-522-4762. Website: www.genovadiagnostics.com
- Another excellent method is known as the Bio Meridian Test for food intolerance and leaky gut, in which a practitioner measures, via electrodes, your reactions to a huge list of foods and substances. For practitioners see www.energetic-medicine.net/practitioners/Category/BioMeridian-Practitioners

GENERAL HEALTH HINTS

- Make time for breakfast, which is the most important meal of the day. You are literally breaking a fast, and to keep your blood sugar level you need to eat, or you will end up craving sugary snacks by mid-morning.
- Oat, quinoa, kamut, amaranth, and low-sugar-based cereals or sugar-free muesli make an ideal breakfast for most people. Gluten is now a problem for many people so try more gluten-free foods. Low-gluten breads are easier to digest; therefore you can try sprouted wheat bread, spelt, or 100% rye breads. Eat cereals and oatmeal with skimmed milk (unless you are intolerant to animal-based milks) or try organic oat, rice, almond, sheep's, or low-fat goat's milk.
- Quality protein really helps wake up your brain, which is why eggs (not fried), grilled fish or lean meat make great breakfasts. Buy organic or free-range eggs. Otherwise, eat some whole-wheat/stone-ground breads, toasted, with a non-hydrogenated spread such as Biona or Olivio or try it with organic raw walnut, hemp seed, coconut, or almond butters with a little honey or low-sugar jam. If you cannot face breakfast, at least take an apple or a couple of bananas and a low-fat, live yogurt with you to eat later.
- Otherwise, make a protein shake the night before and drink it on your way to work. (See recipe, below.)
- Eat as great a variety of foods as possible, preferably locally grown and organic. Locally grown fruit and vegetables are allowed to ripen naturally and therefore contain higher levels of nutrients than foods flown thousands of miles. Unripe fruits and vegetables do not contain as many nutrients from the soil as those that have been allowed to ripen naturally on the vine. The price of organic foods is coming down, and I believe that 100% organic food will help reduce many cancers and greatly alleviate the toxic load on the planet and its inhabitants. Many pesticides, especially the organophosphates (OPs), seep right through the vegetables and fruit and cannot be washed off. They are now linked with many cancers and lowered sperm counts.
- As much as possible, use organic products on your skin and hair. We take in more than 5 pounds of chemicals annually through our skin alone. Also try to eliminate chemical-based cleaners and so on from your home.
- In winter, eat heart-warming cooked foods, and in summer choose lighter meals with plenty of raw foods and fresh fruit. In winter, I make fruit compotes or lightly grill fruits, which are more warming and easier to digest, especially with added freshly grated root ginger to aid circulation.
- Very few people make the effort to drink sufficient clean water, which is vital for good health. Every day we lose around 6.25 pints of water are excreted in urine; 24 fl oz are lost through the skin (more during exercise); 13 fl oz are expelled by simply breathing; and 5 fl oz are excreted with feces. We ingest just under 1.75 pints from food and generate about ¾ pint by burning fats and carbohydrates, so we need to drink at least 2.5 pints, approximately six large glasses, of water every day to simply cover our losses. Under normal circumstances don't drink more than 3.5 pints daily, as this can overburden the kidneys; as in all things, find a balance.Dr Sebagh, a plastic surgeon in London, says that 80% of his patients are dehydrated, and their skin could greatly improve if they would just drink more water. Even the smallest degree of water loss can impair physical and mental function. Also the body siphons what it needs from the colon, and feces can become hard and dry, thus contributing to constipation and increased toxicity in the body. Throughout this book we have re-iterated the need to simply drink more water—it's a quick and easy way to stay healthier.

G

- Cut down on coffee, alcohol, and caffeinated soft drinks, which dehydrate the body. For every caffeinated or alcoholic drink, you need 8fl oz of water.
- The additives, artificial sweeteners (especially aspartame), and sugar in soft drinks and foods can trigger hyperactivity and mood swings. Sugar depletes the body of vital minerals such as chromium. Forget low-calorie drinks: they place a strain on your liver, which slows weight loss. If you find yourself craving sweet foods, take 150mcg of chromium daily. After a few days it will kick in, and you will notice that you crave sugar less. A fair amount of self-discipline is also needed.
- Organic agave syrup (a plant extract), xylitol, and stevia can be used as sugar substitutes, as they have a low glycemic index. Available at all good health stores.
- Remember it's often the foods and drinks you crave the most that are causing the majority of your health problems.
- Drink more herbal teas, especially organic green and white teas.
- Try to eat at least five pieces of fresh, whole fruit and five portions of vegetables daily. Aim to have one salad a day in summer that includes some fresh, steamed or raw vegetables. Otherwise, lightly roast the vegetables, allow them to cool, and then serve in the salad. The darker green the leaves, the more nourishing they are. Three portions of cabbage a week can reduce the incidence of colon cancer by as much as 60%.
- Steam or lightly stir-fry vegetables when possible, as boiling destroys vitamins.
- Keep food simple. Say no to rich foods with rich sauces and to fried, barbecued and burnt foods, which are carcinogenic. (See also *Cancer*.)

G

- Avoid pre-packaged, canned, and fast foods whenever possible, as they often contain plenty of fat, salt, sugar, and additives. Also, a great majority of these foods are packed in aluminum containers, and aluminum is linked to Alzheimer's and senile dementia.
- Do not add sodium-based salt to your food as it can aggravate water retention and cause blood pressure to rise. Our typical diet contains 7–10g of salt a day, and it has been estimated that if we can reduce salt consumption to 3g per person per day there would be between 44,000 and 92,000 fewer deaths in the US each year. There are plenty of magnesium- and potassium-based sea salts readily available from supermarkets and health stores. Try Himalayan Crystal Salt, or try nori or kelp flakes (from seaweed) as a healthy salt substitute.
- Do not become fanatical about fad diets. Remember: everything in moderation because you need to keep a balance of foods at all times for good nutrition. I bake cakes with butter or I use organic olive or coconut oil, which do not become rancid like hard margarines when cooked. You can also try organic walnut, hemp seed, or coconut butters from Artisana, available online from Amazon and at health stores. Use a little organic agave syrup, honey, xylitol, or fresh fruit instead of sugar. Or soak some dried fruits in warm water, drain, chop. and add to the cake mix.
- Use extra-virgin, cold-pressed olive or coconut oil in cooking, and try walnut, avocado, organic sunflower, or sesame oils for salad dressings. These oils have many health benefits, from lowering cholesterol to keeping your skin looking younger.
- Eat your meals sitting down—or at least standing still. Chew your food thoroughly; if you eat too quickly your body will tell you. Aid digestion by eating fruit between meals and not as a dessert. Fruit can ferment when eaten after a large meal, causing wind and bloating.
- Cow's milk is a problem for many people. Skimmed milk is higher in sugar (lactose), and some people are intolerant to this. Try organic oat, quinoa, coconut, almond (try Pacific Natural Foods), or organic rice milks, which are non-dairy. Also try sheep's or goat's milk products and eat plenty of live, low-fat yogurt, which contain beneficial gut bacteria and are rich sources of calcium.

- Throughout this book we have regularly re-iterated how animal dairy products—especially cow's milk—often have a negative effect on many conditions. Firstly cow's milk is difficult for many people to absorb, which can trigger bloating. It is also acid forming after digestion. However, low-fat bio yogurts, which are also low in refined sugars, are somewhat easier to digest as they are fermented. This is why we sometimes recommend avoiding cow's milk, while also advocating that small amounts of yogurt may be okay. Sheep's and goat's milk yogurts are even easier to absorb. We are all unique, and you need to listen to your body and act accordingly.
- Avoid any foods and oils that contain hydrogenated or trans-fats—these are the bad guys.
- Wheat-based cereals, especially wheat bran, trigger bowel problems for many people. Use oat- or quinoa-based cereals, or wheat germ, oat, soy, or rice bran instead. Try lentil-, rice-, corn-, spinach- and potato-based flours and pastas, now available at most health stores.
- Try to avoid red meat, which can putrefy in the gut and may contain antibiotic, hormone, and chemical residues. If you adore meat, gentlemen, please don't eat more than 3.5oz) at one meal, and ladies, keep it to 1.75–2.5oz . Go organic whenever you can to avoid the extra chemicals that non-organic meat contains. Other great proteins are fish, free-range eggs, low-fat cheese, chicken, turkey, tempeh, beans, and lentils.
- Avoid smoking and smoky atmospheres.
- Make time to relax. When we are stressed the body starts pumping out the hormones adrenaline and cortisol, ready for the fight-or-flight response. Eventually this can cause us to blow a fuse. It can be a gastric fuse, leading to ulcers, or a heart fuse, causing heart attacks, and so on. The body and mind are one. If you are stressed, something has got to give in the end, which is why adrenal exhaustion has now reached epidemic proportions. Vitamins, minerals, and diet alone will not keep you healthy. Stress is a major factor in many of today's health problems. Remember, you are special—so give yourself the odd treat and make time for yourself.
- Get plenty of fresh air and learn to breathe deeply; this aids relaxation. Deep breathing also helps alkalize the body. Stress makes it too acid.
- Sunlight is great for your health, and without it you can become very ill indeed. Moderate sunbathing is fine with sunscreen, just stay out of the midday sun. As a general rule, never let your skin go red.
- Learn to laugh regularly, and don't be afraid to laugh at yourself—lighten up.
- Exercise regularly and sensibly, which is one of the best favors you can do for your health. Try brisk walking, cycling, light jogging, swimming, skipping, aerobics and/or aqua-aerobics, as these exercises have the most health-related benefits. You will be amazed at the difference regular exercise can make to your overall wellbeing. If you do nothing else, try to walk for 30 minutes daily, preferably away from main roads.
- Gradual lifestyle changes are of much greater benefits than 2–4-day fad diets.
- Over time, your taste buds will come to love healthier foods.
- Eat when you are hungry and don't let your blood sugar drop too much, as this is when you start filling up on sugary snacks. I tend to eat breakfast, lunch, and dinner, and if I don't snack in between I definitely feel better. Other people find it easier to have small meals at more regular intervals. Listen to your body. Large meals place a strain on the liver and digestive system. Losing weight is easier if you practice this way of eating, which also keeps blood sugar on an even keel, thus preventing mood swings.
- **Breakfast Smoothie Recipe**. Get into blending and juicing. This is a fantastic way to ingest large amounts of nutrients quickly. Buy yourself a blender and learn to love smoothies. For breakfast every day I place all the following items in a blender: one tablespoon of organic

G

sunflower seeds, one tablespoon of non-genetically modified lecithin granules, one tablespoon of linseeds (flax seeds that have been soaked overnight in cold water and drained), one scoop of organic hemp seed green powder protein mix (or a good whey, pea, rice, or soy protein-based powder), half a cup of organic blueberries, a chopped apple (minus the seeds but with the skin), a banana or any fruit you love, especially papaya, pomegranate, pineapple, etc. To this I add a tablespoon of aloe vera juice and a cup or so of organic rice milk. Blend all of this for 30 seconds and drink as a meal replacement (or if it's thick, eat with a spoon or use more milk). It's a tasty combination of fiber, vitamins, minerals, and essential fats.

For added benefits, you can also add a teaspoon of any organic-source green powder such as: Greens Plus, which contains spirulina, chlorella, barley, wheat grass, pectin apple fiber, kelp, broccoli, beets, lactobacillus acidophilus, and more. This is a great way to ingest good nutrients and healthy bacteria and to keep the body more alkaline and help keep you regular.

- With a juicer, you can make yourself fresh raw vegetable juices, again adding any extras such as the aloe, fresh root ginger, a few drops of any herbal tinctures you like. Dandelion and burdock are especially good, as they help cleanse the liver. Drink immediately after juicing while the beneficial enzymes are still active.

GLAUCOMA   (see also Eye Problems and Macular Degeneration)

G

Glaucoma is a group of eye diseases that cause vision loss through damage to the optic nerve. In the US it is estimated that more than 4 million people have glaucoma, but only half of them know it. Experiencing high pressure inside the eyes, without actually having glaucoma, is common and affects 2% of the population between the ages of 40 and 50 and 8% of the population 70 and over. Diabetics are twice as likely to develop glaucoma, which is the leading cause of blindness worldwide. African-Americans also have a greater tendency to suffer from glaucoma, as do people with high blood pressure or a family history of glaucoma. If a family member suffers from glaucoma, it's important that you see an optician annually after the age of 35 to check your eye pressure. Glaucoma can also occur if the eye is injured in any way or suffers chronic inflammation, such as iritis.

The most common type is open-angle glaucoma, which affects more than 90% of Americans with glaucoma. Open-angle glaucoma develops slowly; however, the other type of glaucoma, closed-angle, occurs when the pressure in your eyes rises very quickly. This happens when the drainage angle between the cornea and the iris narrow suddenly, which stops the fluid from leaving the eye, thus increasing intraocular pressure (IOP). This can be very painful and needs urgent medical attention; otherwise your sight can be lost in 2–5 days.

Symptoms of glaucoma differ depending on the type of glaucoma diagnosed. In the majority of cases, typical symptoms would be progressive loss of side vision, followed by reductions in central vision plus watering eyes, headaches, an inability to adjust the eye to darkened rooms, difficulty focusing on close work, and a frequent need to change eyeglass prescriptions. You may also experience nausea, vomiting, pain, and blurred vision, and the whites of your eyes may be inflamed. If you have any of these symptoms, consult an optometrist or an ophthalmologist or go to your local hospital immediately, anyplace where the pressure in your eyes can be tested and immediate action can be taken.

Foods To Avoid
- Reduce or eliminate caffeine and soft drinks, which can contribute to a rise in blood pressure.

- Avoid the artificial sweetener aspartame and greatly cut down on your sugar intake from foods and drinks, as they deplete magnesium, which is often already low in glaucoma sufferers.
- Avoid all mass-produced vegetable oils, including canola oil, and especially margarines. Eliminate deep-fat fried foods from your diet.
- Avoid monosodium glutamate (MSG), which is a potential optic nerve toxin.
- Limit your alcohol consumption. Alcohol interferes with liver function and reduces your levels of protective glutathione, an amino acid.
- Also see diet section under *Eye Problems*.

Friendly Foods
- The flavonoids found in dark purple fruits—red grapes, blueberries, prunes, blackcurrants, blackberries, and cherries—are crucial for supporting your eyes.
- Natural-source carotenes, found in watercress, pumpkin, sweet potatoes, papaya, apricots, and cantaloupe melons, are all great foods to nourish the eyes.
- Eat more flax seeds (linseeds) and oily fish, such as organic salmon, anchovies, trout, mackerel, and sardines, as omega-3 fats are necessary for healthy eyes.
- Eat more avocados and wheat germ, which are rich in vitamin E
- Also see diet section under *Eye Problems*.

Useful Remedies
- Vitamin C is vital, as it helps stabilize intraocular pressure and plays an important role in the prevention and treatment of glaucoma. Take 2–4g daily with food in divided doses. You can take increasing amounts of Vitamin C, up to bowel tolerance, as a way to lower IOP.
- The mineral magnesium has been shown to improve blood supply and visual field, as it relaxes constricted blood vessels. Take 200–800mg per day with food.
- The mineral chromium not only helps balance blood sugar, but also helps the eyes focus. Low levels of vitamin C and chromium are associated with higher IOP. Take 200mcg daily.
- Essential fats, especially fish oils, are also vital for healthy eyes. Take 2g of omega-3 fish oils daily.
- Pycnogenol, pine bark extract, supports healthy collagen. Take 80mg twice daily for one month and then 80mg daily after that.

G

Helpful Hints
- Glaucoma is linked to stress, which thickens the blood and constricts circulation. External pressure increases internal ocular pressure so avoid emotional upsets and upheavals. (See under *Stress*.)
- Make sure you get sufficient sleep.
- According to research from Florida University, contact lenses infused with vitamin E help keep prescription eye drops in the eyes for longer periods of time, making them more effective. Speak to your specialist about this.
- Climates with great temperature variances are thought to be detrimental. Even climates and temperatures appear better tolerated by glaucoma patients.
- Don't smoke, as smoking constricts blood vessels, reducing the blood supply to the eye.
- Avoid prolonged eye stresses, such as long movies, excessive TV viewing or reading, and staring at computer screens for hours on end. Take regular breaks, preferably outside.
- For more help and to find details of where to have laser surgery, visit the Glaucoma Research Foundation's website: www.glaucoma.com

GLUE EAR

(see also Earache)

The Eustachian tube is a pathway that allows for the equalization of air pressure between the middle ear and the back of the throat. However, when a person (usually a child) has glue ear, their middle ear fills up with a glue-like, sticky fluid rather than air. In many cases, glue ear develops after a cough, cold, or ear infection.

Ear infections are one of the most common childhood ailments. They are also likely to re-occur over a relatively short space of time. These infections can be very painful. It is understandable that parents would want to give the child immediate relief; the normal treatment being either antibiotics or the surgical insertion of tubes in the ear. Neither of these treatments is particularly effective. In fact, almost 90% of children with glue ear have food intolerances (see Allergies). Identifying which foods are a problem is important, and the most common culprits tend to be wheat and dairy products from cows. But don't eliminate a whole group of foods and leave the child malnourished. Children who are breast-fed are less likely to develop ear infections. One other odd thing that seems to increase the risk of inner-ear infections is the use of pacifiers when children are very young.

Nutritionist Gareth Zeal has seen many children with glue ear who also suffer from ADHD (Attention Deficit, Hyperactivity Disorder). (See under *Hyperactivity*.)

Foods to Avoid

- Sugar is top of the list, as it weakens the immune system, leaving children more prone to infections. Other than sugar it is very important that any food intolerances or allergies are identified because these are likely to be the primary cause. Typically they would include dairy products from cows, eggs, wheat, and citrus fruits such as oranges, grapefruit, lemons and limes, but it could be any one of a number of other foods.
- Keep your child away from mucus-forming food, such as full-fat cheeses, pizzas, Greek yogurts, white breads and cakes, full-fat milks from any source, soy milk and foods, chocolates, and so on. Mucus will also be formed in response to any foods that the child is sensitive to.
- Remember that many canned drinks and mass-produced desserts and jellies can contain up to 10 teaspoons of sugar. Artificial sweeteners are often a problem for individuals with allergies.
- Try to avoid preservatives and additives in foods and toiletries such as toothpastes.

Friendly Foods

- Fresh fruit and vegetables are rich in vitamin C, which will boost the immune system.
- Garlic helps fight infections, but note that garlic is a common allergen, so keep a food diary and note reactions.
- Chewing gum made with xylitol seems to be beneficial, as children who chew xylitol-sweetened chewing gum have a much lower rate of inner-ear infections. You can also buy xylitol as a sweetener.
- Introduce your child to foods that are low in saturated fats and highly nutritious, such as brown rice, barley, lentils, and pulses; also try rice, amaranth or oatcakes.
- There are numerous health cookbooks that have great recipes for cookies, cakes, and other desserts that are low in fat and sugar.
- There are plenty of low-fat, live fruit yogurts that replenish healthy bacteria in the gut, which helps fight infection.
- Use rice, almond, or oat milk and bake cakes with barley, buckwheat, rice, potato, or spelt flours.
- Use non-hydrogenated spreads such as Olivio, Promise, or Biona.

Useful Remedies

- Colostrum, which is found in breast milk, helps support the immune system and aids healing of a leaky gut, which is normally associated with glue ear. It's also very helpful for babies and children suffering from eczema. Until the age of 2, give a quarter of a teaspoon twice daily on an empty stomach. After that, increase to half a teaspoon twice daily. Only administer this for one month.
- Use echinacea either as a tincture or tablets. An alcohol-free tincture is often easier for children, as it can be added to fruit juice or yogurt. If the child is very small, use one drop per 3lb of body weight. It can be used several times a day while symptoms last. **VC**
- Vitamin C: for children give 250–500mg daily; for adults 1–2g daily. Again, as a lot of children don't like tablets, vitamin C is often available as a chewable tablet or powder; some of them are fairly pleasant tasting. You can find powders that can be added to fruit juice so the child will only be able to taste the juice. Alternatively, use a vitamin crusher. **VC**
- Zinc lozenges and zinc supplements can be given to children. Give 1–2 lozenges a day while the child has an infection. Zinc boosts the immune system and helps fight the infection. Supplement dosages: 25mg daily for adults and 10–15mg daily for children over 8.
- Find a good children's chewable multi-vitamin/mineral. **VC**
- The celloid potassium chloride helps unblock the Eustachian tubes. Take or give 100mg daily. **VC**

Helpful Hints

- It is important to have an allergy test to find your or your child's worst food offenders. Try the YorkTest Laboratories (www.yorktest.com). Another option is the FACT test by Genova Diagnostics, which looks for inflammatory markers indicating that the body is reacting to certain substances. Tel: 1-800-522-4762. Website: www.genovadiagnostics.com
- A humidifier placed in the main living room or the child's bedroom has been found to reduce the risk of inner-ear infections.
- Many nutritional doctors advocate that your child should not be subjected to vaccinations until the cycle of ear infections is cleared, as vaccines place a strain on the child's immune system.
- Try Dr Christopher's Ear & NerveFormula as eardrops. **VC**
- Use ear candles to remove excess wax. This is a pain-free way to reduce some of the aching and must be done by a responsible or qualified adult. Available from most health stores.
- Cranial osteopathy helps as it encourages lymph drainage. (See *Useful Information*.)
- Do not let the child be exposed to cigarette smoke. It increases the incidence of glue ear by 80%.

G

GOUT

(see also Acid–Alkaline Balance and Arthritis)

In the 18th century you were considered fortunate to develop gout, as they believed this prevented you from contracting fatal diseases. It was seen as a rich person's disease, because only those who could afford large amounts of meat, cheese, and wine were likely to suffer. Gout is a form of joint inflammation, which is caused by high levels of uric acid in the blood creating crystal deposits in the joints. It is very common in the big toe, but can also affect other joints and the kidneys. The vast majority of gout sufferers are men but more and more women are beginning to develop gout, which is totally avoidable. An attack can be triggered by ingesting overly rich food and drinks, which would typically include shellfish, cheeses such as Stilton, port, red meat, and red wine. Most people who suffer from gout tend to drink a lot anyway—especially champagne. Occasionally, an accident or trauma to the body can also pre-cipitate an attack.

Foods to Avoid

- Generally, eat a lot less meat, plus reduce beer and cheese consumption, which are the main triggers for gout.
- Avoid any foods that are high in purines, which are found in high-protein foods such as offal, oily fish (including anchovies, herrings, cod, and mackerel), chicken, caffeine, shellfish (including crab, lobster, scallops, and mussels), roe, kidney beans, lima beans, navy beans, yeast-based drinks, oatmeal, and lentils. Once the attack has subsided, you can eat small amounts of these foods.
- Avoid full-fat cheeses, especially Stilton and Brie.
- Most forms of arthritis usually benefit from taking cod liver oil or eating oily fish; with gout, however, these foods would almost certainly make it worse.

Friendly Foods

- Cherries and pineapple should be eaten on a daily basis, cherries in particular. They are one of the easiest ways of keeping gout under control and preventing it, as they increase excretion of uric acid from the body. You can also try diluting pure, low-sugar cherry concentrate in water.
- If you are not a fan of cherries, try blueberries, blackberries, or bilberries. These are very rich in bioflavonoids, which help reduce uric acid levels in the body.
- Prunes, although acid forming, help mobilize uric acid out of the body. Eat daily or try prune juice.

- Eat plenty of fruit and vegetables, especially celery, quinoa, millet, brown rice, and pastas made from corn, rice, amaranth, potato, or buckwheat flours.
- Free-range or organic eggs, cooked soy tofu, and lamb should not cause any problems.
- Make a healthy drink containing a small box of blueberries, some pineapple, frozen or fresh seeded cherries, a pear, an apple, and a banana. Add a teaspoon of any good organic green food powder (which will help alkalize your system), and a tiny piece of fresh root ginger. Put in a blender with half a cup of rice or almond milk, mix for one minute, and then drink immediately.
- Drink at least 6–8 glasses of water every day to encourage excretion of uric acid.

Useful Remedies

- Taking 1–2g of vitamin C a day taken with food will gradually help lower uric acid levels.
- Bromelain is a very powerful anti-inflammatory. Take 500mg twice a day.
- Take a combination of ginger, curcumin, and boswellia supplements—take four capsules, or more, a day. These herbs in combination provide relief from any type of inflammation discomfort.
- Cat's claw (400mg three times a day for 3 months or more) can gradually help lower uric acid levels, as well as improving bowel function. This herb can help protect your gut lining against the negative side effects of anti-inflammatory painkillers—known as NSAIDs. **VC**
- Omega-3 fats found in flax seeds (linseeds), hemp seeds and extracted from oily fish will help dampen inflammation. Although we recommend avoiding oily fish, the proteins that cause the problems have been removed from pure fish oil. Take 2–3g daily with food.

Helpful Hints

- Lose weight, as this is quite often part of the problem. Remember that gout is pretty much self-inflicted and almost entirely caused by a rich diet. Be prepared to make some changes.
- Nettle tea will also aid with excretion of uric acid.
- Massage the painful joint with essential oil of Roman chamomile, juniper, wintergreen, and ginger to help reduce the pain and inflammation.

- Homeopathic Ledum 30c twice daily for 2–3 days will reduce symptoms.
- Do not take aspirin if you are taking anti-gout drugs.

GUMS *(see Bleeding Gums)*

HAIR LOSS *(see also Absorption, Circulation, and Stress)*

The average person loses between 70 and 100 hairs a day, and as we age our hair becomes finer and/or thinner. Most of us tend to associate balding and thinning hair with men, yet many women experience thinning hair as well. In fact many trichologists, who 10 years ago tended to see more men than women experiencing hair loss problems, are now seeing just as many women suffering from hair loss—even Asian and African-American women, who traditionally always have beautiful, thick hair. Our American lifestyle seems to be a major factor.

There are a number of causes for hair loss, such as hormonal changes at menopause or after childbirth, but for the majority of women with hair problems, stress is probably the most likely culprit. Stress robs us of major nutrients that are essential for healthy hair growth. When a person is very stressed the scalp becomes tight, which restricts circulation, and the hair follicles become malnourished, resulting in further hair loss. Adrenal exhaustion, an underactive thyroid and certain prescription drugs are also factors in hair loss.

Naturopath Stephen Langley says: "In Chinese medicine the lung *chi* governs the shine or luster of the hair, and the thickness and strength is governed by the kidney *chi*. Roughly translated, this means that the shine and luster is dulled by our reduced capability to oxygenate our blood cells fully. We can all see evidence of dull-looking hair when we are tired and don't exercise enough, or through anxiety which causes us to shallow-breathe. Smoking will have the same effect.

"The kidney *chi* is depleted through poor nutrient supply that helps make up our essence or primary energy reserves. This happens also when we are run down or our adrenal glands become exhausted through burning the candle at both ends. Our requirements for nutrients under these circumstances will be much greater. (See under *Adrenal Exhaustion*.) We literally feed off our own body, and nutrients will be taken from less important areas (such as the scalp) to supply more important tissues such as the organs. And if tissues are too acid, which they are when we are stressed, then minerals needed for healthy hair, such as iron, magnesium, and zinc, are taken from the hair follicles to buffer this acidity." (See *Acid–Alkaline Balance*.)

Mainly, then, the health of your hair depends on the circulation to the root of the hair and the amount of nutrients present in the blood. Hair is composed of a protein-like substance called keratin and requires a healthy, balanced diet for proper nourishment. Many drugs claim to increase hair growth, but some have negative side effects, which include an inability for men to maintain an erection. So before trying any of these drugs, always discuss any implications with your doctor or a trichologist.

Another important factor is the male hormone testosterone, which is also found in women. Although this hormone is responsible for making men hairy during puberty, it also has a large role to play in hair loss in later life, for both men and women. Some women have too much testosterone, which shows up in excess facial hair and can trigger male-type thinning. In this case, taking the herbs *Vitex agnus castus* or saw palmetto can help reduce testosterone levels.

Hereditary factors are also important. The more hair loss there is/was in your father, uncles, and grandfathers, the more likely you are to lose your own hair. However, dietary supplements and regular daily firm-scalp massage can help slow down hair loss. Hair loss in much younger people is also becoming extremely common, showing that stress is definitely a trigger. Stress and a toxic bowel prevent production of some of the B vitamins that are necessary for maintaining hair color and healthy hair.

Hair loss in women is common after childbirth and menopause, and a lack of protein can trigger thinning hair or even cause it to fall out. Hair loss is also linked to heavy metal toxicity. I have seen several cases of alopecia in young women due to stress, which triggered a leaky gut; when they started taking a digestive enzyme with an easily absorbed multi-nutrient with meals, the hair grew back.

It is thought that men lose hair on the tops of their heads rather than the back and sides because the blood flow to the top of the scalp is reduced in comparison to the sides.

Hair grows faster in summer, and a single hair can live for several years. On average human hair grows between 5 and 6 inches a year.

Foods to Avoid

- Although protein is needed for healthy hair, too much protein such as red meat and cheese, without sufficient fruit and vegetables, leaves the body very acid, which depletes reserves of important alkaline minerals necessary for healthy hair.
- Reduce caffeine from any source. Caffeine increases stress (as it triggers adrenaline and cortisol to be released) and weakens the adrenal glands.
- Avoid sugar and refined carbohydrates, such as pastries, cakes, desserts, pies, and so on, all of which deplete nutrients needed for hair growth.
- Reduce the amount of sodium-based salt in your diet.

Friendly Foods

- Quality protein is the most important food for your hair. Eat organic lean meats, chicken and game, including venison (in moderation), fish, and eggs (particularly egg whites).
- Whey, milk, yogurt, and cheese are also rich in protein. But don't eat too much cheese, as it's very acid forming—like all dairy foods.
- If you cannot tolerate whey protein from cows, then use organic hemp seed protein powders. For a healthy smoothie recipe, see under *General Health Hints*.
- Vegetarian-based proteins are found in seeds, nuts, vegetables, whole grains (such as brown rice and quinoa), and legumes (such as peas, lentils, soybeans, tofu, tempeh, lentils, and peanuts).
- Eat more iron-rich foods, such as egg yolks, green leafy vegetables (like spinach, curly kale, and watercress), wholegrain breads and cereals, meat (especially organic liver), and fish.
- Try adding seaweeds such as kombu, arame, and wakame, to meals. You use them as you would a green vegetable, and they are a rich source of minerals needed for healthy hair.
- Essential fats are vital for healthy hair and a healthy scalp; therefore, eat more oily fish, walnuts, pumpkin seeds, sunflower seeds, and flaxseeds soaked in cold water overnight, drained and then eaten). You can also mix their unrefined oils half and half with olive oil and

use for salad dressings or drizzle over cooked foods. Essential fats help you avoid a dry, scaly scalp and nourish the hair follicles. (See *Fats You Need To Eat*.)

- Cilantro is full of chlorophyll (and selenium), which detoxifies heavy metals from the body, as well as other important nutrients, especially B vitamins. Most organic green food powders contain plenty of chlorophyll. A good version is Greens Plus, containing Hawaiian spirulina, chlorella, lecithin, barley, wheat grass juice, pectin apple fiber, soy and barley sprouts, sea algae, and healthy bacteria. For details visit www. greensplus.com. **VC**
- Muesli, cereals, and oats are all high in B vitamins.
- Eat one avocado a week to help your hair shine.
- Good sources of copper needed for healthy hair are Brazil nuts, almonds, walnuts, and hazelnuts, along with lecithin granules sprinkled over your morning cereal

Useful Remedies.

- Take a good-quality multi-vitamin/mineral daily. Most of the companies listed at the beginning of the book supply specific hair-nutrient formulas. You will need at least 15–30mg of zinc and 1–2mg of copper in your multi, as a lack of copper is linked to graying hair.
- A company called Viviscal makes good multi hair products—www.viviscal.com.
- Romanda Healthcare makes an excellent formula that contains all of the nutrients needed for healthy hair, plus a growth serum and shampoo, which are excellent. (See *Helpful Hints* for contact details.)
- There are blood cleansers available that can help restore hair loss due to stress and mineral depletion like Genesis Today Liquid Super Cleanse. The quality of your scalp depends on the quality of the blood supplying the roots. As we age, the quality of our blood is reduced because of the accumulation of toxins. Once the blood is able to carry more oxygen and nutrients, hair can improve. **VC**

- The B-group vitamins are vital if you want to keep your hair, and many people who take a full spectrum of B vitamins report that their gray hairs disappear. Vitamin B5, PABA, biotin, and folic acid are the anti-graying nutrients, and you would need 1000mcg of biotin daily. Check the content of your multi before taking extra B vitamins.
- Vitamin B6 (50mg per day) is helpful for women taking the contraceptive pill, which can affect hair loss. **You do not need this if your multi contains 50mg of B6.**
- Find out if you are low in iron, in which case take a liquid, easily absorbed formula such as Spatone. Available from health stores worldwide. Don't take iron unless you need it. If you cook in iron pots, you will absorb some of the iron in your food. **NB: Never leave iron supplements near children.**
- Futurebiotics Hair, Skin & Nails supplement provides vitamin C, rutin, hesperidin, cellulose, silica, and vitamins A and D plus much more to strengthen hair and nails. **VC**
- If your hair is thinning because of menopause there are a number of herbs that can help balance hormones naturally, include dong quai, black cohosh, sage, and soy isoflavones. Several of the companies mentioned at the front of this book sell these supplements.
- Thinning hair in men, caused by excess dihydro-testosterone, can be balanced by taking saw palmetto (500mg daily under supervision—it may need to be higher) and zinc (30mg daily).

Helpful Hints

- Exercise regularly, which will stimulate your heart and circulation, thus increasing oxygen flow, reducing stress, and promoting scalp and hair health.
- There is a myth that says the more you brush your hair, the thicker and healthier it will grow—it's not true. Too much brushing pulls hair out, breaks it, and scratches the scalp.
- Don't over-dry your hair, as this makes it more brittle.
- "Women who lose a lot of hair after giving birth should stop panicking," says London- and

New York-based trichologist, Philip Kingsley. "During pregnancy estrogen levels are higher, and this hormone prolongs the natural lifespan of a hair. The average person loses 70–100 hairs a day, but during pregnancy hair falls out less because of the estrogen. Then 4–6 weeks later the woman gives birth and hormones return to normal levels—and all the normal shedding that should have happened during the previous months occurs all at once. As long as these women eat a healthy diet and take the right supplements, the hair should soon get back to normal."

- Philip Kingsley has formulated various hormone drops for men and women that nourish the follicle and help prevent hair loss. They don't make hair re-grow if the hair-loss is permanent, but they help you to keep the hair you have left. For details call 1-212-753-9600. Website: www.philipkingsley.com For more help on hair, read Philip Kingsley's book *The Hair Bible* (Aurum Press).
- Some doctors have noticed that smokers tend to lose their hair faster than non-smokers.
- Shampoo your hair regularly; this helps to re-moisturize the hair.
- Jojoba oil mixed with a little essential oil of rosemary and massaged into the scalp removes dead skin cells and increases circulation. Be firm: you need the skin on your scalp to move so that blood can circulate more freely. Do this before going to bed and leave the oils on overnight.
- Some yogis say that by doing head and shoulder stands they have kept their hair because the circulation to their heads is greatly increased. If, like me, you are not into headstands, simply lie on the floor and put your calves up on a chair or a bed. This not only helps gives your leg veins a rest, but also encourages more blood to flow to the head.
- Chlorine from swimming pools damages your hair and is also linked to asthma and heart disease.
- To find your nearest qualified trichologist visit the International Association of Trichologists' website: www.trichology.edu.au
- Try Romanda lotion and shampoos, along with Romanda hair formula powder supplements. Call Jan Adams on the Romanda Advice Line on 011-44-208-346-0784, or e-mail: jan_romanda@hotmail.com or visit: www.romanda-healthcare.co.uk. Jan is very helpful and formed the company after suffering hair loss. She also helps people with hair loss after chemotherapy, plus alopecia and patchy hair loss.
- Numerous salons offer hair transplants, which are becoming more sophisticated. Many dermatologists and plastic surgeons offer the latest technique called Micro Grafting, which gives a more natural-looking hairline, rather than hundreds of "puncture marks." The surgery is expensive, but the results are amazing.

HALITOSIS (bad breath) *(see also Liver Problems)*

Bad breath is often caused by poor dental hygiene and/or poor digestion, reduced gut function, or a sluggish bowel. A build-up of plaque, infected gums, abscesses, and insufficient brushing and flossing are usually to blame, though. Make sure to see a qualified dental hygienist at least twice a year. Use fluoride-free floss and mouthwash daily, change your toothbrush regularly, and brush your teeth at least twice a day—but not immediately after eating fruit.

Foods such as meat take a long time to digest and can putrefy in the bowel. One of the simplest things you can do is to chew properly, as this enhances carbohydrate digestion and makes it easier for the rest of the digestive process. Try not to eat too much food at one sitting, which overloads the stomach and bowel.

One of the Atkins Diets, which suggests a high-protein, low-carbohydrate way of eating, was notorious for triggering constipation and bad breath. Some people find their digestion improves if they avoid eating proteins and carbohydrates together in one meal. For example, if you are eating a protein meal such as chicken or fish, eat it with vegetables only and not with starches. Conversely, if you are eating rice or pasta, eat it with vegetables only and not with protein. Long-term bad breath can also indicate problems with the liver or kidneys or diabetes, in which case you must consult a doctor. If the bowel is severely congested with impacted matter, the body re-absorbs the toxins into the blood, which eventually makes its way into the lungs where the toxins are then breathed out. (See under *Constipation*.)

Foods to Avoid
■ Avoid too much caffeine, sugar, and low-fiber, high-fat foods, which all weaken digestion and cause sluggish bowel movements. This includes white breads, cakes, cookies, and pastas.
■ Smoking not only causes bad breath directly, but it can also cause it indirectly as it weakens digestion.
■ Cut down on your consumption of milk and dairy products from cows, because they are mucus forming and slow bowel function.

Friendly Foods
■ Leafy green vegetables, such as bok choy, spring greens, kale, watercress, and cabbage are rich in chlorophyll. Chlorophyll is useful for helping clear the bowel and thus improving the smell of the breath.
■ Eat more artichokes, celeriac, radicchio (Italian chicory), and chicory. (See dietary advice in *Liver Problems*.)
■ Eat plenty of fresh whole fruits. Pineapple or papaya, eaten either before or after a meal, are useful, as the enzymes in these fruits can help break down proteins, ensuring proper digestion.
■ Eating a "bio" or live yogurt that contains acidophilus and bifidus for either breakfast or as a dessert improves the quality of the bacteria in the bowel, enhancing digestion and making bad breath less likely.
■ Add more cilantro and fresh mint to foods, and eat fennel or caraway seeds, which help kill the bacteria that cause bad breath.
■ Drink more fenugreek tea and green tea, as they help kill bacteria in the mouth.
■ There are many good aloe vera drinks available. Drink a capful before main meals to further aid digestion.
■ Fructooligosaccharides (FOS)—a powder—can be used as a sweetener and acts like a prebiotic to help the body make more healthy bacteria in the gut, which in turn can help reduce bad breath. Take 5–20g daily sprinkled on cereals or mixed in smoothies. **VC**
■ Drink plenty of water.

Useful Remedies
■ Sprinkle 2–6 teaspoons of flax seeds that have been soaked overnight in cold water and drained into oatmeal or mix in a smoothie. You will find a good recipe under *General Health Hints*. Otherwise, use ready-cracked flax seeds, which do not need soaking.
■ Also use organic sunflower seeds over salads, breakfast cereals, and so on to encourage toxins to move more quickly through the bowel.
■ Taking one capsule of betaine hydrochloride (stomach acid) with main meals improves protein digestion and ensures that foods don't ferment in the bowel. **Do not take this supplement if you have active stomach ulcers, in which case take a digestive enzyme free from stomach acid. VC**

- One to two acidophilus and bifidus capsules with FOS (fructooligosaccharides) taken at the end of a meal can increase healthy bacteria in the bowel and enhance digestion. **VC**
- Take 5–6 drops of chlorophyll daily to help eliminate bad breath.
- Most organic green food powders contain plenty of chlorophyll.
- Try Greens Plus, which contains Hawaiian spirulina, chlorella, lecithin, barley, wheat grass juice, pectin apple fiber, soy and barley sprouts, and healthy bacteria. For details visit www.greensplus.com
- Or try taking Lepicol capsules or powder, which contain both prebiotics and probiotics (beneficial bacteria), daily. Available from most health stores, online retailers, and some pharmacies.
- Make a mouthwash of one capful of hydrogen peroxide mixed with four capfuls of water. Swish it around in your mouth, hold for one minute, and then spit it out. This helps oxygenate the gums and kill off bacteria.

Helpful Hints

- Make up your own healthy mouthwash using a few drops of essential oils of tea tree, peppermint, thyme, and lemon. Mix with warm water and use regularly after meals and before bed. I make mine with boiled water, which I allow to cool, and then I keep the blend in a dark bottle in my bathroom so that it lasts longer.
- Exercise regularly, as this ensures healthy bowel function.
- If bad breath is severe, with your doctor's permission, have a colonic irrigation, which gently washes out the bowel and helps reduce toxicity. (See *Useful Information* at back of this book.)
- Contact the American Breath Specialists through their website: www.breath-care.com
- Ask at your local pharmacist for a tongue scraper and use it regularly to help clear any bacteria off your tongue
- For immediate breath freshening, use a drop of pure peppermint oil on the tongue.

HANGOVERS
(see Alcohol)

HAY FEVER
(see also Allergies, Allergic Rhinitis, and Liver Problems)

Dr Jean Monro, an allergy specialist at the Breakspear Hospital in Hertfordshire, UK, says: "Before the industrial revolution, conditions such as hay fever did not exist. But since then we have done a great job of polluting our atmosphere and thus our bodies, which is why hay fever is actually more common in city dwellers than in people who live in the country. We now know that an accumulation of a variety of pollutants, such as paint sprays or pesticides (there are hundreds of others), acts as the initial trigger; these chemicals became the sensitizers— and in most cases the membranes within the nose and throat begin to react by becoming inflamed. Then the body treats the next thing that comes along, such as grass pollens, as a threatening foreign invader, which increases any inflammation and induces allergic-type symptoms. But it's important to realize that it's the chemicals that sensitize the body in the first place. Chemicals can have a local effect, such as on the skin, and then this effect is communicated to the rest of the body by neural (nerve) pathways, and a sensitivity is born."

This is important news to anyone suffering from hay fever, as Dr Monro and her colleagues have developed vaccines that can help neutralize any reaction to substances found to trigger a response. (For more details, see *Allergies*.)

Meanwhile, symptoms vary from sore, puffy, itchy, watering eyes to continual sneezing and a runny or congested nose. Hay fever is sometimes confused with a condition called allergic or perennial rhinitis, as the symptoms are similar to those of hay fever but occur all year round. Common causes of allergic rhinitis include dust, food allergies, and atmospheric pollution. Many people with hay fever and allergic rhinitis are also likely to have a sensitivity to certain foods, the most common being wheat and potentially dairy products from any source, but some sufferers have problems with anything from eggs to bananas. As this has been linked to digestive problems for some people, see also *Leaky Gut*.

Foods to Avoid
- Greatly reduce your exposure to any foods with additives and/or preservatives, as well as to those that have been sprayed with pesticides and herbicides—eat organic. Keep in mind that non-organic apples, for example, can be sprayed up to 18 times before being sold.
- Avoid any foods that you are intolerant to; typically these would include wheat, dairy products, eggs, and citrus fruits—especially oranges.
- Dairy products are mucus forming and without doubt can exacerbate the problem. While symptoms are acute, avoid milk in any form for at least one week, as well as cheeses, chocolate, and foods high in saturated fats such as croissants, Danish pastries, pies,, and white-flour-based cakes and cookies.
- Many foods high in sugar, such as desserts and candies, are also high in dairy and fats. Too much sugar will greatly lower immune function.
- Reduce salt, caffeine, and alcohol.

Friendly Foods
- Ingesting sufficient fluids is important, as researchers have found that people who are dehydrated tend to suffer more hay fever-type symptoms.
- Garlic and onions are high in the flavonoid quercetin, which can help reduce the severity of allergic reactions.
- Nettle tea helps ease the symptoms of allergic rhinitis.
- Dairy-free alternatives to cow's milk are organic rice, almond, oat, and pea milk. You can also try coconut milk; look for So Delicious (www.turtlemountain.com); it's one of the better-tasting non-dairy milks. If animal-source dairy produce is a problem, try these milks in small amounts and note if they trigger a reaction.
- Drink freshly squeezed vegetable juice, especially one made with beets, artichokes, a little garlic, ginger, apple, and carrot, which boosts the immune system and helps eliminate toxins.
- Bioflavonoids are important protectors of mucous membranes; therefore, eat plenty of blueberries, blackberries, plums, red grapes, strawberries, and cherries.
- Include plenty of fresh vegetables, brown rice, and whole grains in your diet.

Useful Remedies
- Quercetin (400mg three times a day) is a natural antihistamine, which helps reduce puffy eyes and irritation in the nose.
- While symptoms are acute, take up to 2–3g of vitamin C daily in an ascorbate form with food, which also acts like a mild antihistamine.
- Beta Glucans 1–3, 1–6, which are derived from yeast cell walls, are proven to strengthen the body's innate immune system (the one you were born with), making it more resistant to airborne pathogens. It also helps reduce the incidence of food intolerances and can be taken by children. Take 250–500mg daily. **VC** To see good research on Beta Glucans, visit Dr Paul Clayton's website: www.healthdefence.com
- Butterbur, a plant, taken in capsule form can help treat hay fever. Take 500mg twice daily.

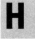

- Taking nettle tablets or tincture three times a day has proven to be effective for allergic rhinitis.
- Garlic, ginger, and horseradish tincture can ease congestion and reduce the symptoms of hay fever.
- D-Hist from Ortho Molecular Products contains vitamin C, quercetin the amino acid cysteine, bromelain, and stinging nettles leaf, which all help if you suffer from seasonal disorders. Take one capsule twice daily. This formula should not to be taken if you are pregnant. Available online at Amazon and other websites.
- If nothing else, take a high-strength multi-vitamin/mineral that contains plenty of the B-group vitamins.
- Take probiotics daily—these healthy bacteria help boost immune function and heal the gut wall, thus reducing the amount of toxins that enter the bloodstream. **VC**
- YS Organic Bee Farms has a bee pollen product with whole granules. Sprinkle daily over breakfast cereals for at least one month prior to the hay-fever season to help reduce the severity or delay the onset of an attack. **VC NB: Do not use if you are highly allergic to bee stings.**

Helpful Hints

- It's well worthwhile checking for food intolerances. See details of the York or Genova Tests under the *Helpful Hints* in *Allergies*.
- Begin subscribing to *Allergic Living* magazine. Tel: 1-888-771-7747 (toll free). Website: www.allergicliving.com

- Buy a pot of honey from your local area, preferably with the honeycomb still in it, and take 2 teaspoons daily for about a month before the onset of the hay-fever season. The pollen in the honey may protect you from developing full-blown hay fever.
- Homeopathy has been successful in treating hay fever with remedies such as allium cepa, euphrasia, or "mixed pollens." Ask for details at your local homeopathic pharmacy or see *Useful Information* to find a qualified practitioner in your area. King Bio, BioAllers, Hyland's, and other brands have convenient formulations for hay fever. **VC**
- Place a few drops of essential oil of basil and melissa on a handkerchief to help clear the sinuses. Massage these oils into the chest and throat once mixed with a base carrier oil, such as almond or jojoba.
- Treat yourself to a good-quality ionizer, and place it near your bed to help reduce any allergens in the air around you.

HEAD LICE
(see Scalp Problems)

HEALING AND HEALERS
(see also Electrical Pollution)

There is now such a huge body of validated independent scientific evidence that hands-on healing and prayer have positive physical effects that the efficacy of healing itself is no longer in doubt. Some health centers and clinics offer healing, and there are hundreds of Reiki healers working in alternative treatment centers around the world. Some people still believe that healing cannot work unless you have a specific religious belief or strong faith that the healing will work, yet there are hundreds of documented cases where young babies, plants, children, and animals have responded positively to healing.

To understand how healing works, it is imperative to first comprehend that we are all electrical beings in a physical shell. If you take a photograph using Kirlian cameras, you can clearly see the energy or auric field surrounding a person, animal, plant or in fact any object; even a stone will have an auric field. Roger Coghill, a bio-electromagnetics research scientist based in Wales, says: "An individual's energy field or aura is as unique to them as their DNA. When we become ill, our field's characteristics change; this was proven by the American neurologist Albert Abrams in 1916."

After my near-death experience in 1998, which is documented in my book *Divine Intervention* (CICO Books), I truly began to comprehend how healing works.

Professor Gary Schwartz at the University of Arizona conducted experiments during 2002 in which a well-known healer, Rosalyn Bruyere, taught 26 doctors and nurses how to give hands-on healing. After the training it was found that the nurses and doctors were able to absorb more gamma cosmic rays (which are the highest frequencies we can measure) and then their bodies acted like transformers, literally "turning down" the cosmic ray frequencies into subtle x-ray frequencies, which they then focused and pulsed into patients' energy fields. There are also machines that mimic this process. Biophysicist Harry Oldfield spent 20 years developing a PIP scanner that can "read" the energies being emitted from our bodies. During his early research at some of the UK's leading teaching hospitals, Harry began to notice that when he compared patients' energy emissions before and after treatments such as chemotherapy, the treatments triggered energy distortions, which eventually manifested as negative symptoms. Over the following 20 years he became an expert at correctly interpreting these energy distortions. He eventually concluded that if these distortions could be treated with correcting harmonic frequencies, this could normalize the person's energy field, which would encourage the body to heal itself. Years later, he designed electro-crystal healing for this purpose.

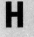

When we become sick, cells begin emitting disharmonic frequencies, which can clearly be seen in our energy field on his specialist scanners. Harry has found that every illness shows up in our energy field before appearing in the physical body. To counteract various medical conditions, he simply pulses the correct tonal frequency back into the patient to encourage the body to heal itself. This is what healers have been doing intuitively for thousands of years. Harry has trained hundreds of therapists in the UK and globally; for more information on your nearest therapist, Harry Oldfield's PIP scanners, and his electro-crystal therapy, visit www.electrocrystal.com

New frequency-based vaccines for allergies work on similar principals (see *Allergies*). This is how dolphins heal. They have been on the planet for 30 million years longer than humans, and their brains are highly developed. They can "scan" someone, much the same as a good healer can, and they then pulse harmonic, healing frequencies back into the patient, which over time can encourage the body to heal itself. And when Harry has scanned healers while they are working, he says the transfer of energy can be clearly seen on his equipment. I have seen film of this myself. Also Harry has said that sometimes the healing energy emanates from inside the healers—usually from within their heart or solar plexus energy centers—while at other times they can clearly see energy from outside the healer being absorbed into the healer and then flowing out through their hands.

However, both Oldfield and Schwartz and other scientists, such as those based at the Institute for Noetic Science in California, make it clear that, in the majority of cases, without a clear intention from the healer, little or no energy transfers take place. They also say it's vital that the healer should be in a positive frame of mind and not be sick themselves when they offer healing to a patient.

Of course, some healers are better than others—just as there are better pianists, computer experts, or surgeons. Recalling that we all emit our own unique range of frequencies, you need to find a healer who is on a compatible range of frequencies to your own, and then you generally receive a more beneficial effect. You will soon know after three or four sessions whether their healing is making any difference. If you are no better, simply find another healer. It is also possible to facilitate a transfer of healing energies over distances—and the science of how this is possible is detailed in my book, *Countdown to Coherence* (Watkins Publishing).

Remember, energy can neither be created nor destroyed—it can only change into other forms of energy. Your thoughts are energy—they go somewhere—and when the intention is done with the whole heart and is for the receiver's greater good, your prayers will reach their destination. And the more people who pray at the same time with the same intention, the more powerful the prayer becomes. According to well-known healers such as Seka Nikolic, it is imperative that we transmit only positive thoughts and visualize the person looking 100% healthy in our mind's eye or imagination. I have also detailed more information on healing and the science of miracles, plus the science behind how spontaneous healing occurs, in my book *The Evidence For The Sixth Sense* (CICO Books).

Helpful Hints

- The human mind is far more powerful than most people can even begin to imagine; therefore, if you also truly believe the healing will work, this really helps. Remember, there is a huge difference between wanting something to work and believing 100% that it will.
- I find healing a great additional therapy when used in conjunction with eating the right diet and so on. It literally recharges your internal batteries, which gives your body more energy to heal itself. Most healers find that the great majority of their patients are looking for a single magic bullet to heal their ills. But if they continue eating junk foods (or foods to which they have an intolerance), don't exercise, and so on, obviously it's like trying to put out a fire while you are still standing in the flames.
- Then again, I have witnessed many miracles. Cancers have disappeared, crippled people have walked again. How can this happen? I firmly believe this is a combination of the power of the sick person's mind believing they are well and the ability of the healer to transmit a strong healing signal. Also, spiritual masters can without doubt effect healing miracles without the person's knowledge. But I also know that if a person believes 100% with their mind and heart they are truly healed, in that instant they are.
- Read *The Biology of Belief* by cell biologist Bruce H Lipton Ph.D., which documents dozens of validated case studies in healing and the mind.
- To find out more about Reiki or to locate a Reiki Master, visit The Reiki Alliance's website: www.reikialliance.com
- Although there are hundreds of good healers in the US alone, there is one I would mention—William Rand, who is a well known Reiki healer, teacher, and author. Tel: 1-800-332-8112. Website: www.reiki.org.
- Diane Stern has written an excellent book on Reiki called *Essential Reiki* (Crossing Press) as well as a number of other books about healing. Visit www.dianestein.net for more information.

HEARTBURN   *(see Acid Stomach, Indigestion, and Low Stomach Acid)*

HEART DISEASE

(see also Angina, Atherosclerosis, Cholesterol, Circulation, and High Blood Pressure)

Heart disease caused more than 425,000 deaths in the United States in 2006, and more than 17.5 million people (about 9.2 million men and 8.4 million women) who are alive today have a history of heart attack, angina, or both. Approximately ever 25 seconds, someone in the US suffers from a coronary event, and every minute someone dies from one. However, the faster you can receive medical attention, the more likely you are to survive. This is because in order to work properly, clot-busting drugs must be given within 30 minutes of arriving at the hospital, and angioplasty needs to be done within 90 minutes.

The majority of younger people who die from heart disease are male. Once women go through menopause, their risk of dying from heart disease increases threefold (see *Menopause*). And symptoms of a heart attack can vary somewhat between men and women.

Your heart is an amazing organ—a simple pump that can beat around 70 times a minute non-stop for 100 or more years, pumping more than 2.6 million gallons (10 million liters) of blood around your 62,000 miles (100,000km) of blood vessels every year. While our hearts are working properly we tend to take them for granted—yet if more people could think of their heart health from their 30s onward, heart and arterial disease would not be the number one killer in the Western world.

For some people, there is a genetic predisposition toward developing heart disease—but if you eat healthily and change any negative and unhealthy lifestyle patterns practiced by your parents and grandparents, then in most cases you can stack the cards in your favor and add decades to your life. The heart, like any other muscle, needs its own blood supply and receives this via three main vessels called the coronary arteries. Over time, one or more of these arteries can become blocked, and if an artery becomes completely blocked, some of the heart muscle may die during a heart attack.

H

Typically, symptoms of a heart attack include a severe pressing band of pain across the chest that can spread up the neck and into the jaw or across the shoulders and down into the left arm. This is often termed a "myocardial infarction" (MI), which means death of the heart muscle due to an interrupted blood supply. The muscle may simply stop beating or, more commonly, it goes into an irregular pattern, which no longer works like a pump. Sweating, breathlessness, and a feeling of nausea can accompany a heart attack, which needs **urgent** medical attention.

A heart attack can be fatal, unless someone can apply immediate cardio-pulmonary resuscitation. (CPR is something everyone should learn, and one day you might save a life with this simple skill). Luckily, many people survive their first heart attack. Specialists may recommend drugs and/or by-pass surgery or other operative procedures, but it's important to consider that none of these medical or surgical treatments attempts to solve the underlying cause of the problem, only the result of the problem.

While some heart attacks appear to strike out of the blue, there are usually warning signs telling us that something is wrong. Some women (and men) report feeling as though they have indigestion, but in women the pain seems to be centered more in the middle of the chest rather than toward the left side, and discomfort or pain is felt between the shoulder blades. Some people report having spasms that travel up their spine and that the jaw pain on both sides can be severe, while others report a sense of "impending doom." **Please take notice.**

And just because you don't have high cholesterol, don't think, "It can't be a heart attack," as myocardial infarctions can be triggered by long-term stress and inflammation in the body. **Call an ambulance.** Do not think, "I'll see how I feel in the morning." It's better to have a false alarm than to die!

Another common warning of heart problems is angina—a constrictive pain in the chest that is provoked by exertion. It's the body's signal that the blood supply to the heart is inadequate due to narrowing of or spasms in the coronary arteries. If you experience angina, it's time to act. You can still turn it around and live another 40 years or more. Some people have gone on to run a marathon after their first heart attack. If you suffer angina or have had a heart attack, then you need to drastically change your diet, increase exercise (gently), and reduce stress.

Other known risk factors for heart disease include smoking, excessive alcohol consumption, high blood pressure, high homocysteine levels (see *High Blood Pressure*), high LDL cholesterol levels, being overweight, having diabetes, doing insufficient exercise, eating a high-fat, -salt, and -sugar diet, insufficient intake of fresh fruit and vegetables, excessive stress, and inflammation. Stress thickens the blood, which in the long term can kill you. Also, people with "Type-A" personalities, who become angry easily, are more prone to heart disease.

There are also links between heart disease and inflammatory conditions caused by the parasite *Chlamydia pneumoniae* and poor root canal treatments. Mercury is also linked to heart disease, as are unbalanced hormone levels—including thyroid hormones, progesterone, and testosterone. Even the statins now used by 24 million Americans to control their high cholesterol levels place a strain on their muscles, including the heart muscle, as they block production of a vitamin-like substance, CoQ10, which is produced naturally in the liver. This is needed for a healthy heart, but as we age production of this vital heart protecting substance slows, and statins exacerbate the problem further.

Foods to Avoid

- Cut down on the saturated fats found in meats, butter, cheese, cream, and hard margarines. Keep in mind that many low-fat foods are high in sugar, which will convert to fat in the body if not burned off during exercise.
- Reduce the amount of concentrated store-bought fruit juices, soft drinks, desserts, cakes, and pastries you eat.
- Reduce your intake of dairy, especially milk. Research published in *The Lancet* medical journal in 1999 showed how changes in a country's milk-consumption pattern, either up or down, accurately predict changes in coronary deaths 4 to 7 years later.
- Especially avoid any foods and mass-produced oils containing hydrogenated or trans-fats, which are found in most mass-produced cookies, pies, cakes, and so on.
- Don't eat too much fried food, as frying damages fats and turns them into the dangerous fats that heart surgeons find in your arteries.
- Cut down on sodium-based table salts. Use a low-salt alternative or a little magnesium- or potassium-rich sea salt, available from all good health stores and most supermarkets. Try nori flakes or kelp flakes, which are rich in minerals and do not cause the damage that sodium-based salts do.
- Greatly reduce your intake of mass-produced burgers, pies, sausages, pastries, cakes, and desserts.
- Avoid excessive alcohol consumption, even though a moderate intake—that is, 1 glass a day—is slightly protective. Drinking large amounts of alcohol over time is a known risk factor for heart disease. Red wine, such as Pinot Noir, seems to confer the most health benefits, as it's high in polyphenols and bioflavonoids that help protect the arteries. Aim for around no more than 6 drinks a week on average. See *Alcohol*.

Friendly Foods

- Pomegranate has been proven in several trials to disrupt the formation of plaque and has shown some benefit in reducing blood pressure. I eat at least a tablespoon daily. Otherwise, drink the juice daily. Studies done in the US found when patients drank pomegranate juice daily for a year, atherosclerosis was reduced by as much as 25%. The most potent form to take includes pomegranate whole fruit, flower and seed extracts. See www.lef.org for details.
- Oily fish are rich in omega-3 essential fats. Farmed organic salmon, black cod, sardines, pilchards, red snapper, mackerel, trout, and herrings are good sources, as are flax seeds. Try to eat oily fish two or three times a week.
- Generally, eat more fish of any kind in preference to meats.
- Unrefined, unsalted seeds, such as pumpkin, flaxseed, sesame and sunflower seeds, and their unrefined oils, are also good sources of essential fats. Use unrefined organic flaxseed oil for salad dressings, as people who consume more flaxseed oil, which contains omega-3 essential fats, have a lower risk of developing heart disease.
- Lean meats such as venison, boar, buffalo, rabbit, chicken (preferably breast meat with skin removed), and turkey are fine in moderation.
- Avocado oil contains monounsaturated fats and is great for salad dressings, as is walnut oil. Make them organic and always keep cool. Never cook with these oils.
- Eat plenty of fruits and vegetables that are high in carotenes and antioxidants, such as carrots, asparagus, French beans, broccoli, Brussels sprouts, watercress, pumpkin, papaya, cabbage, spinach, sweet potatoes, spring greens, apricots, mangoes, and tomatoes, which help lower your risk of heart disease.

- Include brown rice and pastas, oatmeal, beans, whole-wheat/stone-ground bread and other grains, such as quinoa, amaranth, and barley in your diet.
- Eat more garlic and onions, which help thin the blood naturally.
- Fiber derived from fruits and vegetables is very protective, and additional fiber from flax seeds, oat or rice bran, or psyllium husks all help lower your risk.
- Eating pistachios, walnuts, pecan nuts, and macadamia nuts on a regular basis has been shown to help lower LDL cholesterol.
- Wheat germ and soybeans are rich in natural vitamin E, which has been shown to reduce the risk of heart disease. This is particularly true for people who have stickier blood, such as those with Type A or AB.
- Use non-hydrogenated spreads such as Biona or Olivio. There is nothing wrong with a little butter, as long as you are eating sufficient omega-3 essential fats. Otherwise, try organic raw walnut, hemp seed, or almond butters, which are available from health stores.
- A vegetarian diet that includes a lot of beans, vegetables, grains, and pulses dramatically lowers your risk of developing heart disease.
- Sprinkle 2 teaspoons of soy lecithin granules over breakfast cereals and desserts, which really helps to break down the "bad" LDL fats and, as a bonus, nourishes your brain. **SVHC**
- Olive oil raises HDL (the good cholesterol) levels, lowers bad LDL cholesterol, and contains antioxidants that protect LDL from damage.
- Drink more fluids.

Useful Remedies

- One of the most important nutrients for your heart is Co-enzyme Q10, which is a vitamin-like substance that your body manufactures naturally in the liver. As we age, we make less, and if we take statins, they block production of CoQ10. Therefore, to protect your heart and maintain good energy levels, take 100mg daily with either breakfast or lunch. If you have already had a heart attack, you need 200mg daily in a divided dose.

- Take a multi-nutrient formula to support your heart. Most of the companies featured at the beginning of this book can help you. Otherwise try Solgar's Cardiovascular Support. **SVHC**
- There are several formulas that contain pure cocoa, concentrated pomegranate, and either blueberry extract or super oxide dismutase, an enzyme known to defend the body against oxidative stress. The Life Extension Foundation makes a good one called Endothelial Defense. Take as directed. **LEF**
- Otherwise take a pomegranate concentrate formula. **VC**
- Take a garlic capsule such as Allimax daily, which helps thin the blood naturally.
- After the age of 50, unless you have a medical condition that requires iron, do not take extra iron supplements as excessive iron in the body is linked to heart disease. This applies more to men than to women.
- Vitamin C and the amino acid lysine can help reverse arterial blockages. You need approximately 3g of each per day. Take the vitamin C with meals and the lysine 30 minutes before meals. **VC**
- Take a high-strength B complex or homocysteine formula such as the ones from NSI, Kal, Country Life, and Source Naturals. You may not need this if you are on a high-strength multi that contains a full spectrum of B vitamins; it depends how high your homocysteine level is. **VC, VS**
- Include a good-quality multi-vitamin/mineral for your age and gender that contains at least 400IU of natural-source vitamin E, 150mcg of selenium, 30mg of zinc, 100mcg of chromium, and 400mg of magnesium. Almost all the vitamin companies listed on pages 15–16 supply such formulae.

- Try taking the herbs hawthorn (100–500mg of standardized extract) and ginkgo biloba (60–120mg of standardized extract) daily, as tea, tincture, or capsules. Both are known to improve circulation. Nature's Answer makes a formula called CardioNutriv containing hawthorn, motherwort, linden flower, and cayenne fruit to help balance the heart and circulation. **VC NB: Always tell your doctor if you decide to take hawthorn, because it can lower blood pressure.**
- Several studies have demonstrated that a lack of vitamin K2 *accelerates* arterial calcification, whereas taking K2 daily (approximately 100mcg) can help keep excess calcium in the bones and out of your arteries. **NB: People on Warfarin should not take vitamin K without a doctor's advice.**
- Carnitine is an amino acid that helps remove fat deposited in the arteries. Take 500mg three times daily, at least 30 minutes or so before food.
- Research from the University of Colorado has demonstrated a link between low vitamin D levels and an increased risk of heart disease, even in younger people. As low vitamin D levels are associated with numerous problems, from cancers and high blood pressure to osteoporosis and depression, most nutritional physicians now state that everyone should take 1000IU daily and make the effort to expose their skin to sensible amounts of sunshine.
- Take 2g of omega-3 fish oils daily.

Helpful Hints

- People who are generally happy, positive, and enthusiastic are less likely to develop heart disease than their unhappy counterparts.
- Make sure you get a good night's sleep, as research has shown that women who are chronically short of sleep are more at risk of heart problems.
- If you are overweight, lose weight. (See *Weight Problems*.)
- Gentlemen, unless you are very tall, a good rule is to not let your waist exceed 39in; for ladies, the figure is 35in, if you want to avoid heart problems.

- Learn to test your heart health. What's your resting pulse? For 1 minute place your first two fingers on the vein crossing the bony protuberance on the thumb side of your inner wrist and check your pulse. While your blood pressure tells you about the health of your arteries, your pulse is a measure of your heart health. If your heart is strong and able to pump blood easily around the body, it will pump slowly and rhythmically, around 60–70 beats per minute. If it's weak, and therefore can't pump as much blood as it should with each beat, it will have to beat more often to keep your cells properly oxygenated, so your pulse will be higher. This is why your pulse goes up when you exercise—your cells need more oxygen, so the heart pumps more rapidly. In time, this strengthens the heart, and it will be able to pump more blood with each beat, so your resting pulse will slow down. A raised pulse is now considered a "normal" result of aging, although there is no reason you can't have a pulse of 70 when you're over 70.
- Under medical guidance, try chelation, an intravenous therapy that has saved thousands of people from undergoing major heart surgery. It helps to clear clogged arteries, which reduces the likelihood of strokes and heart disease. There are naturopathic clinics around the country that offer this procedure.
- Reduce stress in your life, because stress is now proven to increase coronary arterial disease. (See *Stress*.)
- There is now an easy test to discover your plasma homocysteine levels. Made by YorkTest Laboratories and backed by the British Cardiac Patients Association, it's a simple pinprick method that can be done through the mail. For details call visit www.yorktest.com

- Get some exercise. If you have a heart condition then, with your doctor's permission, start walking for 30 minutes every day and gradually build up to an hour a day. Join a gym and go regularly. If you don't have access to a gym, walking, swimming, jogging, or cycling along quiet roads or nature trails are good alternatives. A little exercise every day is far more effective than a lot of exercise once a week. Even though exercise raises your heart rate while you're doing it, the overall effect is to strengthen the heart and slow your resting heart rate. Research has shown that even moderate exercise after having a heart attack is a very effective way of preventing a second one. If you have had any heart problems, undertake an exercise program only under professional supervision.
- Stop smoking and avoid places where you will be exposed to second-hand smoke. The chemicals in cigarette smoke damage your arteries, oxidize the cholesterol that forms plaque in your arteries, and increase the likelihood of clotting.
- Reduce your exposure to toxic metals such as lead, cadmium, and mercury. Eat more cilantro, which helps eliminate toxic metals from the body – as does chelation (see above).
- People who are angry and argumentative suffer more heart problems. Millions of people are dying because they don't get things off their chest. Learn to deal with anger and internal emotions. See a counselor; your life may depend on it.
- Contact the American Heart Association, 7272 Greenville Ave., Dallas, TX 75231. Tel: 1-800-242-8721 (English), 1-888-474-8483 (Spanish). Website: www.heart.org
- Read Patrick Holford's *Say No to Heart Disease* (Piatkus), which is an excellent book that explains the causes of arterial damage and what you can do to prevent or correct high blood pressure and heart disease.
- Another good book is *Put Your Heart in Your Mouth* by Natasha Cambell-McBride.
- See *High Blood Pressure* for more information about protecting your entire cardiovascular system.

HEMORRHOIDS   *(see Constipation and Piles)*

HEPATITIS A, B, and C *(see also Liver Problems)*

Hepatitis A

Hepatitis A is the most common of the seven known types of hepatitis and is caused by a virus that triggers inflammation of the liver. It is 100 times more infectious than HIV. The hepatitis A virus is found in the feces of someone who is infected and can easily be passed from one person to another with poor personal hygiene if even a fraction of feces residue gets into another person's mouth. Hepatitis A is common in countries where sanitation and proper sewage is poor. You can become infected by eating foods that have been washed in contaminated water or drinking contaminated water. It can also be passed on sexually, but washing the genital area and using condoms can help prevent transmission.

Symptoms may include flu-like symptoms, nausea, vomiting or diarrhea, loss of appetite, weight loss, yellowing of the skin and of the whites of the eyes, and abdominal pain. Symptoms are not always present when a person is infected, but the virus is still active and can still be passed on. If you suspect that you have hepatitis, it is important that you visit your doctor or local sexual health clinic, where a simple blood test can confirm the presence of hepatitis.

If you are run down before the onset of the virus, you may feel fatigued for some months afterward. There is no standard medical treatment for hepatitis A, but once the virus is cleared from the body you are immune from repeated attacks for life. Hepatitis A immunization offers effective protection against the virus and is worth considering, especially if you are going to travel out of the country or are living with someone who is infected.

Foods to Avoid

- Do not drink any water if you have any doubts about its purity, especially in places such as and the Far East.
- When you go abroad, avoid eating salads that have been washed in local water. (See *Food Poisoning*.)
- Avoid raw or partially cooked shellfish.
- Stay away from **all** alcohol, as this adds to liver damage.
- Avoid foods that are full of saturated animal fats, as well as red meat and dairy products (cheese, cream, butter, and milk), as these add an additional burden on the liver. Also avoid deep-fried foods, such as French fries, fried chicken, fried breakfasts, and potato chips.
- Simple carbohydrates such as white rice, pasta, bread, cakes, and pastries give the liver extra work to do, so keep them to a minimum.
- Caffeine, from tea, coffee, cola-type energy drinks, and some painkillers, adds to the overall load of the liver, so they are best avoided.
- Try not to consume excessive amounts of preserved meats such as pizza meats, jerky, salami, provolone, sausages, hot dogs, or hamburger meats, as these are often high in unfriendly bacteria, which the liver has to clear from the body.
- Toxicity is linked to aspartame so avoid artificial sweeteners; look out for aspartame that is hidden in hundreds of foods, drinks, and chewing gums.
- A high-potassium, low-sodium diet is known to have a positive effect on the liver. Avoid salt and salty foods, such as potato chips, sauces, TV dinners, pretzels, and other savory snacks, to reduce your salt intake. Increase your consumption of fresh fruits and vegetables to increase your potassium intake.

Friendly Foods

- Eat more organic food, as non-organic food often contains antibiotic, steroid, hormone, and pesticide residues, all of which place a strain on the liver.
- Include salads in your diet—made with fresh raw vegetables such as tomatoes, shallots, sliced red onion, cucumbers, broccoli, lettuce, endives, radicchio, celery, red radish, avocado, shredded cabbage, carrots, beets, grated horseradish, ginger, and so on. You can use a dressing of cold-pressed oil, apple cider vinegar and/or lemon and lime juice. Try to have a salad 4 to 5 times a week, or ideally every day.
- Drink several cups of antioxidant-rich green tea daily. Green and white teas are also rich in polyphenols, which have strong anti-viral properties.
- Make yourself raw vegetable and fruit juices regularly. Ideally, you should do this every day; however, even if you make raw juices only two to three times a week, you will see tremendous benefits. A basic juice to improve liver function can be made with equal parts of apple, carrot and/or beets, as well as cabbage of different colors; one week use a purple–red cabbage and the next week, a green cabbage.
- Flaxseed oil is essential for improving liver function. It is beneficial for damaged liver cells and reduces inflammation. Use instead of butter on baked potatoes and for salad dressings.
- Sprinkle a tablespoon of non-GM lecithin granules over cereals, fruit salads, oatmeal, etc., which helps the liver metabolize fats and lowers LDL cholesterol. It also nourishes the brain. **SVHC**
- Wholegrain foods such as brown rice, millet, brown pasta, and rye contain a lot of B vitamins that are needed for the liver to work effectively.
- Sulfur-rich foods, including onions, garlic, and leeks, enhance liver function, so try to eat a little of one of these daily.
- Globe artichoke, celeriac, kale, and beets are all great liver foods.

Useful Remedies

- Flaxseed oil is a good source of omega-3 and -6 essential fats, which help repair damaged liver cell membranes and reduce inflammation. This helps cell walls become more resistant to infection. Use with olive oil in salad dressings or take flaxseed oil capsules (one capsule, three times per day with meals). **VC**
- Otherwise, take 1–3g of pure omega-3 fish oils daily.
- Licorice is known for its anti-viral and immune-enhancing actions, as well as for being beneficial to the liver. Take 1–2g of powdered whole root once a day or 250mg of solid root extract once a day. If you are taking licorice for long periods of time, increase the amount of fresh fruit and vegetables you are eating to address your potassium balance, which can be upset by licorice. **VC**
- Milk thistle extract is highly protective for the liver as it boosts levels of glutathione, a very important amino acid for liver function, which is often low in hepatitis patients. In all cases of hepatitis, take 500mg three times daily.
- Methionine is an amino acid that hugely supports liver function. Take 500mg three times per day, 30 minutes before meals.
- Take selenium (200–500mcg per day), as selenium is strongly anti-viral. Do not take more than 500mcg daily for more than a month; then reduce to 200mcg.
- Taking a high-strength B vitamin complex will improve clearance of toxins from the liver.
- Vitamin C has strong anti-viral properties. Take to bowel tolerance levels (5–10g per day). Any vitamin C (ascorbate) powder can be added to a bottle of water and drunk throughout the day. **VC**
- Lipoic acid, a major antioxidant, helps protect the liver from oxidative damage. Take 200mg daily.

Helpful Hints

■ Avoid using chemical cleaning products in your home, as it's the liver's job to break these down. Instead, opt for natural products. Look out for the Ecover range, which is available in most supermarkets.

■ People who travel to areas such as Asia, Africa, India, Haiti, Eastern Europe, and Central and South America are at high risk. While traveling, drink only boiled or bottled water, avoid eating all raw fish and shellfish, and use disinfectant soaps for your hands. (For more help see *Food Poisoning*.)

■ If you have hepatitis A, get plenty of rest and above all practice good hygiene.

■ Cigarettes weaken your immune system, compromising its ability to fight the virus; do your best to give it up. (See *Smoking*.)

Hepatitis B (Hep B)

The hepatitis B virus (HBV) is very common worldwide, and more than 350 million people are infected. The virus can survive on dry surfaces for up to 7 days, making it one of the most communicable diseases and the ninth most common cause of death worldwide. Ninety percent of sufferers recover but 10% are chronically infected, meaning they could develop liver damage, which can be fatal. This virus can be spread via blood or other bodily fluids. The most common routes of infection are via unprotected penetrative sex—especially if blood is produced—or by sharing contaminated needles during drug use. Hepatitis B is also contracted by blood transfusions and the use of non-sterile needles, which may be used in hospitals in certain developing countries. (All blood used in the US is tested for hepatitis B.) Non-sterile equipment used for tattooing, acupuncture, or body piercing is also a risk. It can also be passed from an infected mother to her unborn child, usually during delivery. Hepatitis B cannot be spread via sneezing, coughing, or coming into contact with feces of an infected person. Symptoms are the same as those of hepatitis A (see above) and may need hospital treatment. As vaccination is 95% effective, it's worth considering if you are traveling abroad or living with an infected person.

Foods to Avoid

■ See dietary advice for *Hepatitis A*.

Friendly foods

■ See dietary advice for *Hepatitis A*.

Useful Remedies

■ Selenium reduces hepatitis B infection by 77%, as well as helping prevent liver cancer, a secondary complication common in chronic hepatitis B sufferers. Take 200–500mcg daily. Do not take more than 500mcg daily for more than one month; then reduce to 200mcg daily.

■ See *Useful Remedies* for *Hepatitis A*.

Helpful Hints

■ If you are planning to travel outside the US to developing countries, it is possible to get a small first-aid kit that contains sterile needles to prevent infection. Sterile first aid kits are available online, as well as at most outdoors stores or pharmacies.

■ See also *Helpful Hints* for *Hepatitis C*.

Hepatitis C (Hep C)

Hepatitis C is a cancer-causing, infectious, blood-borne virus that often goes undiagnosed. As many as 3 to 5 million people may be infected in the US alone.

It can take from 15–150 days or more to develop, and around 8 out of 10 people are unaware that they have it. Unlike hepatitis A and B, there is no vaccine for hepatitis C. Infection occurs from blood transfusions, needle-sharing (including acupuncture, piercing, and tattooing), sharing of bills used to snort cocaine, working in a medical environment, and sexual contact—especially if a woman is having her period or genital sores are present and bleeding. Hepatitis C is usually passed from the male to the female if internal tissue is damaged. On very rare occasions it can be passed from an infected mother to her baby, mainly during delivery. If you have ever received a blood transfusion in a country where blood is not tested for the hepatitis C virus (many developing countries), or if you received a transfusion in the US before 1990 (all blood for transfusion in the US is now tested), or if you have received medical or dental treatment abroad where equipment may not have been sterilized properly, you may want to have a blood test. As with all types of hepatitis, symptoms may not occur but the virus can still be passed on. Evidence suggests that about 20% of individuals who have hepatitis C appear to clear the virus from the blood, while about 80% will remain infected and can pass on the virus to others. If a person continues to be infected over a number of years, he or she may develop chronic hepatitis, liver cirrhosis, or liver cancer. The hepatitis C virus is not spread by sneezing, hugging, coughing, food or water, sharing eating utensils or drinking glasses, or casual contact.

A simple blood test can detect hepatitis C.

Foods to Avoid
- See dietary advice for *Hepatitis A*.

Friendly Foods
- See dietary advice for *Hepatitis A*.
- Drink plenty of water; try to drink 8 full glasses a day. If you vomit a lot, you should drink more clear liquids.
- Include salads in your diet. Make them with fresh raw vegetables such as tomatoes, shallots, sliced red onion, cucumbers, broccoli, lettuce, endives, radicchio, celery, red radish, avocado, shredded cabbage, carrots, beets, grated horseradish, ginger, and so on. You can use a dressing of cold-pressed oil, apple cider vinegar and/or lemon and lime juice. Try to have a salad 4 or 5 times a week, or ideally every day.

Useful Remedies
- Keep iron levels to a minimum and do not take an iron supplement. Approximately 30% of hepatitis C sufferers have high iron levels due to the massive amounts of oxidative stress in their livers. Ask your doctor to investigate this possibility. Alpha-lipoic acid, a potent antioxidant, reduces oxidative stress by raising levels of glutathione in the liver. Take 200mg twice daily.
- Take four green tea extract capsules daily with food, which will help block iron absorption. **VC**
- See also *Useful Remedies* for *Hepatitis A*.

Helpful Hints
- Blood spills should be wiped up with bleach, and all cuts and wounds should be covered with adhesive dressings. Bloodstained tissues, sanitary napkins, and so on must be disposed of safely.
- Tell your healthcare provider and dentist that you have the virus to avoid infecting them.

- Do not share toothbrushes, razors, nail files, nail clippers, scissors, or any object that may come into contact with your blood.
- Do not share food that has been in your mouth and do not pre-chew food for babies.
- Tell sexual partners you have the virus, and advise them to see their doctor. In the meantime, use a condom.
- For more help call the Hepatitis C Association on their toll-free support line: 1-866-437-4377.
- An informative Hepatitis C website can be found at www.hepatitis-central.com
- To find details about your local STD clinic, go to www.hivtest.org (a service of the CDC).
- See also *Helpful Hints* for *Hepatitis A*.

HERPES

(see also Cold Sores)

There are two types of herpes simplex virus: Type 1 (HSV-1), which causes cold sores, and Type 2 (HSV-2), which is sexually transmitted and is the most common. HSV-2 can cause extreme pain and swelling of the genital area and is sometimes accompanied by fever. You never eradicate the virus once you have it, but you can keep attacks under control by using supplements and eating a healthier diet.

There can be a stigma associated with herpes, suggesting that the person must be promiscuous, but nothing could be further from the truth! It is very common, and millions of people in the Western world suffer from it. The virus needs only a depressed immune system to take hold and can spread most easily through sexual contact.

Lack of sleep, poor nutrition, too much alcohol and cigarettes, as well as allergies to certain foods, will all encourage the virus to multiply. In addition, sunburn, over-exercising, or excessive sexual activity can also lead to a recurrence.

Those with sensitive nervous systems, and who are prone to anxiety or depression, are more vulnerable to recurrence. The virus will lie dormant and resides in a nerve center or ganglia. When activated, the virus moves down the nerve and can show up anywhere in the genital area (depending on which nerves are involved), as well as the buttocks, back, or legs. Vegetarians may be more prone to attacks because they do not eat enough foods rich in the amino acid lysine, which helps starve the virus.

Foods to Avoid
- Avoid alcohol, especially fortified wines such as sherry and port, as well as wine and beer.
- Caffeine and smoking should also be curtailed.
- During an attack, avoid all foods high in arginine, which feed the virus. This includes chocolate, nuts (especially peanuts, almonds, cashews, and walnuts), seeds (especially sunflower and sesame), coconut, and grains such as wheat and oats.
- Avoid all foods high in sugar and pre-packaged junk foods, as they will greatly deplete your immune function.

Friendly Foods
- Foods high in lysine will help suppress arginine, which tends to feed the virus. So eat more fish (especially halibut), milk, eggs, chicken, turkey, lamb, and potatoes,.
- Vegetarians should eat more corn and soy-based foods, which also contain good amounts of lysine.
- Make sure your diet is rich in all fruits, vegetables, eggs, brown rice and breads.
- Eat more garlic and onions, as they are highly anti-viral.

Useful Remedies

- Take 1g of vitamin C for prevention and between 2 and 3g daily with meals during an attack.
- The amino acid lysine inhibits replication of the virus. If you suffer from attacks regularly, take 500–1000mg daily as a preventative measure and up to 3g daily 30 minutes before food while suffering an attack.
- Beta Glucans 1–3, 1–6, which are derived from yeast cell walls, are proven to strengthen the body's innate immune system (the immune system you were born with). Nutritionist Gareth Zeal says, "Within two days of taking Beta Glucans, which are highly anti-viral, most patients say that genital pain is hugely reduced." This supplement can also be taken by children with cold sores. Take 250–500mg daily. **VC**
- Propolis cream is highly anti-viral. Use daily on affected areas.
- Olive leaf extract acts like a natural antibiotic and boosts immune function. Take 2–3 capsules daily.
- Take a daily multi-vitamin/mineral that contains around 30mg of zinc.
- Lemon balm (*Melissa officinalis*) helps stop the spread of the virus and speeds up the healing process. Available in capsules and liquid drops. You can also dilute the liquid drops and gently bathe the affected areas. **VC**

Helpful Hints

- Avoiding sexual intercourse when you have an attack of HSV-2 is very important, as the virus is extremely contagious. If you must have sex, then use a condom, but you may well find it is too painful and need to wait until the sores have either healed or completely disappeared.
- Avoid oral sex when you have an attack of HSV-1 or -2. Remember that oral sex is one way of transferring a cold sore and turning it into genital herpes.
- For further help contact the American Social Health Association's STI Resource Center Hotline at 1-919-361-8488 or visit www.ashastd.org

HIATUS HERNIA

(see also Acid–Alkaline Balance, Indigestion, and Low Stomach Acid)

The gullet, or esophagus, takes food from the mouth to the stomach and passes through a sheet of muscle called the diaphragm. A hiatus hernia occurs when a part of the stomach pushes up through the diaphragm and allows acid to escape into the gullet, causing heartburn, reflux of food, and indigestion, especially when lying down. It can also cause a fair amount of chest pain, which obviously needs looking at quickly by a doctor. Most hiatus hernias can easily be seen on an x-ray. Being overweight is a common factor for hiatus hernia. Believe it or not, too much exercise—especially jogging or weight lifting to excess—can trigger this problem on occasion.

Sometimes people think that they have excess stomach acid because they are experiencing acid reflux, but low stomach acid is far more likely to be the problem. (See *Low Stomach Acid*.) But if you suffer from indigestion-type pain after eating for several weeks and find that you wake up at night with heartburn, then please see a doctor.

Foods to Avoid

- Generally avoid large meals, especially ones containing red meat, fried foods such as French fries, and creamy-type sauces, which can trigger an acid reflux attack. Melted cheese is especially hard to digest, so keep away from pizzas.
- Alcohol, strong tea, coffee, soft drinks, sugar, chocolate, dairy products, and all high-fat

foods can sometimes cause an "acid" rebound reaction, as they are all acid-forming foods within the body.

- Chew food thoroughly and don't drink too much fluid while eating.
- If symptoms are acute, avoid eating for a short time, or, at most, just eat small lightly cooked meals regularly.
- Avoid artificial sweeteners, such as aspartame, and artificial additives, which can aggravate symptoms.
- Chewing gum causes the body to produce stomach acid by making it think that food is on its way. This depletes levels of stomach acid (needed for digestion) when you finally eat a meal.
- Eating pasta with a glass of wine can be a lethal combination for people with this condition.

Friendly Foods
- Aloe vera juice really helps soothe symptoms. Take one capful in a little water 20 minutes before food. If stomach acid has damaged the back of your throat, the aloe will also help soothe this problem.
- Slippery elm and licorice both soothe the esophagus, as well as providing a gentle fiber that can reduce discomfort. Ask at your health store for deglycyrrhized licorice, and chew 20 minutes before each main meal. Licorice works as well as many drugs without causing negative side effects.
- Try decaffeinated beverages, and drink more herbal teas such as chamomile, licorice, and peppermint.
- Try dandelion root coffee.

- Food combining has proved very useful to people who have this condition. The basic rule is to avoid eating proteins, such as meat or fish, with potatoes, pasta, rice, or bread. And when eating potatoes, pasta, rice or bread, do not eat proteins, but eat vegetables and salads instead.
- Generally eat a low-fat diet, but see *Fats You Need To Eat* and *General Health Hints* to ensure that you get all of the essential nutrients you need.
- Steam, boil, poach, stir-fry, roast, or grill your food.
- Eat more wheat germ, soybeans, alfalfa and dark green vegetables (especially cabbage, watercress, and kale), because they are rich in glutamine, which helps heal the gut. Also eat a little avocado, which is rich in vitamin E, to aid soft tissue healing.
- Sprinkle lecithin granules over a low-sugar breakfast cereal daily to help emulsify fats.
- Eat more garlic and fresh root ginger.

Useful Remedies
- Taking two tablets of slippery elm at the end of each meal can help reduce discomfort.
- L-glutamine, found in cabbage, helps heal any ulceration in the gut. Take 1–2g daily before food for 6 weeks. **VC**
- Take a good-quality multi-vitamin/mineral for your age and gender.
- Taking calcium fluoride tissue salts (four a day) will help strengthen the diaphragm.
- Healthy bacteria, known as probiotics, are essential for healthy digestion and gut function. Jarro-Dophilus EPS is a good formula. Take one daily with meals for a couple of months. **JF**
- Prebiotics are certain foods that encourage healthy bacteria in the gut to multiply. These are good to use, as levels of good bacteria in hiatus hernia patients are likely to be low. They are also a great way to stay "regular" and thus avoid any discomfort from straining on the toilet. I have found a great prebiotic based on the agave plant called Agave Digestive Immune Support, which I take every morning in my breakfast shake. Or you can dissolve one scoop of this powder in water. It really helps keep you regular! **LEF**

Helpful Hints

- Eat smaller meals, which are easier to digest. Avoid large, rich meals at any time.
- Try to relax as much as possible and avoid lying down immediately after eating.
- Do not smoke near meal times. Smoking and alcohol relax muscles, thus allowing food from the stomach to return more easily up to the esophagus.
- Go for a gentle walk after meals, but do not get involved in heavy exercise.
- Many people report relief from symptoms after seeing a chiropractor. (See *Useful Information*.)

HIGH BLOOD PRESSURE

(see also Atherosclerosis, Circulation, Stress, and Stroke)

High blood pressure makes you more susceptible to heart disease, strokes, and kidney disease. Blood pressure of 140 over 90 or more is classified as high. A normal reading is less than 120/80, but 139/89 or less is considered raised, but acceptable. There is no reason why you shouldn't have a blood pressure of less than 120/80 when you're 80 if you take good care of your arteries.

While your pulse is a measure of your heart health, your blood pressure tells you about the health of your arteries. High blood pressure, also known as hypertension, is often considered a "normal" part of aging, but the fact that something is common doesn't mean it's normal. It's important to remember that high blood pressure is a symptom of a problem, not the problem. The problem is that your arteries are too constricted to properly relax when your heart pumps blood through. As a result, narrower arteries make you age faster because this reduced oxygen supply to tissues makes the heart works harder, which raises your blood pressure even more, exposing arterial walls to even more damage. This triggers further hardening, and the problem gets worse still.

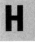

Think of your arteries as being like a complex system of garden hoses leading from a single pump—your heart. Every time your heart beats, it's sending oxygen and nutrient-rich blood around your body via your arteries to nourish each of your trillions of cells. These gushes of blood, which are forced through your arteries with every heartbeat, exert pressure on the walls of your arteries, and this pressure can damage the delicate cells lining your arteries. To reduce the pressure and ensure smooth blood flow rather than blood flow in spurts, the arterial walls are flexible and are surrounded by smooth muscle that is able to expand and contract in response to the pressure being exerted on the arterial walls by the pumped blood. Over time, many peoples' arteries become gradually harder and narrower, a process called arteriosclerosis; if the arteries are thickened with plaque deposits, the condition is called atherosclerosis.

Arteriosclerosis is a major recognized cause of dementia in the elderly. (See *Alzheimer's Disease* and *Atherosclerosis*.) The kidneys, liver, and other organs suffer reduced blood flow, too, so they cannot detoxify the body as effectively. Lumps of thickened matter (called "plaques") build up in the artery wall and reduce the diameter of the vessels that the blood flows through. We now know why this occurs, and it all starts with damage to the arterial wall. This can occur due to abrasion (from high blood pressure), viral or bacterial infection, high homocysteine levels (a toxic amino acid formed as a byproduct of the metabolism of proteins) or free radical damage. Once the damage is done the body tries to repair the area, forming scar tissue, and this is made worse by high levels of low-density lipoprotein (LDL— "bad cholesterol"), which can pass into the walls of the artery where it is oxidized by free radicals into dangerous rancid forms. This in turn is gobbled up by macrophages (part of your immune system), which become engorged "foam cells." The whole area attracts more and more oxidized cholesterol, more immune responses, more inflammation, and inevitably the arteries grow stiffer and narrower.

Homocysteine is now thought to be one of the key agents involved in damaging the arterial walls. This harmful compound is produced in the body but is normally recycled or broken down by vitamins B6, B12, and folic acid—nutrients often deficient in overly refined foods.

Another key cause of raised blood pressure is a lack of the mineral magnesium. Magnesium is needed for muscles to relax after they've contracted (muscle cramps or eye ticks are a symptom of magnesium deficiency), and research has shown that arteries are considerably narrower in those who are deficient in magnesium. In some countries, paramedics inject magnesium directly into the heart of heart-attack victims to relax the muscle and the blocked arteries supplying it. Many heart attacks and strokes are now thought to be due to arterial spasms blocking blood supply to the heart or brain, rather than a clot.

Stress and excessive exercise are known to deplete magnesium, which may be deficient if you don't eat enough dark green leafy vegetables, whole grains, and seeds. This may explain why apparently healthy people sometimes die suddenly from a heart attack or stroke.

A dangerous side effect of arteriosclerosis is an increased risk of developing blood clots. This is especially true for those with A or AB blood types. Turbulence in the blood caused by rough areas in the normally very smooth arterial walls can increase clotting. Also the plaques can break off and travel along the artery until they get stuck in a narrower blood vessel; this is commonly known as "thrombosis." If these clots reach an area sufficiently narrowed by arterial plaques, they can block the vessel completely and starve the tissues "down stream" of blood, oxygen and nutrients. If this happens in the vessels supplying the heart or brain, a heart attack or stroke can occur.

Eighty-five percent of all cases of high blood pressure can be treated without drugs if the person is willing to change their lifestyle and diet. For example, in societies where salt is virtually absent, hypertension is equally absent. Too much caffeine, alcohol, and smoking, when combined with high blood pressure, greatly increases your chances of suffering from heart disease or stroke. Stress is another **major** factor in the development of high blood pressure, because the adrenaline released into the bloodstream during times of stress increases your heart rate, breathing, and blood pressure, but also constricts your arteries.

Foods to Avoid

- Reducing or eliminating wheat grains, cornstarch, and sugars can really help reduce blood pressure. This includes white bread, pasta, cookies, pre-made pies, and so on.
- Avoid all highly refined hydrogenated oils and fats found in mass- produced cooking oils, margarines, cookies, pastries, and cakes.
- One-third to a half of people with high blood pressure benefit from lowering salt intake. Therefore, eliminate sodium-based table salts because sodium causes more water to be retained by the kidneys. More water means more blood volume, and therefore higher blood pressure. There are plenty of magnesium- and potassium-based salts, such as Solo Sea Salt and Himalayan Crystal Salt available from health stores and on the Internet. Use sparingly on the food that's on your plate.
- Reduce stimulants. Blood pressure has been shown to drop as much as 20 points when all caffeine is eliminated, because caffeine ultimately causes arteries to constrict. Some decaffeinated drinks contain formaldehyde, so look for coffee and other decaffeinated drinks that have been decaffeinated using the more natural water method.

- Sugar is also a problem, since sugar converts into fat in the body if it is not used up during exercise. Also be aware that many low-fat foods are high in sugar so you must always check the labels.
- If you have eliminated all of the above and still have a tendency toward high blood pressure, it might be worth consulting a nutritionist who can check for food intolerances, particularly if you are a migraine sufferer. (See *Useful Information*.)

Friendly Foods

- Eat more pomegranate, which helps prevent arteries from becoming clogged in the first place. Also eat plenty of blueberries, blackberries, strawberries, and raspberries, which all help to balance blood pressure.
- Eat green vegetables, fresh fruit, unprocessed and unsalted nuts, fresh fish, and whole grains such as brown rice, breads and pastas, to increase your intake of the B vitamins B6, B12, and folic acid, which are involved in breaking down homocysteine.
- Lima beans, currants, dried figs, apricots, almonds, black treacle, and sunflower seeds are all rich in minerals such as magnesium and potassium.
- Use nori flakes or kelp flakes, which are rich in minerals, as a salt substitute. They are great over fish and in stir fries. Available from most health stores.
- Another useful salt is A. Vogel Herbamare Organic Herb Seasoning Salt. It is made from organic sea salt, dried celery, leeks, cress, parsley, kelp, garlic, and basil and sold online, as well as in health stores and supermarkets.
- Try Solo Sea Salt (www.soloseasaltusa.com) instead of table salt, which is potassium- and not sodium-based. Potassium can help lower blood pressure because it balances sodium.

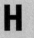

- Two bananas or four sticks of celery a day (rich in potassium) have been shown to help lower blood pressure over time.
- If you are not a fan of eating fresh fruit and vegetables, at least drink a couple of glasses of freshly made fruit or vegetable juice. You will miss out on the fiber, but you will still get much of the nutrient content.
- Try switching to a more vegetarian-based diet, as the more fruit, vegetables, bean,s and lentils you eat, the greater your potassium intake and, generally speaking, the lower your sodium intake. Vegetarians also tend to have much lower blood pressure.
- Chickpeas and soybeans contain isoflavones, which can help reduce LDL.
- Eat more garlic, onions, and broccoli (which are antioxidant, anti-viral and antibacterial) and celery (which is a diuretic).
- Use unrefined organic virgin olive, walnut, pumpkin, flaxseed or sunflower oil for your salad dressings, and eat oily fish three times a week. (See *Fats You Need To Eat*.)
- As high levels of toxic metals, such as lead, can contribute to high blood pressure, buy a good-quality water filter. The fiber in apples (pectin), plus cilantro and seaweed, which are high in chlorophyll, help detoxify metals from the body.
- Natural-source vitamin E helps thin blood naturally; therefore, eat more soybeans, wheat germ, alfalfa sprouts, dark green vegetables, hazelnuts, almonds, and avocados. This is especially important for those with type A or AB blood.
- Add more cayenne paper to your food, or take one capsule three times daily to help lower your blood pressure. Check with your doctor if you are taking drugs such as Warfarin.
- See also *Friendly Foods* under *Constipation*, as constipation can aggravate blood pressure.
- The lycopene in tomatoes and watermelon has been found to slow the accumulation of arterial plaque.
- Try hibiscus tea, which has been shown to lower blood pressure.

Useful Remedies

- If you are taking blood-pressure medication, tell your doctor about any supplements you are taking. In time your prescription drugs may be able to be reduced because these supplements help lower blood pressure naturally, and you don't want your blood pressure to go too low.
- Take 500–1000mg of magnesium with 400mg of calcium daily. Both of these minerals have been shown to lower blood pressure.
- Taking pycnogenol, pine bark extract, regularly has been shown to help patients lower their medication. Take 125mg daily. **VC**
- The spice turmeric contains curcumin, which has highly anti-inflammatory properties. As atherosclerosis is basically inflammation of the arteries, taking this spice daily in a concentrated form with meals can greatly reduce plaque formation. Take around 1g daily in divided doses with food. **LEF**
- Essential fats thin the blood and reduce inflammation in your arterial walls. Take 2g of fish oil daily or 2g of flaxseed oil, both of which contain omega-3 fats. (See *Fats You Need To Eat*.)
- Take 900mg of garlic a day. When used long term, garlic can help gently lower blood pressure and thin the blood.
- Hawthorn, either as tincture or as tablets, is a gentle way to bring blood pressure back down to normal. Take 1–3ml of tincture or 1–2g of the tablets. **NB: You must tell your doctor if you want to try hawthorn, as your blood-pressure medication may need to be reduced.**
- Begin taking 100IU of natural-source, full-spectrum vitamin E and gradually increase to 500IU a day. Vitamin E thins the blood, protecting you from clotting, and also prevents LDL cholesterol from oxidizing.
- Include a high-strength multi-vitamin/mineral in your program, as the B vitamins help support your nerves, controlling muscle contraction and improving your tolerance to stress.
- If your homocysteine level is high, take an extra 10–50mg of vitamin B6, 400–1000mcg of folic acid, and 10mg of B12. To find your plasma homocysteine levels, use a simple pinprick method that can be done through the mail. For more information visit Test Laboratories' website: www.yorktest.com

Helpful Hints

- High blood pressure can occur during pregnancy, in which case seek medical attention.
- Cigarettes, plus the chemicals in cigarette smoke, damage your arteries and make the blood more likely to clot, raising your risk of developing heart disease.
- Reduce stress, which in the long term can kill you. Try to find a method of relaxation that you enjoy whether it's meditation, tai chi, yoga, exercising, walking, or swimming. (See under *Stress* and *Adrenal Exhaustion*.)
- Have regular aromatherapy massages using relaxing essential oils such as rosewood, ylang ylang, clary sage, lavender, and marjoram.
- Get a pet. Researchers from the State University of New York at Buffalo have shown how having a pet can protect against the effects of stress better than drugs designed to lower blood pressure.
- Exercise is vital for reducing blood pressure. With your doctor's permission, start walking briskly for 30 minutes a day. People who are overweight and don't get much exercise are much more likely to suffer from high blood pressure.
- Breathe deeply regularly. This helps re-alkalize the body and helps you stay calm.
- Toxic metals in the body are also linked to high blood pressure. If you have tried all of the dietary guidelines list above without much improvement, have your metal levels checked.

- Have a hair mineral analysis done. This test costs upwards of $100 and determines your level of calcium, magnesium, and other important minerals, as well as identifying any raised levels of heavy metals in your system. ARL Analytical Research Labs in Arizona does this test. www.arltma.com
- Have your doctor obtain an ordinary cardiac risk blood profile. This will check your total cholesterol, HDL (good cholesterol), LDL (bad cholesterol), and triglycerides. There is no doubt that raised triglycerides put you in the high-risk category, although this does not mean that triglycerides are necessarily to blame. If you're prescribed cholesterol-lowering drugs, get a second opinion. (See *Cholesterol*.)
- Have your homocysteine level checked. Because it is not tested routinely, you will need to ask for the test. Your level should be below 8; above 10 is poor; above 12 is definitely not great. Homocysteine levels rise with age and can be controlled by supplementing vitamins B6, B12, and folic acid. If your homocysteine is high, you need higher levels of these vitamins than you can get in your diet alone. There is an easy test to discover your plasma homocysteine levels (see above).
- Many men who suffer arteriosclerosis have low levels of testosterone; therefore, men over the age of 45 should ask their doctor to test their hormone levels.
- Patrick Holford's, *Say No to Heart Disease* (Piatkus) is an excellent book that explains the causes of arterial damage and what you can do to prevent or correct high blood pressure. He has also written *The H Factor*, which gives all of the details of homocysteine. Website: www.patrickholford.com

HIRSUTISM
(see Body Hair, Excessive)

HYPERACTIVITY
(see also Allergies)

Hyperactivity is also often referred to as Attention Deficit Disorder (ADD) or Attention Deficit Hyperactivity Disorder (ADHD), and they are all closely related. These conditions occur predominantly in children, but sometimes symptoms can continue into adulthood. There is no hard-and-fast definition of this disorder, and consequently children who are merely rebellious, find it difficult to pay attention for great lengths of time, or find it difficult to learn may tend to be labeled as having ADD. And children who are constantly fidgeting and are always on the go may well be diagnosed as having ADHD.

Typical symptoms include an inability to concentrate or sit still for any length of time, rapid and severe mood swings, and the need for very little sleep. Children who are affected often find themselves in trouble and are passed from school to school. They can become delinquent teenagers and often end up using drugs and alcohol.

Nutritionist Gareth Zeal says: "In clinical practice, it's been noted that children with eye problems such as short-sightedness, astigmatism or a "lazy eye" are more likely to be genuine ADHD cases. We encourage all pregnant women to take 3–5g of omega-3 fish oils during pregnancy, as they are crucial for healthy brain and eye development."

All of these conditions are associated with an excessive intake of artificial sweeteners, colorings, and preservatives that are found in prescription medicines and thousands of foods and drinks. Sensitivities to various foods also play an enormous role in hyperactive children and adults. Other substances, such as bubble bath, air fresheners, spray deodorants, perfumes, and toothpastes have also been known to trigger these types of behavioral problems. Far too many children still eat huge amounts of junk foods that are devoid of vitamins, minerals, and essential fats. Junk foods deplete nutrients from the body, and tests have shown that these children are malnourished. The lack of proper nutrients can have devastating effects not only on their bodies, but most importantly on their brains. Also, exposure to neurotoxins, such as lead from water pipes and car fumes, plus cadmium from cigarettes, can make the problem even worse, as can over-exposure to these chemicals during pregnancy.

The normal drug therapy is Ritalin, from the amphetamine family, which initiates changes in brain structure and function that remain long after any therapeutic effects have dissipated. Ritalin may also increase the incidence of depression and addiction to other substances such as cocaine and smoking in later life. Understandably, many parents don't feel comfortable giving this drug to their child; however, others feel it is the only way to making their child controllable or easier to teach.

There is a growing body of negative evidence against this drug, and nutritionists such as UK-based Patrick Holford have shown time and again that if artificial additives and foods to which the child is sensitive are removed from the diet, and proper nutrition is practiced, these children improve tremendously. In prisons in the US and the UK, it has also been shown that when violent prisoners are given a healthier diet, plus the right vitamins, minerals, and essentials fats, they become calmer and "kinder" people.

Foods to Avoid

- It is very important to discover which foods and/or substances are triggering the hyperactivity. (See under *Helpful Hints* for York and Genova Tests.)
- Any foods containing large numbers of additives, particularly strong colorings such as tartrazine (FD&C Yellow 5). Candies that are bright and rainbow colored should be completely avoided.
- Greatly reduce or eliminate soft drinks, and any foods or drinks that contain the artificial sweetener aspartame. Look out for hidden sources such as chewing gum.
- Generally cut down on foods containing sugar, such as cakes, cookies, chocolates, and snack bars. One specialist once told me that giving sugar to hyperactive children was "like putting rocket fuel in a Mini." The odd treat is okay, but try to buy organic, low-sugar snack bars that have been sweetened with apple juice or honey. Most of the mass-produced refined foods (white bread, pasta and rice; packaged TV dinners, and so on) should go. As an occasional treat, allow the child to eat a small amount of organic chocolate. Sugar depletes the mineral magnesium needed to stay calm, and B vitamins, which support the nerves and brain function. Sugar also depletes essential fats that are crucial for healthy brain function.
- Citrus fruits and juices are often a problem.
- If your child has a favorite food, be it cheese, eggs, wheat-based foods, cow's milk, or orange juice, try cutting these out for 1–2 weeks and see if behavior improves. It is usually the foods they eat and crave the most that are triggering many of their symptoms.
- Buy a book that gives you all the food dye levels in foods and note which foods have the highest amounts, then avoid them like the plague.

Friendly Foods

- As much as possible feed your child organic foods, free from pesticides and herbicides.
- Try buying corn-, lentil-, rice- and spinach-based pastas.
- Introduce more whole foods and grains, such as brown rice, millet, oats, quinoa, lentils, and vegetables into your child's diet.

- Nature's Path and Barbara's Bakery make healthier breakfast cereals that are sweetened with apple juice. Any health food store sells ranges of wheat-free and/or low-sugar organic cereals, mueslis, and snack bars these days. Add a chopped apple or banana to the cereal for additional fiber and nutrients.
- Use sunflower and pumpkin seeds or flaxseeds, plus nuts such as pecans or hazelnuts, as they are high in essential fats and minerals like zinc, which are also vital for healthy brain function.
- Add pumpkin seeds to a salad. They are delicious and rich in magnesium and zinc.
- Try organic rice, oat, hemp, almond, or goat's milk or yogurt, which are less likely to cause a problem.
- Give your child diluted sugar-free pear, apple, or even grape juice, which are less likely than the citrus fruits to cause problems.
- Encourage the child to drink water instead of soft drinks, and try to encourage fresh fruit rather than sugary sweets.
- Add low-sugar fruit yogurts to colorful fruit for tasty desserts. I make gelatins with a base of low-sugar cranberry or freshly squeezed orange (or mango) juice, chamomile tea, or fresh grapes. I chop fresh fruit into the gelatin liquid and allow it to set for a wonderful low-sugar treat.
- Give your child a serving of quality protein, such as chicken, fresh fish, eggs, tempeh, lentils and beans, nuts and seeds, with each meal of the day.
- Essential fats found in oily fish are really important for controlling this type of behavior. (See *Fats You Need To Eat*.)
- Ensure plenty of iron-rich foods are included in their diet, as a lack of iron can decrease attentiveness and narrow attention span. Good choices are cooked tofu, lean meats, beans and pulses, spinach, eggs (unless your child has an intolerance to eggs), cabbage, prunes, dates, apricots, and pumpkin seeds. Eat them along with some strawberries or papaya, which are rich in vitamin C, to enhance absorption.
- Use unrefined, cold-pressed, preferably organic olive, sunflower, hemp, walnut, or sesame oils for salad dressings, or drizzle over cooked foods. Cook only with olive oil or use coconut oil instead, which is in most supermarkets.
- Make dessert bars using oats, raisins, sunflower and pumpkin seeds, chopped organic apricots or dates with olive or sunflower oil; then add organic agave syrup (which has a lower glycemic index than refined sugar). Or use a little melted butter. Bake weekly and keep in an airtight container.

Useful Remedies
- Magnesium is known as nature's tranquillizer, and many children are low in this vital mineral. Give them 400mg daily. Dr Bernard Rimland, the director of the Autism Research Institute, has found that combining vitamin B6 and magnesium is up to 10 times more effective than Ritalin. 50mg of B6 can be taken in a high-strength B-complex.
- Essential fatty acids are vital. Eskimo makes a flavored omega-3 fish oil supplement, and Barlenes make a lemon version for children. These are available online or at health stores like GNC.
- Give your child a good-quality chewable multi-vitamin/mineral that is free from artificial additives. Solgar's chewable Kangavites are flavored with natural fruit (avoid if citrus is a problem for your child). Nature's Plus also makes a great children's range of nutrients.
SVHC, NP

Helpful Hints
- Try to avoid smoking and drinking during pregnancy, as both have been linked to an increased likelihood of your child becoming hyperactive.

- If the child has allergies or food intolerances, explain to the child how they affect their behavior. Also tell everyone who might be giving the child food or drinks, such as people at their school or relatives, so they know the effects of these foods that they probably think are perfectly harmless.
- For some children natural compounds found in food, called salicylates, can cause problems. (See *Autism*.)
- Homoeopathy has a great track record of dealing with ADD and hyperactivity so, if you can, get your child to see a good homoeopath. Be prepared to be patient, as it may not be an overnight success. (See *Useful Information*.)
- It is really important to avoid exposure to air fresheners **of all types**, spray deodorants, potpourri, perfumed fabric softeners, and laundry detergents. Try Ecover products, which contain far fewer chemicals. They are available in all major supermarkets and health stores.
- As children with ADHD are seven times more likely to have food intolerances than other children, get these checked out. Genova Diagnostics (www.genovadiagnostics.com) has an in-depth food intolerance test, and you can also request that they add food additives to the test. Otherwise you can contact YorkTest Laboratories, who can test for a large range of intolerances via a simple at-home test kit. For details visit www.yorktest.com.
- Links have been found between hyperactivity and high levels of heavy metals, namely mercury, lead, copper, and aluminum. Many vaccines still contain mercury. (See under *Fluoride*.) You can check your child's heavy metal levels with a simple, non-invasive, hair mineral analysis test. For more information, call ARL Analytical Research Labs Inc. on 1-602-995-1580. E-mail: information@arltma.com. Website: www.arltma.com
- Read Patrick Holford's book, *New Optimum Nutrition for the Mind*.
- ADD and ADHD are complex conditions, and because it is important that children do not become deficient in any nutrients, enlist the help of a qualified nutritionist. Contact the National Association of Nutrition Professionals at 1-800-342-8037 or visit their website: http://nanp.org
- A great site for additional resources and support is www.chadd.org CHADD (Children and Adults with Attention Deficit/Hyperactivity Disorder) is a non-profit organization that was founded in 1987 to help parents and their children with ADHD combat the frustration and sense of isolation that often accompanies this disorder.
- For help finding an ADD/ADHD support group, the Attention Deficit Disorder Association has an excellent database on its website: www.add.org

HYPOGLYCEMIA   *(see Low Blood Sugar)*

I

IBS

(see Irritable Bowel Syndrome)

IMMUNE FUNCTION

(see also Adrenal Exhaustion, MRSA, and Stress)

With new strains of bacteria and viruses mutating with alarming speed, the challenge for our immune systems has never been greater. Our immune system is made up of a network of cells, organs, and fluids that help defend us against the millions of bacteria, viruses, and fungi that bombard us in our daily lives. And one of the most important things you can do to stay healthy, throughout your life, is to keep your immune system in good shape. For example, when I was younger I did not realize how diet and lifestyle affected my ability to fight off illnesse—so when I was under pressure, not getting sufficient sleep, and eating the wrong foods, I was always ill. At times when I felt horrible, I would turn to a sugary snack to keep me going, and I could literally feel my immune system going "over the edge." Stress alone can suppress immune function by up to 60% (see also *Adrenal Exhaustion* and *Stress*).

These days I recognize my limits; I know when to stop and get more sleep. I eat a cleaner diet and try as much as possible to keep my stress levels within limits. You need to listen to your body and take notice! Often the first signs of an immune system under threat are a chronic sore throat, regular colds, or niggling infections. If this is the case with you, it's time to take action.

Meanwhile, most people don't think of their skin as being part of the immune system, but it forms a physical barrier against attack. The immune system is in charge of cell regeneration within your skin, so the more efficient your immune system is, the fresher your skin will look.

Then comes your stomach acid, which helps to destroy harmful organisms, but as we age and get stressed, stomach acid levels fall and more bacteria can get through (see *Low Stomach Acid*).

Within a child's bone marrow there are "stem cells" that, as we grow, develop into various types of immune cells, some of which mature in the thymus gland where they become known as T-cells. The spleen also contains immune cells that manufacture antibodies; and the lymphatic system, often called the master drain, is also a major player in immune function. The lymph system removes toxins and microbes from the body's tissue and, along with bone marrow, manufactures lymphocytes (a specific kind of white blood cell that comes in three types—B-cells, T-cells, and natural killer cells—which keep your immune system in good shape). Lymph nodes are found all over the body, but the ones most people are aware of are situated in the neck, groin, and arm pits. During an infection, the lymph glands can swell as they produce more white blood cells; this is very common in throat conditions, for example. If the lymphatic system becomes congested, the fluid thickens and becomes more gel-like, which inhibits proper drainage and detoxification and puts more pressure on the liver and kidneys. This is why a fully functioning lymph system helps you fight off invading bacteria and viruses. The liver and thymus gland also play a huge role in immune function (see *Liver Problems*).

Unfortunately, as we age our immune system becomes less effective at protecting us, and more viruses and bacteria get through our defenses. Conversely, our immune system can also overreact, which produces chronic inflammation when we eat certain foods or are exposed to pollen, pollutants, and so on. In conditions such as lupus and rheumatoid arthritis, the immune system may even begin attacking the body's own tissue; this is called an "autoimmune response."

High cholesterol levels are also linked to a lowered immune response because cells containing high levels of cholesterol can disrupt our cells' ability to communicate with each other, which is vital for proper immune response (see *Cholesterol*).

Lowered immune function is also linked to chronic fatigue, allergies, parasite infections, and some forms of heart disease. Many women also have low iron levels, which can reduce immune function—so have a blood test to check iron levels if you think this may be a problem. Prostaglandins, which are hormone-like substances, become more out of balance as we age. This suppresses the immune system and affects important processes such as body temperature and metabolism. Essential fatty acids, such as EPA (from fish oil) and GLA (from evening primrose, blackcurrant, and borage oils) help restore healthy prostaglandin ratios, thereby supporting the immune system (see *Fats You Need To Eat*).

Foods to Avoid

- As a person with a sweet tooth, I'm sorry to say that refined sugar greatly compromises our immune systems. If you are run-down and then you eat, let's say, one mass-produced sugary breakfast bar, it can literally send your immune system into free-fall. Then the next thing you know, you have a cold or develop cold sores or whatever. So if you know that you are under stress, stay away from products that are high in refined sugars and allow your immune system time to regroup. Use a little organic agave syrup or organic brown rice syrup as healthier alternatives to refined sugar, and generally cut down on pies, cookies, candy, and store-bought sugary snacks and drinks.
- Reduce your intake of caffeine and alcohol, which place an extra burden on the immune system.
- Avoid any foods that contain lots of preservatives, additives, and especially the artificial sweetener aspartame, which places an extra burden on your liver.
- Avoid all smoked foods and cheeses.
- Reduce your intake of saturated fats found in red meat and full-fat dairy products, including milk, cheese, Greek yogurts, and chocolates, as well as hydrogenated and trans-fats. (See *Fats You Need To Eat*.)

Friendly Foods

- When the body is under attack it requires more protein, so eat fresh fish, organic tofu (cooked), fresh chicken, turkey, and lean organic meats. Lentils, beans, and pulses are also excellent sources of low-fat, healthy protein.
- Eat organic as much as possible. Make sure your diet is high in all fresh fruits and vegetables, which are packed with nutrients.
- Eat more fresh fish, broccoli, cabbage, cauliflower, parsley, green beans, apples, green salads, pumpkin, buckwheat, watercress, papaya, mango, quinoa, soybeans, and millet.
- Eat sprouts such as alfalfa, brown rice, and algae such as spirulina and chlorella. Otherwise use Greens Plus, which contains Hawaiian spirulina, chlorella, lecithin, barley, pectin apple fiber, soy and barley sprouts, and lactobacillus acidophilus. This is a great all-around way to ingest good nutrients and healthy bacteria, keep the body more alkaline, and help keep yourself regular. Add a teaspoon of this powder to a breakfast smoothie to boost immune function (recipe under *General Health Hints*). **GP**

- Eat more purple, red, and orange foods. Blueberries, bilberries, and blackberries are high in immune-boosting nutrients, as are sweet potatoes, apricots, pumpkin, papaya, and red peppers.
- Nuts and seeds are packed with essential fats and minerals, such as zinc and selenium. (See *Fats You Need To Eat*.)
- See also *General Health Hints*.
- Eat more freshly made soups. Many supermarkets and restaurants now sell freshly made organic soups. They are easy on the digestive system and full of nutrients. Add barley, brown rice, lentils, and more cabbage to soups.
- Alternatives to refined sugars are organic agave syrup or xylitol (found in fruit fibers), which have a low glycemic index and thus a minimal impact on blood sugar levels. A number of xylitol-based sweeteners are available for purchase on www.amazon.com and from Vitacost (**VC**). Otherwise, try muscovado sugar, a totally unrefined sugar that is rich in minerals. It is available through a number of online retailers, as well as specialist chains like Whole Foods.

Useful Remedies
- Take a good-quality, high-strength multi-vitamin/mineral and an antioxidant formula daily.
- Use organic-source hemp seed protein powder (available from all good health stores) or MuscleMeds Carnivor Beef Protein powder, which is free from lactose but contains plenty of easy-to-absorb protein. **VC**
- Add organic-source green food powders to your breakfast cereals, smoothies, or vegetable juices, and drink daily. They are packed with nutrients that help keep your immune system in good shape. See details of Greens Plus, above.
- Drink more pau d'arco herbal tea, which can boost immune function.
- A combination formula of echinacea and astragalus, which can be taken in capsules or as a fluid extract, really helps boost immune function if taken daily for 3 months. Astragalus has been shown to increase white blood cell counts. Nature's Way has an Echinacea Astralagus capsule formulation. **VC**
- Drink more alkaline water, as the immune system is weakened when the body becomes too acid. (See *Acid–Alkaline Balance*.) Life Ionizers supply alkalizing water filters for your home. Their number is 1-888-688-8889 or visit www.lifeionizers.com
- Colostrum is the pre-milk fluid produced by all mothers after giving birth. It arrives before breast milk and contains 37 natural immune-boosting factors and 8 growth factors, which support the immune system and regeneration of all types of cells. Recent studies have shown it to be extremely beneficial, not only for the newborn, but for people of all ages. Dose: 2000–4000mg per day. Take for one month. **VC** This supplement is great for young children as it boosts immune function and reduces the likelihood of suffering from food intolerances.
- Astragalus is a traditional Chinese herb used to strengthen the immune system. At least one clinical trial in the US has shown astragalus to boost T-cell levels to close to normal in some cancer patients, suggesting the possibility of a synergistic effect of astragalus with chemotherapy. Dose: 250mg twice a day.
- Sunlight and vitamin D are absolutely crucial for good immune health. Get sensible amounts of sunshine, and take 1000IU of vitamin D3 daily.
- Beta Glucans 1–3, 1–6, which are derived from yeast cell walls, are proven to strengthen the body's innate immune system (the immune system you are born with), making it more resistant to pathogens from food and air. Take 250–500mg daily. It can also be taken by children and reduces the likelihood of food intolerances triggered by a weakened immune system. Dr Paul Clayton, based in the US and the UK, is a medical pharmacologist. His website (www.healthdefence.com) contains tons of research into Beta Glucans and is well worth a look. **VC**

Helpful Hints
- One of the simplest ways to boost immune function is to get more sleep and relax more. Take a day off to call your own; take a vacation; walk out in the countryside breathing the fresher air—and see how that alone lifts your spirits.
- Laugh a lot. Watch films that make you laugh and/or make friends with people who make you laugh. Laughter and having some fun strengthen immune function.
- Stress alone can suppress immune function by up to 60%. Stress triggers the release of the hormone cortisol, which is thought to shrink the thymus gland (which is where T-cells mature and is situated in your upper chest area, just below the hollow in your neck). Therefore, keep your stress levels in check. (See also *Adrenal Exhaustion* and *Stress*.)
- Learn to say no and not feel guilty.
- Greatly reduce your exposure to external pollutants, such as cigarette smoke, car exhaust, chemical-based sprays, and heavy metals.
- If possible take regular vacations to someplace sunny, which helps boost your immune system.
- Think positively. People who are cheerful and who look on the bright side have stronger immune systems.
- Exercise regularly but not to excess. Don't over-exercise if you are truly exhausted.
- To help decongest your lymphatic system, apply therapeutic grade essential oils along the spine, under the arm, and in the neck, breast, and groin areas—anywhere that is congested. Try a blend of three drops of cypress, one of orange, and two of grapefruit.
- See *General Health Hints* for more help.

IMPOTENCE

(see also Libido Problems)

There are many reasons why a man may lose either his desire for sex or his ability to get and maintain an erection. Both problems are often linked to long-term stress and, by dealing effectively with stress, sexual desire and function can, in many cases, be restored. The related problem of "brewer's droop" is mainly due to excessive alcohol consumption, which can interfere quite severely with the ability to maintain an erection. Stress and an imbalance of male hormones such as testosterone, DHEA, and cortisol are also linked to this condition. Dr Shamin Daya says: "When men's (and women's) energy levels are compromised, then libido is almost always also affected. Statins and many prescription drugs, including beta blockers, will also affect libido."

Smoking has been linked with reduced ability to maintain an erection; this is because smoking constricts the blood flow that is essential for erectile function. Anyone with erectile problems should also consider a cholesterol-lowering diet.

Foods to Avoid
- See *Circulation* and *Libido Problems*.

Friendly Foods
- See *Circulation* and *Libido Problems*.

Useful Remedies
- Taking the herb ginkgo biloba regularly improves circulation.
- Take 2g of the amino acid L-arginine daily (unless you are suffering from an attack of cold sores at the time, as arginine will make them worse). This amino acid has been shown to improve impotence. Or you could try ArginMax (www.arginmax.com), which contains L-

arginine, ginseng, gingko, vitamins, antioxidants, and minerals that all help to support sexual function.

- Stress reduces B vitamins in the body; therefore, also include a good-quality multi-vitamin/mineral for men that includes a full range of B vitamins.
- Muira Puama, a South-American herb, is considered nature's most potent Viagra. A daily dose of 1g of a standardized extract has been shown to be effective as it raises testosterone levels. In one study of 100 men with impotence problems, 66% had increased frequency of intercourse, while 70% reported intensification of libido. The stability of the erection was restored in 55% of the patients, and 66% reported a reduction in fatigue. The herb is suitable for both men and women. Solaray makes a good one. **VC**
- Pycnogenol, pine bark extract, increases nitrous oxide production, which relaxes blood vessels, thereby increasing blood flow to the sexual organs. Take 100mg daily. **VC**

Helpful Hints

- Have your hormone levels checked by a qualified doctor, as testosterone patches are known to help increase libido in both sexes. Once hormones are balanced, sex drive often returns. (See *Menopause*.)
- Testosterone creams that are applied directly to the genital area are also available. These have been shown to increase libido and erectile function in most patients. For more help, visit www.centreformenshealth.co.uk
- Measures to alleviate stress are often very effective. Exercise regularly and learn to laugh more. This releases natural endorphins, which lowers stress levels and helps you feel more positive. Learn to breathe more deeply.

- People who use a large amount of marijuana or take steroids may also find their erectile function diminished.
- By constantly worrying about your lack of sex drive you often make the situation worse.
- Studies have shown that a lack of vitamins C, E, A, and B, plus the minerals zinc and selenium, can cause a low sperm count and lack of sex drive. Anyone taking regular antidepressants or sleeping pills may be lacking these nutrients. Supplement has been shown to quickly increase libido and erectile function. For more details contact The Male Health Center at 1-972-420-8500 or visit www.malehealthcenter.com
- If the condition continues, or you are worried about infertility as well as impotency, see a doctor who is also a nutritionist. (See *Useful Information*.)
- Acupuncture can help with impotence by unblocking energy channels within the body that help increase blood flow.
- To help get you in the mood, try watching a sexy movie. This works for most people.

INCONTINENCE *(see also Cystitis, Leaky Gut, and Prostate Problems)*

Incontinence can cause urine to leak out when the bladder is put under pressure, such as when you laugh, cough, sneeze, or exert yourself. It can also occur when you have eaten to excess and the bloated bowel starts to puts pressure on the bladder. This type of problem is referred to as stress incontinence and is usually associated with a weakness in the pelvic floor muscles.

Exercise can help keep the pelvic floor strong, but childbirth tends to weaken it, so it is a good idea to do plenty of pelvic exercises after giving birth. I suffered this problem during my twenties after giving birth to my daughter. It became so embarrassing that in my early thirties I found a gynecologist who specialized in bladder repair and had surgery. It has really made a huge difference, and I can now exercise without the embarrassment. Non-chronic but acute urinary incontinence is usually caused by an infection (see also *Candida* and *Cystitis*).

Also if you suffer from a leaky gut, you may also be prone to a leaky bladder. (See under *Leaky Gut.*)

Foods to Avoid
- Any food that you have an allergy or intolerance to can aggravate incontinence. The worst offenders are usually wheat and cow's milk.
- Avoid fluoridated water, toothpastes, and mouthwashes. I have received many letters from people saying that when fluoride is eliminated, the problem stops. It also seems to help with children who wet the bed.
- The biggest culprits are usually yeast, wheat, dairy, alcohol, and sugar.
- Don't overeat because when your bowel becomes full, pressure is exerted on the bladder.
- See also *Stress* because when your adrenals are at their limit you often need to urinate far more often.

Friendly Foods
- Add a little cayenne pepper to your foods. It may initially aggravate the problem but it usually helps in the long term.
- See *General Health Hints* and this section under *Leaky Gut*.

Useful Remedies

- A high-strength, multi-vitamin/mineral for women.
- 500mg of calcium with 250mg of magnesium to help muscle control. After 6 weeks you should see benefits.
- The mineral silica—take 75mg daily.
- The herb horsetail, which contains silica, is very useful for strengthening the bladder. You can take 5ml daily.
- Cantharis is a homeopathic remedy for frequent urination associated with any burning. Causticum and equisetum arvense (horsetail) help reduce symptoms when there is a weakness in the bladder.
- Azo Cranberry contains cranberry concentrate, vitamin C, and acidophilus and helps fight any infection (such as cystitis). Available at most pharmacies and online retailers.

Helpful Hints
- Check with your doctor, who will soon tell you if you have an infection that is causing this problem.
- Women can try using a set of vaginal cones containing weights to help strengthen the muscles. For information on the Aquaflex system, call 1-941-492-4110 or visit www.aquaflexvaginalweights.com
- Also there are progressive resistance exercisers called pelvic exercisers that have proven to be very useful in improving muscle tone, which can help cure or greatly relieve this problem. Available online at Amazon.
- An osteopath or chiropractor can check the alignment of bones in the pubic area. This can help because if the bones are out of balance, urine flow in both men and women can be affected.
- Acupuncture has proven helpful to some people. (See *Useful Information*.)
- Contact the National Association for Continence on 1-800-BLADDER (1-800-251-3337) or visit their website: www.nafc.org

INDIGESTION   *(see also Flatulence, Hiatus Hernia, and Low Stomach Acid)*

Indigestion covers a wide variety of symptoms from cramping in the stomach to heartburn, wind, belching, and even pain in the bowel. It is usually a sign that the digestive system is having difficulty coping with food, and this is frequently due to a lack of stomach acid and digestive enzymes in the small intestine. The problem can be made worse if you eat too quickly and don't chew food thoroughly. Overeating, drinking to excess, eating poor food combinations, or eating when stressed all exacerbate indigestion.

Many people who suffer from chronic indigestion have the bacterium *Helicobacter pylori*. Ask your doctor about a blood, breath, or stool test because it is worth investigating this possibility. If you test positive, you need to remove gluten, cow's milk, and soy milk from your diet.

Severe indigestion-type symptoms in the center of the chest may indicate a heart problem. If you are distressed in any way, call a doctor. Better to be safe than sorry!

Foods to Avoid

- Red meat and fatty cuts of meat are hard to digest, as is cheese (especially melted cheese). Keep these foods to a minimum.
- Chocolate can be hard for some people to digest, and any foods that you are not digesting properly can trigger indigestion and bloating.
- Generally, reduce your intake of sugar and sugary foods, such as cakes, cookies, and rich desserts.
- Coffee, tea, chocolates, caffeine in any form, alcohol, peppers, citrus fruits, onions, and sometimes garlic can be difficult to digest.
- Salt hinders digestion and assimilation of proteins, so cut down on sodium-based salts.
- Don't drink too much liquid with meals as this dilutes stomach acid, which you need for digestion.
- Avoid fruit immediately after a large meal, unless it's a small chunk of pineapple or papaya.
- As much as possible, avoid rich, creamy foods and heavy desserts.
- Avoid antacids that neutralize stomach acid, the very substance you need to digest your meals.
- Many people with indigestion have problems digesting wheat. Try whole grain and low-salt crisp breads, rice cakes or amaranth crackers, which are available from health stores. Especially avoid warm croissant-type treats, as freshly cooked "dough" is really hard on your digestion. I know they are delicious, so if you are desperate, just one a week!

Friendly Foods

- Drink some ginger or dandelion root tea with or before meals to stimulate digestion.
- Small meals made from whole foods and small quantities of meat or fish are much easier to digest.
- Try eating small amounts of pineapple or papaya before a meal. They contain enzymes that can enhance digestion.
- Add more fresh root ginger to foods, as it is very calming.
- If you like beans and pulses but they give you wind, soak them overnight and/or cook them with a strip of kombu seaweed, which helps pre-digest the beans.
- Eat more live, low-fat yogurts.

Useful Remedies

- Take one capsule of betaine hydrochloride (HCl; stomach acid) with main meals. If you have active stomach ulcers, or the HCl causes a burning sensation, take a digestive enzyme that is free from HCl.

- Chew 1–2 tablets of deglychyrrized licorice before a meal. This soothes any symptoms of heartburn or indigestion.
- Acidophilus and bifidus are healthy bacteria that encourage better digestion and elimination. Take 1–2 capsules at the end of a meal.
- Sip peppermint tea after meals.
- Bitters stimulate the production of stomach acid and therefore improve digestion. Dr Theiss Swedish Bitters and A. Vogel (Bioforce) Centaurium tincture work very well when taken before meals.
- If symptoms are at the bowel level, try a good colon cleanser, such as psyllium husks. Lepicol powder or capsules contain both psyllium husks and probiotics.
- Aloe vera is a very good digestive system healer. Take twice a day between meals. To find see a store near you that stocks it, visit www.lakewoodjuices.com.

Helpful Hints
- Digestive enzyme production is greatly inhibited when you are stressed; therefore, your ability to digest and absorb foods is severely impaired. Try not to eat when you are stressed—but if you have to, especially avoid glutens in breads and cereals, plus cheese and rich foods.
- Sit down and eat food in a relaxed setting.
- Go for a walk after eating, which really aids digestion.
- Eat fruit between meals, but avoid fruits you know are a problem such as oranges and grapefruit.

- If symptoms are acute, avoid eating for a short time, or at most, eat only lightly cooked, small meals at regular intervals.
- Sometimes when people suffer from indigestion it is because they are unable to digest some information or something going on in their lives. If this were the case, it would be worth seeing a homoeopath who might be able to resolve the underlying issues. (See also *Stress*.) Meanwhile, the homeopathic remedy Nux Vomica 30c helps reduce the symptoms of indigestion.
- Consult a nutritionist who will help re-balance your system. (See *Useful Information*.)

INFERTILITY

(see also Adrenal Exhaustion, Polycystic Ovarian Syndrome, and Stress)

Sperm counts have dropped dramatically during the last 50 years, and around 25% of couples planning to have a baby will have problems conceiving. In four out of every ten cases the problems are on the male side, with 30% of men being sub-fertile while 2% are totally infertile. If male sperm count is low this can sometimes be a result of an infection such as mumps.

A low sperm count can be due to a poor diet, nutrient deficiencies, and/or environmental toxins, such as lead, mercury, and cadmium. Food additives, smoking, alcohol, food intolerances, urinary tract infections, and stress can all affect fertility. Common organisms such as *Mycoplasma hominis, Ureaplasma, toxoplasma or chlamydia* can infect the urinary tracts of men and women. They don't always cause infertility, but there seems to be a higher number of these organisms in the secretions of couples who have unexplained fertility problems. Smoking and alcohol can also reduce sperm count. Many scientists now openly state that sperm counts in the Western world are dropping because of overuse of herbicides and pesticides, which have an estrogen-boosting effect within the body that counteracts male testosterone.

Female infertility may be due to blockages in the fallopian tubes, which can be triggered by an infection such as thrush or cystitis or by chlamydia and other sexually transmitted diseases. Whatever the cause, diagnosis requires a medical examination.

Sometimes there is a problem with ovulation, usually due to a hormone imbalance. Other conditions, such as endometriosis, polycystic ovarian syndrome (see that section), low thyroid function, a diet deficient in nutrients especially zinc, magnesium and vitamin D, and/or environmental toxins are also common causes of infertility in women.

When women are under a lot of stress the body releases adrenaline, eventually exhausting the endocrine system and affecting hormone levels, which can prevent conception. (See under *Adrenal Exhaustion*.) Candida, a yeast fungal overgrowth, is also linked to infertility.

Foods to Avoid

- Coffee, chocolate, and soda, which all contain caffeine, have been shown to affect impotence and reduce the chance of conception.
- Sugary snacks, deserts, and candy provide empty calories and in turn upset hormone balance. Keep these to an absolute minimum; see below for healthy, fertility-boosting snacks.
- Alcohol alone can reduce your chances of fertility, and the more you both drink, the more your chances of conceiving are reduced. Alcohol affects zinc levels, reduces sperm count, causes malformation of sperm, and impairs sperm motility in men, while preventing implantation in women. The effect is worse when combined with caffeine.
- Avoid foods high in saturated fats, junk foods, pre-packaged meals, sugar, and salt, which deplete the body of the nutrients needed for conception.
- Avoid dairy products from cows, which can lead to malabsorption of essential nutrients if you are intolerant. (See *Allergies*.)
- Wheat is high in phytates, chemicals that block absorption of some minerals. Avoid foods containing wheat as much as possible. This includes, bread, cakes, spelt-based foods, cookies, pasta, and pizza crusts.
- Refined soy products, including soy milk, may well have a negative effect on fertility.
- Avoid food additives, preservatives, and artificial flavorings and sweeteners. Tartrazine (FD&C Yellow F) is known to lower zinc levels, and other additives lower magnesium. The London Food Commission found that of 426 chemicals listed, 35 were found to individually cause reproductive problems ranging from impotency to birth defects. No one knows the real effect of a chemical cocktail on fertility or the fetus.
- Non-organic food is high in pesticides and other hazardous substances that have a hormone-disrupting effect. Offspring in cattle exposed to high levels of pesticides are known to be born with higher levels of malformation.
- When a woman's tissues are more alkaline, this helps with conception since the body functions more efficiently when the pH is alkaline. For full information, see *Acid–Alkaline Balance*.

Friendly Foods

- Good-quality protein is needed for hormone health and sperm synthesis. Choose from lean organic poultry and meat, eggs, fish, and vegetable sources, such as seeds, nuts, and beans.
- Fiber found in whole grains—brown rice, millet, quinoa, barley, and oats—helps reduce excess estrogen levels and eliminate hormone residues.
- Make sperm stronger by eating more brown rice, lentils, beans, organic nuts, and seeds—all rich in fertility-boosting zinc. Enzymes on the sperms' heads need zinc in order to push through the egg to fertilize it. Zinc has a huge impact on women's fertility, too.
- Eat oily fish, such as mackerel, organic-farmed salmon, trout, sardines, pilchards, or herrings, at least once a week as they are rich in omega-3 essential fats needed for hormone health.

- Add some sunflower seeds, pumpkin seeds, and flaxseeds to any low-sugar breakfast cereal, as they are high in minerals and essential fats.
- A lack of selenium in the diet has been shown to reduce egg production in females and leads to stunted testicular growth and problems with sperm maturation in men. Eat more brown rice, seafood, oats, barley, and garlic.
- Nuts, barley, rye, oats, and brown rice are also rich in the mineral manganese, a lack of which leads to defective ovulation and testicular degeneration, as well as affecting libido in men.
- Fresh fruit and vegetables are rich in vitamin C, which helps sperm motility. Choose from papaya, mango, strawberries, broccoli, sweet potatoes, pumpkin, watercress, cabbage, red and yellow peppers, peas, blackcurrants, and oranges.
- Carry a small bag of mixed seeds around for a fertility-boosting snack. These are full of the minerals zinc, manganese, and chromium, as well as essential fats.
- Use organic olive, sunflower, walnut, and flaxseed oils for your salad dressings.
- If you have an iron deficiency, eat more lean meats, especially calves' liver, turkey, and chicken, plus eggs and dried apricots.
- Leafy green vegetables, cereals, honey, beans, and nuts are all good sources of magnesium, which may also be deficient. An alkaline diet is important for conception. (See *Acid–Alkaline Balance*.)
- Try caffeine-free alternatives to coffee and tea, such as dandelion tea or dandelion root coffee, as these can have beneficial effects on the liver and consequently enhance hormone production.

Useful Remedies

- The most important supplements are folic acid (which can prevent spina bifida), vitamins B12, B6, C, and E, zinc, selenium, essential fats, and natural-source carotenes.
- In order to produce testosterone at optimal levels, any multi-vitamin for men needs to contain at least 30mg of zinc, 200mcg of selenium, and 250mg of magnesium.
- Daily Wellness has researched and developed a natural treatment plan for couples to help them take control of their reproductive health. FertilityBlend for women and FertilityBlend for Men contain nutrients and other ingredients that are vital for conception and your baby's healthy development. Tel: 1-866-222-9862. Website: www.fertilityblend.com
- Many companies now make special multi-vitamin/mineral formulas for women who are trying to conceive. Try Fertilizer-Hers by Maximum International or the herbal formula called Christopher's Female Reproductive Formula. **VC**
- New Chapter makes an Organic Perfect Pre-Natal formula balanced with nutrients needed for any woman wanting to become pregnant. **VC**
- Men should also take a multi-vitamin/mineral formula.
- Both partners should take a B-complex plus 3000IU of vitamin A, which are needed for egg and sperm production. Once pregnant, the vitamin A should be reduced to 3000IU daily. **NB: If you are taking a pre-natal multi, then you should not need extra vitamin A or B.**
- Full-spectrum, natural-source vitamin E (200IU a day) has been shown to help reduce both male and female infertility by helping balance hormone levels and enabling egg and sperm to fuse. This should be included in most multi-vitamins for men and women.
- Both partners should take 1–3g of vitamin C daily with meals.
- Essential fats are crucial for healthy hormone function in both partners. Take a 1g omega-3 capsule daily. (See under *Fats You Need To Eat*.)
- 150mg of the celloid mineral complex potassium chloride can help clear the fallopian tubes. Or try the tissue salt Kali Mur. **VC**
- L-arginine and carnitine are two amino acids that are needed for sperm production and to

prevent sperm from becoming too "sticky," which can interfere with conception. You can take 1.5–3g of each daily. Avoid arginine if you have herpes (cold sores) or shingles.

■ Dr Marilyn Glenville also recommends the herb agnus castus, which has been shown to help restore hormone balance in women. It also helps regulate periods and increases the ratio of progesterone to estrogen. **NB: Not to be used by anyone using drugs treatments or IVF to conceive.**

Helpful Hints

■ Anyone wishing to become pregnant should have a full health check-up to make sure that hormone and nutrient levels are all in balance and to rule out conditions such as blocked fallopian tubes, PCOS, endometriosis, thyroid imbalances, and diabetes.

■ For more help read *Natural Solutions to Infertility* (Piatkus) by Dr Marilyn Glenville, one of the leading alternative doctors in this field. For more information on Dr Glenville's work log on to www.marilynglenville.com This site also includes an online personalized supplement assessment with action plans based on your results.

■ Another good book for women struggling with their health and fertility issues is *Women's Encyclopedia of Natural Medicine* by professor of gynecology, Tori Hudson.

■ Anthony Porter, a reflexologist since 1972 who went to China and other parts of the Far East to teach reflexology during the 1980s, found that their methods, combined with his own, gave even better results. He has taught his advanced techniques to thousands of reflexologists internationally and says: "With ART we can not only balance various parts of the body (which is what happens with normal reflexology), but we can also feel more subtle changes within the 7,000 nerve endings or reflex areas of the feet, and after working on them, this has a profound therapeutic effect." Medical research with a leading gynecologist has shown huge success using ART to help women conceive. To find an ART therapist in your area, visit www.artreflex.com

■ Eat organic and get more nutrients, as hormone and antibiotic residues are known to affect fertility in both men and women.

■ Your weight can affect your fertility, so check out your body mass index (BMI)—a measure of your weight in relation to your height. A BMI of 20–25 is ideal. Below 20 is underweight and above 25 is overweight.

■ Hypnotherapy has been proven to be an effective aid in dealing with infertility. Studies have shown that it can also increase conception rates for couples undergoing IVF treatment. (See *Useful Information*.)

■ Regular acupuncture has been proven to be very successful for many couples. (See *Useful Information*.)

■ Cigarette smoke is high in the toxin cadmium. This toxin competes against zinc, which is vital for fertility. This is one of the reasons why smokers are less likely to conceive. Stop smoking, and avoid alcohol.

■ Ask to be screened for any urinary infections and sexually transmitted diseases, many of which lay dormant and are often symptom free. 69% of couples screened have an infection.

■ Much of the water in the US is contaminated with high levels of fluoride, aluminum, copper, and cadmium, which compete with essential minerals in the body. Pesticide residue and traces of the contraceptive pill (which can have hormone-disrupting qualities) are excreted via urine, which eventually find their way into the water system where they can affect fertility. Pure Water Systems offers a broad range of water filters. Call them toll free at 1-866-444-9926 or visit www.purewatersystems.com

■ Limit the amount of chemicals in your home and garden, such as wood preservatives, perfumes, insect sprays, and so on. Use eco-friendly products.

- Avoid too much exposure to cellular phones, computers. and electrical equipment.
- If either partner is taking prescription drugs or regular over-the-counter remedies, check for known side effects.
- Deal with stress, as stress in either partner can lower the chances of conception. I have received letters from many couples who, when they gave up trying so hard to conceive, bought a pet, or adopted a child, found that a baby was on its way!
- See supplements to help reduce stress under *Adrenal Exhaustion*.
- Sitting for long periods raises the temperature in the testicles, which may reduce male fertility. If you are deskbound, for example, or a long-distance driver, wear loose-fitting underwear and trousers, and get plenty of exercise.
- Most hospitals provide or can recommend where to get pre-conception counseling that gives couples information about how to plan for a healthy pregnancy and increase fertility naturally. The service usually includes nutritional advice as well.

INSECT BITES (and repellents)

Apart from the obvious discomfort that they cause, insect bites can occasionally transmit serious disease and cause severe allergic reactions, such as anaphylactic shock. If you know that you or a family member has a particular sensitivity to stings and bites, it is important to discuss this with your doctor to make sure you take the appropriate medication away with you. You may also find the *Allergy* section very useful. People who suffer from anaphylactic shock need to carry adrenaline injections with them at all times.

For anyone traveling to tropical countries where malarial mosquitoes live, take precautions seriously. In Africa a child dies every 30 seconds from malaria. In the Caribbean both my husband and myself have suffered dengue fever from mosquito bites, and I would never want to feel that ill again. The key, as always, lies in prevention.

If you are unfortunate enough to be attacked by a swarm of bees, immediately close your eyes and mouth and wait for help. If you happen to be near water and can swim, then jump in.

Foods to Avoid
- Sugar makes your blood taste sweeter, especially to mosquitoes. If you are visiting the tropics, greatly reduce refined sugar at least a week before you travel. Otherwise use small amounts of organic agave syrup or xylitol (found in plant fibers), which have a lower glycemic index.

Friendly Foods
- Eating garlic on a regular basis may make you smell less appetizing to stinging insects. You could also take a one-a-day garlic tablet, such as Allimax.
- Malaria-carrying mosquitoes are attracted to the smell of human feet. Limburger cheese or other strong cheeses smell just like your feet so by putting a bit of the cheese in your room at least 5ft (2.5m) away from you, you can distract the mosquitoes.

Useful Remedies
- Take 300mg of thiamine (B1) and 50mg of zinc per day. When these are excreted in our sweat, they give off an odor that repels insects. As all of the B vitamins work together, also take a B-complex.
- Brewer's yeast, either as tablets or powder, is a rich source of vitamin B1, which changes the smell of your sweat, making you less attractive to insects. Take 6–8 tablets daily for a week

prior to travel and during your stay. However, if you are suffering from candida, don't take this supplement.

- Some people have found that taking feverfew, the herb that contains pyrethrum (an effective insecticide), really helps. The herb catnip also repels mosquitoes.
- Use Bug-Ban by NOW Foods. Apply the non-sticky cream liberally as needed. **NOW**
- Quantum Buzz Away is DEET-free and made from a combination of essential oils, such as cedarwood, eucalyptus, lemongrass, and peppermint. Website: www.quantumhealth.com
- Try a calendula, arnica, and echinacea spray to reduce the inflammation and itching associated with bites. A good one is Biofreeze Pain Relieving Spray with Ilex; available online from Amazon.

Helpful Hints

- Use lemongrass or citronella candles at dusk to repel insects.
- Try an essential oil preparation for repelling insects. Mix 10 drops of lavender oil, 10 drops of orange oil, 5 drops of eucalyptus, 5 drops of citronella, and 10 drops of neem oil into a base of 50ml apricot or almond oil. Apply sparingly on exposed areas of skin, especially ankles and wrists. Most good health food stores will carry these oils. If you do not have the time to do all this, the Herbal Armor range of products contains a combination of five natural essential oils that are recognized by the EPA as insect repellents. Call 1-800-246-7328 or go online to www.allterrainco.com
- Try adding some essential oils to an unscented body lotion, such as the herbs melissa, geranium, lavender and other essential oils that have been proven to help repel insects.
- Avoid wearing any perfumed toiletries at night and wear cotton pajamas that cover the arms and wrists.
- Use a mosquito net. In Africa, studies with children showed that the incidence of malaria was cut by 80% when nets were used at night. These are easy to buy at travel stores.
- Homeopathy World (www.homeopathyworld.com) offers a general travel kit, which includes items for bites and stings, food poisoning, sunstroke, as well as malaria. Another useful homeopathic remedy for bites is Caladium, which changes the smell of your sweat, making you less attractive to insects.

INSOMNIA

(see also Adrenal Exhaustion and Stress)

If there is truly one subject I could fill a book on, it's this. I have suffered from chronic insomnia for almost 30 years, and I really do know what it's like not to be able to get to sleep because your mind is racing, and then when you do drop off, to be wide awake again at 3 or 4am. Thanks mainly to our modern way of life—open-all-hours, stress and anxiety—one in every four people experiences problems with irregular sleep. In order to go to sleep, you need to switch your brain from its normal busy, or beta-brainwave, state to a more relaxed alpha state. The best way to achieve this is by regular meditation, self-hypnosis, or relaxation tapes.

No one functions well when they are short of sleep, as it not only compromises your immune system but also can severely affect your day-to-day performance. Studies have shown that, when it comes to driving, lack of sleep can have almost as drastic an effect as drinking alcohol. Lack of sleep has also been shown to increase inflammation in the body.

Many people, including myself, when absolutely desperate, resort to prescription sleeping pills. The problem then can become chronic and addictive. This is why it's best to use sleeping pills only on the odd or occasional night, as a precaution, to stop the body and brain from becoming overtired, which often makes it even harder to get to sleep. In the long term, pre-scription sleeping pills can affect your memory and upset delicate brain chemistry. It's worth noting that if you tend to wake up regularly between 3 and 5am you are likely suffering from adrenal exhaustion. (See under *Adrenal Exhaustion*.) If you regularly wake up between 1 and 3 a.m., then it's likely that your liver is struggling. In this case you need to cut down on fats, coffee, and alcohol, and eat lightly for a few days. (See also *Liver Problems*.)

People who suffer from muscle twitching or restless legs also tend to suffer from sleep deprivation. (See *Restless Legs*.) There can be many explanations for not getting enough sleep, such as noise or bladder problems, but if you can get to the root cause of the problem and deal with it, this often helps you let go of the fear of not sleeping.

Foods to Avoid

■ Avoid eating large meals late at night, as this promotes a high insulin release that could, later in the night, lead to low blood sugar. When this happens, adrenaline is released into the bloodstream to compensate for the low blood sugar, which usually wakes us up and leaves us unable to go back to sleep.

■ Don't go to bed hungry, either, as this will affect your ability to fall asleep. See below.

■ Caffeine is one of the most important substances to avoid after around 5pm. Having said that, I have friends who can drink espresso and sleep like a log. I'm not one of them; if I drink filter coffee after 4pm I can be awake until the early hours. Remember that caffeine is not just found in tea and coffee, it's also in soda, chocolate, caffeine energy-type drinks, cocoa, and some over-the-counter cold remedies.

■ If you drink a fair amount of alcohol you tend to feel sleepy—but unfortunately, because of the way it is metabolized in the body, you might sleep for 2–3 hours and then wake up again and find it very difficult to get back to sleep.

■ Food intolerances can make the problem considerably worse. In one study cow's milk appeared to be the problem, but it can be any food that you have a sensitivity to. Keep a food diary. (See under *Allergies*.)

■ Avoid red meat and too much protein in the evenings, which tend to wake up the brain. Eat protein for breakfast and/or lunch.

■ Avoid cheese at night. It contains amino acids that can keep you awake and is very hard on your digestion.

Friendly Foods

■ Try to eat your last meal of the day before 8pm, and if possible, make it carbohydrate-based using small amounts of pasta, potatoes, or brown rice. These starchy foods can have a slightly soporific effect. Eating carbohydrate-rich foods before sleep also encourages the body to produce a brain chemical called serotonin, which can help reduce anxiety and improve the quality of sleep.

■ Serotonin is made from a constituent of protein called tryptophan, so include more foods such as fish, turkey, chicken, cottage cheese, beans, avocados, persimmon (Sharon fruit), bananas, and wheat germ in your diet.

■ Sprinkle wheat germ over a healthy breakfast cereal. Nature's Path makes a healthy cereal from spelt, quinoa, and kamut called Heritage Flakes that is available from Vitacost. **VC**

■ Eat more lettuce at night, as it contains the natural sedative lactucarium, which encourages deeper sleep. You can also heat crisp lettuce in stir-fries and so on—it's delicious.

■ Some people find that eating a banana or an oatcake half an hour before they go to sleep helps them to sleep longer as bananas and oats are a good source of tryptophan, which is calming.

- Many people have oatmeal for breakfast, but often having it for dinner or as a late-evening snack made with organic rice milk and a chopped banana encourages sound sleep. If I wake at night or cannot fall asleep, I often have a small bowl of gluten-free oatmeal with a chopped banana, a few sunflower seeds, and raisins, made with a little organic rice milk and water, which helps me to get to sleep almost immediately. Otherwise, use any low-sugar cereal and only eat a small amount.
- If you are a regular tea or coffee drinker, gradually switch over to the decaffeinated varieties. Don't do this too quickly, as caffeine withdrawal headaches can be quite unpleasant.
- Drink chamomile tea (or any night-time formulas) before going to bed.
- If you suffer low blood sugar problems, eat a banana with an oat- or amaranth-based cookie or a cracker spread with something like humus just before going to bed. (See also under *Low Blood Sugar* and *Adrenal Exhaustion*.)

Useful Remedies

- Calcium and magnesium are nature's tranquillizers. Take a two-in-one formula with your evening meal that includes 600mg of calcium and 300–400mg of magnesium. **SVHC**
- If, like me, you are a Type A person —always on the go with a "busy" mind that you find you often cannot "switch off" at night—try the supplement Cortisol Manager. It's a blend of ashwagandha, L-theanine (from green tea), magnolia bark extract, and phosphatidlyserine. This blend can be used during the day if you find yourself becoming very stressed and are producing cortisol and adrenaline. It really helps calm you down. If you take this supplement just before bed, it can help you wind down. It is available from Integrative Therapeutics, Inc. Tel: 1-800-931-1709. Website: www.integrativeinc.com **NB: If you are suffering from total adrenal exhaustion then you are probably not producing sufficient cortisol; therefore, you would not need this blend. To check your adrenal function, you can have a simple saliva test. (See under *Adrenal Exhaustion*.)**
- Otherwise the Life Extension Foundation makes an L-theanine and lemon balm blend. The amino acid theanine is found in green tea and produces calming effects within the brain without making you drowsy or groggy. It helps you relax by increasing alpha-brainwave activity. It also increases levels of dopamine, a brain chemical that improves mood. Try 100mg twice daily. **LEF**
  NB: Drinking green tea during the day is a great boost to your health, but it also contains caffeine, so avoid drinking it at night. Otherwise buy a decaffeinated version.
- Take a B-complex every morning to support your nerves and keep you calmer.
- Published research in 2010 demonstrated that pure jasmine oil enhances production of GABA, a neurotransmitter in the brain that induces relaxation and reduces anxiety. Jasmine oil has been found to be as effective as sedatives and sleeping pills. Dab a tiny amount on your wrists at night.
- As we age, production of melatonin declines, which means we sleep less and sometimes have more problems getting to sleep. Melatonin is one of the most efficient known antioxidants and helps protect DNA. Bioelectromagnetic research scientist Roger Coghill says: "If you take melatonin supplements that you can buy on line…, most synthetic tablets contain thousands of times the natural dose that your pineal gland normally produces at night." Roger suggests a supplement called Asphalia, which contains natural melatonin extracted from certain grasses, which mimics the normal dose made by your pineal gland to induce sleep at night rather than the larger doses that are found in mass-produced tablets. You should take 1–2 capsules 30 minutes before bed. The exclusive distributor of Asphalia in the US is Diva Marketing, Don't Disturb Me!, 2612 Sleepy Hollow, Pearland, TX 77581. Tel: 1-713-221-1873 or 1-866-692-8037. Website: www.dontdisturbmesite.com

- The Life Extension Foundation makes a Natural Sleep Melatonin formula that also contains co-factors such as calcium and B vitamins. **LEF**
- Try Neurexan, a homeopathic mix of oats, passiflora, valerian, and coffee (Coffea). Put one pill under your tongue three times during the evening. For more information about Neurexan, visit www.heelusa.com

Helpful Hints

- Aim to be in bed by 10:30pm at the latest.
- Turn off all electrical devices near your bed. (See *Electrical Pollution*.)
- One of the most important factors in sleep management is to get up at the same or a similar time every morning, regardless of when you go to bed.
- To help your body make more melatonin naturally, get out in the sun during the day, and then sleep in a fully darkened room at night—the darker the better.
- Noise is a problem for many people. I wear earplugs, which are at times a godsend.
- If you tend to be near or work with electrical equipment every day, particularly computers, then try walking barefoot in grass for 5 minutes each evening in the summer. This helps disperse any electromagnetic radiation that you have built up during the day.
- Warm your feet before going to bed. In the winter, wear socks to bed if your feet tend to get cold.

- Try reading a novel before switching off the lights. This takes your mind away from the day's activities and helps you wind down. If you can't get to sleep, don't panic. Get up and do something relaxing, like reading a few more pages of the novel, until you start to relax and let go; then go back to bed. Don't try to make yourself go to sleep; allow yourself to fall asleep naturally. Eat the breakfast cereal I suggested on the previous page—it works every time for me. You can also try taking another Cortisol Manager (see above).
- Exercising on a regular basis can often improve sleep patterns, but don't exercise too late in the day as the endorphins released by the brain can be quite stimulating.
- Find a way to reduce stress levels, as stressed individuals definitely have worse sleep patterns.
- Meditation is particularly useful, as it helps you clear your mind and get rid of all those extraneous thoughts. People who meditate on a regular basis enjoy better-quality sleep.
- Smoking can also be a factor in insomnia so if you want another reason for quitting, poor sleep patterns might be the last push you need.
- Massage your chest with a mixture of essential oils of lavender, clary sage, marjoram, and basil, or add them to a relaxing bath. Or, buy a burner and let the aroma fill your room.
- NSI Sleep Complex is an herbal remedy with melatonin that promotes natural sleep. **VC**
- Don't read anything related to work too close to bedtime. It stimulates your mind.
- Turn your alarm clock to the wall, so you will not panic about the time.
- Advanced reflexology, homeopathy, acupuncture, and hypnotherapy have all proved useful in restoring natural sleep patterns. (See *Useful Information*.)
- InnerTalk also makes some very good tapes. For details call 1-800-964-3551 toll free or visit www.innertalk.com
- Persistent insomnia can also be exacerbated by food intolerances, in which case it would be wise to consult a doctor who is also a qualified nutritionist. (See *Useful Information*.)
- Invest in a really comfortable mattress. Simply being cozy, and not too warm and not too cold, will really help you. In winter buy a sheepskin mattress cover, and in summer use cotton sheets.
- Read *Alternative Medicine—A Definitive Guide to Sleep Disorders* by Herbert Ross.

INSULIN RESISTANCE

(see also Adrenal Exhaustion, Candida, Diabetes, Leaky Gut Syndrome, and Low Blood Sugar)

Thanks to our over-consumption of refined sugary foods, stress and eating in a hurry, blood-sugar problems are truly reaching epidemic proportions. If any blood-sugar imbalance is not addressed, over time it can develop further into insulin resistance, which is also known as metabolic syndrome, or metabolic syndrome X, and finally into full-blown diabetes.

Insulin is a hormone secreted by cells in the pancreas. Its major function is to lower blood sugar levels and promote the storage of sugars as fats. Its release is stimulated by the consumption of any type of carbohydrate, from fruits and grains to cakes and starchy vegetables like potatoes. It also slows the breakdown of any stored fats.

Of all the hormones associated with aging, insulin is the key player. Dr Shamin Daya of the Wholistic Medical Centre in Harley Street, London, UK says: "High insulin levels trigger inflammation, hormone imbalance, and deterioration of virtually every body system. This problem is closely associated with adrenal function—mainly adrenal exhaustion." (See under *Adrenal Exhaustion*.)

According to US diabetes expert, Dr Ron Rosedale, MD, almost everyone who eats a typical Western diet is overproducing insulin. Bread, rice, potatoes, pasta, and so on are digested into simple sugars, such as glucose, when they enter the gut. Eating large amounts of carbohydrates, such as cakes and cookies, can result in a "sugar rush." Basically, insulin makes cells more receptive to glucose so they can either metabolize it or store it for future use as glycogen or fat. This takes glucose out of your blood and into your cells, lowering your blood sugar levels.

"However," adds Dr Daya, "when this process has been abused for many decades, it's liable to break down. Eventually, the body ceases to respond to glucose as it should and despite ever-increasing levels of insulin, glucose in the blood begins to rise. The cells can no longer utilize it properly. Insulin receptors on the surface of cells seem to have switched off and stopped listening to the signal from insulin, hence the term for this condition. Insulin resistance is dangerous. Apart from the obvious risk of progression into Syndrome X and eventually diabetes, high insulin levels result in excess sympathetic nervous system activity, which means the individual is prone to fatigue. What's more, because insulin is usually only released when there's an excess of blood sugar, conversion of fat back to sugar for use as fuel is blocked by the hormone, so weight loss becomes increasingly difficult. Insulin resistance is also an important factor in polycystic ovarian syndrome." A real giveaway symptom of insulin resistance is weight gain around the waist and midriff—as in becoming more "apple shaped" rather than "pear shaped."

Foods to Avoid

- White flour, white sugar, corn syrup, white potatoes, and other refined starch-rich foods will increase blood-sugar problems, as will breads, cakes, cookies, pasta, pastries and other dessert items, French fries, food-thickeners, coffee creamer, white rice, and skimmed milk (milk with the fat reduced has proportionately more sugar).
- Avoid refined sugar and foods containing sugar, such as soft drinks, chocolate, candies, and many processed foods (check labels), plus reduce your intake of honey, dried fruit, and juices, as they are all rich in fast-releasing sugars. Healthier alternatives to refined sugars are organic agave syrup or xylitol, which have a low glycemic index. Also try diluting fruit juices.
- Artificial sweeteners may seem like a good solution, but they do nothing to reduce your sweet tooth. Also, because they place a strain on the liver, they can add to weight gain and other health problems.

- Caffeine, found in coffee, tea, and soft drinks, is a powerful stimulant. A cup of coffee contains around 100mg of caffeine, soda 50mg, tea 60mg, green tea 25mg, a slice of chocolate cake 25mg, and 1oz (25g) of dark chocolate 30mg. Stimulants encourage sugar to be released into the blood stream, so replace chocolate with fresh fruit. Replace coffee and tea with coffee alternatives available in all health stores. Try green or white teas, peppermint, or fruit teas.
- Alcohol is such a refined carbohydrate that much of it is converted to fat in the body. We are not suggesting that you eliminate it altogether, but just be aware that it is fattening.
- Note that many foods advertised as being low in fat are often high in sugar, which if not used up during exercise will turn to fat in the body and live on your hips!

Friendly Foods

- Eat more lentils and beans. Dr Jeffrey Bland and fellow researchers at the Functional Medicine Research Center in Gig Harbor, WA, have found that legumes create a very low insulin response. As a result, increased intake of lentils, chickpeas, beans, and peas is desirable in the management of blood-sugar problems.
- In general, vegetables have a beneficial effect on blood sugar and insulin, but certain vegetables appear to be even better at maintaining blood sugar and insulin levels than others, including members of the brassica family (cabbage, cauliflower, and broccoli), plus sweet potatoes and other green leafy vegetables.
- Soy products, especially fermented soy products like tempeh, help balance blood-sugar levels. Soy helps improve glucose transport, as well as containing soluble fiber that slows down the absorption of glucose from the gut.
- See also the dietary guidelines under *Diabetes*.
- Make time for breakfast, because this meal "kick starts" your metabolism for the rest of the day and is crucial for better energy balance. "In 11 years of advising people on how to improve their energy levels," says nutritionist Shane Heaton, "I've never met anyone who skips breakfast and has good energy levels for the rest of the day." He recommends a piece of fruit followed by muesli or oatmeal with added pumpkin, sunflower, or amaranth seeds. Oats rich in B vitamins and fiber are ideal, as they provide good, slow-burning energy; however, the most important thing is to choose breakfast foods you enjoy. By eating breakfast, your energy will improve throughout the day. Any cravings for stimulants will decline, you'll sleep better, and you'll wake feeling more refreshed in the morning.
- Protein helps wake up the brain and keeps you feeling full for longer. Eggs, tofu, quinoa, lean meats (preferably organic), and fresh fish are all great proteins. Otherwise, make yourself a delicious breakfast smoothie (recipe under *General Health Hints*) that includes hemp seed protein powder.
- Eat more foods in their natural state. Include complex carbohydrates and whole foods, which contain higher levels of nutrients and fiber, such as brown rice, basmati rice, quinoa, buckwheat, amaranth, stone-ground or rye bread, oatmeal, fruits, and vegetables. These foods also tend to have a low glycemic index.
- Choose more foods with a low glycemic index. The glycemic index is a guide that measures how much and how quickly sugar is released from certain foods compared to pure glucose, which measures at 100 on the scale. Some foods are fast, while others are slow. For example, white bread scores 70, while rye bread is just 41. Bananas are 62, whereas apples are 39. You don't have to stick to low glycemic index foods all the time, but where possible, choose alternatives with lower scores. And when you do eat high glycemic index foods, mix them with protein or low glycemic index foods to slow the release of sugar. Read *The Low GL Diet Bible* (Piatkus Publishing) by Patrick Holford, which is a godsend for anyone with this problem. Website: www.patrickholford.com

- Drink more fluids, as dehydration is a key cause of fatigue and can make you crave fast-energy foods that contribute to blood sugar imbalance.
- If you are desperate for sugar, use small amounts of xylitol sweeteners or organic agave syrup.

Useful Remedies

- Find a high-strength, multi-vitamin/mineral complex that provides a good range of antioxidants, chromium, and plenty of B vitamins.
- The mineral chromium is the main constituent of "glucose tolerance factor," a substance that helps with the delivery of sugar to cells. It is widely used by nutritional therapists to help balance blood sugar levels and reduce cravings. Take 100–200mcg twice daily with meals. US researchers have found that when people who tend to eat a high-carbohydrate diet are given 200mcg of chromium daily, this one action helps reduce the incidence of diabetes by 50%. Most multis contain around 150mcg.
- Fish oil supplementation has been found not only to improve insulin sensitivity in diabetic animals, but also to prevent diabetes-induced nerve damage. Take 2g of omega-3 fish oils daily.
- Antioxidant nutrients have also been found to improve insulin sensitivity. Try taking a good-quality antioxidant formula that contains 100–400mg of natural-source, full-spectrum vitamin E and 50–100mg of alpha-lipoic acid, both of which are known to improve insulin response. VC
- Ultrameal Plus 360 is a specially fortified, vegetarian, powdered beverage mix designed for the nutritional support of glucose metabolism and insulin regulation. For more information, visit www.metagenics.com
- Vitamin C is involved in energy production so if your energy levels are low and your stress levels are high, take 1000mg of vitamin C twice a day with food.
- If stress is a real problem in your life, consider trying the herbs rhodiola or Siberian ginseng. They're both adaptogenic herbs so they will help you adapt to stress and can really help improve your tolerance to stress of all kinds. Take 200–300mg of a standardized extract of either herb daily with meals. (See *Adrenal Exhaustion* for more adrenal support.)
- Metagenics (www.metagenics.com) make a formula called Insinase—a formula of acacia and hops, whose unique action helps reverse insulin resistance. Take one tablet three times a day.

Helpful Hints

- As well as eating sensibly, another way to improve glucose control and insulin sensitivity is through regular aerobic activity. This doesn't have to be intense exercise and can be as moderate as a regular walking program. Even 20 minutes a day will help.
- Moderate alcohol consumption is OK.
- Reduce stress. Stress is a major barrier to stabilizing blood sugar levels because the fight-or-flight mechanism, which is linked to cortisol and adrenalin production, floods your blood with sugar so that it is ready to act. If we constantly suffer from low blood sugar, we can sometimes learn subconsciously to use stress as a way to keep us going. We might stay in a stressful job, make situations more stressful than they need to be, seek out stressful situations, take too much on, do things at the last minute, be late everywhere we go, and so on. Blood sugar imbalance itself is a major stress on the body and at the same time lowers your stress tolerance, so by improving your blood sugar balance, your tolerance to other stresses in your life should improve. Try yoga, tai chi, meditation, massage, or having "down time" every week. Also learn how to relax. (For more help, see *Stress.*)
- Stop smoking. Cigarettes are a stimulant that many people use to keep themselves going. If you find smoking relaxing, you're addicted. The feeling of relaxation is very likely the alleviation of withdrawal symptoms (commonly anxiety, stress, tension, nervousness, and so

on). Those who stop smoking and gain weight do so because they usually replace cigarettes with other stimulants, such as sugar or sugar-containing foods or drinks.

■ The worst thing you can do if your energy levels are low is go long hours without eating. Eat small, frequent meals throughout the day (every 2–3 hours or so) and avoid skipping meals. People who miss meals often experience hypoglycemic (low blood sugar) symptoms. Healthy snacks throughout the day can include fruit, nuts, seeds, rice or oatcakes with humus or other spreads, raw vegetables (such as carrots), rye crackers with lentil pâté and so on.

INTERMITTENT CLAUDICATION

(see also Angina, Atherosclerosis, Circulation, and Heart Disease)

This condition is characterized by a pain in the legs, usually in the calves, when walking. It is caused by blockages in the arteries that supply blood to the legs and is due to hardening of the arteries in the lower body. To successfully deal with intermittent claudication you need to resolve the hardening of the arteries. Diets and natural therapies that help reduce the build-up of deposits in the arteries are the most important treatments. (See under *Atherosclerosis*.)

Dr Shamin Daya says: "Statins, drugs used to lower LDL cholesterol levels, can contribute to this problem, and also food intolerances (particularly to gluten and wheat), lack of exercise, and dehydration. Smokers are more likely to develop these types of circulation problems."

Foods to Avoid
■ Greatly reduce your intake of animal fats and saturated fats, including margarine and highly refined, mass-produced cooking oils. Avoid red meat, chicken skin, too much butter, full-fat milk, and most mass-produced pies, sausages, cakes, and so on.
■ All fried foods should be avoided.
■ Cut down alcohol to less than two drinks a day.
■ See under *Atherosclerosis*.

Friendly Foods
■ Oily fish is rich in omega-3 fats that help thin the blood naturally.
■ Use garlic and onions liberally as they help lower LDL cholesterol levels.
■ Adopt a diet rich in soluble and insoluble fibers from fruits and vegetables, nuts and seeds, flaxseeds, oat or rice bran, and psyllium husks.
■ Eggs are fine as long as they are boiled, poached or scrambled, and not fried.
■ Use plenty of fresh root ginger in cooking, in teas or with fruits to aid circulation.
■ Look for non-hydrogenated spreads in the supermarket such as Biona and Olivio. Use olive oil instead of butter.
■ You can also use hemp, pumpkin seed, walnut or coconut oil butters that are available from most health stores.
■ Drink at least 6–8 glasses of water daily.
■ Eat more cilantro, which helps detoxify heavy metals from the body, as does chlorella.
■ See *Friendly Foods* in *Atherosclerosis* and *Circulation*.

Useful Remedies
■ Take 400IU a day of a natural-source, full-spectrum vitamin E supplement. This has been shown to improve walking distance and decrease the discomfort of intermittent claudication. The supplement needs to be taken for a minimum of six months to be effective. **NB: Check with your doctor if you are on blood-thinning drugs, as vitamin E will thin your blood naturally.**

- Take 2g daily of vitamin B3 in the form of inositol hexaniacinate for at least three months. This form of B3 can help lower cholesterol, and studies have shown that it is very effective for intermittent claudication. **NB: Niacin produces an intense short-term flushing of the skin, so start with 100mg daily with food and work your way up from there. It's very effective as it increases blood flow and lowers LDL, but many people are put off by the flushing effect.**
- Make sure to include a B complex supplement, as all the B vitamins work together in the body.
- Omega-3 fish oils help support circulation; take 2g daily.
- Ginger drops, taken three times daily in water, or ginger tea can aid circulation. **VC**

Helpful Hints
- Discuss chelation therapy with your doctor. This process involves a doctor giving you an IV that, over time, will help clear your arteries. There are several clinics in the US—for details search on www.holisticnetworker.com or do your own searches on Google.
- Don't smoke, as there is a strong link between smoking and the development of intermittent claudication.
- Gentle exercise is definitely beneficial, even though it may be uncomfortable. Talk to your doctor before starting any exercise program. People who exercise regularly are much less likely to develop intermittent claudication.
- Acupuncture and reflexology (especially advanced reflexology) are great for improving circulation and reducing pain. (See *Useful Information*.)

IRRITABLE BOWEL SYNDROME (IBS)

(see also Colitis, Constipation, Crohn's Disease, Diverticular Disease, and Leaky Gut)

Nutritional physician Dr Shamin Daya based in Harley Street, London, UK says, "Virtually all the above conditions have their root cause in food intolerances and a leaky gut, and when these issues are addressed the gut can, in the majority of cases, heal itself."

Approximately 60–100 million Americans suffer from some type of digestive complaint, and irritable bowel syndrome accounts for 30–35 million. Worldwide, 20–25% of people in the western world are believed to suffer from IBS—to varying degrees—and this condition is three times more common in women than in men. IBS is an umbrella term used to describe a range of gut-related symptoms such as abdominal pain, constipation, or diarrhea—or both alternating from day to day. Bloating, gas, headaches, nausea, blood and/or mucus or undigested food in the stool, anxiety, cramps, and depression are also often associated with IBS.

The most commonly offending foods known to trigger IBS and all gut problems are gluten, wheat, dairy from animal sources, refined carbohydrates (white foods full of refined sugar), coffee, alcohol, tea, and citrus foods—although it is possible to have an intolerance to the most innocuous foods that you would never suspect.

Stress is a major factor in gut problems, as the digestion shuts down during stressful times. These digestive juices then don't get to do their job properly, which leaves incompletely digested particles of food to irritate the gut. A lack of digestive enzymes and stomach acid (see *Acid Stomach* and *Low Stomach Acid*) can also lead to incompletely digested food irritating the gut.

Parasites are a growing and often overlooked factor. Twenty percent of all people tested have parasites. In those with IBS, 49% are known to have the parasite *Blastocystis hominis*, and 20% have the parasite *Dientamoeba fragilis*. If you have ever had food poisoning (either while on vacation or in the US), allow pets to walk on food-preparation surfaces, eat raw fish (sushi) or insufficiently cooked meats, or store meat above vegetables in your fridge, then parasites could be a factor.

You and your doctor should also consider dysbiosis—an imbalance of good to bad bacteria in the gut. Any yeasts such as candida (see *Candida*), parasites, and bad bacteria present in the bowel upset this delicate balance and can cause symptoms of IBS. This imbalance of bacteria can also be triggered by a poor diet that has insufficient fiber and is high in alcohol, fatty foods. and/or sugar. Antibiotics will also upset this balance.

Occasionally, the symptoms of IBS can reflect a more serious underlying condition, so it is very important to see your doctor in case you have Crohn's disease, ulcerative colitis, or diverticulitis, which are often mistaken for IBS. People with IBS need to support their liver by watching their intake of fats, caffeine, and alcohol. (See also *Liver Problems*.)

Foods to Avoid

- Refined carbohydrates are generally high in gluten; therefore, avoid wheat, barley, oats, and rye and look for gluten- and wheat- free foods.
- Avoid yeasts, vinegar, mushrooms, and refined sugars. Also most fruits other than berries, mango, and papaya ferment easily. (See under *Candida*.)
- All dairy products from animal sources, including milk, chocolate, cheese, cream, ice cream, and yogurt, should be avoided.
- Soy can be a problem for some people. Keep a food diary and note when symptoms are worse.
- Other problem foods are often eggs and citrus fruits, especially oranges; and foods with a high tyramine content, such as cheese, port, red wine and sherry, beef, liver, herring, sauerkraut, and yeast extracts.
- If you suspect candida, see *Foods to Avoid* under *Candida*.
- Melted cheese is very hard for the body to digest so it avoid at all costs.
- Refined foods such as white rice and pasta, as well as cakes and pastries, alcohol, fried foods, high-sugar foods, and foods high in saturated animal fat (found in meat and dairy) all deplete good bacteria in the gut and help feed the bad guys.
- Avoid heavy, rich meals, and especially avoid fried foods.

Friendly Foods

- There are plenty of alternatives to wheat and gluten. Ask at your health store for wheat-free breads; millet-, buckwheat-, quinoa- and/or corn-based crisp breads; and rice and corn cakes.
- You can now buy lentil-, corn-, millet-, rice-, buckwheat- and potato-based pastas and/or noodles.
- Try organic rice, almond, or quinoa milk.
- Eat more brown rice, as it cleanses and heals the digestive tract. Also eat more potatoes, fish, lean (preferably organic) poultry and meats, fresh fruits and vegetables.
- Peppermint, fresh mint, fennel, chamomile, and rosemary teas can all enhance digestion and ease discomfort.
- Instead of orange juice, try diluting low-sugar apple, pear, or pineapple juice.
- Add more ginger to your food, which soothes your gut and has anti-parasitic properties. This is why Japanese sushi—raw fish, which can contain parasites—is often served with ginger. (See also *Leaky Gut*.)
- Pumpkin seeds have anti-parasitic action, so munch on some daily.
- Eating pineapple, which contains bromelain, helps digest protein—so, eat pineapple in between meals.

- In order to make stomach acid for efficient digestion, you need vitamin B6 and the mineral zinc. These are found in sunflower seeds, soybeans, walnuts, lentils, lima beans, peas, buckwheat flour (this is a grass and is not related to wheat), avocados, chestnuts, brown rice, lentils, pumpkin and sesame seeds, almonds, and cooked tofu.
- Eat lighter meals. Soup and fish-based meals are easier on the digestion than a pizza with melted cheese! Avoid rich sauces.

Useful Remedies

- See all remedies under *Leaky Gut*.
- Take one acidophilus or bifidus capsule twice a day to replace healthy bacteria in the gut and improve digestion. Nature's Way Primadophilus and other enteric coated probiotics have been shown to survive stomach acid and make it to the gut where they can to do their job. **VS**
- Take a high-strength B-complex to make sure you have all of the nutrients necessary to digest carbohydrates, proteins, and fats. Look for a supplement that contains 50mg of most of the B vitamins.
- Aloe vera juice, 20ml taken before meals, has helped a lot of people, as it helps increase stool bulk, enhances digestion, and eases the discomfort of IBS. Lakewood Organic Juices make a good pure aloe juice. Available from most supermarkets and health stores.
- Take 2–6 teaspoons (10–20g) of organic flaxseeds daily, building up slowly, one teaspoon at a time. The mixture of soluble and insoluble fibers in flaxseeds helps stimulate the bowel gently, while providing stool bulk, thus enabling the bowel to function normally and comfortably. Flaxseeds have also been successful in alleviating both constipation and diarrhea, but they must be taken with plenty of water. Generally, soak the flaxseeds overnight in cold water, drain, and use on cereals, in oatmeal, or in smoothies. Or use a ready-cracked variety.
- See remedies under *Constipation* and *Diarrhea* if either is your main problem.
- As absorption of nutrients is often a problem for people with IBS and you may also be low in stomach acid (see *Low Stomach Acid*), dilute 1 teaspoon of apple cider vinegar in water and drink with each meal. If symptoms persist, try taking a hydrochloric acid supplement plus a digestive enzyme supplement with pancreatin along with meals. This will provide some stomach acid mixed with digestive enzymes. Take it after the first few mouthfuls, but do not chew it. Also, never take it on an empty stomach. **NB: Avoid all of these remedies if you have active stomach ulcers or if they create a feeling of warmth in your stomach. Instead, take a pancreatic digestive enzyme formula without the HCl, which can irritate the gut.**
- Zinc helps the body produce its own stomach acid; therefore, if you know that you are suffering from low stomach acid, take 30–60mg zinc daily with food.
- Try a combination of cayenne capsules (which help stop any bleeding), pure slippery elm tea (which soothes and heals the gut), and Botanical Colitis Symptom Reliever capsules of wild yam, an anti-spasmodic, plus bayberry and agrimony, which tighten and heal the tissues. Take 3–9 capsules daily depending on the severity of the symptoms. Available from www.bontemedical.com or 1-877-426-9253.

Helpful Hints

- Chew, chew, chew, and chew again. As you chew, you send signals to the digestive system to produce its digestive enzymes. Thoroughly chewed food also gives the enzymes less to do, making them more effective.
- Drink more alkaline water, as the gut heals more quickly if it is more alkaline. Purification Filters supplies alkalizing filters for your home. Visit www.purificationfilters.com for more information.
- Consider using Kangen Water—a water system unit that attaches to your kitchen faucet and

ionizes and greatly alkalizes water. It has been used in Japanese hospitals with highly beneficial health results. For full details, visit www.kangenwaterusa.com

- Oil of peppermint has anti-spasmodic properties so massage it on your abdomen and drink peppermint tea after meals. Fennel tea is another herb that aids digestion.
- Gentle exercise on a regular basis enhances bowel function. Yoga, Pilates, swimming, and walking are all good forms of exercise that do not overtax the system and enhance relaxation.
- Remember to eat in a relaxed fashion; being stressed while you eat makes it very difficult for your digestive system to work at its best. Sitting down for 10 minutes before and after a meal is advised. Try to avoid eating food on the run.
- Remember, if you have an intolerance to one food, you are actually likely to be intolerant to more than one. Very few of us react to just one food, and in most cases we react to four or five. Genova Diagnostics does a thorough food intolerance test and can be contacted at 1-800-522-4762 or through their website: www.genovadiagnostics.com
- Another excellent method is known as the Bio Meridian Test for food intolerance and leaky gut. During this test a practitioner measures, via electrodes, your reactions to a huge list of foods and substances. For practitioners see www.biomeridian.com
- Professor Roland Valori, a gastroenterologist at Gloucester Royal Hospital in the UK, has found that 90 out of 100 of his patients who were treated with hypnotherapy experienced significant improvements. (See *Useful Information*.)
- Contact the IBS Treatment Center, which is the first clinic in the US to focus solely on treating this condition. They will test for all of the most common IBS triggers, including food intolerances, candida overgrowth, and parasites. Tel: 1-888-546-6283 or 1-206-264-1111. E-mail: info@ibstreatmentcenter.com. Website: www.ibstreatmentcenter.com
- For more information, visit www.aboutibs.org

J

JET LAG

(see also Deep Vein Thrombosis)

Jet lag is a disturbance of the body's natural sleep/wake cycle that is triggered by air travel across time zones and has become a part of modern living. It's obvious that if you travel for many hours across various time zones, your whole system is going to be affected. Usually, the more time zones you cross, the worse the symptoms will be. These symptoms include difficulty falling asleep at the "new" local bedtime and sleepiness and fatigue during the day. In addition, your circulation can become sluggish, triggering problems such as leg, ankle, and foot swelling or in extreme cases DVT. (See under *Deep Vein Thrombosis*.)

Also, as you are breathing recycled air along with myriad bacteria and viruses while you are on the plane, you are at risk of contracting a whole host of diseases from a simple cold to something more serious, such as tuberculosis, which has made a comeback. You are also exposed to considerable amounts of radiation, which can lower immune function; your pineal gland can become confused, thus affecting melatonin production (the hormone that controls the sleep/wake cycle), which plays havoc with your internal body clock.

Scientist Roger Coghill says, "Because you are moving between local magnetic fields, while your body adjusts, you can feel very disorientated indeed." (See *Helpful Hints* for more about magnetic fields.) Children under the age of 3 seem to suffer little jet lag, as they are not set in their ways and therefore are more adaptable. Also the less rigid you are in your everyday life, the less likely you are to suffer from jet lag.

Foods to Avoid
- On long flights eat smaller meals and reduce your intake of caffeinated teas, coffee, alcohol, and soft drinks, which all dehydrate the body. Caffeine can contribute to poor sleep patterns, so ask for decaffeinated varieties.
- Sugar depletes minerals and lowers immune function, which can be a real problem since bacteria and viruses spread quickly in airless airplane cabins. (See *Immune Function*.)
- Alcohol is 2–3 times more potent when you drink it in the air.
- Also see this section under *Circulation*.

Friendly Foods
- Try to eat light, healthy foods the day before you leave, and drink plenty of water. I realize that airline food can leave a lot to be desired, but eat at regular intervals on the flight to help balance blood sugar levels.
- Foods that help calm you down and aid restful sleep are turkey, cottage cheese, avocados, pasta, bananas, and skimmed milk.
- Chamomile, lemon balm, or passiflora teas are great for relaxation. Take a few tea bags with you.
- Ask the cabin crew to give you a few bottles of mineral water and drink it throughout the flight.
- Eat more garlic during the week or so before flying. It's antibacterial, anti-viral, and thins the blood naturally.

Useful Remedies
- Take 1g of vitamin C with bioflavonoids every 2–3 hours with meals.
- Take a high-strength multi-vitamin/mineral.
- Try Emergen C, a powdered vitamin C and electrolyte formula that helps replenish depleted minerals. Sold at all good health stores and pharmacies.
- The amino acid L-theanine (extracted from green tea) helps the brain produce more alpha waves and helps you relax without making you groggy. (See under *Insomnia*.)
- Melatonin, which is produced in the pineal gland at night, has proven highly effective for reducing jet lag. However bioelectromagnetics scientist Roger Coghill says: "When you take melatonin supplements that you can buy on line..., most synthetic tablets contain thousands of times the natural dose that your pineal gland normally produces. If you only take small amounts for jet lag this should be fine; 0.5mg taken as you get off the plane and one more at bedtime in the short term would be fine." Roger has developed a supplement called Asphalia that is extracted from certain grasses that contain natural melatonin, which mimic the normal dose made by your pineal gland at night rather than the larger dose you get in mass-produced tablets. Take 1–2 capsules 30 minutes before bed. Roger's exclusive distributor in the US is Diva Marketing, Don't Disturb Me!, 2612 Sleepy Hollow, Pearland, TX 77581. Tel: 1-713-221-1873 or 1-866-692-8037. Website: www.dontdisturbmesite.com
  NB: Asphalia should not be taken by severe asthmatics, children under the age of 1 and pregnant women in their third trimester.
- A homeopathic mixture called Jet Lag, which contains arnica and cocculus, reduces symptoms of jet lag by helping the body readjust to local time. Available from www.nojetlag.com

Helpful Hints

■ Get a good night's sleep before your flight, which will help reduce jet lag. When you arrive, if practical, exercise a little by taking a walk or a swim.

■ Try to stay up until the local time to go to bed. When I travel west from the UK to the US, I usually manage to stay up until the local bedtime (around 8pm), but if I'm going east I find this harder and often take a nap. Basically, the sooner you get on to local time the better.

■ Get as much sunlight as you can as soon as you arrive by going for a walk. This will help re-set your body clock.

■ Also, to help reset your body clock, attach a Super Magnet to the top of your head for 15 minutes before landing. One of the reasons you get jet lag is because your body clock is trying to adjust to the new magnetic field. By using the magnet you can reset your body clock to the local magnetic field.

■ If you have a long wait for a connecting flight, try to take a shower, which will help relax your muscles and get your circulation moving again.

■ Walk and stretch as much as you can on board the plane and in the airport.

■ Have a light, healthy snack when you arrive to help you sleep, otherwise low blood sugar can cause you to wake in the middle of the night.

K

KIDNEY STONES

(see also Acid–Alkaline Balance)

Your kidneys filter the plasma of your blood and extract all the waste and unwanted toxins, which are then excreted in the urine (a sterile liquid). The residues of antibiotics, prescription drugs, and hormones, as well as vitamins and minerals, are also excreted in the urine. The kidneys maintain the acid–alkaline balance of your blood within very narrow limits, and if the blood becomes too acid or too alkaline, life is not possible. Without functioning kidneys you would not survive for very long.

These remarkable organs weigh just a few ounces each and yet, if they cease to function (known as kidney failure), they must be replaced with a dialysis machine. Two of the main threats to our kidneys are high blood pressure and toxins. If you tend to have a poor diet or do little to no exercise, it's likely that you may develop hypertension, which, sooner or later, plays havoc with the kidneys. (See also *High Blood Pressure*.) Other toxins that affect the kidneys are found in our air, water, and food. Mercury, arsenic, pesticides, and a huge amount of chemical pollutants all pose potential problems to the kidneys. Cadmium from cigarette smoke is a major kidney poison, and the accumulation of this metal in the kidneys is one of the reasons why smokers often succumb to illness sooner than average—they simply cannot clear their bloodstream of harmful waste products as efficiently as non-smokers. If the kidneys have to work harder, they may weaken under the strain.

If we eat a poor diet, kidney stones, miniscule crystals that look like gravel, can start to form over time and can damage the delicate tubules in the kidneys, impeding proper urine flow. Kidney stone episodes are more common in the summer, when urine becomes more concentrated as we tend to sweat more. The stones are generally made from minerals such as calcium, phosphates, and deposits of uric acid, the most common component of which is calcium oxalate. Kidney stones can cause excruciating pain as they try to move out of the kidneys and into the bladder. Passing a kidney stone is one of the worst pains you can experience in all of medicine. So, try to make sure this never happens to you.

Vegetarians have a 40–60% lower chance of developing stones than meat-eaters; and voracious meat-eaters tend to develop more stones because of their higher uric acid production. Having kidney stones in the body also makes bladder infections much more likely. If you ever pass blood in your urine or have persistent back pain, then it's very important to see your doctor. People with high homocysteine levels also tend to suffer from more kidney problems. (See *Cholesterol* and *Heart Disease*.) You can lower homocysteine levels through your diet and by taking B vitamins.

Foods to Avoid
- Refined sugar is the worst food for your kidneys, as it stimulates the release of insulin from the pancreas, which in turn stimulates calcium excretion through the urine. Over time, this can increase the risk of kidney stones.
- If you tend to eat a lot of foods that are high in oxalic acid, such as chocolate, cocoa, tea, spinach, rhubarb, and chard, don't eat these foods too regularly.
- Beets, instant coffee, grapefruit, oranges, gooseberries, peanuts, and strawberries also contain oxalic acid, so you should reduce your intake of these foods if you suffer from kidney stones.
- Also reduce or avoid high acid-forming foods, such as red meat, full-fat dairy products, refined sugar, and sweets.
- Cut down on all soft drinks and reduce your intake of alcohol and caffeinated drinks.
- Antacids, excessive animal-based milks, and carbonated drinks such as soda water can all add to the problem.
- Avoid sodium-based salts. Ask at your health store for magnesium- and potassium-based sea salts instead. However, use them sparingly.
- Also see dietary advice under *Gout*, as you also need to avoid high-purine foods.

Friendly Foods
- Drink cranberry juice, parsley tea, dandelion leaf tea, mullein tea, and barley water, which all help break down any stone formation.
- Drink plenty of pure water, and increase to 8 glasses daily in summer. Distilled water works best for removing and preventing kidney stones. This is one of the most important things you can do to prevent stone formation and/or breaking down stones.
- Eat black cherries, which help remove uric acid crystals from the body.
- Drink carrot, celery, and parsley juice or make "smoothies" with them. Celery does contain a little oxalic acid, but it makes a great kidney cleanser, as it is rich in potassium, which helps to flush the kidneys.
- Eat plenty of garlic, horseradish, asparagus, parsley, watermelon, apples, cucumber, kale, parsnips, turnip greens, and mango, which are all great kidney foods.
- All magnesium- and calcium-rich foods help you avoid kidney stones and encourage healthier kidneys. Try green leafy vegetables plus apricots, blackstrap molasses, raw honey, curried vegetables, watercress, soy flour, yogurt, muesli, and sesame seeds. Raw wheat germ is high in magnesium and vitamin E.
- Asparagus is great for breaking down kidney stones.
- Try rice, oat, almond, quinoa, or coconut milks as non-dairy alternatives to cow's milk.
- Use organic, unrefined olive, walnut, or flaxseed oils in salad dressings.
- Use olive and coconut oils for cooking.

- Vegetable-source proteins are less likely to trigger this problem. Try tofu, quinoa, beans, lentils, peas, or hemp seed protein powders.
- If you like animal protein, choose white fish in preference to meat.
- Sprinkle non-GM lecithin granules over your food. These help emulsify saturated fats that can contribute to stone formation. Lecithin also contains choline, which helps protect the kidneys from damage due to arteriosclerosis and hypertension. Take 2 tablespoons a day. See *General Health Hints* for a healthy breakfast smoothie recipe.
- Kelp and all seaweeds are a great source of calcium, magnesium, and trace minerals. Use nori flakes as a healthy salt substitute.
- Try spelt, amaranth, or millet breads and crackers, as spelt, millet, and amaranth are alkaline foods.
- Eat more barley- and lentil-based dishes.

Useful Remedies

- A great remedy for kidney stones is hydrangea root, made into an herbal drink with water, and consumed over the course of a day. Often one treatment can make a big difference. **VC**
- Take a high-strength B-complex, especially if you are under stress. B vitamins are usually in any good multi-vitamin/mineral formula, which you also need.
- Vitamin C (2g daily with food) is a good detoxifier.
- Take vitamin D3 in a halibut liver oil capsule.
- Choline protects the kidneys from inflammation. It is available as the amino acids methionine and s-adenosyl methionine (SAMe), which is super-strength methionine. Take 500mg a day of methionine, by Allergy Research, or 50g of SAMe.
- Drink more organic green or white tea, which help re-alkalize the system.
- New Era tissue salts, silica, and calcium fluoride help break down kidney stones. Take four of each daily.
- The herb horsetail acts as a diuretic, which promotes kidney function. It can be taken either as capsules or as a tincture to help reduce stones, but do not use it if your kidneys are already damaged.
- Drink one cup of nettle tea three times a day. It is best made with the dried herbs available in tea bags or as loose tea from good health stores.
- Include either a liquid multi-mineral, such as Fulvic Mineral Complex from Vital Earth Minerals, or a multi-mineral tablet in your regimen. **VC**
- Take calcium citrate, 500mg, with each meal as the calcium binds to the oxalate and reduces the likelihood of kidney stone formation.
- The amino acid lysine helps decrease urinary calcium. Take 500mg twice daily before meals. **VC**
- Magnesium citrate helps keep calcium in the bones and out of the arteries. Take 600mg daily in divided doses.

Helpful Hints

- Lemon juice (citric acid) helps break down stones and also smooth out irregular stones. Take 1 teaspoon of neat lemon juice every half an hour during the day for two days, away from food.
- Skin-brushing and lymphatic drainage massage also help remove toxins. However, reflexology, massage, manual lymph drainage, and other therapies that encourage toxins to move out of tissues can temporarily overload the kidneys. Warn your therapist to be gentle if you have a kidney problem. Drink plenty of distilled water afterward.
- If you need painkillers, avoid acetaminophen (Tylenol), which has a negative effect on the kidneys.
- Some homeopathic remedies are excellent for strengthening kidney function. Populus and

Solidago are well-known kidney remedies. HEEL also does Mucosa compositum, which helps the healing process. Available from a number of online retailers.

■ Avoid excessive sweating, which may mean you need to moderate your exercise routine and stay out of the midday sun. Do not consume strong (concentrated) drinks, which means no sodas or alcohol-containing sodas. If you do drink alcohol, make sure that you swallow plenty of water with it. Avoid dehydration at all costs, so also eat less salt.

■ Stress can make you produce more sweat, too! Stay calm.

L

LEAKY GUT

(see also Adrenal Exhaustion, Allergies, Candida, Eczema, Irritable Bowel Syndrome, Low Stomach Acid, and Lupus)

If you have a leaky gut, you are unlikely to absorb enough of the essential nutrients from your food that your body needs for good health. If this leaky gut is not healed, then the long-term implications for your health are serious indeed.

Thanks to many people's stressed lifestyles, eating too many of the wrong foods, often in a hurry, leaky gut syndrome has now reached epidemic proportions. Dr Shamin Daya, a nutritional physician based at the Wholistic Medical Centre in Harley Street, London, UK says: "In my clinical experience, leaky gut is a major contributing factor in all autoimmune conditions. This is because the gut lining is an important defense mechanism within the body that protects the internal organs against pathogens and undigested food particles. Once the gut becomes leaky, not only are you not absorbing sufficient essential nutrients, but the body is then compromised and at risk from fungus and other infections, which in turn triggers inflammation elsewhere in the body, thus self-perpetuating the autoimmune process.

"Osteoporosis, recurrent candida, IBS, colitis, Crohn's disease, eczema, and even autism are, in my opinion, all linked to chronic malabsorption problems."

At any age the small villi (small finger-like protrusions) in the small intestine can become irritated or eroded, which allows larger, undigested food molecules and toxins to pass through our gut wall into the blood stream, affecting both the liver and the lymphatic system and also placing a greater strain on our immune system. These undigested food molecules are treated as foreign invaders and provoke an immune reaction. Our bodies then begin reacting to food as if it were an infection entering our system and send out antibodies to fight it. Leaky gut is now recognized as a major trigger for most food intolerances and allergies and, in some people, migraines.

Various toxins accumulate in our body, especially in the small intestine (gut) and large bowel. The accumulation tends to be a combination of undigested food, impacted feces, bacteria, fungi, parasites, and dead cells. As the toxins build up, the gut wall can become irritated and damaged, which enables partly digested food molecules to cross it and make their way into the blood stream.

Generally, if you suffer from bloating, constipation and/or diarrhea, crave sugary, refined foods, feel tired all the time and/or notice that your food comes out the other end looking fairly much the same as it went in, you may have a leaky gut. You may also have unexplained weight loss and skin rashes, and if the leaky gut is chronic, then you may also suffer from conditions such as rheumatoid arthritis or lupus. Candida, a yeast fungal overgrowth, is also a common cause or results of a leaky gut. (See also *Candida*.) Most people with a leaky gut also tend to have low zinc levels.

Foods to Avoid

- Avoid gluten found in wheat, rye, spelt, oats, and barley, as it hugely contributes to a leaky gut and triggers bloating. Eating gluten- and wheat-free foods should make a considerable difference.
- Refined sugar encourages fermentation and growth of unfriendly bacteria in the bowel, so keep refined sugary foods and drinks to an absolute minimum.
- If you tend to bloat a lot after eating, avoid eating fruit directly after a large protein meal, as fruit likes a quick passage through the gut. If it gets stuck behind proteins such as meat, the fruit will ferment, which adds to the problem. Alcohol, vinegar, and most pickled foods contribute to fermentation.
- Any foods that you have an intolerance to will only aggravate the problem, the most common culprits being wheat, citrus fruits, and cow's milk/products. Chocolate should also be avoided.
- Melon is particularly bad for a leaky gut. This should only be eaten on its own.
- Generally fruits such as apples, grapes, bananas, and pears can cause bloating because they ferment rapidly. Cut down or eliminate them if you usually bloat after eating these fruits. Keep a food diary and note when symptoms are worse.
- Avoid heavy, fatty, large meals, which place a strain on the digestive system and the liver.
- Cut down on low-fiber foods, such as gelatin, ice cream, burgers, cookies, cakes, pies, pastries, and so on.

Friendly Foods

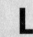

- As an alternative to refined sugars, use a little xylitol, sold online and in health stores. It contains 40% less calories than refined sugar and only has a minimal impact on blood sugar levels. You can also use small amounts of organic agave or brown rice syrup.
- Pineapple and papaya are rich in enzymes that improve protein digestion, making it less likely that undigested proteins will end up in the bowel. Eat before or in between meals.
- Mango, papaya, pineapple, pomegranate, and berries do not tend to ferment as rapidly as most other fruits. Eat them between meals.
- Try almond, rice, quinoa, or coconut milk as non-dairy alternatives.
- Beets, Jerusalem artichokes, peas, radishes, celeriac, and dandelion are all good liver cleansers, which also improve digestion. Beans, pulses, and lentils are also good gut foods. They contain inulin, which helps encourage the growth of bifidus within the large bowel. This helps reduce the load on the liver in the long term. (See *Liver Problems*.)
- Unsalted sunflower, pumpkin, and sesame seeds, flaxseeds (soaked overnight in cold water, then drained, and eaten), and nuts are all rich sources of fiber. A great way to get more nuts and seeds into your diet is to place 1 tablespoon each of sunflower, pumpkin, hemp, and sesame seeds, as well as walnuts, hazel, or Brazil nuts in a coffee grinder or food mixer and pulse for a few seconds. Keep them in a screw-top jar in the fridge and sprinkle over cereals, salads, desserts, fruit, yogurts, and so on. The mixture will stay fresh for about a week.
- Drink plenty of water—at least 6–8 glasses a day.
- Garlic and onions help fight infection and encourage growth of friendly bacteria in the bowel.
- Organic-source chlorella is a great way to detoxify the system. Stir into smoothies or juices, or sprinkle over cereals and fruit salads.

- Use fresh root ginger in your cooking, which soothes and heals the gut.
- Green cabbage is rich in the amino acid L-glutamine, which helps to heal a leaky gut. Eat more raw or steamed cabbage, and use the liquid left over after cooking to make gravy and sauces.
- Eat plenty of fresh vegetables, and if you eat fruit, eat it between meals or for breakfast.
- Try quinoa, buckwheat, millet, and plenty of brown rice.
- Most health stores sell pastas made from soy, millet, buckwheat, amaranth, or rice flour.
- Sprinkle rice bran over cereals.
- Drink more organic green and white teas, which are high in antioxidants.
- Try The Gluten-Free Bakeshop, Food For Life, EnerG, Glutino, and Kinnkinnick breads, which are wheat- and gluten- free. All health stores (and some supermarkets) now sell wheat- and gluten-free crackers and cookies as well.
- Amaranth crackers or rice cakes should be fine.

Useful Remedies

- Take a digestive enzyme capsule with meals.
- Multi formulas specifically designed to heal a leaky gut are LGS-Zyme, Gastro-ULC, and Perma-Clear. All are available from a number of online retailers.
- The amino acid L-glutamine helps heal a leaky gut. Take between 1 and 4g a day, on an empty stomach, for the first month and then reduce to 1g daily. Children can take colostrum—a quarter teaspoon twice daily on an empty stomach. **VC** (See under *Allergies* for more details.)

- Take a high-strength, easily absorbed multi-vitamin/mineral supplement daily. There are so many brands of liquid multis. **VC**
- Add 2–6 teaspoons of raw, ready-cracked flaxseeds to your cereals or yogurts every day. Keep the seeds in the fridge. Otherwise soak a tablespoon of flaxseeds overnight in cold water, drain, and use in a breakfast smoothie. (See *General Health Hints* for breakfast smoothie recipe.)
- Use a good green powder daily in smoothies to help alkalize your system, as the gut heals faster when it's more alkaline. Greens Plus, which contains Hawaiian spirulina, chlorella, lecithin, barley, pectin apple fiber, soy and barley sprouts and lactobacillus acidophilus, is a great all-around way to ingest good nutrients, healthy bacteria, keep the body more alkaline, and help keep you regular. **GP**
- Half a teaspoon of baking soda twice daily in warm water, well away from food, will really help re-alkalize the body and therefore help it heal faster.
- After changing your diet and taking these supplements for three months, your gut should be in better shape, and you can then reduce this regimen to a good multi-vitamin/mineral plus a digestive enzyme daily.

Helpful Hints

- A urine test via Genova, called a Gut Permeability Test, can detect a leaky gut (see below).
- It is really important to have an allergy test to find foods that are a problem. One of the best I have found is available from YorkTest Laboratories (www.yorktest.com). Another option is a FACT test from Genova Diagnostics, which looks for inflammatory markers that indicate the body is reacting to certain substances. Tel: 1-800-522-4762 or 1-828-253-0621. Website: www.genovadiagnostics.com
- Another excellent method is known as the Bio Meridian Test for food intolerance and leaky gut, in which a practitioner measures, via electrodes, your reactions to a huge list of foods and substances. For practitioners, see www.biomeridian.com
- It is vital that you chew your food thoroughly and more slowly, which helps break it down

more effectively. Many people with a leaky gut swallow large food particles in a hurry, which places a huge strain on their already laboring digestive tract.

- Smoking increases the toxic load on the body and can make the situation worse.
- Make sure you get plenty of regular exercise and always walk for at least 15 minutes after a meal to aid digestion.
- Lower your stress levels (see *Stress*), as stress greatly contributes to a leaky gut (see *Adrenal Exhaustion*). Also, only eat light meals when you are under stress.
- Drink more alkaline water as the gut heals faster if it is more alkaline. Purification Filters supplies alkalizing filters for your home. Website: www.purificationfilters.com
- Remember not to eat on the move. As much as possible, eat in a relaxed, comfortable environment, but if nothing else, always sit down to eat.

LEG ULCERS *(see also Cholesterol, Circulation, and Diabetes)*

This is a very common problem in people over 60 and is caused by restricted circulation and a lack of oxygen and nutrients reaching the skin. Leg and foot ulcers are more common in diabetics because of changes in circulation and the nerve endings near the skin. As leg ulcers can be related to diabetes, ask your doctor for a blood test to rule this out.

Foods to Avoid
- Avoid foods that impede circulation, including animal fats (especially red meats), sausages, burgers, full-fat cheeses and dairy products, as well as hard margarines made from refined vegetable oils.
- Avoid all fried foods and don't use mass-produced vegetable oils.
- Cut down on alcohol and on low-fiber foods, such as gelatin, ice cream, white breads, and mass-produced pies and cakes.
- See dietary advice in *Circulation* and *Cholesterol*.

Friendly Foods
- Eat more leafy green vegetables, especially cabbage, kale, celery, bok choy, spinach, and broccoli, which contain high levels of carotenes and minerals.
- Eat more salads and sprinkle sunflower, pumpkin, and sesame seeds over them, as these seeds are high in essential fatty acids, minerals, and fiber.
- Oily fish are rich in omega-3 fats, which thin the blood naturally and aid healing.
- Cook with a little organic butter, olive oil, ghee, or coconut oil. Never heat oil to smoking, which turns it rancid. Coconut oil, ghee, and butter are more stable at higher temperatures.
- Sprinkle wheat germ and lecithin granules over breakfast cereals to lower "bad" cholesterol.
- Add almonds, Brazil nuts, hazelnuts, and walnuts to fruit dips as they are all high in zinc, which aids skin healing.
- High-protein foods, such as hemp seed or whey protein, are a very rich source of glutamine, which speeds the healing process. You can buy these at all health stores.
- Eat more garlic and onions, which are antibacterial.
- Drink more organic green or white teas to help boost your immune system. They are delicious with a small amount of organic agave syrup or xylitol (instead of refined sugars).

Useful Remedies
- Take 30mg of zinc 1–2 times a day with meals. This is absolutely essential if you are suffering from slow wound healing.
- Take 500mg of gotu kola three times a day with meals. This herb has been used historically for

wound healing and when combined with zinc can be very successful. It helps increase circulation in the lower limbs and can have a slight laxative effect—for many people, this is a bonus!

- Vitamin C, 2g daily in divided doses with food, is essential for healing connective tissue.
- If the ulcers are superficial and not too deep, applying aloe vera gel topically can speed healing, ease the discomfort, and protect the wound from infection.
- Many elderly people are often not concerned about cooking nutritious meals. In these cases, an easily absorbed, high-quality multi-vitamin/mineral is essential.
- Try Solgar's horse chestnut seed extract, which contains the active ingredient aescin. Aescin has been shown to effectively support venous problems and has the ability to strengthen capillaries and enhance circulation. **SVHC**

Helpful Hints

- Try Bach Rescue Remedy cream once the skin starts to heal. This is available from good health stores.
- Ultra Vein-Gard Leg Therapy Cream contains an herbal combination that includes horse chestnut, butcher's broom (an anti-inflammatory), and more. It helps circulation in the legs and feet.
- Place raw manuka honey on the site of the ulcer, which will speed the healing process. You can also buy honey-containing dressings (made by Advancis) that are easier to use. Available from www.benefitsofhoney.us
- Raise your legs above hip level while resting and slowly move your feet backward and forward to increase the circulation in your lower legs. Try to walk for at least 15 minutes twice a day.
- Regular acupuncture and reflexology will greatly help improve your circulation. (See *Useful Information*.)
- Accu-band makes magnet-filled dressings to place directly over wounds, which have been shown to heal faster with the magnet therapy. Available online from Amazon and other online retailers like www.acu-market.com

LIBIDO PROBLEMS *(see also Adrenal Exhaustion, Impotence, and Stress)*

It is important to remember that everyone has different appetites, and you should not assume you have a "libido problem" just because you do not want sex as often as your friends or people in the media. Moreover, it is quite normal to experience a decline in desire as the years go by. Other pleasures shared with your partner, equally fulfilling, may take the place of sex, which then occasionally surfaces at moments of great tenderness, romance, or nostalgia.

Libido is only a problem, as such, when an otherwise harmonious couple has sexual needs that are wildly different. As always, a compromise is a good solution—one partner trying harder to get in the mood and the other trying to reduce high demands.

Impotence in men and frigidity in women are extreme cases of lowered libido, where one or the other partner cannot or does not wish to perform.

Dr Keith Scott-Mumby, a British doctor living in Los Angeles, says: "Without doubt, the single biggest factor that impairs sexual performance is poor general health. Conditions as varied as obesity, hypertension, stress, digestive disorders, depression, and alcoholism will all result in lessened interest in sex. The number one turn-off for everyone is stress. Living a life full of worry, with an uncertain or threatening future, is bound to result in lowered libido."

Certain prescription drugs, such as statins and drugs for high blood pressure, are also known to affect libido. Dr Mumby also points to the natural age-related decline in sexual function: "Hormone levels fall off slowly at first, but by the fifth decade this natural slow-down process accelerates. Women experience a dramatic shift at menopause. Men suffer a more gradual process that is widely overlooked, known as the andropause. Beyond menopause, lowered estrogen levels for women may result in vaginal dryness and soreness. This obviously interferes with sexual desire and performance. The onset of andropause for men is an indicator of diminishing testosterone levels, and this leads to loss of libido. Interestingly, healthy women also need low levels of natural testosterone that drives their libido."

Foods to Avoid

- If you have become overweight, make an effort to lose weight, as it helps men and women feel sexier and look better. (See *Weight Problems*.)
- Avoid refined carbohydrates, refined sugars, high-sodium foods, and the saturated fats found in red meat, full-fat dairy products, sausages, chocolates, and other manufactured and pre-packaged foods.
- Eliminate caffeine and drink only organic decaf or, better still, herbal teas, and low-sugar or diluted fruit juices.
- Reduce your alcohol intake to 14 drinks a week or less for men and 7 drinks or less for women. Remember Shakespeare's words: "Alcohol promotes the desire but takes away the performance." (See under *Alcohol*.)

Friendly Foods

- Pumpkin and sunflower seeds, Brazil nuts, flaxseeds, and oysters are rich in zinc, which is vital for a healthy sex life.
- Include garlic and onions in your diet to improve circulation and lower LDL, the "bad" cholesterol.
- Sprinkle cayenne pepper and turmeric over your food to add spice to your life; you can also take them in tincture or capsule form.
- Eat more fresh fruits and vegetables, and replace red meat with fresh fish and chicken.
- See *General Health Hints*.

Useful Remedies

- Take 80mg of pycnogenol, pine bark extract, daily plus the amino acid arginine (500mg twice daily away from food), as both encourage nitrous oxide production that relaxes blood vessels and improves blood flow to the reproductive organs. **NB: If you suffer from regular cold sores, arginine may trigger an attack.**
- The above formula, if taken over time, acts as a natural form of Viagra. Prelox from Life Extension contains both. **LEF**
- Taking 500–1000mg of Korean ginseng a day helps reduce the underlying stress that is often linked to this problem. This is shown to be more effective when taken for a month, then stopped for a month and so on. (See under *Stress*.)
- Several brands like make NSI make libido formulas containing ashwagandha and other herbs known to help libido. **VC**
- Damiana, an herb from Mexico and India, is a natural aphrodisiac for men and women. Planetary Formulas makes a Damiana-Sarsaparilla formula called Damiana Male Potential that is available through a number of online retailers
- Stress reduces B vitamins in the body; therefore, also include a good-quality multi-vitamin/mineral for men that includes a full range of B vitamins.
- Zinc and magnesium are often low in young men with libido problems.
- Muira puama, a South American herb, is considered nature's most potent Viagra. A daily dose

of 1g of a standardized extract has been shown to effectively raise testosterone levels. In one study of 100 men with impotence problems, 66% had increased frequency of intercourse, while 70% reported intensification of libido. The stability of the erection was restored in 55% of the patients, and 66% reported a reduction in fatigue. The herb is suitable for both men and women.

- The herb maca has been found to improve libido in men and women, as it helps balance hormone levels, so if the problem is hormonal try taking one capsule three times daily (500mg).

Helpful Hints

- Measures to alleviate stress are often very effective, so exercise regularly and learn to laugh more. This releases natural endorphins, which lower stress levels and help you feel more positive. Learn to breathe more deeply.
- If there is a problem, you must talk about it openly with your significant other. If one partner's needs are not being met it, can lead to frustration and even hostility. It is unfair to put your partner in a position where he/she has no ethical means of satisfying his/her physical desires.
- Quit smoking. Smoking has been linked with a reduced ability to maintain an erection, because it constricts the blood flow that is essential for erectile function.
- Ylang ylang, rose, and jasmine therapeutic oils applied to the lower abdomen area can help revive a flagging sex drive in men and women.
- Men who use a large amount of marijuana or take steroids may also find their erectile function diminished.
- By constantly worrying about your lack of sex drive, you often make the situation worse.
- Studies show that a lack of vitamins C, E, A, and B and the minerals zinc and selenium can cause a low sperm count and lack of sex drive. Anyone taking regular antidepressants or sleeping pills may be lacking in these nutrients.
- Have your hormone levels checked via blood or saliva tests. Testosterone patches are known to help increase libido in both sexes. Once hormones are restored sex drive often returns. (Also see *Menopause*.)
- If the condition continues, or you are worried about infertility as well as impotency, see a doctor who is also a nutritionist. (See *Useful Information*.)
- For help contact The Male Health Center at 1-972-420-8500 or visit www.malehealthcenter.com
- Acupuncture can also help with poor libido by unblocking energy channels within the body, which helps increase blood flow. (See *Useful Information*.)
- Discuss whatever turns you on with your partner. If you find that difficult, discuss sex in general until you are more comfortable with this topic. To help get you in the mood, try watching a sexy movie, which works for many people!
- Try reading *His Needs Her Needs—Building an Affair-Proof Marriage* by Willard F Harley, Jr or take a look at the website: www.marriagebuilders.com
- Try reading *Maximize Your Vitality and Potency: For Men Over 40* by Jonathan V. Wright, MD or visit the website: www.tahoma-clinic.com

LICHEN PLANUS

(see also Immune Function)

Lichen planus is a chronic condition of the skin and mucous membranes, typically the lining of the mouth. This is thought to be caused by a virus and has some features in common with other skin problems, such as eczema and psoriasis. Sores on the skin are often localized to the wrist and ankles, but they can be widespread. Basically, the more you can support your immune system, the less likely you are to suffer from this problem.

Foods to Avoid

- Anything that weakens the immune system, such as concentrated sugars, refined carbohydrates, concentrated fruit juices, and any food that you have an intolerance to, should be strictly avoided.
- Foods that are a problem for many sufferers are tomatoes, pineapples, mushrooms, coffee, red meat, chocolate, and ice cream. Keep a food diary and note when symptoms are worse so you can identify and remove those foods from your diet.
- Alcohol, vinegars, and oily, spicy foods can make the problem worse—avoid them.
- Avoid dairy products from cows as much as possible, as this can create an inflammatory response in the gut because they are hard to digest.

Friendly Foods

- Eat more fresh fish of any kind, but try to make it oily fish, such as organic-farmed salmon, black cod, pilchards, sardines, or mackerel. Oily fish are rich in omega-3 essential fats and vitamin A. Aim for twice a week.
- Natural-source beta-carotene converts naturally to vitamin A in the body and aids soft tissue healing. Therefore, eat plenty of carrots, green vegetables, French beans, watercress, spinach, cantaloupe melons, spring greens, sweet potatoes, papaya, apricots (fresh and dried), pumpkin, butternut squash, parsley, and mangoes. A little butter is also fine since it is rich in vitamin A, but organic is best.
- Organic unrefined and unsalted nuts and seeds, such as sunflower seeds, pumpkin seeds, sesame seeds, flaxseeds, Brazil nuts, and walnuts, are high in zinc, which can speed up healing.

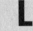

Useful Remedies

- Take 10,000IU of vitamin A daily for up to 1 month, as there is speculation that lichen planus is due to a vitamin A deficiency. After this, change to a natural-source carotene supplement that is non-toxic and will convert naturally into vitamin A in the body. **NB: If you are pregnant or planning to become pregnant, only take 3000IU daily**.
- Take a good-quality multi-vitamin/mineral.
- Olive leaf extract is anti-viral and boosts immunity. Take 500mg twice daily with food.
- Take 30mg of zinc in addition to the multi once a day. Zinc and vitamin A are complementary in their actions. Zinc is essential for wound healing and a healthy immune system.
- Organic aloe vera juice, taken before every meal, speeds up healing and reduces discomfort, as well as boosting the immune system.
- Other anti-viral herbs are echinacea, licorice, and St John's wort.

Helpful Hints

- Try to rest as much as possible. Don't overwork and don't over-stress your system, as it is much harder for the body to heal.
- Use laundry detergents that are suitable for sensitive skin.
- Ultraviolet light often brings relief, but only try this under proper supervision.
- Moderate amounts of sunshine can help, too, but avoid sunbathing between 11am and 3pm.
- Chickweed ointment has been useful to some people.
- Homeopathy has helped many sufferers. (See *Useful Information*.)

LIVER PROBLEMS

Your liver is the most overworked organ in the body, having to break down all of the ever-increasing amounts of toxins found in our environment (including our air and water) and our food. The liver is, in essence, the chemical factory of your body, building or recycling substances you need for good health and breaking down those you don't. If your liver isn't functioning properly, toxins that would normally be filtered out by the liver accumulate in the body. Most people's livers work only at around 35–40% of their potential capacity because of the large amount of toxins we ingest. When it's working properly, though, the liver can clean up to 99% of bacteria and toxins from the blood. Around 4 pints (2.25 liters) of blood pass through the liver every minute for detoxification, and every day the liver manufactures about 2 pints (1 liter) of bile to help carry away toxins via the bowel.

The liver's capacity to eliminate toxins effectively varies widely between individuals. Part of this may be genetic, or linked to exposure to a wide range of pollutants, viruses, and parasites. The rest is due to lifestyle and diet.

Typical symptoms of a sluggish liver are: feeling constantly tired even though you have slept, nausea (especially after a fatty meal or alcohol), skin disorders (such as acne, eczema and psoriasis), muscle and joint pain, age spots on the skin, and/or regular infections. Also, most people don't associate being constipated with poor liver function, but blood from the bowel first goes to the liver, via the portal venous system, hence a bowel loaded with junk is going to overwork the liver.

Other symptoms of poor liver function can include yellowing of the whites of the eyes, yellow-looking skin, fever, nausea, difficulty digesting fatty foods, and an increased sensitivity to cigarette smoke, strong perfume, gasoline, and other chemicals.

Because the brain is unable to disarm a wide range of toxins, it relies on the liver to clean the blood before it gets there. So, over the long term, an under-performing liver can have dire consequences for the brain and nervous system, including memory loss, Parkinson's disease, and Alzheimer's disease.

While detoxification is the key function of the liver, it also produces bile to aid fat digestion (as well as eliminate toxins), manufactures and balances hormones, stores various vitamins and minerals, assembles amino acids, makes cholesterol, controls glucose and fat supplies, and plays a key role in immunity.

Your digestive system is closely involved in the health of your liver, as the blood from your digestive system, where nutrients are absorbed from your food, goes directly to the liver for filtering before it goes anywhere else in the body. If your diet is good and your digestion and absorption are working well, then the nutrients needed for good health will make it to the liver and then into the body. However, if your digestive system is generally toxic, thanks to a poor, low-nutrient, high-fat diet, constipation, poor gut flora, a leaky gut and so on, these toxins and any others you ingest will similarly be delivered directly to your liver, adding to its workload.

The good news is that the liver is capable of regenerating itself, so with a good diet and lifestyle and the right supplements there is no reason why you can't maintain liver function at an optimal level at any age. And if you look after your liver, your skin literally glows with health.

Begin by eliminating as many unnatural chemicals as possible from your home and environment. Keep in mind that many man-made chemicals (especially in plastics and pesticides) have a hormone-like effect within the body. That is why the incidence of hormone-related cancers (including breast, ovarian, testicular, and prostate cancer) are all increasing. These chemicals are commonly found in plastic food packaging, non-organic food, plastics and laminates, synthetic fabrics (clothes, carpets, and furniture), dry-cleaning chemicals, air "fresheners" (a misnomer as most of them poison the air), cosmetics, paints, glues, food additives, medicines, household cleaning products, and wallpaper… but the list is virtually endless, and they are all around us.

You could drive yourself crazy trying to avoid all these things, but you would be surprised to learn how many healthier, safer alternatives to all the above are available if you are willing to seek them out.

Foods to Avoid

- Avoid excess alcohol, which is a liver toxin. One to two drinks per day are generally considered not harmful, although the best gauge is how you feel afterward or the next day. If you feel worse than you should, your liver is probably struggling to detoxify the alcohol.
- Reduce your consumption of non-organic foods as much as possible, as certain foods (such as lettuces) are often sprayed up to 11 times with pesticides and/or fungicides before they are harvested.
- When you can't avoid non-organic fruits and vegetables, wash them thoroughly.

If you're trying to detox or suspect your liver is under-functioning, avoid eating or drinking grapefruit. It contains naringenin, a compound known to slow liver detoxification. A glass of grapefruit juice can significantly affect the action of some medications, which explains why some very expensive medications are prescribed with grapefruit juice: it slows down the body's ability to remove the drug, thus increasing its efficacy.

- Avoid eating excessive protein, as protein metabolism gives the liver a lot of work to do. Generally reduce your animal-protein (meat, chicken, dairy) intake, and increase the amount of vegetable protein in your diet from beans, lentils, nuts, seeds, and fermented soy products, such as tempeh or miso, plus whole grains, such as brown rice.
- Reduce your intake of saturated fats, especially hydrogenated or trans-fats, as well as fried and highly processed foods. Don't avoid all fat, as essential fats found in oily fish and seeds are vital for proper liver function. (See *Fats You Need To Eat*.)
- Refined foods that contain fructose should be avoided.
- Caffeine, acetaminophen (Tylenol), aspirin, and most other medications place a strain on the liver. A good alternative to coffee is dandelion coffee, available in health food stores.
- Melted cheese is very difficult for the liver to process, so avoid it as much as possible. This unfortunately means that pizza should also be avoided.
- Eggs are an excellent source of nutrients, but they are hard to digest for anyone with liver problems. Keep it down to two a week.
- Avoid eating heavy meals and/or fried foods with alcohol at all costs.

Friendly Foods

- Increase your intake of all fruit and vegetables, especially those rich in antioxidants, such as organic carrots, sweet potato, pumpkin, papaya, mangoes, alfalfa sprouts, and watercress.
- Eat more berries, grapes, Brussels sprouts, and kale. Aim for 40% of your diet to be raw during the summer. This is not nearly as hard as it sounds if you eat plenty of fresh fruit and salads.
- Eat more globe artichokes, radicchio, black cherries, pears, and celeriac, all of which help support the liver.
- Eat more raw or cooked beets. They are one of the best vegetables for the liver because they aid digestion, improve liver function, and reduce constipation.
- Also include sulfur-rich foods in your diet, such as garlic, onions, leeks, asparagus, cabbage, and broccoli.

- Sprinkle 2 teaspoons of lecithin granules over breakfast cereals, fruits, and yogurts, as lecithin helps the body digest fats, which eases the burden on the liver.
- If you know that your liver is a problem, eat lighter meals regularly and avoid heavy, rich meals. If you eat too much at one sitting, especially fatty or fried foods and alcohol, then you place an enormous burden on your digestive system and liver, which could make you feel nauseous.
- Foods that naturally raise glutathione levels in the body are fresh asparagus, avocado, and walnuts. Spinach and tomatoes are also great foods for raising glutathione, but they need to be eaten raw.
- Curcumin, the pigment that gives the spice turmeric its yellow color, has been shown to greatly increase glutathione production. Found in curries and mustards, curcumin also has anti-inflammatory properties. For the best effect, toast the curcumin seeds and then lightly grind them before adding them to foods. Otherwise take pure curcumin capsules. **LEF** Curcumin may reduce the effectiveness of Phase 1 liver detoxification processes in some people. If you are unsure, take a urine or saliva Sensitive Liver Pathway Test available through Genova Diagnostics. Tel: 1-800-522-4762 or 1-828-253-0621. Website: www.genovadiagnostics.com
- Eat organically produced food as much as possible. The US Department of Agriculture acknowledges that pesticide residues are considerably lower in organic food than in conventional produce.

Useful Remedies

- As always, start with a good-quality multi-vitamin/mineral, which provides a nutrient foundation you can then add to. Make sure it contains the 15–30mg of zinc needed to make liver enzymes. Many multi-vitamins now also contain most of the nutrients below.
- Take 1g of vitamin C plus bioflavonoids daily.
- Take 1g of fish oil or one flaxseed oil capsule daily. Make sure the fish oil you buy is free from toxins such as PCBs and dioxins.
- Magnesium is required by literally hundreds of enzymes throughout the body, many of which work to aid detoxification. Take at least 500mg daily in divided doses; twice that if you have a backache, twitching, and/or can't sleep.
- The best-known remedy for the liver is the herb milk thistle, which contains the bioflavonoid silymarin. This promotes cell regeneration in the liver, increases levels of glutathione, and has been shown to repair liver damage from alcohol. For optimum effects, you will need to take 600mg of standardized extract daily in divided doses with food.
- The most powerful antioxidant and detoxifying compound in the liver is glutathione, a naturally occurring amino acid combination. Unfortunately it is not particularly well absorbed via capsules; however, by taking alpha-lipoic acid (50–100mg a day) and N-acetyl cysteine (500mg a day in between meals), you can help increase the natural production of glutathione in the liver. Your body also needs B vitamins and selenium to make glutathione.
- Another key nutrient needed by the liver is sulfur. It can be supplemented as MSM or the amino acids cysteine and methionine. Take 500mg of all three daily. Also include sulfur-rich foods in your diet, such as garlic, onions, leeks, asparagus, cabbage, and broccoli.
- The B-group vitamins choline and inositol prevent the accumulation of fat in the liver, thereby enhancing general liver function. Take 300–400mg of each, 1–3 times per day.

Helpful Hints

- Standard tests for liver function (see above under Genova Tests) involve measuring levels of key enzymes. If they are raised, it means that your liver is struggling. This indicates a chronic problem and, while it's useful for letting you know that a problem exists, it doesn't tell you the best way to recover. A better, non-invasive test that is available through nutritionists is a comprehensive Liver Detoxification Profile. This urine test tells you exactly which detox phases and pathways in the liver are under-performing, and you can then be advised which nutrients are needed to restore normal function. To find a qualified nutritionist, see *Useful Information*.

■ Stop smoking, and reduce the amount of time you spend in traffic. There can be more pollution inside your car than outside! If you are walking or cycling, avoid busy roads whenever possible.

■ Indoor air pollution is now recognized as a real problem, and the availability of more natural household-cleaning products, paints, and fibers has improved dramatically in recent years. Visit your local health food store for natural cleaning products such as Ecover.

■ Use a water filter to remove unwanted chemicals from your drinking supply. Reverse osmosis (RO) filters remove 99.999% of all known chemicals. RO water will even filter anthrax spores. For details about RO water, visit www.freedrinkingwater.com (Tel: 1-800-880-4808) or www.waterfiltersonline.com

■ Otherwise, consider using Kangen Water—a filtering device that attaches to your kitchen faucet and ionizes and greatly alkalizes water. It has been used in Japanese hospitals with highly beneficial health results. For full details, visit www.kangenwaterusa.com

■ Another good option is to drink bottled natural mineral water. Volvic or Fiji bottled water are the preferred choice of many nutritionists. A filter jug containing a simple carbon filter is the bare minimum, but don't forget to change the cartridges regularly.

■ Because the liver is responsible for balancing hormones, if it's not working efficiently, hormones can accumulate inappropriately or become unbalanced, triggering problems such as facial hair. Also many women who take the contraceptive pill and orthodox HRT put on weight, which could be because these hormones place a greater strain on the liver.

■ According to traditional Chinese medicine, the liver does most of its work between 1 and 3am. Liver dysfunction will often wake a person up at these times.

■ The liver detoxes more efficiently when we are lying down and relaxed, so make sure you are getting sufficient sleep.

■ Don't eat large meals late at night or drink alcohol after 11pm if you know your liver is in trouble.

■ Repressed anger and resentment affects liver function, so deal with any stress-type issues.

■ Coffee enemas have long been known to stimulate liver function, as they increase bile flow from the liver and gallbladder and aid detoxification. A great book to read is *Tired or Toxic?* by Sherry Rogers (Prestige Publishing).

LOW BLOOD PRESSURE (hypotension)

(see also Adrenal Exhaustion, Low Blood Sugar, Panic Attacks, and Stress)

The most classic symptom of low blood pressure is a feeling of light-headedness on standing, especially from the ground up. It is more common in women. It may be triggered by hereditary factors whereby the blood vessels may have lost their integrity. (This is basically the opposite of high blood pressure, in which the arteries become stiff.)

Orthodox doctors in the US do not think low blood pressure is a problem; however, in certain European countries the condition is often treated. Because the blood is responsible for carrying oxygen and nutrients to the body's tissues and organs, low blood pressure can often trigger problems with energy levels and mental function. The condition is frequently a sign of weakness in the adrenal glands (see under Adrenal Exhaustion). These glands sit on top of your kidneys and play an important role in your hormonal system. Adrenal weakness is often a result of being over-worked and excessively stressed and is compounded by dietary deficiencies. Far too many of us have a lifestyle that over-stresses our adrenal glands. We work too many hours, don't get sufficient sleep, and tend to rely on coffee, sugar, and refined carbohydrates to get us through the day or to pick us up when our energy levels drop off. In the long term, all of these factors weaken adrenal function.

One of the most common complaints received by staff in health food stores these days is of "feeling tired all the time." The first question you need to ask yourself is: do you start the day with a good breakfast, or do you find that you can't face breakfast and the only thing that gets you going is two or three cups of tea or coffee? What you are doing is putting a stimulant into your body that adds more stress on your adrenal glands.

Foods to Avoid
- Caffeine and refined sugar in any form will particularly deplete the adrenal glands. Remember that tea, coffee, chocolate and soda all contain caffeine. You might remember not to put sugar in your tea or coffee, but are you having several cookies with it?
- Refined foods, such as mass-produced breads, cookies, cakes, pizza, burgers, and pies, all deplete the body of the B vitamins necessary to keep the adrenal glands in good shape.

Friendly Foods
- Eat more quality protein, such as fresh fish, chicken, lentils, beans, pulses, and tempeh. Protein helps normalize blood sugar, which will in turn help stabilize blood pressure. (See under *Adrenal Exhaustion*.)
- Hemp seed proteins or whey protein are useful sources of quality protein. (See *General Health Hints* for a great breakfast smoothie recipe.)
- Whole grains, which include brown rice, quinoa, spelt, buckwheat, millet, and amaranth, are highly nutritious.
- Eat plenty of fresh fruit and vegetables, particularly fresh juices. If you are feeling low on energy, rather than reaching for a coffee, try a glass of carrot, beet, apple, and ginger juice.
- Green tea has a small amount of caffeine, which will give you a boost, and contains many health benefits. Or you can try ginseng or licorice teas, which will support your adrenal glands.
- Eat more avocados and wheat germ, which are rich in vitamin E.
- Use potassium- and magnesium-based salt, such as Solo Sea Salt, in your diet. BioForce (A. Vogel) also makes excellent herbal salts. Nori flakes or powered kelp from health stores are high in easy-to- utilize minerals.
- Licorice is one of simplest ways to restore your adrenal glands to their normal function. Look for pure licorice sweetened with molasses; sold in most health stores.

Useful Remedies
- An advanced stress formula by Jarrow—Adrenal Optimizer—contains licorice, Siberian ginseng and more, which can help nourish the adrenals. Take 1.5 teaspoons daily in a little water. **JF**
- Take a high-potency B-complex twice daily with meals. Take B vitamins with breakfast and lunch, not with supper, as they keep you more alert.
- Ginseng (1–3g a day for 60 days) helps balance the body. If your blood pressure is low, ginseng can help to bring it back up. Ginseng also has the added benefit of being an excellent adrenal restorative.
- Try Dr Christopher's Blood Circulation capsules (www.drchristophers.com), which contain ginger, cayenne, and hawthorn. These help normalize blood pressure (high or low); take 1 or 2 capsules three times daily with meals. **NB: Anyone suffering from heart problems must check with a doctor before taking any supplement containing hawthorn.**

Helpful Hints

- Do sensible amounts of exercise, but also make sure you are getting sufficient rest.
- See *General Health Hints*.
- See *Adrenal Exhaustion and Stress*.

LOW BLOOD SUGAR (hypoglycemia)

(see also Adrenal Exhaustion, Insulin Resistance, and Low Blood Pressure)

Low blood sugar, also known as hypoglycemia, is something that 95% of us experience at some time if we go without food for too long. The most common cause is skipping breakfast. I have met a number of young women who suffer from occasional blackouts, fainting spells, and dizziness that their doctor cannot explain. But when they tell me about their diet of missed meals and sugary drinks and snacks, I know almost immediately what the problem is. As these symptoms are also common with *Adrenal Exhaustion*, see this section as well.

The level of sugar in the blood is critical to how you feel. If it is too low, you may feel very tired, find concentration difficult, become shaky, feel very hungry and drowsy, possibly have headaches, and feel anxious. These myriad symptoms can simply result from skipping breakfast. If you are one of those people who won't eat breakfast for the sake of an extra 15 to 20 minutes in bed, or simply can't face it in the mornings before rushing off to work, by mid-morning you are going to feel even hungrier than you did when you left the house. Most people then reach for coffee, tea, snacks, and cookies, something that will quickly raise blood sugar levels. Unfortunately, not long after consuming this type of food, our blood sugar drops even lower than it was before. This is a result of the body producing an excess of insulin to compensate for the sugar load. One of the problems with skipping breakfast is that even if your first meal of the day (lunch) is a good wholesome one, your blood sugar levels are still likely to remain erratic. This can cause you to become irritable with your colleagues or extremely emotional in response to even small problems.

Other people with low blood sugar will find it crucial to have their meals at regular times. If their lunch hour is normally midday and someone asks them to wait until 2pm, they may feel weak, suffer memory problems, or simply find it hard to concentrate.

The brain's only food source is pure glucose and, if you have not eaten for a while, the hypothalamus area within the brain will just demand more sugar. Basically, if your hypothalamus is not happy, no amount of willpower will stop you from craving something sweet. Nutritionists have known for years that the easiest way to control blood sugar is to eat small, healthy, low-glycemic meals more regularly, but most people don't do this. The average person in the West eats 35lb of snacks a year, which causes weight gain and very unstable blood sugar levels. The result is a huge increase in diabetes. As symptoms of low blood sugar are similar to those of high blood sugar (diabetes), have a check-up with your doctor. However, a single blood test is unlikely to show any problem with low blood sugar because, unless you are actually suffering a dip in blood sugar at the time of the test, the results will probably come back normal. (See also *Insulin Resistance*.)

Foods to Avoid

- Most people with low blood sugar rush from one sugar fix to the next. In extreme cases they might eat 6–8 chocolate-type snacks a day. Cravings for caffeine, sugar, and refined carbohydrates, such as croissants, cookies, pastries, and pizza are all common. Not only do all of these foods have a negative effect on blood sugar, they are also low in fiber, vitamins, and minerals.

- See under *Adrenal Exhaustion.*

Friendly Foods

- Fiber helps slow down the release of sugars, and if absent, the sugars in any foods get into the bloodstream too quickly. Great fibers are flaxseeds (soaked overnight in cold water and drained), oat or rice bran, sunflower seeds, and psyllium husks.
- Begin the day with a good breakfast, such as low-sugar muesli or cereal, oatmeal, or eggs.
- Eat more raw foods, such as carrots, cucumbers, tomatoes, celery, fruits, and so on, because they are high in insoluble fiber.
- If you have time for only a small meal, try to make sure it is high in protein rather than carbohydrates, which will keep you more satisfied in the long term. (See *General Health Hints* for a delicious smoothie recipe made with hemp seed protein powder.)
- If your blood sugar drops too low, not only can you feel faint, but you are also more likely to suffer a panic-type attack. At the very least, eat a banana with a handful of sunflower or pumpkin seeds (to slow the sugar rush) and a low-fat fruit yogurt. Carry almonds with you to munch on.
- Eat more brown rice, barley, oats, lentils, buckwheat, sweet potatoes, amaranth, spelt and whole-wheat bread and pastas; also try corn, spinach, and rice pastas. *The Lo-GL Diet* by Patrick Holford (Piatkus Publishing) lists low glycemic foods.
- As more natural alternatives to refined sugars, use small amounts of organic agave or brown rice syrup, or try xylitol-based sweeteners.

- Make sure you eat a portion of good-quality protein with each meal—such as fish, lean meats, chicken, turkey, cooked tofu or eggs—or use whey or hemp seed protein powders.
- Eat smaller meals more regularly.
- Snack on fresh fruit, such as apples, apricots, cherries, pomegranate, berries, and papaya, or on low-sugar snack bars available from your local health store. You can also try low-fat humus, avocado, or goat's cheese on an amaranth cracker or rye crisp bread.
- Drink freshly made or organic vegetable juices.
- Snack on low-fat yogurts with added sunflower or pumpkin seeds to reduce sugar cravings.
- Have a piece of whole-wheat toast or an amaranth cracker with a little low-fat spread and low-sugar jam.
- Drink more herbal teas and pure dandelion coffee. **NB: Some brands contain 50% lactose, which is a form of sugar.**
- Drink more water.
- Make salad dressings with a combination of any unrefined organic oils, such as sesame, walnut, olive, or sunflower.
- Essential fats help sustain energy levels and help balance blood sugar. (See *Fats You Need To Eat.*)

Useful Remedies

- Lipoic acid helps stabilize blood sugar (take 200mg daily) while also supporting brain function, which can be a problem with low blood sugar.
- US studies have shown that when people who eat a refined Western diet are given 200mcg of the mineral chromium twice daily, the incidence of late-onset diabetes is halved. Chromium is greatly depleted in the body by sugar and junk foods. Once you cut down on sugar and white carbohydrates, you may crave sweet foods. Therefore, begin taking 400mcg of chromium daily. It takes a few days to kick in, but it really does help reduce cravings. After two weeks reduce to 200mcg.

- Take 200–500mg of magnesium spread throughout the day with food. Magnesium helps regulate blood-sugar levels.
- Take a strong B-complex with 30mg of niacin (B3). **NB: Make sure it's a no-flush-type niacin, as niacin can cause skin flushing.)** Vitamin B3 is essential for the control of blood-sugar levels.
- Take full-spectrum, natural-source vitamin E (400IU daily). Vitamin E has been shown to help improve insulin response in the body.
- NSI makes Synergy GlucoPower, which contains all the above nutrients and much more in one formula. **VC**

Helpful Hints

- If you suffer from acute symptoms such as fainting spells, blackouts, extreme weakness, and trembling, it is important to restore blood-sugar levels as quickly as possible. In an emergency, you need to get glucose into your body. While I would generally not recommend high-sugar foods and drinks, this is one occasion when you can use them. Drink Gatorade or something similar, or eat a sugary snack. This is definitely not a long-term solution!
- Talk to a doctor who is also a qualified nutritionist. (See *Useful Information*.)

LOW STOMACH ACID

(see also Acid Stomach, Indigestion, and Leaky Gut)

When we eat food, particularly protein-based foods, our stomachs should produce a lot of gastric juice in response. This juice is a mixture of mucus, which protects the stomach lining, and a very strong acid, hydrochloric acid (HCl). High levels of hydrochloric acid are needed for the production of pepsin, which is essential for proper digestion, before the food moves into the small intestine and the nutrients start to be absorbed. Due to various aspects of our diet, lifestyle, and age, the amount of acid we produce over time tends to decline. Low levels of stomach acid are associated with poor digestion and, more importantly, poor absorption of the nutrients we need for good health.

Conditions strongly linked with low stomach acid levels are asthma, allergies, leaky gut, and gallstones, and low stomach acid can also be a factor in stomach ulcers. When many people have indigestion they blame it on having too much stomach acid; however, in reality, they often produce too little. A lot of people will take an antacid, which neutralizes what little acid was available, making digestion even harder. Undigested foods can end up leaking into the bloodstream, causing food allergies. Undigested food also rots in the bowel, causing gas, bloating, and overgrowth of unhealthy organisms such as candida (see *Candida*).

An easy way to find out if you have low stomach acid is to take a level teaspoon of baking soda, dissolve it in some lukewarm water, and drink well away from food. If sufficient quantities of acid are present in the stomach, the soda mixture will be converted into gas, producing significant bloating and belching within 5–10 minutes of drinking it. Little to no belching signifies low stomach acid levels.

Foods to Avoid

- Cut down on alcohol, sugar, caffeinated drinks, and dairy products made from cow's milk, which all can cause an acid reflux.
- Don't eat in a rush, and keep heavy, rich meals that contain red meat and creamy sauces to a minimum.
- Avoid all fried foods, which are hard to digest.

- Avoid eating proteins, such as fish or meat, with carbohydrates, such as potatoes, rice, or pasta, because the body uses different enzymes for each food group.
- Avoid eating fat and protein together—such as fish and chips—as the fat slows protein digestion, which is the problem with low stomach acid.
- Stop chewing gum. This makes the stomach think that food is about to arrive, which triggers stomach-acid production.
- Avoid eating large amounts of fruit directly after a large meal.

Friendly Foods
- Generally eat fruit in between meals or include a little papaya and pineapple with meals, which are packed with digestive enzymes.
- Bitter-tasting vegetables are great for stimulating digestion. Eat more arugula, artichoke, radicchio, and celeriac, as well as ginger. These foods encourage gastric-juice production.

Useful Remedies
- As levels of stomach acid production tend to drop as we age or when we are under prolonged negative stress, take one betaine hydrochloride (stomach acid) capsule with a glass of water just before your main meals. If you have active stomach ulcers or taking this causes you any discomfort, use a good-quality digestive enzyme that is free from HCl instead. One option is 500mg of bromelain a few minutes before main meals.
- Try taking 10–20 drops of peppermint oil before a meal. If you feel bloated and uncomfortable after eating, take 10–20 drops after finishing your meal. **VC**
- Acidophilus and bifidus are the healthy bacteria in your gut that help regulate digestion. Take one capsule daily at the end of your main meal. I recommend Jarro-Dophilus EPS made by Jarrow Formulas. **JF**
- B vitamins and zinc are needed to help the body naturally produce more stomach acid. Take a multi-vitamin/mineral formula daily for your age and gender that contains at least 30mg of zinc.

Helpful Hints
- Chewing food thoroughly really helps improve the digestive process. Don't eat on the run.
- Some people have found that not eating proteins and carbohydrates together in the same meal has improved their digestion tremendously.
- Eat small meals regularly; try four snack-type meals daily. Avoid eating while stressed.
- If you have pronounced longitudinal ridges in your nails, this is a common sign of poor nutrient absorption and is often due to low stomach acid
- Drink peppermint, fennel, or fresh mint herbal teas to aid digestion.
- The herb meadowsweet helps regulate low stomach acid. **VC**
- Walking for 30 minutes each day aids digestion.

LUPUS

(see also Adrenal Exhaustion, Leaky Gut, Sjogren's Syndrome and Stress)

Lupus is an autoimmune condition that triggers inflammation in multiple sites around the body. This condition can take years to manifest and is often missed until symptoms become more apparent. Typical symptoms might include arthritis-type joint pains, skin rashes (especially a "butterfly-like" rash on the face around the nose and cheeks that comes and goes), lowered immune function, and low white and/or red blood cell counts. Lupus sometimes causes "flare ups" of inflammation in the tissues that surround the heart, lungs, and even the brain, but there are widely varying degrees of lupus. The most common and serious form is systemic lupus erythematosus (SLE). Fatigue, depression, low-level fever, eye or gut problems may also be involved. Some people also develop Raynaud's disease (see under *Raynaud's Disease*).

Symptoms usually come and go in a series of flare-ups and remissions and are hugely dependent on the patient's stress levels. An attack can also be precipitated by over-exposure to ultraviolet light or exposure to certain chemicals, such as those found in hair dyes.

A blood test is needed to confirm a diagnosis of lupus. One of the most common forms of orthodox medical treatment is steroid therapy, which can weaken the immune system as well as further exacerbating the osteoporosis that is also seen as a result of lupus.

Lupus requires specialist help from a nutritional physician. However, there are many things you can do to help yourself. As this is a highly multi-factorial condition, it is more than likely that you have eaten foods that you have an intolerance to for years and that was what triggered the initial inflammatory responses. (See under *Candida* and *Leaky Gut*.)

If this situation continues in tandem with an on-going highly stressed lifestyle (or personality type that reacts negatively to stress), then the stress hormones cortisol and adrenaline would, over time, add to the inflammatory burden on the body and contribute to the osteoporosis. Eventually, a combination of these situations could cause the immune system to start attacking itself and conditions such as lupus can arise.

Foods to Avoid

- The most likely trigger for your food intolerances are any foods containing gluten, but it may be cow's milk.
- Oranges, orange juice, and tomatoes may also be a problem.
- Avoid foods from animal sources that are high in saturated fat.
- If you tend to eat lots of "white," refined foods that are high in sugar, these need to be cut down to a minimum since sugar triggers inflammation in the body.
- Alfalfa sprouts and mushrooms are known triggers for some people.
- Avoid refined sugars in any form, including maltose, dextrose, and fructose, which are found in mass-produced cookies, cakes, pies, and so on.
- As your immune system and your gut work more efficiently in an alkaline environment, you need to re-alkalize your system. (See under *Acid–Alkaline Balance*.)
- Certain foods are high in arachidonic acids, which tend to increase inflammation in the body. These include as meats, eggs, and dairy products from animals.
- Cut down on alcohol and caffeine, which encourage cortisol production.

Friendly Foods

- Generally eat more oily fish, such as organic-farmed salmon, sardines, pilchards, mackerel, anchovies, and black cod, for their anti-inflammatory properties.
- Eat more vegetable-based proteins, such as lentils, quinoa, organic tofu, peas, beans, and pulses.
- Use organic-source hemp seed protein powders.
- Eat more brown rice, buckwheat, and non-wheat-based pastas.
- Try non-dairy sources of milks, such as almond, quinoa, rice, and coconut.
- Try avoiding all foods that contain wheat and gluten for a month, and I'll bet that your symptoms will begin to subside. Many supermarkets and health stores now sell gluten- and wheat-free foods.
- Use a little organic agave or brown rice syrup, which have a lower glycemic index, or use xylitol-based sweeteners such as XyloSweet from Higher Nature. **VC**
- Eat more foods rich in carotenes, which are needed for tissue healing. These include pumpkin, watercress, papaya, sweet potato, apricots, mango, spinach, all green vegetables, and carrots.

- White fish, chicken, and turkey are preferable to red meats.
- Eat more nuts and seeds that are high in omega-6 and -3 fats, such as flaxseeds, sunflower seeds, pumpkin seeds, and hemp seeds. You could also use their unrefined oils for salad dressings.
- Drink more green and white teas because they are rich in antioxidants

Useful remedies

- Quercetin, a polyphenol found in garlic, has shown great promise in reducing chronic inflammation because of its effects on C-reactive protein. Lupus sufferers tend to have high levels of C-reactive protein, so take 250mg twice daily with food.
- Gamma-linolenic acid (GLA) is found in evening primrose and borage oil. Take 2–4 500mg capsules daily. **VC**
- Fish oils are essential to dampen inflammation. Take 2–3g of omega-3 fish oil daily.
- Take 400IU of full-spectrum, natural-source vitamin E to help neutralize free radical damage caused by inflammation.
- If you have long-term adrenal exhaustion, you probably need to supplement your levels of the hormone DHEA. Ask your doctor for a blood test to confirm if you have a deficiency, and if so, your doctor will tell you how much you need to take a day. **LEF**
- Include a high-strength multi-vitamin/mineral for your age and gender that includes a full spectrum of the B-group vitamins to support your nerves.
- You will also need a multiple bone support formula that contains calcium, magnesium, D3, boron, K2, and silica. **VC**

- To help re-alkalize your body, try Greens Plus, which contains Hawaiian spirulina, chlorella, lecithin, barley, pectin apple fiber, kelp, soy and barley sprouts, and lactobacillus acidophilus. It is a great all-around way to ingest good nutrients, healthy bacteria, keep the body more alkaline, and help keep you regular. Add it to your breakfast smoothie or just take in water. **GP** (See *General Health Hints* for a healthy smoothie recipe.)
- L-theanine, found in green tea, really helps reduce feelings of stress. (See *Adrenal Exhaustion*.)
- Co-enzyme Q10 will help raise your energy levels. Take 100–200mg daily with breakfast and/or lunch.
- Healthy bacteria known as probiotics help keep the immune system strong and keep candida in check. Take one Jarro-Dophilus EPS capsule daily after a meal. **JF**
- In numerous studies from the US, Hungary, Israel, and Russia a fermented wheat germ extract known as AWGE has demonstrated remarkably beneficial immune-modulating effects. Take one sachet daily in water at least an hour before breakfast. It must be kept refrigerated. Also available in capsules, but you would need quite a few; therefore, the powder is easier to take once a day. For further information visit www.avemarwge.com or e-mail office@biropharmausa.com
- Take a high-strength antioxidant formula that contains vitamin C, carotenes, and bioflavonoids daily.
- Collagen is a vital component of healthy joints, skin, hair, nails, cartilage, ligaments, and tendons, which also improve bone strength. It is the most widely distributed protein in the body and helps signal the body to reduce inflammation. Take one scoop of NeoCell Super Collagen drink daily in a glass of water or diluted juice 30 minutes before a main meal. **VC**

Helpful Hints

- A urine test supplied by Genova Diagnostics (called a Gut Permeability Test) can detect a leaky gut (see below).
- It is really important to have an allergy test to identify any foods/substances that are a

problem. One of the best I have found is available from YorkTest Laboratories; visit www.yorktest.com for more details. Another is a FACT test from Genova Diagnostics, which looks for inflammatory markers that indicate the body is reacting to certain substances. Tel: 1-800-522-4762. Website: www.genovadiagnostics.com

■ Exercise is important, but don't exercise if you are truly exhausted as this can be counterproductive. Gentle walking would be fine.

■ Get some sleep and go to bed before 10pm. Sleep is the best way to heal the body.

■ Deal with negative long-term stress and your reaction to it. (See *Stress*.)

■ Be sensible when it comes to sun exposure.

■ Have your hormones checked, as you may also need progesterone, estrogen, and testosterone as well as DHEA. (See *Menopause*.)

■ Also see *Osteoporosis*.

MACULAR DEGENERATION (see also *Eye Problems*)

Macular degeneration (also known as AMD—aged-related macular degeneration) is the slow deterioration of cells in the macula, a tiny yellowish area in the central part of the retina that is responsible for visual sharpness. More than 10 million people in the US are affected. Macular degeneration is now the leading cause of blindness in people over the age of 55, and 30% of people in the West over the age of 70 have symptoms of AMD—symptoms that increase over time, thus affecting your ability to read, write, drive, and so on.

There are two types of macular degeneration: wet and dry. Ninety percent of people with macular degeneration have the dry type, in which small, yellow spots called drusens form underneath the macular. Drusens are waste products that accumulate because there are not enough antioxidants to clear them from the eyes. The drusens slowly break down the cells in the macula, causing distorted vision. In the wet type, abnormal blood vessels begin to grow toward the macula, causing rapid and severe vision loss.

Scientists believe that AMD is triggered by oxidative stress caused by free radical reactions in the body, especially in the retina because of its high consumption of oxygen. Free radical reactions occur as the normal by-products of living, eating, and breathing, but are also triggered by over-exposure to ultra-violet radiation, smoking, a poor diet ,and a compromised immune system. This condition is also linked to hardening of the arteries and poor circulation (see *Atherosclerosis, High Blood Pressure*, and *Circulation*).

A high homocysteine level (see under *High Blood Pressure*) and low B vitamin intake are associated with an increased risk of AMD, and women with light-colored irises are also more at risk.

Foods to Avoid

■ Cut out full-fat dairy products, plus meats, hamburgers, mass-produced pies, sausages, cheeses, chocolates, and sugary, fatty foods—all the usual suspects.

■ Definitely avoid too many fried foods and hydrogenated or trans- fats, which are found in most margarines and mass-produced vegetable oils. (See *Fats You Need To Eat*.)

- Cut down or eliminate sodium-based salt; instead use natural mineral-based salts, which are available from all good health stores.
- Avoid monosodium glutamate (MSG), which is a potential retinal toxin.
- Avoid excessive alcohol, but the occasional glass of wine is fine. Too much alcohol interferes with liver function and reduces protective glutathione levels in the eyes. (Because glutathione is so important, see *Liver Problems* for more details.)
- Avoid foods and drinks that contain the artificial sweetener aspartame at all costs.

Friendly Foods

- The most important foods for preventing AMD and reducing symptoms are those containing carotenes (especially lutein and zeaxanthin). Lutein is found in all dark green leafy vegetables, such as spinach (raw is best), kale, broccoli, spring greens, watercress, cabbage, and so on. Zeaxanthin is found in yellow and orange fruits and vegetables, such as carrots, peaches, persimmons, pumpkins, sweet potatoes, mangoes, apricots, and cantaloupe melons.
- Saffron is also wonderful as it is high in zeaxanthin. So eat more curries.
- Other great eye foods are onions, apples, green tea, cherries, pears, grapes, cranberries, red onions, garlic, mustard greens, alfalfa sprouts, asparagus, and butternut squash.
- Generally, eat more whole foods, such as stone-ground whole-wheat bread, brown rice, quinoa, and buckwheat.
- Eat more oily fish, and choose white fish over meats.
- Eat more blueberries, bilberries, and blackcurrants.
- In addition, green drinks made from organic grasses, blue-green and sea algae, herbs and other nutrients are very helpful. Most health stores sell excellent organic green-food-based powders.

- Vitamin-E-rich foods help reduce the risk of developing AMD. These include hazelnuts, almonds, cod liver oil, raw wheat germ, avocado, and tomato paste.
- Chicken and turkey (the dark parts of the meat) are high in the amino acid taurine, which is good for the eyes.

Useful Remedies

- Take a high-strength multi-vitamin/mineral daily to create a strong foundation. Make sure your multi contains a full spectrum of B vitamins to control high homocysteine levels, 200mcg of selenium, 30mg of zinc, 100IU of full-spectrum vitamin E, and at least 100mg of vitamin C.
- Vitamin C helps make collagen, which strengthens the capillaries that nourish the retina and protects it from UV light. The eye contains the second highest concentration of vitamin C in the body next to the adrenal glands. Take 1g daily in an ascorbate form with food.
- Bilberry has been called the vision herb for its powerful effect on all types of visual disorders. British Royal Air Force pilots during World War II reported improved night vision after consuming bilberry. The fruit supports the structural integrity of the tiny capillaries that deliver oxygen and nutrients to the eyes. Take 200–300mg daily.
- Bioflavonoids, such as quercetin and rutin, are plant pigments rich in antioxidants that protect the eyes from sunlight damage. Take 1000mg daily of a mixed bioflavonoid supplement.
- Glutathione is essential for vision. This antioxidant is found in large concentrations in the eyes, and if you take 200mg of lipoic acid twice daily, it will help raise your levels of glutathione.
- Cysteine is important for a healthy retina. Taken as N-acetylcysteine (NAC), it also increases production of glutathione. Take 500mg daily half an hour before a meal.
- Taurine is another potent antioxidant that is highly concentrated in the eye, normally within the retina. A deficiency of this amino acid alters the structure and function of the retina. Taurine also helps prevent cataracts. Take 500mg daily.

- If you don't eat plenty of carotene-rich foods, you definitely need to take a high-strength, natural-source carotene complex.
- Most of the companies listed on pages 15–16 make an all-in-one eye formula that contains most of the above.
- Macushield contains good levels of natural-source carotenoids from marigold that are known to support eye health. For more information, contact Douglas Laboratories through their website (www.douglaslabs.com) or by calling 1-800-245-4440.

Helpful Hints
- Make sure to get sufficient exercise, which helps increase circulation.
- Acupuncture can help increase circulation to the eye area, as can Advanced Reflexology. For a therapist near you, visit www.artreflex.com
- When you are out in bright sunshine, always wear a hat or cap and good sunglasses, preferably wrap-around —even when young.
- Don't smoke, which can increase the likelihood of developing AMD by more than 2.5 times.

ME (myalgic encephalomyelitis)

(see also Adrenal Exhaustion, Candida, Leaky Gut, and Low Blood Sugar)

Somewhere between 1 and 4 million Americans are recognized as having chronic fatigue or ME, but I, and my fellow co-authors, believe that hundreds of thousands more go undiagnosed. Many people feel tired all the time and just struggle on, but only when the crushing exhaustion becomes incapacitating do people seek medical help.

Symptoms range from chronic, debilitating tiredness to depression, muscle and joint pain, headaches and decreased concentration, poor sleep quality, low blood pressure, low blood sugar, food cravings, bloating, chemical sensitivities, and night sweats to name but a few. In writing this book I now firmly believe that virtually all ME-type symptoms are linked either to a severe leaky gut and candida or adrenal exhaustion. If you read these three sections, you will be left with no doubt in your mind as to why they appear to mirror virtually all the symptoms associated with ME. And once these issues are addressed, then the ME is often alleviated. Also, if you have suffered from a viral illness, such as the flu, herpes, or mono, are exposed to a lot of electrical equipment, or have running water under your home, any or all of these factors may play a role. ME is also linked to heavy metal toxicity (especially mercury), liver congestion, food intolerance, and deficiencies in minerals such as magnesium. There is also a possible link to parasites.

What helps one person may not work for another, but without a doubt, eating the right diet and taking the right supplements will make a difference. If you contract a viral infection, you must give your body a chance to rest and recover, which gives you more chance of avoiding long-term illness.

Foods to Avoid
- Avoid any foods and drinks that contain caffeine, refined sugar, and alcohol, all of which lower immune function, weaken the adrenal system, and play havoc with blood-sugar levels. Also, most pre-packaged foods that are high in sugar are also high in saturated fats, salt, additives, and preservatives.
- Most mass-produced, canned foods and fast food are lacking in magnesium. Forty percent of ME patients have low levels of this vital mineral.
- Some people mistakenly use guarana (or drinks like Red Bull) as an energy source when they

are very tired. Unfortunately, the primary reason they give you energy is the caffeine content, which will only serve to weaken your adrenal glands in the long term. Never mix Red Bull with alcohol.

- If you find yourself constantly craving foods such as wheat, sugar, and snacks, are bloated, have an urgency to urinate, suffer from mood swings, and are always tired, you may well have candida. (See *Foods to Avoid* under *Candida*.)
- Almost everyone with chronic fatigue will have multiple food intolerances, the most common being gluten from wheat and dairy products from cow's milk. (See under *Allergies*.)

Friendly Foods
- Also see *Insulin Resistance*.
- Essential fats are vital because they support the endocrine system, boost immunity, and help balance blood sugar. Eat more organic sunflower, hemp, pumpkin, and flaxseeds. (See *Fats You Need To Eat*.)
- It is vital that you eat good-quality protein, such as organic lean meat, chicken, fresh fish, or beans, at least twice a day. Protein helps balance blood sugar for longer periods of time.
- Also try organic hemp seed proteins, which are easy to absorb.
- Include plenty of vegetables and fruits in your diet, but don't eat too much fruit if you have candida.
- Generally eat more low-glycemic foods, such as lentils, beans, pulses, millet, quinoa, barley, gluten-free oatmeal, buckwheat, and sweet potato. Nutritionist Patrick Holford's book *The Low-GL Diet Bible* (Piatkus Publishing) offers good lists of low-GI foods,.

- Replace animal-source milks with organic almond, rice, oat, quinoa, pea, or coconut milk.
- Remember to include plenty of cabbage, kale, watercress, spring greens, bok choy, broccoli, celery, wheat germ, Brazil nuts, walnuts, almonds, curries, blackstrap molasses, unprocessed honey, and beans in your diet, as they are rich in magnesium.
- Drink plenty of pure water, even if you are not thirsty, to help detoxify your system.
- Eat sunflower, pumpkin, hemp, sesame, and flaxseeds, which are packed with essential fats and fiber. Also use extra-virgin unrefined olive or sunflower oils for salad dressings.
- Sprinkle cilantro over your food to help detoxify heavy metals from your body. Chlorella does this as well.
- Green tea is high in L-theanine, which helps you relax. Make sure to buy decaffeinated organic green teas.
- Replace refined sugars with organic agave syrup or xylitol, which have minimal impact on blood sugar levels. **VC, VS**

Useful Remedies
- L-carnitine, an amino acid, has been shown to help reduce symptoms of chronic fatigue. Take 500mg twice daily before food spread throughout the day.
- L-carnitine works well with the antioxidant lipoic acid to raise energy levels in the body. Take 200mg of lipoic acid daily.
- Jarrow's advanced stress formula called Adrenal Optimizer contains licorice, Siberian ginseng, ashwaganda, and gotu kola, which help support the adrenal system. **JF**
  NB: This supplement is not suitable for children, pregnant or breast-feeding women, or those with high blood pressure.
- Take magnesium citrate, 600–1000mg per day, which helps reduce muscle soreness. Take in divided doses throughout the day, making sure to take the last 200mg before bed.
- Take a high-strength multi-vitamin/mineral twice daily.
- Beta Glucans 1–3, 1–6, which are derived from yeast cell walls, are proven to strengthen the body's innate immune system (the immune system you are born with), making it more

resistant to pathogens from food and air. Take 250–500mg daily. It can also be taken by children and reduces the likelihood of food intolerances triggered by a weakened immune system. Dr Paul Clayton, based in the UK and US, is a medical pharmacologist. His website contains a great deal of research about Beta Glucans and is well worth a look—www.healthdefence.com **VC**

- Because the body heals more quickly if it is alkaline, take an organic-source green food powder daily, such as Greens Plus powder, which is available from health stores. (See *General Health Hints* for a delicious smoothie recipe.) **GP**
- Co-enzyme Q10 is a vitamin-like substance that is naturally made in the liver; however, it is often depleted in ME patients. Take 100–200mg with breakfast or lunch to give you extra energy. **SVHC**

Helpful Hints

- Get some quality rest; it's nature's way of healing. Go to bed by 10pm.
- Do some gentle exercise. One study found that people with chronic fatigue were able to walk for 3 minutes and then rest for 3 minutes until they had walked for a total of 30 minutes, without any negative effects.
- Try a gentle stretching program to tone your muscles gradually and help drain the lymph system, which is often overloaded.
- Learn to relax. Meditation is a great way to give the body and brain a complete rest.
- If you want more information about being checked for parasites, which are often linked to ME, see details of Genova Laboratory's tests under IBS (*Irritable Bowel Syndrome*).

- Have a friend massage your aching muscles with a mix of thyme and lemongrass essential oils. To help lift depression, try a mix of neroli and rose in a good base oil.
- For a free introductory brochure, or for more help, contact the CFIDS Association of America by calling 1-704-365-2343, e-mailing cfids@cfids.org, or visiting www.cfids.org
- If your symptoms persist, try having your house dowsed for electrical or geopathic stress. To find a dowser, contact the American Society of Dowsers (www.dowsers.org).
- Cranial osteopathy has helped many people with ME, as it frees up nerve endings, which releases energy in the body. (See *Useful Information*.)
- Hands-on healing, such as Reiki, has proven very successful for many ME patients. (See *Healing and Healers*.)
- If you have ME it is best to consult a doctor who is also a qualified nutritionist, as you may need injections of magnesium and B12. (See *Useful Information*.)

MEMORY

(see also Alzheimer's Disease, Atherosclerosis, Circulation, Parkinson's Disease, and Stress)

At the age of 61 I regularly forget people's names and where I left certain objects—we all do. And just because you forget a few things doesn't automatically mean that you have Alzheimer's or dementia, so don't panic. Most people think that once a brain cell dies, it's gone for ever, but it's now known that brain cells can and do regenerate.

Just like our muscles, the brain needs regular use—and if you don't use it, you lose it. The secret to improving your memory is to keep your brain active and to eat less junk food and more super-brain foods. However, your brain also requires quality and sufficient sleep in order to function at an optimal level. Anyone who has experienced jet lag or lost a night's sleep knows how this can affect your ability to stay sharp.

There really is no need for your memory or brain function to decline with age. My mother-in-law died at 95, and her brain was as sharp as a razor, as she had spent 30 years regularly completing crosswords.

Temporary memory loss is not uncommon after drinking alcohol, if your blood sugar level is low, after a high fever, following surgery, after an epileptic seizure, or when you are under stress. Depression and acute anxiety can also cause temporary memory loss. More serious memory loss can occur after an accident, brain injury, or stroke. Senile dementia involves progressive loss of short-term memory until the individual is unable to remember what they did or saw only a few moments before. The long-term use of many prescription drugs, such as statins, sleeping pills and/or drug "cocktails" (like those used by people who are taking pills for high blood pressure, cholesterol, and so on), affect memory. External influences, such as poor eyesight and hearing, can also inhibit our ability to learn—thus affecting memory.

However, the vast majority of cases of poor memory are caused by years of eating too much of the wrong foods, especially saturated fats, which clog the arteries until the small capillaries are affected, preventing sufficient fresh, red blood from reaching the brain, depriving it of oxygen. Simply taking a deep breath every 20 minutes or so can help improve brain function.

Lead is well known for its effects on memory, which is why unleaded gasoline was introduced on both environmental and health grounds. Mercury fillings are also linked to memory loss (see *Mercury Fillings*). A high level of homocysteine, a by-product of protein metabolism, can trigger memory loss-type problems. (See under *Alzheimer's Disease* for full details.)

Foods to Avoid

- If you want to keep your memory sharp, you need to cut down on high-fat foods, such as meat and full-fat dairy products. Also avoid mass-produced pies, cakes, cookies, white bread, pizzas, burgers, and so on, which not only deplete nutrients but also contribute to clogging your arteries. Research shows that people who eat high-fat, nutrient-poor foods, such as burgers and fries, are less intelligent and have poorer memories than those who eat a low-fat, nutrient-dense diet. (See under *Atherosclerosis*.)
- Alcohol depletes the body of vital nutrients.
- Avoid excess sodium-based table salt, and don't add salt to food once it has been cooked.
- In some people, excess wheat triggers "brain fog." This is usually due to the gluten content, but any food that you are intolerant to can trigger this problem. (See *Allergies*.)
- Avoid too much refined sugar, which ages your brain.
- Avoid aspartame and monosodium glutamate (MSG), as they are brain toxins.

Friendly Foods

- Always eat breakfast. Low-sugar cereals, such as muesli or oatmeal, are rich in B vitamins that are often lacking in dementia patients (especially B12).
- Low blood sugar levels can easily trigger "brain fog" symptoms, such as memory loss. Make sure to eat small meals regularly to balance your blood sugar. (See *Low Blood Sugar*.)
- Omega-3 essential fats are vital brain nutrients. Salmon, sardines, pilchards, black cod, herrings, and mackerel are all rich in both EPA and DHA.
- Use unrefined, preferably organic, olive, sunflower, walnut, or sesame oils for salad dressings and to drizzle over cooked foods. (See *Fats You Need To Eat*.)
- Fresh coffee is often criticized, but in terms of memory function it seems to help it, particularly in the elderly. Two cups a day is fine.
- Green leafy vegetables, particularly spinach, watercress, cabbage, bok choy, celery, broccoli, and spring greens, as well as red and purple fruits, such as strawberries, pomegranate,

blueberries, blackberries, and cherries, are all rich in antioxidants that will help to slow memory decline.

- Eat more apples, papaya, pineapple, grapes, prunes, and raisins.
- Eat more wholegrain foods, such as brown pasta and rice, whole-wheat bread and flour, and barley and buckwheat.
- For those with a sweet tooth, use a little unprocessed honey, brown rice syrup, organic agave syrup, or xylitol.
- Phosphatidyl choline is a vital brain nutrient found in egg yolks and fish, especially sardines.
- Non-genetically modified lecithin granules are a great brain food that also reduces the amounts of LDL (the "bad" cholesterol) in your body. Taking this nutrient during pregnancy can result in brainier children. Sprinkle a tablespoon of the granules over your breakfast cereal or into salads or yogurts. Available from all health stores.
- Eat more ginger and live, low-fat yogurt to aid digestion.
- Add freshly chopped sage to your salads and meals as it has been shown to improve memory and brain function.

Useful Remedies

- Take a high-strength multi-vitamin/mineral/antioxidant formula for your age and gender.
- Include a vitamin B-complex, as B vitamins are essential for normal brain function and for keeping homocysteine levels in check. (These should already be in your multi.)
- The herb ginkgo biloba is proven to increase memory by improving blood flow to the brain. **VC**

M

- Vinpocetine by Life Extension Foundation is derived from an extract of the periwinkle plant which, like ginkgo, is an herb that helps improve circulation. It is especially useful when blood flow to the brain is diminished, as occurs with hardening of the arteries or minor strokes, and it also helps some people with tinnitus (ringing in the ears). Take 20–40mg daily. **LEF**
- Phosphatidyl serine (100mg up to three times a day) has been shown to improve mental function. Take early in the day, as taking it at night can increase dreaming.
- Taking 100mg of co-enzyme Q10 a day can improve energy production within the brain
- The amino acid L-glutamine also makes a great brain food, as it is the most abundant amino acid in the fluid surrounding the brain. Take 250mg twice daily on an empty stomach 30 minutes before food.
- Acetyl L-carnitine, an amino acid, helps slow the progression of early dementia as well as slowing brain deterioration. Take 500mg three times daily before meals.
- Glutathione is a vital brain nutrient. (See *Liver Problems*.)
- More than 15 years of research by Dr Hirokazu Kawagishi of Shizoka University in Japan has demonstrated that a pure extract of the Lion's Mane Mushroom has the remarkable ability of increasing Nerve Growth Factor (NGF) in the brain, which in turn helps make more neurons. Take daily for at least 3 months, as nerves do not grow overnight! Mushroom Science sells a Lion's Mane supplement. For details visit www.mushroomscience.com or Tel: 1-888-283-6583.

Helpful Hints

- Regular exercise is vital for preserving your memory. The more oxygen you get to the brain, the less likely you are to lose your memory.
- Make sure you are getting sufficient quality sleep.
- Common sage contains thujone (a naturally occurring substance that gives sage its flavor), which can trigger fits in sensitive individuals if used as sage essential oil. However, Spanish sage contains almost no thujone. Regular head massages with Spanish sage essential oil (diluted in a base oil) have been shown by Dr John Wilkinson at Middlesex University in the

UK to increase memory. Available online from Amazon and other retailers. **NB: All sage is safe for cooking.**

- Rubbing the essential oil of basil and/or rosemary, diluted in a base of almond oil, into the scalp will help increase circulation to the scalp and clear your mind, thus aiding concentration.
- Chelation therapy helps unclog your arteries, which increases the amount of blood and oxygen that reaches the brain. Chelation therapy also helps remove deadly metal toxins from the body. I give full details of this treatment in my book *500 of the Most Important Ways to Stay Younger Longer* (CICO Books). There are many chelation clinics. Search for one near you on www.holisticnetworker.com or on Google.
- Play more word games and complete crossword puzzles. During long car rides, when traveling, on an airplane or standing in line at the supermarket, add or multiply random numbers in your head.
- Minimize your exposure to aluminum. This includes many deodorants, cooking pans, some cheeses, and so on. (See *Alzheimer's Disease*.)
- Meditation helps improve memory.
- Minimize your exposure to mercury. (See *Mercury Fillings*.)
- Avoid using your cell phone for more than 10 minutes at a time and avoid using it in cars and trains, which amplify the negative effects. (See *Electrical Pollution*.)
- Stop smoking because smoking narrows blood vessels, thus depleting the brain of much-needed oxygen.
- If, after trying these remedies for three months, you are still experiencing memory problems, consult a doctor who is also a nutritionist.
- For further help read *New Optimum Nutrition for the Mind* by Patrick Holford (Piatkus).
- Also see *Helpful Hints* under *Alzheimer's Disease*.

MÉNIÈRE'S SYNDROME *(see also Tinnitus and Vertigo)*

This is a little-understood problem of the inner ear that causes recurrent attacks of vertigo, nausea, and ringing in the ears, as well as progressive deafness. People with this problem tend to feel unsteady and suffer from headaches and neck pains. Causes are suggested as being linked to salt retention, food intolerances, nutritional deficiencies caused by poor absorption, or even spasms in the walls of small blood vessels. If you have food intolerances, this can trigger leaky gut syndrome, which occurs when toxins leak through the gut wall into the body, triggering these types of symptoms. (See under *Leaky Gut*.)

In Chinese medicine, the ears are linked to the kidney and adrenal area, which iswhy stress can greatly exacerbate this problem.

Foods to Avoid

- Many people with this problem react to soy-, wheat- (gluten is usually the culprit), corn- and yeast-based foods.
- Avoid sodium-based salt.
- Generally avoid any foods containing gluten, salt, and caffeine, as well as fried foods and alcohol.
- Reduce your consumption of full-fat milk and dairy products from all animal sources.
- See also *General Health Hints*.

Friendly Foods
- Eat more ginger, garlic, leeks, and onions, which are very cleansing.
- Papaya and pineapple contain digestive enzymes that aid in the absorption of nutrients from your food.
- Add 2 teaspoons of organic apple cider vinegar to water and sip. This mixture is rich in potassium, which may be low in people with this condition.
- See *Friendly Foods* under *Leaky Gut* and *Vertigo*.
- Cherries, blueberries, blackberries, and plums are all rich in flavonoids, which help support ear function.
- Eat more wheat germ, pecans, Brazil nuts, almonds, buckwheat, spinach, peas, and beans, which are all rich in manganese, as a lack of this mineral is linked to this condition.

Useful Remedies
- Take a high-strength multi-vitamin/mineral.
- The herb ginkgo biloba helps increase circulation in the ears.
- Take a digestive enzyme capsule with main meals. **VC**
- Taking 5–10mg of manganese may be useful. A deficiency in this mineral has been linked to Ménière's Syndrome. Most multi formulas will contain this amount.

Helpful Hints
- It is important to consult a chiropractor or cranial osteopath, who can check for any cranial, spinal or neck misalignments.
- Acupuncture has proven very useful for this condition because it helps increase circulation to the ears. (See *Useful Information*.)

MENOPAUSE (see also Adrenal Exhaustion, Low Blood Sugar, and Osteoporosis)

As a woman in her early sixties, I am writing this section from a place of experience. Many women believe that menopause is an illness for which you need a drug (orthodox HRT), but it's not. Menopause is part of the normal cycle of a woman's hormonal life when menstrual cycles cease and it is also a time of great potential.

Menopause generally occurs between the ages of 45 and 55, although it can occur as early as 35 or as late as 65 years of age. Chemotherapy and excess exposure to hormone-altering chemicals such as pesticides and herbicides can also trigger early menopause.

Dr Marilyn Glenville, a UK-based expert on menopause, says: "At the time of menopause, a woman still produces estrogen but not sufficient to prepare her womb for pregnancy. Levels of progesterone plummet or disappear completely. The ovaries continue to produce small quantities of estrogen for at least 12 years after the onset of menopause."

For most women, menopause happens in three phases. First comes peri-menopause, when you still have periods, but they may become heavier or lighter, and symptoms such as hot flashes can appear. Then comes menopause, when ovarian function declines and periods stop. The last phase is called post-menopause, which begins 12 months after your last period.

Throughout this time, many signs associated with aging can appear as your hormonal balance alters with the dropping levels of estrogen and progesterone. Skin is more likely to wrinkle, and there can be an increased growth of facial hair or a thinning of the hair in the temple region. Muscles lose some of their strength and tone, and many women suffer from hot flashes and insomnia. Your joints may begin to ache, and bones can become more brittle, increasing the risk of osteoporosis. Vaginal dryness often results from these hormonal changes. The vaginal wall also becomes thinner, and blood flow is restricted. Dryness can make sexual intercourse painful or uncomfortable and can lead to irritation and increased risk of infection. You will be happy to note that regular sexual intercourse increases blood flow into the vagina.

Loss of bladder tone, which can result in stress incontinence (leaking urine when you cough, sneeze, laugh, or exercise), can also result (see *Incontinence*). Orthodox chemical-based HRT has now been linked to an increase in urinary incontinence, and studies have shown that conditions such as Alzheimer's and memory loss may also be sped up by orthodox HRT.

You may also experience a whole host of emotional ups and downs—one minute feeling on top of the world and the next in the pits of despair. The good news is that by eating the right diet, taking the right supplements, exercising, and using natural hormone replacements, virtually all of the symptoms of menopause can be avoided or alleviated.

I do not advocate taking orthodox HRT because of the increased risk of high blood pressure, blood clots, weight gain, and gallbladder and liver problems, not to mention breast and endometrial (uterine) cancers. The increased health risks of orthodox HRT have now been shown to far outweigh the benefits. Yes, it does slow the rate of bone loss, but only while you are taking it. Also, if you are under a lot of stress at this time, adrenal function is greatly affected. And if you are stressed, then your adrenal glands are kept busy pumping out stress hormone like cortisol, disrupting the endocrine system and potentially causing estrogen levels from the ovaries to fluctuate.

I had a hysterectomy at the age of 31, and at that time no one warned me that I might need more estrogen to protect my bones. If you keep your ovaries after surgery, you will produce some estrogen for a time, but often not enough to prevent osteoporosis, which crippled my mother. I have always taken bone supplements, but these alone could never make up for the years of insufficient estrogen, which is why I now have osteoporosis. Therefore, if you have an early menopause, which is becoming more common thanks to our stressful and toxic environment, or if you have a hysterectomy (even if you kept your ovaries), **please** make sure that your hormone levels are checked every year...otherwise you could end up like me!

Also, on the subject of estrogen, only a few women are aware of the condition known as estrogen dominance. This is when the amount of estrogen in the body is not balanced by the right amount of progesterone. This can happen because of failed ovulations or over-exposure to environmental chemicals found in herbicides, pesticides, and plastics called "xenoestrogens" that have an estrogen-like "building" effect within the body. These chemicals accumulate in our fatty tissue and greatly increase our risk of hormonal cancers.

When you have too much estrogen activity compared to progesterone, you can exhibit symptoms such as water retention, bloating, and menstrual irregularities. Globally we are living in a dangerous ocean of hormone-disrupting chemicals that are causing animals and fish to change sex—and we, too, are seeing sexual mutations and lowered sperm counts.

One problem with conventional HRT is that it does not contain natural progesterone; it contains synthetic hormone-like substances called progestins (or progestogen) instead. These artificial hormones have side effects such as irritability, liver dysfunction, vaginal bleeding, blood clots, and so on, and they reverse the positive effects of estrogens on the heart. Conventional HRT also uses much higher levels of estrogen than bio-identical HRT. For this reason, I prefer to use natural HRT (see below for details).

If you have had a partial hysterectomy (that is, your ovaries are remaining) before menopause, you will still have hormonal changes similar to the normal menstrual cycle. If you need supplemental hormones and are told that you only need estrogen because you do not have a uterus, you should also take a bio-identical (natural) progesterone. If you have had a total hysterectomy and need HRT, use the lowest dose of estrogen possible for you and always use bio-identical (natural) progesterone with it.

Some women go through early menopause, which can happen for many reasons, ranging from estrogen-like chemicals in the environment to smoking, drinking heavily, or being severely malnourished. Whatever the cause, it is important to make sure that your bones remain healthy. So it is important to have a bone scan periodically and a urine (deoxypyrodi-noline) test to measure bone breakdown. If bone loss is occurring then you need to take the appropriate measures. (See *Osteoporosis*.)

Also, nutritional scientist and naturopath Robert Jacobs at the Society for Complementary medicine in London, UK, says: "Many women younger than 50 may have not yet gone through their menopause and therefore may still have high levels of estrogen in their blood that is thought to be heart protective. After menopause, estrogen levels drop and can thus contribute to an increased risk for heart disease—which is why balancing one's hormones is really important after menopause, as well as living a healthy lifestyle."

Foods to Avoid

- Make the effort to cut down on "white" foods such as cakes, cookies, breads, and pastries. Also reduce your intake of pre-packaged refined foods, full-fat dairy from animal sources, and fatty meats.

- Although dairy products from animals contain calcium, they are also proteins that have often been exposed to hormones and pesticides.
- Avoid chemicals that mimic estrogens (xenoestrogens), found in pesticides or herbicides, by eating more organic foods.
- Minimize your exposure to foods stored in plastic containers, and never heat or microwave food in plastic containers. These containers will leach xenoestrogens into your food.
- Cut down on caffeine, soft drinks, refined sugar, and chocolate, and avoid drinking too much alcohol, as all of these act as stimulants and trigger blood sugar problems. Caffeine and/or alcohol can trigger a hot flash on their own. (See *Low Blood Sugar*.)

Friendly Foods

- Increase your intake of fresh, locally grown and preferably organic fruits and vegetables.
- Fermented soy-based products are truly one of the best foods for managing the symptoms associated with menopause. Soy contains isoflavones (phyto-estrogens) that have estrogen-like effects on the body and block the harmful effects of xenoestrogens. But there has been much misinformation written about soy. Dr Glenville says: "Soy foods in their traditional forms of miso, soy sauce, and tempeh (a fermented form of soy) and natto are all rich in isoflavones, which have been proven to reduce the risk of developing cancers. But they are best eaten cooked."
- Isoflavones are also found in chickpeas, soybeans, lentils, alfalfa, fennel, kidney beans, sunflower, pumpkin, hemp, and sesame seeds, Brazil nuts, walnuts, and flaxseeds. All seeds and their unrefined oils are rich in essential fatty acids, which also help reduce joint pain and the risk of heart disease, as well as helping lubricate the vagina. (See *Fats You Need To Eat*.) For a great breakfast smoothie recipe, see *General Health Hints*.
- Brazil nuts and sesame seeds are good sources of calcium.
- Foods from the brassica vegetable family help protect against estrogen-sensitive cancers (including breast cancer and cancer of the cervix), balance hormones, and can greatly alleviate menopausal symptoms. Vegetables in this family include cabbage, watercress, broccoli, bok choy, Brussels sprouts, cauliflower, kale, mustard, rutabaga, and turnips.

- Live, low-fat yogurt increases healthy bacteria in the gut, which aids absorption of nutrients from your diet.
- Vitamin B12 has been shown to reduce the irritability, bloating, and headaches associated with menopause and is found in oily fish, eggs, and lean meats.
- Potassium and pantothenic acid (vitamin B5) help to support adrenal function. They can be found in whole grains (such as brown rice, amaranth, and buckwheat), kelp, raisins, wheat germ, barley and quinoa, as well as salmon, peanuts, mushrooms, sweet potatoes, tomatoes, broccoli, cauliflower, avocados, dried apricots, banana, cantaloupe melon, oranges, and fish.
- Use dried seaweeds such as kombu, in your cooking (particularly in stir-fries), as seaweed is rich in iodine (which supports the thyroid) and calcium (see also *Thyroid*). Try nori seaweed flakes or kelp flakes instead of salt (available from most health stores).
- Eat organic foods, including lean meat, chicken, vegetables, and fruits, to avoid ingesting too many toxic herbicides and pesticides.
- The folic acid found in wheat germ, eggs, leafy greens, calves' and chicken liver, dried yeast, and beets is very important for protecting the bones during menopause.
- Include garlic, onions, and leeks in your diet, which help keep cholesterol levels in check.
- Sprinkle lecithin granules over cereals and add to smoothies to nourish your brain and lower LDL cholesterol.
- Drink more spring water, which helps regulate body temperature.
- Avoid very hot drinks and spicy foods.
- If you have trouble sleeping, try valerian and passionflower teas.
  (Also see *Insomnia* for some great natural sleep aids.)

- Drink more organic decaffeinated green teas, which contain L-theanine, an amino acid that helps increase alpha wave activity in the brain, helping induce feelings of calmness. You can also take L-theanine capsules. **SVHC**
- Try organic almond, oat, rice, and quinoa milks as non-dairy alternatives to animal-source dairy products.

Useful Remedies

- Because cruciferous vegetables help regulate estrogen in the body and help the liver remove potentially harmful by-products of excess estrogens, take one Triple Action Cruciferous Vegetable Extract daily. **LEF**
- Try Menopause Support (formerly Women's Balance 40+), which includes herbs such as blessed thistle, squaw vine, and Siberian ginseng, which all help cleanse the reproductive organs and balance hormones. Available on Amazon
- If you dislike soy foods, then take a soy isoflavone capsule daily.
- Take a women's multi-vitamin/mineral such as New Chapter's Every Woman II. Any women's multi that you choose should contain boron, vitamin K, selenium, folic acid, vitamin D, vitamin E, calcium, and magnesium to support you throughout menopause.
- A vitamin B complex will help relieve stress, depression, and mood disorders and is needed for energy production. (This should be included in your multi.)
- A remedy extracted from a Peruvian root vegetable called maca has been used for centuries to help alleviate hormonal-based symptoms. Research shows that maca helps stimulate the pituitary gland into producing hormone precursors, which eventually raise estrogen and progesterone levels naturally, as well as balancing the adrenal glands, the thyroid, and the pancreas. Taken regularly, this root has been shown to reduce the hot flashes and other menopause-related symptoms. **VC**
- Taking a full-spectrum, natural-source vitamin E (400IU per day) can help reduce hot flashes.

- Take an EFA formula that contains omega-3 and -6 oils; take at least 1g daily. (See *Fats You Need To Eat*.)
- Taking 100mcg of vitamin K2 per day can reduce the heavy menstrual bleeding that is common in the peri-menopausal years. It is also needed to keep calcium in the bones and out of the arteries. **NB: Avoid vitamin K2 if you are on blood-thinning drugs.**
- Black cohosh can relieve hot flashes and other menopausal symptoms after 4 weeks of use. Other herbs for reducing menopausal symptoms include agnus castus, hops, licorice root, dong quai, and wild yam. These herbs can be taken individually or in a combination formula. Nature's Sunshine has a formula called Natural Changes containing all these herbs and more. www.naturessunshine.com
- As sleep can be a problem for many women, try a natural-source melatonin supplement each night before bed. It really helps. (For details of Asphalia, see under *Insomnia*.)
- Omega-7 fats from sea buckthorn have been found highly effective for supporting mucosal membranes. Take daily to reduce a dry vagina. **VC**
- For more details about the bio-identical hormones progesterone and estrogen plus DHEA, see below.

Helpful Hints

- If your doctor suggests that you use orthodox pessaries for a dry vagina, then avoid ones containing estradiol, which is a stronger estrogen and can increase the risk of hormone-related cancers. Ask for estriol-based creams and pessaries, which are a weaker form of estrogen.

- If you are suffering from heavy bleeding, you must have this checked by your doctor or gynecologist.
- Regular weight-bearing exercise not only helps raise levels of DHEA, a vital anti-aging hormone (see below), but also reduces stress, which makes symptoms and hormone imbalances worse. Also our waistlines tend to expand in mid-life. Exercise keeps you trim and increases bone density. It also makes you feel more positive and cheerful about life, and women who exercise regularly tend to have fewer hot flashes.
- Use relaxation techniques, such as meditation or yoga.
- Add essential oils of geranium, chamomile, and jasmine to your bath to aid relaxation.
- If you suffer from night sweats, wear loose-fitting cotton nightwear and have a change of nightwear ready. Use cotton blankets and keep the room cool.
- Homeopathic Sepia 30c (one per day for a week) helps reduce hot flashes.
- To further help prevent vaginal dryness and painful intercourse, avoid using deodorant soaps or scented products in the vaginal area.
- Try the KY Silk vaginal lubricant, which contains aloe vera. There are many creams containing wild yam available in health food stores, which can be used topically as a vaginal lubricant.
- Read *Natural Alternatives to HRT* and *Healthy Eating for the Menopause*, both by Dr Marilyn Glenville (Kyle Cathie).
- Marilyn's website (www.marilynglenville.com) is packed with useful information.
- If you want more information about natural progesterone and about finding a doctor, visit www.natural-progesterone-advisory-network.com

Hormones associated with menopause

Don't use hormones in any form unless blood and/or saliva tests show that you need them. If you have good bone density and no hormonal-type symptoms, there should be no need for extra hormones.

- **Progesterone** Natural (bio-identical) progesterone is made from an extract of wild yams and then converted into the hormone progesterone, which is bio-identical to the hormone you made in your body prior to the menopause. This progesterone is often needed to balance excess estrogen activity that is linked to hormonal cancers. Natural progesterone can also greatly reduce or alleviate many of the side effects associated with menopause. Natural progesterone most often comes as a cream that you rub on the skin. PharmWest makes a product called Pro Body Cream. Tel: 1-310-301-4015. Website: www.pharmwest.com

  Many women believe that if they have gone through menopause they only need estrogen and not progesterone, but Robert Jacobs says, " The latest breakthroughs have shown that progesterone and estrogen need to be balanced in the body, and estrogen alone, unopposed by progesterone, increases the risk for hormonal-type cancers."

- **Natural estrogens** are synthesized from soybeans and are identical to the estrogen that you make in your body. If you have mood swings, depression, bone thinning, or insomnia you may need natural estrogens as well as the natural progesterone. Many companies now make these in a duo formula, such as PhytoEstrogen Body Cream by PharmWest.

  These creams can be applied to the inner arms or thighs or to the stomach, breasts, or face. Regularly change the areas on which you apply the cream, otherwise tissues can become saturated, thus affecting absorption.

- **Cortisol** You can find out more about how this stress-related hormone affects menopause and hugely contributes to osteoporosis under *Adrenal Exhaustion* and *Osteoporosis*.

- **DHEA** Around the time of menopause, women often undergo rapid age-transformation, and while most doctors suggest some kind of HRT, very few prescribe DHEA. DHEA helps reverse many of the unfavorable effects of excess cortisol. If your DHEA levels are low, you are likely to feel tired all the time, have "brain fog" and PMS-like symptoms, and your skin will age faster. Lack of DHEA can also be a factor in some autoimmune conditions such as lupus.

  This hormone is produced by the adrenal glands and is the most abundant steroid hormone in the body. It is made from cholesterol and can be converted into estrogen or testosterone. By the age of 65, we make only 10–20% of the amount of DHEA we made at age 20. One 20-year study found that DHEA levels were far lower in men who died of heart disease than in healthier men. Low levels of DHEA have also been found in Alzheimer's patients. In fact, there is now little doubt that DHEA may help prevent the ravages of brain aging. It protects against Alzheimer's and dementia as well as increasing a sense of wellbeing, which scientists have linked to increased levels of endorphins (the chemicals we make naturally when we are happy and during exercise). Tests have also shown that DHEA can help prevent some cancers, heart disease, and bone and skin degeneration. It helps maintain brain function and gives powerful support to the immune system. In addition, it helps protect against infections, autoimmune disorders, obesity, diabetes, and stress.

  DHEA has also been shown in numerous studies to improve mood and energy levels in both men and women, and therefore is a valid treatment for depression and long-term negative stress. This effect was found to be particularly noticeable for post-menopausal women. One German study showed that DHEA considerably increased libido and sexual satisfaction in the women taking part.

  DHEA is easy to supplement in tablet or liquid form, and serum levels can be controlled with ease. But, as always, before you begin taking hormones, have a blood, saliva, or urine test to find out if your hormone levels are depleted. In women, anything more than modest dosages may trigger increased facial hair growth, pimples, or in some cases greasy skin.

  NB: Because DHEA can be metabolized into testosterone and estrogen, DHEA use should be avoided by anyone who currently has prostate or breast cancer. Also do not take this hormone if you are pregnant, nursing, or have had prior ovarian, adrenal, or thyroid tumors. Women should avoid DHEA just prior to menopause because their levels typically increase naturally around that time anyway.

Where to buy DHEA

DHEA is available over-the-counter (and online) in the US, and there are a wide variety of doses and combinations for both men and women. However, it's important to remember that it's impossible to know what your DHEA levels are without having a blood and/or saliva test, so make sure to talk to a doctor before starting any type of hormone therapy.

Numerous nutritional physicians, health professionals, and doctors work with DHEA and other natural hormones. To locate a qualified practitioner in your area, contact:

1. American Board of Integrative Holistic Medicine. Tel: 1-218-525-5651. Website: www.holisticboard.org
2. American Association of Naturopathic Physicians. Tel: 1-866-538-2267 (toll free) or 1-202-237-8150. Website: www.naturopathic.org
3. Professional Referral Network. Website: www.healthreferral.com
4. Women in Balance. Tel: 1-866-972-8249. Website: http://providers.womeninbalance.org

For more information, read DHEA—Unlocking the Secrets to the Fountain of Youth by Ley and Ash (BL Publications).

■ **Testosterone** If levels of this hormone are low, extra testosterone may be prescribed for men to restore libido and endurance, and in women small amounts may also be required not only to help restore libido but also for healthy bones. Women who tend to suffer from very dry eyes after menopause often need small amounts of this hormone. Like progesterone and estrogen, testosterone is also available in creams, but you should only use them under the guidance of your doctor or other healthcare professional.

MERCURY FILLINGS

There is now a huge body of evidence to show that mercury fillings are detrimental to health. Mercury is one of the most toxic substances known to man and is an accumulative poison. Originally, it was thought that mercury vapor could not escape if it was locked into solid metal fillings, but we now know this is not the case. Mercury vapor is now proven to pass through the blood–brain barrier; it deposits in the brain, affecting both structure and function. At least 2% of the US population is estimated to suffer from mercury sensitivity—that is, around 4.5 million people. To put this in perspective, when the same ratio of people has, say, the flu, this is considered to have reached epidemic proportions. Yet amalgam fillings are still widely used in the US and other countries like the UK.

There is now good evidence from researchers at the University of Calgary in Canada that shows mercury causes brain cell degeneration. This research and many more facts on mercury are available via www.iaomt.org—The International Academy of Oral Medicine and Toxicology. More than 14,000 papers have been published suggesting that mercury is toxic and should not be used in fillings.

Currently the FDA has issued no restrictions on the use of amalgam fillings, but many countries have. For example, mercury fillings are banned in Japan, Norway, and Sweden and are not allowed in women and children in Austria and Germany. Even the UK Department of Health advises all dentists not to remove or replace amalgam fillings in pregnant women. Now why do you think that is, if mercury fillings are not dangerous?

Dr Jack Levenson, a dental surgeon who has passed away, spent almost 20 years investigating the effects and potential dangers of dental amalgam. He told me a few years ago: "Eighty percent of the mercury vapor that we inhale from mercury fillings enters our bloodstream, and there is a strong body of research linking mercury toxicity to heart disease, Alzheimer's, Parkinson's, multiple sclerosis, motor neuron disease, thyroid problems, migraines, chronic fatigue, digestive disorders, infertility in men and women, antibiotic resistance, joint and muscle pain, impaired immune function, autoimmune diseases, hair loss and excessive hair growth, visual disturbances, numbness, tingling, and tremors."

Are you nervous? When Jack tested my teeth, two of my amalgam fillings were 10 times over the supposed safe limit of mercury emissions. I had them removed on the spot. It would seem that the government continues to refuse to back safer, composite white fillings in order to save the healthcare system millions of dollars. If they were to admit that amalgam had poisoned millions of people, the litigation bill would be huge and health insurance companies would then be forced to pay for the fillings' removal and replacement. Money, not health, seems to be the bottom line here.

Many people suffering mercury toxicity have also been found to have candida. (See under *Candida*.)

Foods to Avoid
- If you have mercury fillings, avoid Spanish- or Gulf-sourced mackerel, marlin, shark, swordfish, Chilean sea bass, tuna, and swordfish, which often contain high quantities of mercury. (Around 20 tons of industrial mercury plus lead, cadmium, and copper is dumped into the North Sea alone every year.) For state and local fish advisories, visit the Natural Resources Defense Council's website: www.nrdc.org

Friendly Foods
- Generally eat more organic vegetables, fruits, and grains, as mass-produced fruits, grains, and vegetables are often treated with a mercury-based fungicide.
- Cilantro and chlorella detoxify mercury from the body.
- Generally drink more pure filtered water.
- Currently, in 2010, low levels of mercury can be found in anchovies, catfish, clams, domestic crab, crayfish, Atlantic haddock, hake, North Atlantic mackerel, plaice, pollock, fresh salmon, sardines, scallops, tilapia, freshwater trout, and whiting.

Useful Remedies
- If you have mercury fillings, take a good-quality multi-vitamin/mineral to help support your immune system.
- You need a full spectrum of B vitamins. (These should be in your multi.)
- Mercury depletes the mineral selenium, which is known to reduce the incidence of cancer and heart disease. Take between 100 and 200mcg of selenium daily.
- Vitamin E increases the effectiveness of selenium; take 200IU of full-spectrum, natural-source vitamin E daily.
- Lipoic acid, an important antioxidant, helps eliminate mercury from the body. Take 200mg daily.
- Take 2g of vitamin C daily with food in divided doses.
- The amino acid N-acetyl cysteine (NAC) really helps detoxify the liver. Take 500mg twice a day at least 30 minutes before food.
- Pure Encapsulations makes an HM Chelate Formula that contains vitamin C, chlorella, zinc, selenium, lipoic acid, NAC, and pectin. Take 3–6 daily away from food for optimum results. Available from a number of online retailers.

- Take any organic-based chlorella green food powder daily, such as Greens Plus, which contains Hawaiian spirulina, chlorella, lecithin, barley, pectin apple fiber, soy and barley sprouts, and lactobacillus acidophilus. This is a great all-round way to ingest good nutrients and healthy bacteria, keep the body more alkaline, and help keep you regular. And the more regular you are, the fewer toxins like mercury you will store in your body. **GP**

Helpful Hints

- Many vaccines use mercury as a preservative.
- To find a list of dentists in the US who specialize in safe removal of amalgam fillings, visit http://mercuryfreedentists.com or call 1-870-576-9635.
- Contact IAOMT—The International Academy of Oral Medicine and Toxicology—at 8297 ChampionsGate Blvd, #193, ChampionsGate, FL 33896. Or call 1-863-420-6373. You can also visit their website (www.iaomt.org) to read the latest research on mercury. The Academy gives lots of information on mercury fillings and holistic dentistry.
- For a list of holistic dentists in your area, you can contact the Holistic Dental Association by calling 1-619-923-3120 or by visiting www.holisticdental.org
- www.melisa.org also carries the latest research into the links between mercury and Parkinson's and mercury and multiple sclerosis.
- The Henry Spink Foundation at www.henryspink.org has published great fact sheets about mercury.
- Read *Toxic Bite* by Bill Kellner-Read (Credence) or *The Toxic Time Bomb* by Sam Ziff (Aurora).

MIGRAINE   *(see also Allergies, Leaky Gut, Low Blood Sugar and Liver Problems)*

More than 30 million Americans suffer from regular migraines, but three times as many women are affected as men. However, more than half never consult their doctor as to what might be causing their migraines. Sufferers on average experience around thirteen attacks annually and roughly 10% of school-age children suffer from migraines, with more boys getting migraines before puberty than girls.

In the US alone, the cost of migraines is more than $13 billion a year, which is why prevention is always preferable to cure. Migraines usually occur on one side, at the back or front of the head, and an attack can be precipitated by flashing lights or partial blindness. Others suffer from tingling sensations, sensitivity to light or noise, vomiting, and so on. Some people are debilitated for a few hours, others for several days, and in addition an attack can often be accompanied by nausea and vomiting.

Migraines are, in many cases, linked to intolerances to foods such as wheat or cow's milk, internal toxicity, and sometimes to the menstrual cycle. "In fact," says nutritionist Gareth Zeal, "as many as 90% of migraine cases I see are linked to food intolerance. In addition, 40% of migraine patients also have the bacterium *Helicobacter pylori* (see *Stomach Ulcers*). Migraines can also be a sign of liver congestion, so you really need to cut down on alcohol, caffeine and fats—and keep your diet clean. (See also *Leaky Gut, Constipation, Liver Problems*, and *Low Blood Sugar*.)

Weather changes, negative stress, or lack of sleep can also trigger migraines.

Foods to Avoid

- The foods most commonly known to trigger an attack are cheese, animal-based dairy products, red wine, peanuts, chocolate of any type and color, corn, coffee, wheat, and citrus fruits and juices.

- Avoid refined sugars, which are found in most cakes, cookies, pastries, snacks, and soft drinks.
- Avoid food additives, colorings, preservatives, alcohol, and caffeine as much as possible.
- Avoid hard margarines, shortenings, and any foods that contain hydrogenated fats and oils.
- Cut down on red meat, full-fat dairy products, and eggs if you know that you have an intolerance (see below). People who eat a low-saturated-fat diet tend to suffer from fewer migraines.
- If you are constipated on a regular basis, certain bacteria in the bowel can convert tyrosine (found in high amounts in peanuts) to tyramine, which again is thought to be a trigger. Cheese is also high in tyramine.

Friendly Foods
- Eat more fresh pineapple and papaya, which aid digestion.
- Include more turmeric (curcumin) in your diet, as it has great anti-inflammatory properties. You can also take this in capsule form.
- Eat more flaxseeds; they can be soaked in cold water overnight, drained, and eaten. Sunflower, pumpkin, hemp, and sesame seeds all help keep your bowels regular. Sprinkle them over a low-sugar breakfast cereal or use in yogurts, as a snack, in smoothies, and in salads.
- Drink at least 6–8 glasses of water daily. Dehydration can trigger a migraine, especially in the summer.
- Eat more healthy grains, brown rice, quinoa, buckwheat, lentils, and barley, and try amaranth, oat, and rice crackers as a change from wheat.

- Try The Gluten-Free Bakeshop, Food For Life, EnerG, Glutino and Kinnkinnick wheat-free breads.
- Eat plenty of fruits and vegetables, preferably organic.
- Make sure to eat quality protein, such as fresh chicken or cooked tofu, once a day.
- Otherwise use organic hemp seed protein in smoothies. (See recipe in *General Health Hints*.)
- Use unrefined walnut, sesame, avocado, sunflower, and olive oils in salad dressings.
- Live, low-fat, non-dairy-based yogurt contains healthy bacteria that aid digestion and keep the bowel healthy.
- Oily fish is rich in omega-3 fats that naturally thin the blood and reduce the severity of migraines. Eat more organic-farmed salmon, sardines, pilchards, anchovies, mackerel, and black cod.
- Drink vervain tea to help reduce head pain, and add the essential oil to your bath.

Useful Remedies
- Levels of the mineral magnesium are often low in migraine sufferers. Magnesium helps relax blood vessels so that oxygen and nutrients can get to the brain. Taking magnesium citrate (600mg in divided doses throughout the day) should help. Remember to take the final 200mg just before bed.
- Ginkgo biloba helps prevent blood vessels from constricting. Take 120mg of standardized extract daily.
- As all the B vitamins are vital for preventing headaches, particularly folic acid, B2 and B6, take a high-strength B-complex daily.
- Include 1g of vitamin C with bioflavonoids daily. **VC**
- As digestive problems are heavily associated with migraines, take a digestive enzyme with main meals.
- If you crave sweet foods, take 200mcg of the mineral chromium for at least 1 month to reduce food cravings. (See under *Low Blood Sugar*.)

- Taking 500mg of omega-3 fatty acids (fish oils) twice daily should help relieve migraine headaches.
- Minovil contains vitamin B2, magnesium citrate, butterbur, ginger, and feverfew—a herbal anti-inflammatory with natural calming effects. Take two tablets daily. www.minovil.com
- The herb butterbur has been shown to help reduce the duration of migraines. Take 500mg twice daily during an attack. You can also use it for prevention.
- Co-enzyme Q10 helps encourage energy production and has been shown in trials to help lower the incidence of migraines. Take 100mg daily.
- Several studies have shown that taking small doses of melatonin, the hormone produced in the pineal gland in the brain to induce sleep, can help reduce the occurrence of migraine attacks and also can help treat an existing migraine. Bioelectromagnetic research scientist Roger Coghill says: "If you take melatonin supplements that you can buy online..., most synthetic tablets contain thousands of times the natural dose that your pineal gland normally produces at night." Roger has developed a supplement called Asphalia, which contains natural melatonin extracted from certain grasses that mimics the normal dose made by your pineal gland to induce sleep at night, rather than the larger doses that are found in mass-produced tablets. Roger's exclusive distributor in the US is Diva Marketing, Don't Disturb Me!, 2612 Sleepy Hollow, Pearland, TX 77581; Tel: 1-713-221-1873 or 1-866-692-8037; website: www.dontdisturbmesite.com

Helpful Hints

- Low blood sugar can trigger an attack, so eat healthy meals regularly. (See *Low Blood Sugar*.)
- Migraines are often triggered by food intolerances, especially to wheat and cow's milk, as well as by liver congestion or hormonal problems. Keep a food diary to see if you can identify any foods that trigger an attack.
- Take a food intolerance test to check which foods/substances are your specific triggers. Try YorkTest Laboratories (www.yorktest.com). Another option is the FACT test offered by Genova Diagnostics, which looks for inflammatory markers indicating that the body is reacting to certain substances. Tel: 1-800-522-4762. Website: www.genovadiagnostics.com
- Regular aerobic exercise has been shown to reduce migraine attacks, and yoga helps reduce stress levels.
- Taken regularly, rosemary or fresh ginger tea can help bring relief from some of the symptoms.
- Grinding the teeth over many years often causes the jaw to slip out of alignment. This causes blood flow to the head to be restricted, triggering regular headaches and/or migraines. Problems with vertebrae in the neck can also disrupt blood flow to the brain. See a chiropractor or a cranial osteopath, who can re-align the neck and head. (See *Useful Information*.)
- Alternate warm and cold packs. Use each for 10 minutes on the back of the neck to help increase blood flow to the head.
- Contact the National Headache Foundation by calling 1-888-643-5552 or 1-312-274-2650. There is also a wealth of information on their website: www.headaches.org
- For further information or to connect with other sufferers, visit the Migraine Research Foundation's website (www.migraineresearchfoundation.org) or call 1-212-249-5402.

MONONUCLEOSIS (mono)

(see also Adrenal Exhaustion, Candida, Immune Function, and ME)

Mono is caused by the Epstein Barr virus. It is most common in younger people, between the ages of 15 and 25, when the immune system is developing, hence the nickname the "kissing disease." Symptoms include a severe sore throat, fever, swollen glands in the neck, and a feeling of overwhelming exhaustion. Initially it can appear similar to a bad case of the flu, but after a few days it becomes obvious that it is not the flu, and the symptoms can continue for several months. The liver can also be affected, and some sufferers develop mild hepatitis caused by the virus. (See also *Hepatitis* and *Liver Problems*.)

Antibiotics are inappropriate for treating mono because it is a viral infection, and certain types of antibiotics can actually make this illness much worse. Bed rest and good nutrition are essential to help prevent a relapse, but unfortunately the illness often coincides with stressful points in the academic year (like finals), making life rather difficult. It is one of those diseases where you can appear to make a full recovery and then experience a relapse a month later. For some individuals, this can lead to chronic fatigue syndrome or ME. The more you rest when the problem is first diagnosed, the more likely you are to make a complete recovery. The yeast fungal overgrowth candida often occurs with mono (see *Candida*) because the immune system is compromised from lymphatic congestion.

Adrenal exhaustion may result from mono. (See this section.)

Foods to Avoid

- Sugar is the most important food to avoid, as it lowers immune function and adds to adrenal exhaustion. Soft drinks often contain up to 10 teaspoons of sugar, and sugar in any form will greatly diminish immune function.
- Avoid all pre-packaged, ready-made meals, which are usually low in nutrients and high in additives, fats, and sugar. Many stores now sell organic soups and other healthier alternatives.
- Try to eliminate hamburgers and sugary snacks.
- White bread, croissants, Danish pastries, cakes, chocolate snacks, potatoes chips, chicken nuggets, hotdogs, and all these instant-type foods should be avoided for a few weeks.
- If you know you have problems with certain foods, the most common being gluten from wheat and dairy from cow's milk, then eliminate them for two weeks.
- Stimulants such as caffeine and alcohol can overload the body, giving brief bursts of energy, but actually reducing it in the long-term. (See *Insulin Resistance*.)
- See *General Health Hints*.

Friendly Foods

- Try to eat plenty of fresh fruit and vegetables that are rich in magnesium and natural-source carotenes, such as spring greens, cabbage, artichokes, kale, sweet potatoes, pumpkin, watercress, papaya, pineapple, dried apricots, parsley, broccoli, spinach, and all orange fruits.
- If you have a juicer, try a mixture of carrots, raw beets, apple, and small amounts of garlic and onion. Garlic and onions are highly anti-viral.
- Cook with garlic and onions.
- Make rich soups and stews and add some fresh ginger.
- Plenty of good-quality, high-protein foods, such as fresh fish, chicken, tempeh, beans, lentils, and free-range eggs, all help support the immune system. If you are really low, then add hemp seed or whey protein powders to breakfast cereals and smoothies. (A good smoothie recipe can be found in the *General Health Hints*).
- Eat more whole-wheat/stone-ground breads and pastas, as well as baked potatoes, brown

rice, quinoa, and amaranth. Make oatmeal with organic rice, almond, or low-fat goat's or sheep's milk and look for low-sugar cereals.

- Eat more low-fat, live yogurts to help replenish healthy bacteria in the gut.
- Drink plenty of fluids.
- Cilantro and parsley are packed with nutrients.
- Drink licorice tea to help support your adrenal glands, which are usually exhausted.

Useful Remedies

- Beta Glucans 1–3, 1–6, which are derived from yeast cell walls, are proven to strengthen the body's innate immune system (the immune system you were born with), making it more resistant to pathogens from food and air. It also helps fight viruses. Take 250–500mg daily. Also safe for use by young children.
- Vitamin C is anti-viral and antibacterial. While symptoms are acute, take 5–6g daily in divided doses with food. Use an ascorbate or esther form, and after a couple of weeks reduce your intake to 1g daily for several months. If this causes loose bowels, reduce the dose to just below bowel tolerance. **VC**
- A high-strength, multi-vitamin/mineral is important when fighting an infection, as we are often depleted in minerals such as calcium, magnesium, and zinc.
- Because vitamin A is vital for immune function and for fighting viruses, take 30–60mg of natural-source beta-carotenes daily while symptoms are acute, as they naturally convert to Vitamin A in the body. When you start to improve, reduce the dose to 15mg daily. **VC**

- Herbs such as echinacea, olive leaf extract, goldenseal, astragalus, wild indigo, and Siberian ginseng are all anti-viral. Take 3g of either the single herbs or a combination formula daily. The astragalus and goldenseal also support liver function, which is often impaired in people with mono. (See *Liver Problems*.)
- Co-enzyme Q10 is a vitamin-like substance that the body naturally makes to help produce energy. Take 100mg twice daily until you improve, then take 100mg with breakfast daily.
- Propolis has been shown to be highly anti-viral; try taking 1–3g daily for the duration of your illness. **NB: Avoid this remedy if you are severely allergic to bee stings**
- If for any reason you end up taking antibiotics, then take probiotic capsules for a month. **VC**
- A powder of fructooligosaccharides (FOS)) can be used as a sweetener and as a prebiotic, which helps the body make more healthy bacteria in the gut and, in turn, boosts immune function. **VC**

Helpful Hints

- A gradual return to normal life is necessary, because doing too much too soon can provoke a relapse.
- Gentle exercise is really important to get you moving again.
- Homeopathic Ailanthus Glandulosa 6c or Gelsemium 6c (three times daily for 10 days) should help dramatically reduce symptoms.
- Check for possible iron deficiency with your doctor, and take iron if necessary. (See under *Anemia*.)
- You should also ask your doctor to check for parasites. (See under *Irritable Bowel Syndrome*.)
- If, after two months, your energy and appetite have not returned, contact a qualified nutritionist. (See *Useful Information*.)

MOUTH PROBLEMS
(see also Halitosis)

Burning mouth syndrome

(see also Candida, Leaky Gut, Low Stomach Acid, and Liver Problems)

This is most common in women, especially after menopause, and may be triggered by decreased hormone production, nerve damage, stress, or sensitivity to certain foods. It may also be linked to digestive problems. In rare cases it can be due to a lack of vitamin B12 and folic acid. Symptoms can include a swollen tongue, metallic taste, soreness, and a dry mouth and tongue, even when the tongue looks normal. It can also be triggered by low stomach acid (see *Low Stomach Acid*). If you have a cold or the flu, symptoms are usually worse. This condition also denotes that your liver is under stress (see *Liver Problems*). Excessive talking can exacerbate the problem. Conditions such as a leaky gut and candida can also trigger burning mouth, as can a lack of zinc and essential fats.

Foods to Avoid
- Burning mouth syndrome is usually made worse by highly spiced or acidic foods, such as vinegar, oranges, or pineapple.
- Avoid too much alcohol, black tea, and coffee, which are all acid forming in the body
- Red meat, cheese, and chocolate are especially acid forming and could make symptoms worse.

Friendly Foods
- Keep your diet clean (see *General Health Hints*) and drink plenty of water.
- Eat more organic nuts, seeds, and fish, which are high in zinc.
- Cereals, oats, alfalfa, eggs, liver, brown rice, skimmed milk, and fish are all rich in B vitamins.

Useful Remedies
- A swollen tongue can be a sign of an iron deficiency so have a blood test.
- A dry mouth is a specific sign of potassium phosphate deficiency; take NuAge Kali Phos daily. **VC**
- Take 1g of vitamin C per day to prevent deficiency.
- Take 30mg of vitamin B6 per day.
- Take 800mcg of vitamin B12 in a sublingual tablet daily to prevent deficiency.
- Take 400mcg of folic acid per day.
- As all of the B vitamins work together, take the recommended amounts of B6, B12, and folic acid in a B-complex daily.
- Take 30mg of zinc per day, as a lack of zinc is linked to this problem. Because zinc depletes copper, make sure your zinc supplement also contains about 1–2mg of copper.
- Gamma-linolenic acid (GLA) is an essential fat found in evening primrose oil; take 250mg of GLA per day to prevent deficiency. **VC**
- Sea buckthorn is an omega-7 fatty acid that helps supports soft tissue; therefore, take four capsules daily for one month and then two capsules daily after that for maintenance. **VC**
- Bromelain, extracted from pineapples, will help reduce the inflammation. Take 250mg twice daily with food.

Helpful Hints
- Mouth problems often reflect issues in the gut and digestive system. See a nutritionist who can re-balance your diet and suggest supplements to boost your immune system.
- Suck on ice cubes if the pain is severe.

- This problem is exacerbated by stress, so learn to meditate and practice some form of relaxation.
- Sodium lauryl sulfate thins the lining of the mouth; therefore, use an SLS-free toothpaste such as those from Waleda or Burt's Bees.
- As nitrates and other chemicals found in our drinking water are known to make symptoms worse, install a water filter. You can find a wide variety on waterfilters.net
- As an over-acid system may be triggering this condition, you may want to consider using Kangen Water. This is a water system unit that attaches to your kitchen faucet and ionizes and greatly alkalizes water. It has been used in Japanese hospitals with highly beneficial health results. For full details visit kangenwaterusa.com

Canker sores   *(see also General Health Hints and Immune Function)*

Canker sores are quite common and usually occur on the inside of the cheek, tongue or gums. They denote that the body is run down or under stress, but can also be caused by accidentally biting the side of the mouth, excessive tooth brushing, eating food that is too hot, eating acidic and spicy foods, or smoking. Many people get canker sores after eating oranges, pineapple, and/or tomatoes, while others find that ill-fitting dentures or braces are the problem. Any chronic dental problem can trigger an outbreak. If the sores do not clear up within three weeks, see your doctor or dentist.

Sodium lauryl sulfate, a foaming agent used in numerous cosmetics, particularly toothpaste, can also trigger this problem. You might also be deficient in B vitamins and iron. Have a blood test to confirm if your iron levels are low.

Foods to Avoid
- Sugar, vinegars, pickles, tomatoes and tomato sauces, peanuts, strawberries, pineapple, plums, rhubarb, kiwi fruit, oranges, and grapefruits are problem foods for those who suffer from canker sores.
- Avoid really hot and spicy foods.
- Reduce your intake of sugary snacks and white-flour-based breads, cakes, and cookies, all of which lower immune function.
- Avoid really salty foods, such as potato chips, peanuts, and salted meats and fish.

Friendly Foods
- Low-sugar licorice tablets or sticks can be chewed to speed up sore healing. You can also drink licorice tea.
- Eat more manuka honey with an activity level of 10+, as this honey is very healing.
- Drink more green and white teas, which help boost immune function.

Useful Remedies
- Vitamin C and zinc are often deficient in people who suffer from canker sores. Take 1g of vitamin C daily, plus 30mg of zinc.
- Taking a vitamin B complex will help prevent and heal canker sores.
- Take a good multi-vitamin/mineral (which should include all the B vitamins, some vitamin C, and zinc, in which case you do not need to take any extra).
- Omega-7 fats from the sea buckthorn aids healing of mucosal membranes. Take four capsules daily while the sores are acute, and then reduce to two daily. Chew the capsules so the oil goes directly onto the sore.

Helpful Hints
- Stop smoking.

- Rinse your mouth out with a warm salt solution several times a day. Add 1 teaspoon of salt to a glass of cooled, boiled water. Add a few drops of goldenseal or licorice tincture to aid healing.
- If stress is the culprit, exercise and relaxation may be the long-term solution.
- Try Albadent herbal mouthwash, which contains bee propolis, calendula, and St John's wort, all of which are great for canker sores. Available online at Amazon.
- Tea tree oil is a natural antiseptic and makes a wonderful mouthwash when a few drops are mixed with warm water.
- Some people have found that they are allergic to the materials that false teeth are made from. Ask your dentist to test you for an allergy. Porcelain can be used as an alternative material.
- I find that using toothpaste that contains fluoride gives me canker sores. Try to avoid all fluoride.
- Mouth problems often reflect problems in the gut and digestive system. See a nutritionist who can re-balance your diet and suggest supplements to boost your immune system. (See *General Health Hints*.)

Cracked lips

Lips that are sore and cracked, especially at the corners of the mouth, are usually a sign of a deficiency of B vitamins, vitamin B2 in particular. Very rarely, cracked lips can be a sign of vitamin A toxicity. You would need to have taken thousands of units of vitamin A for more than a month for this to happen, but nevertheless, if you have been taking extremely high doses of vitamin A, have a blood test.

Friendly Foods
- Vitamin B2 is found in milk, eggs, liver, green vegetables, and most other fresh vegetables.
- B vitamins are also found in wholegrain rice, quinoa, and buckwheat.
- This problem is also linked to lack of natural-source vitamin E and essential fats. So eat more wheat germ, avocados, oily fish, seeds and their unrefined oils.
- Generally, eat more foods high in natural carotenes such as pumpkin, carrots, papaya, apricots, and watercress.
- Since dehydration is also a major cause, drink more water.

Useful Remedies
- Take a high-strength vitamin B complex.
- Take a multi-vitamin/mineral that contains at least 30mg of zinc, 1–2mg of copper, 200IU of full-spectrum vitamin E, and 500mg of vitamin C.
- Rub pure vitamin E cream onto your lips at night.
- For two weeks only, take 30,000IU of vitamin A. After that, switch to natural-source beta-carotenes, which will naturally convert to vitamin A in the body and are non-toxic. **SVHC**

Helpful Hints
- Use a lip balm made from vitamin E and aloe vera.
- Take homeopathic Nat Mur 6x twice daily for 3–4 days.

Dry Mouth
(see also Sjogren's Syndrome)

If you have ever been extremely nervous then you know that your mouth automatically goes dry. This is because saliva, which contains enzymes for digestion, is not required when we are under extreme stress. In contrast, if you are really hungry and see tempting food, you automatically produce more saliva.

If you have dry mouth you may simply be thirsty, but if it is chronic, you may have digestive problems such as a leaky gut. Also, one of the classic symptoms of the autoimmune condition Sjogren's syndrome is an extremely dry mouth (and eyes). A consistently dry mouth can also be a sign of a potassium phosphate deficiency.

Foods to Avoid
- Flour and dense grain-based foods tend to draw water away from the body into feces in the bowel and make you feel more thirsty. Therefore, keep breads, cereals, cookies, cakes, and "drying" foods to sensible levels.

Friendly Foods
- Fresh fruits are packed with easy-to-absorb minerals that you may be lacking. Eat more melon, especially watermelon.
- Drink plenty of water.
- Essential fats found in nuts, seeds, oily fish and their unrefined oils help nourish a dehydrated system.

Useful Remedies
- Omega-7 fats extracted from the sea buckthorn really help support soft tissue in the mouth. Take two capsules daily for the long term. **VC**
- Take at least 1g of omega-3 fish oils daily.
- Include a multi-vitamin/mineral in your regimen.
- A dry mouth can be a sign of a potassium phosphate deficiency. Take NuAge Kali Phos. **VC**
- Xerostom products, based on olive oil, vitamin E, xylitol (to help protect the teeth), and betaine, all help soothe and moisturize the mouth. They include mouth gels, toothpastes, capsules, and chewing gum. Order from www.docsimon.com
- Begin taking liquid hyaluronic acid (HA) daily in water. HA is a naturally occurring protein in the body that helps it hold more water. HA is what makes young skin look plump and supple. Unfortunately, as we age levels of HA in the body decline, resulting in dry skin and joint problems. Take 1ml daily in water on an empty stomach to help re-hydrate the body. **VC**

Helpful Hints
- You will need to be careful about dental hygiene because the less saliva you make, the more likely you are to accumulate plaque and have various dental problems. Clean your teeth regularly and see a dental hygienist at least twice a year. If the problem becomes severe, you may need to use fluoride-containing toothpaste once a day and a more natural toothpaste the rest of the time.

MRSA AND SUPERBUGS

(see also Antibiotics and Immune Function)

One of the unhealthiest places you can find yourself these days is in certain hospitals, where infectious microbes such as *Acinetobacter* are found. According to the CDC, an estimated 1.7 million people are infected by a healthcare-associated infection each year, and at least 99,000 people die as a result.

Two of the most virulent and deadly infections are *Clostridium difficile*, which triggers acute diarrhea, followed by MRSA. In recent years strains of pathogenic bacteria that are resistant to all known antibiotics, including methicillin, have given rise to the condition's technical name, MRSA, standing for methicillin-resistant *Staphylococcus aureus*. The secret to avoiding becoming one of the 1 in 20 patients who contract a serious hospital-acquired infection is to boost your immune function and take sensible precautions.

MRSA produces symptoms no different from any other type of *Staphylococcus aureus* ("Staph") infection. A patient may experience redness and inflammation around wound sites on their skin, but once it enters the body, symptoms can be more serious and include fever, lethargy, headache, urinary tract infections, pneumonia, toxic shock syndrome, and even death.

Staph infections, including MRSA, occur most frequently among people in hospitals and healthcare facilities (such as nursing homes and dialysis centers) who have weakened immune systems. However, there have been cases in which people have become infected with MRSA without having a medical procedure or spending time in a hospital. In these cases it is known as CA-MRSA—community-associated MRSA.

The media term "superbug" has distracted from the fact that MRSA is a man-made problem that is avoidable. Overuse and abuse of antibiotics have led to the emergence of resistant strains. The key to fighting any infection (regular or super) is to support and enhance natural immunity rather than relying on medication. This can be done through proper diet, supplements, and specific safe remedies, such as herbs and homeopathy. If you do have to go to a hospital for any reason, make sure to boost your immune system beforehand. MRSA rarely affects really healthy individuals. (See *Antibiotics* and *Immune Function*.)

Foods to Avoid
- Eliminate refined sugar, which has been scientifically shown to slow the performance of the white blood cells needed to isolate and destroy infectious invaders. This means stay away from all manufactured and "junk" foods because sugar is often an unsuspected ingredient. Also limit your intake of sweet fruit juices and fruits such as dates and grapes.
- Also avoid artificial sweeteners such as aspartame.
- Keep in mind that honey, brown rice syrup and maple-type syrups are all sugar—although somewhat healthier.
- Also see *Food Poisoning*.

Friendly Foods
- Also see *Immune Function* and *General Health Hints*.
- Garlic is especially useful, as it has antibacterial and anti-viral properties.
- You can eat small amounts of manuka pure honey with a UMF level of 15, which has been shown to kill MRSA bacteria. The higher the UMF, the more antiseptic the honey. If the MRSA causes open sores, then honey-containing dressings (made by Advancis) are also available. Visit www.benefitsofhoney.us for more information.
- Healthier forms of sugar with a lower glycemic index are xylitol and organic agave syrup. **VC, VS**

Useful Remedies
- See this section under *Antibiotics* and *Immune Function*.
- Bee propolis is a substance that bees manufacture to sterilize their hives, which has been shown in three studies to kill MRSA bacteria. You would need to take 3g a day before any hospital stay and continue for at least a month afterward. **VC NB: If you severely allergic to bee stings, avoid propolis.**
- *Astragalus membranaceus*, or Chinese root, is widely used throughout Asia. Scientific studies from the University of Texas Medical Center in Houston have shown that it boosts immune performance by enhancing white-cell activity, stimulating interferon, and reducing infection times. (Because of this, astralagus could also be beneficial for cancer and AIDS patients.) **VC**

- Herbs such as pau d'arco and St John's wort have been shown to help destroy MRSA. You would need 3–4g of St John's wort and 1–3g of pau d'arco daily. **NB: If you are taking blood-thinning medication, avoid St John's wort.**
- Beta Glucans 1–3, 1–6, which are derived from yeast cell walls, are proven to strengthen the body's innate immune system (the immune system you are born with), making it more resistant to pathogens from food and air. Take 250–500mg daily. Beta Glucans have also been shown to reduce post-surgical infections by as much as 50%, and they help the body fight off any bacterial infection. Dr Paul Clayton, based in the UK and US, is a medical pharmacologist who has done a lot of research on Beta Glucans, much of which you can find on his website: www.healthdefence.com **VC**
- If you are placed on high doses of antibiotics, make sure to take a course of healthy bacteria (probiotics) afterward. (See *Antibiotics*.)
- Oregano is a powerful antibacterial and anti-viral herb. Try taking oregano oil capsules while you are in the hospital. **VC**

Helpful Hints

- Make sure to ask all nurses, doctors, and anyone else who has contact with you in a hospital to wash their hands thoroughly in warm soapy water before they touch you. You can also take antibacterial wipes with you and wear sterile gloves (available from all pharmacies). Keep your visitors to a minimum, and as much as possible, make sure that your room or the area around your bed is cleaned really thoroughly. Ask a relative to take your towels and so on to wash in a very hot wash. Simple measures like these can save lives.

- You can buy oregano essential oil as a spray and use it to coat any surfaces, as it has potent anti-viral and antibacterial properties. You can also inhale steam with a little added oregano oil, apply a little of the pure oil to the spine, or dilute it in a base of almond oil for massage.
- Researchers at the University of Leeds in the UK have shown that using ionizers in hospitals can greatly reduce *Acinetobacter* infections. They believe the negative ions that are emitted remove bacteria from the air, thus stopping the transmission of many infections. Take an ionizer into the hospital with you and place it near your bed!
- If you have a severe infection, look into the possibility of having hydrochloric acid injections. In 1927 Dr Burr Ferguson, MD of Birmingham, Alabama began injecting patients suffering from severe infections with very dilute concentrations (1:1,000) of hydrochloric acid. This is a substance that occurs naturally in human stomachs in far higher concentrations. Ferguson's results were published in the journal *Medical World* in 1932. One of the most sensational cases was a woman at the point of death from puerperal sepsis. William Howell, a doctor who had read Fereguson's findings, injected the woman with hydrochloric acid. Within an hour her temperature had dropped from 106°F to 103°F, and the woman said she felt much better. Except for feeling a bit weak, the following day all trace of the infection had disappeared! These were dramatic pioneer days. Find more details visit www.tldp.com/issue/11_00/martin.htm

MULTIPLE SCLEROSIS (MS)

(See also Adrenal Exhaustion, Candida, and Leaky Gut)

Multiple sclerosis (MS) is a chronic, progressive, disabling disease that affects the central nervous system (the brain and spinal cord). Inside your brain and spinal cord there are two types of matter, gray and white, which are made up of millions of nerve cells. The white matter contains nerve fibers that are coated with a myelin sheath (similar to an electrical cord with the wire covered by a white outer-insulating case). The job of the myelin is to speed up nerve transmissions and allow for the easy passage of electrical signals. When the myelin breaks down or becomes inflamed, nerve transmission is disrupted, thus resulting in the damage seen in MS.

MS is also an autoimmune disease, which means that the body's own immune system is attacking the myelin. Initial symptoms may be tingling; numbness; weakness affecting a hand, foot, or one side of the body; double vision; or a loss of sensation in various parts of the body. Difficulty walking, slurred speech, tremors, and inflammation of the optic nerve are found in around 55% of sufferers, and these symptoms serve as one of the early warning signs of MS. Also, a decline in cognitive function is sometimes a symptom, such as not being able to find a word that you use regularly in conversation, or impaired reasoning ability. Dizziness and vertigo are common symptoms, as are feelings of light-headedness. (See *Adrenal Exhaustion*.)

Bladder dysfunction occurs in more than 80% of cases. More women than men suffer from MS, which can begin at virtually any age but most commonly appears between the ages of 20–40. Depression is also common among MS sufferers.

MS is not a hereditary disease although in rare cases it can strike members of the same family. People living closer to the equator seem to be less at risk of developing MS, and in countries such as Malaysia and Ecuador, it is virtually unknown. This thought to be linked to vitamin D levels (see *Useful Remedies,* below).

There are four main types of MS, but each sufferer has a unique set of symptoms and disease pattern, making it very difficult to diagnose. For this reason it may be missed by doctors for several years, leading to considerable frustration.

M

Type 1—Benign MS This usually starts with a small number of mild attacks followed by complete recovery. It does not worsen over time, and there is no permanent disability. The first symptoms are usually sensory. It is only possible to classify people as having benign MS when they have little sign of disability 10–15 years after the onset of the disease. Around 20% of people with MS have the benign form.

Type 2—Relapsing-Remitting MS This is the most common form of MS. Periods of remission are interrupted by periods of attacks. The attacks can range from mild to quite debilitating. In the early stages of the disease, complete recovery between relapses is common, but over time remissions may result in residual symptoms caused by the damage done to the myelin during the attack. Around 25% of people with MS have this relapsing-remitting form.

Type 3—Secondary Progressive This type starts out as relapsing-remitting MS; however, after repeated attacks, remissions stop and the condition moves into a progressive stage. The time it takes to move into the progressive phase varies, but it usually happens within 15–20 years from the first onset of MS.

Type 4—Primary Progressive Some people with MS have no distinct relapses and periods of remission. From the beginning they experience steadily worsening symptoms and progressive disability. This may level off at any one time or may continue to get worse. Around 15% of people with MS have this type, which is also known as "chronic progressive."

The onset of MS has been attributed to having a weak nervous system that is then aggravated by trauma, shock, infection, or toxic metals, especially mercury. Dr Patrick Kingsley, who before he retired was one of Britain's leading alternative nutritional physicians specializing in cancer and MS, told me: "Many of my patients had high levels of mercury in their spinal fluid, and the first thing I recommend is that they have the emissions measured from any mercury fillings." Dr Kingsley also says that "MS symptoms can also mimic those of candida, so this possibility, plus a leaky gut, would also need to be eliminated." Parasites are another consideration. (See also *Candida* and *Leaky Gut*.)

Up to 70% of people with MS have problems absorbing nutrients so deficiencies are common, especially in B vitamins, vitamin D, and the essential fats (EFAs) needed to make up myelin. EFAs play a critical role in MS (see the "Swank" diet below). For this reason, therapeutic doses of some supplements are needed. Many patients also have multiple sensitivities to certain foods, the most common being gluten and cow's milk and dairy products. In fact, these foods are now considered a major trigger. However, individual patients may react to almost any food so sensitivities need to be identified on an individual basis. Many patients benefit when they follow a strict anti-candida and gluten-free diet. (See *Allergies*.)

Exciting work is being carried on by Dr Paolo Zamboni in Italy, who has found that most MS patients have a narrowing or twisting of the veins in the neck (known as CCSVI). This prevents blood in the brain from draining properly so it "refluxes" back up, triggering a host of problems. By surgically unblocking these veins, many MS patients are experiencing fewer MS-type symptoms. You can contact Dr Zamboni via the Department of Surgery at the University of Ferrara in Italy. E-mail: zmp@unife.it

Trials at Georgetown University and the University of Buffalo have left little doubt that CCSVI is a causal factor in the majority of, but not all, MS cases. Therefore, if CCSVI is detected after a scan, researchers recommend it should be treated as soon as possible.

Meanwhile, other research is also ongoing using stem cells to help MS (and cancer) sufferers. Professor Shimon Slavin is one of the world's leading experts in this field and runs a state-of-the-art center that people from all over the world come to for treatment. Contact him via The International Center for Cell Therapy & Cancer Immunotherapy, Tel Aviv Medical Centre, 14 Weizman Street, Tel Aviv 64239 Israel. E-mail: slavin@CTCIcenter.com

Nutrition is a very important factor in managing MS. The most common diets are:

The Swank Low-Saturated-Fat Diet
Professor Swank started his research in the 1940s in North America. He noticed that MS was higher in countries in which the diet was rich in animal fats and where lots of dairy products were consumed. Therefore, he recommended a low-saturated-fat diet that was high in essential fats from fish oils (DHA and EPA), as well as GLA found in evening primrose oil. (See under *Fats You Need To Eat*.) For more information visit www.swankmsdiet.org

Stone Age Diet or "Best-Bet Diet"
Research done by Canadian scientist Dr Ashton Embry has resulted in the "Best Bet Diet." The thinking behind this diet is that certain people are especially sensitive to "modern" foods. Therefore, he advocated excluding all "new" foods as well as foods that may have been around during the Stone Age but have changed significantly since then. For example, modern wheat is bred to increase its gluten capacity so that cakes, breads, and pastries can gain added structure, thereby increasing their appearance and shelf life. The "Best Bet Diet" excludes all gluten grains, animal dairy produce, beans, legumes, eggs, margarine, refined oils, yeast, refined sugar, and saturated fat. Embry has an excellent website at www.direct-ms.org

Foods to Avoid

- Cut down on saturated fats. Especially reduce or avoid those from animal sources, including meats and all full-fat dairy products (butter, cheese, milk, chocolates, and cream). Be careful of curries as these are generally cooked using ghee, a clarified butter. Especially avoid cow's milk, yogurt, and even quark.
- Avoid all oils and hydrogenated or trans-fats. These are found in many meat-substitute meals, margarines, cookies, cakes, pastries, and most mass-produced vegetable oils. (See *Fats You Need To Eat*.)
- Avoid fried food, potato chips, French fries, burgers, and so on as they can lead to inflammation. Instead grill, stew, poach, steam, and bake.
- Avoid all refined carbohydrates and any foods containing gluten, such as white bread and rice, pies, pastries, pizza, cakes, and cookies.
- As refined sugar also triggers inflammation in the body, avoid it as much as you can.
- Avoid caffeine found in tea, coffee, sodas, chocolates, some painkillers, and many energy drinks.
- Avoid alfalfa sprouts. Although these are an excellent food source for most people, they should not be eaten by people with autoimmune diseases.
- Avoid alcohol, which can cause nerve damage and depletes essential B vitamins known to help MS.
- It is crucial that you identify and eliminate any foods that you have an intolerance to. (See under *Allergies*.)

Friendly Foods

- Great alternatives to caffeine drinks are herbal and fruit teas and diluted organic fruit and vegetable juices. Homemade is best. Drink immediately after juicing for optimum results.
- Instead of cow's milk try oat, rice, quinoa, almond, or skimmed coconut milk. These are all available from health stores and some supermarkets.
- Juices, soups, and stews are easy-to-absorb, nutritious foods.
- Eat plenty of oily fish like organic salmon, mackerel, herring, sardines, and anchovies. (See *Mercury Fillings* for a list of fish that should be avoided as they are high in mercury). Fish oils reduce inflammation and also provide the raw materials for making myelin.
- Eat plenty of fresh, preferably organic, leafy green vegetables, as they are full of B vitamins and antioxidants, which help protect good fats from damage.
- Gamma-linolenic acid (GLA) is found in sunflower seeds and safflower oil and helps nourish nerve endings. Use unrefined, organic seeds and oils. Always keep them in the fridge.
- Pumpkin, sunflower, sesame, and flaxseeds and their unrefined oils are all rich in essential fats that are vital for people with MS.
- Eat organic foods as much as possible.
- People on vegan or gluten-free diets often experience some relief from symptoms, but the diet would need to be maintained for at least two years. Vegan diets are rich in the essential fats needed for nerve function and are low in saturated fat.
- Eat more brown rice, quinoa, kamut, lentils, barley, and whole grains.
- Substitute sodium salts with mineral-rich seaweeds such as nori flakes. Available from all health stores.
- Eat plenty of GM-free, organic lecithin granules, which are very important for the structure of the myelin sheath.
- Blueberries are a particularly good source of antioxidants, which protect myelin from free-radical damage. Eat daily.
- Add more curcumin (from the spice turmeric) to foods. This helps slow the erosion of the myelin sheath. In countries where people eat plenty of curcumin, MS is very rare.

Useful Remedies

- Take a good-quality multi-vitamin/mineral to cover your basic needs.
- Also take a full-spectrum beta-carotene complex. **SVHC**
- Take 100mg of vitamin B1 (thiamine) daily, which is an essential component of myelin, as is vitamin B12. Take 1000mcg per day. Also take 50mg of vitamin B6.
- If you prefer not to take three pills, since the B-group vitamins work together, you can take a high-strength B complex daily instead.
- You can take up to 3g of vitamin C daily. Take it with meals in an ascorbate formula spread throughout the day.
- If muscle aches are a problem, take 200–600mg of magnesium spread throughout the day to help relax muscles.
- Omega-3-rich fish oils help support nerve endings and are needed for normal functioning of the brain and nervous system, as well as for the production of myelin. Take around 2–4g daily, more on days when you don't eat oily fish.
- Taking 2g of GLA daily will help suppress autoimmune reactions and help provide the building blocks needed rebuild the myelin sheath.
- Take a digestive enzyme with main meals to help increase the absorption of nutrients from your food.
- Co-enzyme Q10, a vitamin-like substance, is a potent protective antioxidant and also plays an important role in energy production. Take 100–200mg daily taken in divided doses with breakfast and lunch. **SVHC, VC, VS**

- Take a probiotic (healthy bacteria) supplement daily to help keep your digestion and bowel in top condition. Try Jarrow-Dophilus EPS. **JF**
- Studies have shown the amino acid acetyl L-carnitine to be more effective and better tolerated than the medication Amatadine, which is given to improve energy. Take 1000mg twice a day at least 30 minutes before meals. **VC**
- Lipoic acid is a powerful antioxidant that helps protect the myelin sheath. Take up to 400mg twice daily.
- Vitamin D regulates immune function. Countries with the lowest levels of vitamin D have the highest levels of MS. During a day in the sun your body can make 20,000IU of vitamin D; therefore, with your doctor's permission, take 5,000IU of vitamin D3 daily for a month and then stay on a maintenance dose of 600–800IU daily. **NB: Only take higher levels of D3 under the guidance of a health professional and/or doctor.**
- In numerous studies of autoimmune conditions from the US, Hungary, Israel, and Russia, fermented wheat germ extract known as AWGE has demonstrated remarkably beneficial immune-modulating effects. Take one sachet daily in water at least one hour before breakfast. Keep refrigerated. Also available in capsules, but you would need quite a few; therefore, the powder is easier to take once a day. For more information visit www.avemarwge.com

Helpful Hints

- To discover which foods you are intolerant to, contact Genova Diagnostics at 1-800-522-4762 or visit their website: www.genovadiagnostics.com
- Vitamin D helps regulate immune function and lift mood. Ask your doctor to run a 25(OH)D test to look at your levels. Optimal levels are 45–50ng/ml or 115–128nmol/l. If your levels are out of this range, contact a nutritional therapist who can help you address this issue. Any levels below 20ng/ml are considered serious deficiency states and will increase the risk of autoimmune diseases.
- Check the possibility of excess mercury in your diet or environment.

- Consider having a hair mineral analysis to check your body levels of mercury. This is a non-invasive test that only requires a small sample of hair. Contact ARL Analytical Research Laboratories Inc. at 1-800-528-4067 (toll free) or 1-602-995-1580. Website: www.arltma.com
- Vitamin B12 injections may help some patients.
- Take three 10–20 minute rest periods every day, spaced throughout the day. Also do some form of exercise every day, such as walking, doing push-ups, or weight lifting. Start slowly and build up gradually.
- Cranial osteopathy is a whole-body treatment that works with the central nervous system and the rhythmic pulsation that it produces. It has been very beneficial for some people with MS. Find a practitioner at www.cranialacademy.com or www.naturalsolutionsmag.com/find-practitioner
- Have a look at www.melisa.org—a medical network that gives the latest research linking mercury fillings to MS. (See also *Mercury Fillings*.)
- There are a number of organizations and societies that provide educational resources, support and advice. These include:
  1. The National Multiple Sclerosis Society. Tel: 1-800-344-4867. Website: www.nationalmssociety.org
  2. The Multiple Sclerosis Association of America. Tel: 1-800-532-7667 (toll free) or 1-856-488-4500. Website: www.msassociation.org
  3. The Multiple Sclerosis Foundation. MS Helpline: 1-888-673-6287. Website: www.msfocus.org
  4. MS Moms. Website: www.msmoms.com

- Susie Cornell, MS sufferer and director of Under Press, the UK's leading MS Clinic, has written a great book called *The Complete MS Body Manual* (Under Pressure Publications). Susie leads the field with a revolutionary approach in the natural treatment of MS. For more information visit www.susiecornell.com
- For more help read *Multiple Sclerosis* by Judy Graham (Thorsons), the founder of the Multiple Sclerosis Resource Centre. She also has written a very informative book called *Multiple Sclerosis and Having a Baby* (Healing Arts Press).

N

NAIL PROBLEMS

(see also Absorption, Leaky Gut, and Low Stomach Acid)

Nails are mostly made up of keratin, a protein-like substance, which is also found in your hair. There are fat and water molecules in between the keratin, which help keep nails healthy and supple.

Your nails are a great barometer of your health. For example, if you are stressed or have poor digestion, then stomach acid levels often fall and you may notice longitudinal (top to bottom) ridges in your nails. Ridges across the nails (from side to side) can denote stress, as well as a lack of calcium and/or magnesium. White spots can show that you are either ingesting too much sugar, alcohol, and junk foods, or have insufficient zinc in your body. Brittle, transparent, and flat-looking nails that curl up at the edges are a common problem that is associated with low iron levels. However, as excessive iron intake after the age of 50 is linked to heart disease, don't take too much iron unless a blood test shows that you need it.

Brittle, splitting nails are a sign of a silica deficiency, while soft, peeling nails often indicate a calcium deficiency. Excessively curved nails (like an upside-down spoon) can indicate a potassium deficiency.

Anyone who has their hands in water for long periods of time usually has weaker nails, and biting your nails is an obvious cause of poor nail appearance. Fungal infections turn the nails white, or at the very least, cause discoloration and deformity. Nails can thicken if you eat too much protein or when the immune system is weak. If your nail beds are red, your liver may be congested from too much fat and alcohol, and you should have your cholesterol levels checked.

Foods to Avoid
- Avoid junk foods, soft drinks, white bread, cookies, and pastries. All of these foods deplete the body of nutrients, especially B vitamins.
- Reduce your intake of caffeine and alcohol.
- Keep sugar to a minimum.
- Hard, thick nails can be a sign that you are eating too much fat and excess protein. Avoid hydrogenated or trans-fats. Also avoid too much fat from animal sources, including full-fat milk, cheeses, chocolates, pies, desserts, and so on.

Friendly Foods

- Make sure to eat good-quality protein at least once a day, as nails are made from protein. Try chicken, fish, quinoa, cooked tofu, or a little organic lean red meat.
- Eggs, blackstrap molasses, almonds, red meats, and spinach are rich in iron.
- Oily fish and unrefined nuts and seeds (especially hazelnuts, Brazil nuts, walnuts, sunflower seeds, pumpkin seeds, sesame seeds, and flax seeds) are rich in zinc and essential fats. Use their unrefined oils over salads and cooked foods to nourish your nails.
- Drink plenty of fluids.
- Eat more pumpkin, apricots, papaya, green leafy vegetables (especially kale, watercress, and spinach), cantaloupe melons, and sweet potatoes for their vitamin A content.
- Cereals, brown rice, buckwheat, amaranth, oats, organ meats, eggs, lentils, peas, nuts, and leafy green organic vegetables are all rich in B vitamins, which are vital for healthy nails.
- Eating a small amount of pineapple and papaya before or after meals aids digestion.
- Eat one avocado a week and sprinkle organic wheat germ over cereals and desserts, as they are rich in vitamin E.
- Silica-rich foods are lettuce, green and red peppers, cucumbers, bean sprouts, and asparagus, as well as all other high-fiber foods, vegetables, and whole grains.

Useful Remedies
- Take a comprehensive multi-nutrient vitamin/mineral formula that includes essential fats. All of the companies listed on pages 15–16 have in-house nutritionists who can help you choose the right multi for your age and gender.
- Take a B-complex plus 2.5mg of biotin, a lack of which is linked to brittle nails. Vegetarians and vegans often also have low levels of B12, which is found in meat, fish, and eggs; therefore, make sure that your B-complex contains at least 50mcg of B12. (Most multi formulas will include all B-group vitamins.)
- The mineral silica is important for healthy nails. Take 75mg daily.
- If you have a fungal infection, the herbs pau d'arco (two 500mg capsules twice daily) and cat's claw (two 500mg capsules twice daily) will reduce fungus in the body and nails. Also follow a low-sugar diet.

- NuAge Tissue K helps reduce brittle nails, and Combination L helps reduce fungal problems.
- MSM, an organic form of sulfur, helps strengthen nails. Take 1000mg daily.
- White blobs (more than tiny spots) on the nails can signify a lack of selenium. Take 200mcg daily.
- Collagen is a vital component of healthy joints, cartilage, ligaments, and tendons, and it also helps build nails. Take daily in a glass of water or diluted fruit juice 30 minutes before a main meal. Super Collagen drink is available from NeoCell. **VC**

Helpful Hints

- Massage jojoba, neem, and lemon oil into your nails to nourish and prevent splitting. **VC**
- Nail-polish remover contains solvents that are notorious for drying out nails and making them more brittle. Most nail salons and beauty counters sell oils specifically for the nails, which can be used after painting. Always use a base coat.
- To remove yellow stains from your nails, soak them in a cup of warm water that contains the juice of one lemon for 15 minutes daily.
- Massage your nails regularly with jojoba, olive, or almond oil.
- If you have a fungal infection, soak your nails in white distilled vinegar for at least 10 minutes twice a day. You can also use diluted tee tree oil or neem oil on the nails. ICI Natural makes a neem and tea tree cream that can be used on hands and nails. Available online from Amazon.
- Bacteria, viruses, and superbugs can breed under the nails, and being in close contact with someone who has dirty nails is a great way to pass on infections. Also if you shake hands with someone who has a cold, this too will spread the virus. Keep your nails clean.
- If your nails are constantly in water, then wear surgical or rubber gloves. Wear gloves while gardening.
- Only use nail salons that keep their instruments scrupulously clean.

NAUSEA

(see Vomiting)

NUMBNESS/TINGLING SENSATIONS— FINGERS AND TOES

These types of symptoms are usually a sign of poor circulation (see *Circulation, Diabetes*, and *Raynaud's Disease*) but can also be caused by pressure on a nerve. These sensations are common if you sleep or sit in an awkward position but may also be a symptom of cervical spondylosis (pressure on nerves in the neck, causing numbness in the hands, a stiff neck, or headaches) or carpal tunnel syndrome (numbness in the thumb-side of the hand and sharp pain at night). If you continually have really cold fingers and toes during the winter, you may well be suffering from Raynaud's disease (see *Raynaud's Disease*). Any conditions that reduce circulation to the nerves in the skin will produce these types of symptoms. If symptoms continue have a check-up, as numbness is also linked to multiple sclerosis, ME, and Sjogren's syndrome.

Foods to Avoid

- See this section under *Atherosclerosis* and *Circulation*.
- Generally avoid caffeine, animal fats, and smoking.

Friendly Foods

- See also *Circulation*.
- You are likely to be lacking essential fats, which are found in oily fish, flaxseeds, and sunflower and pumpkin seeds and their unrefined oils. (See *Fats You need To Eat*.)
- Eat more blueberries, blackberries, sweet potatoes, cherries, apricots, spinach, watercress, kale and all leafy green vegetables. These are all rich in flavonoids, which help strengthen capillaries.
- Wheat germ and avocados are rich in vitamin E, which thin the blood naturally.
- Garlic is great for circulation, while ginger will warm you.
- Lecithin granules help repair nerve endings. Sprinkle them on breakfast cereals or mix them into yogurts.

Useful Remedies

- Take a high-strength vitamin B-complex daily. B vitamin deficiencies can cause tingling in the nerve endings.
- Older people may also benefit from a B12 injection or a 1mg B12 tablet; a lack of this vitamin is linked to tingling in the extremities.
- Take 1–2g of vitamin C with bioflavonoids daily spread throughout the day with meals to help repair nerve endings.
- Lipoic acid, a powerful antioxidant, has been shown to improve diabetic neuropathy. It is also a great nutrient for the brain and helps balance blood sugar levels. Take 200mg daily with food.

- Essential fats are needed for good circulation and well-toned blood vessels. Omega-3s (found in fish oils) have been shown to reduce blood-vessel spasms; omega-6s (in nuts and seeds) inhibit blood-vessel constriction.
- Fish oil is a great source of omega-3 fatty acids (EPA and DHA). Taking pure fish oil such as Krill Oil is more beneficial than flaxseed oil for this condition. Omega-6 fatty acids (GLAs) are found in evening primrose and borage (starflower) oils. (See *Fats You Need To Eat*.)
- As this problem can denote a calcium deficiency, take 600mg of calcium daily, plus a multi-mineral that includes 400mg of magnesium.
- The herb gotu kola taken over time (3 months) helps increase circulation to the extremities. 500mg twice daily.

Helpful Hints

- If, after taking these supplements for 6 weeks, you still have numb/tingling fingers or toes, see your doctor.
- Walking for half an hour each day or skipping, jumping on a small trampoline, and swinging your arms full circle regularly will help get your circulation going.
- It is also helpful to massage your hands and feet. Obviously, it is easy to massage your own hands, but if you find it difficult to massage your own feet, ask your partner, a relative, or a friend to do it for you. Use essential oils of geranium, ginger, black pepper, and lavender in a base oil. If you have no one to massage your feet, put a few drops of the oils in the bath and soak your feet for 10 minutes.
- Reflexology and acupuncture often help reduce or eliminate this type of problem. (See *Useful Information*.)
- You may have a trapped nerve, in which case consult a chiropractor or an osteopath.

OBESITY

(see Weight Problems)

OSTEOARTHRITIS

(see Arthritis)

OSTEOPOROSIS

(see also Acid–Alkaline Balance, Adrenal Exhaustion, Leaky Gut, Menopause, and Stress)

Osteoporosis silently threatens men and women—and, thanks to our highly stressed lifestyles, over-consumption of sugary refined foods, and a host of other factors, we are now at huge risk from a health time bomb. An estimated 8 million women in the US alone have been diagnosed with osteoporosis, and at least 33 million more are at risk of developing the disease. Because of this disease, nearly 300,000 hip fractures occur every year in US, costing $13–18 billion annually in medical bills, rehabilitation, extended care facilities, and lost productivity, as well as costing 20% of those with fractures their lives. One in two women and one in four men over the age of 50 will break a bone because of osteoporosis during their lifetime.

Your bone mass peaks in the your mid-twenties, but if you live a fast- paced lifestyle and tend to become stressed easily, then you seriously need to start looking after your bones now. Excess production of the stress hormones adrenalin and cortisol can hugely deplete minerals from your bones. In addition, if you also tend to eat in a hurry, eat plenty of refined sugary or pre-packaged foods, and have taken antibiotics, then you may have a leaky gut. This is an often overlooked problem that also contributes to your risk of developing osteoporosis and a host of other health problems later in life, because you may not be absorbing sufficient nutrients from your diet. Therefore, before reading on, please read the *Absorption, Acid–Alkaline Balance, Adrenal Exhaustion*, and *Leaky Gut* sections.

Although osteoporosis still tends to be thought of as a disease of old age, there is now no doubt that its roots lie in adolescence. Many young people love soft drinks that are high in the industrially altered version of the mineral phosphorous, and too much can deplete bone minerals. I reiterate that junk foods, alcohol, too much caffeine, and refined sugar also deplete minerals—as does stress.

Genetics and other hormones besides cortisol and adrenalin also play an important role in osteoporosis developing. For example, when I was in my early thirties I had a hysterectomy, and at that time no one warned me that I might need to use prescription estrogen to protect my bones. If you keep your ovaries after surgery, you will produce some estrogen for a time, but often not enough to prevent the osteoporosis that crippled my mother. I have always taken bone supplements and done plenty of weight-bearing exercise, but I now know that these alone did not compensate for the years of insufficient estrogen, which is why I now have osteoporosis. My Type A personality of always being in a rush and having plenty of stress in my life, which at times I did not deal with effectively, plus antibiotics in my teens and twenties, which at times have triggered leaky gut issues, have also contributed to my osteoporosis.

Therefore, if you have an early menopause, which is becoming more common thanks to our stressful and toxic environment, or you have a hysterectomy (even if you keep your ovaries), please make sure that your hormone levels are checked every year.... otherwise you could end up like me. Make no mistake—osteoporosis can kill you. I beg of you to take heed, because prevention is absolutely better than cure.

Osteoporosis is also associated with a lack of weight-bearing exercise, excess animal protein in the diet, low body weight, and lack of skin exposure to sunshine (being out in the sun increases vitamin D levels in the body). My mother undoubtedly suffered from osteoporosi—partly due to her poor diet, but also because she never exposed her skin to the sun. When she died at 78, her skin was amazingly wrinkle free, but her bones were in a dreadful state. I firmly believe that women who are fanatical about staying out of the sun would definitely benefit from exposing their skin regularly to 15 minutes of early-morning or late-afternoon sunshine to boost their vitamin D levels. Everyone, including children, should also supplement extra vitamin D3.

Other risk factors are a family history of osteoporosis, premature menopause, some cancers, long-term use of certain drugs (such as tranquillizers and steroids), a thin body-frame (which I have), and smoking. Women who suffered from anorexia when they were younger and those who exercise to the point where their periods stop are also at risk because of lowered hormone levels. As always, a sensible balance is needed.

Traditionally osteoporosis is prevented and treated by hormone replacement therapy (HRT), but nutritional scientist and naturopath Bob Jacobs says: "Women who have taken orthodox HRT for 10 years or more may have a greater bone density than those who have not taken it, but they lose any increased bone density rapidly when the HRT is stopped, and end up with only 3.2% higher bone density than women who took nothing. When women exercise regularly, eat a healthy diet, and take the right vitamins and minerals, bone density can be maintained and even increased, without having to endure the potential side effects of conventional HRT, which are an increased risk of breast and endometrial (womb) cancers, thrombosis, and strokes. If extra hormones are required, it is far better to use bio-identical hormone therapy." (See *Useful Remedies*, below.)

Other hormones, such as DHEA and testosterone, also play a part in good bone health.

My co-author, naturopath Stephen Langley, adds: "Calcium is relatively easy to get (and absorb) in our diet, as it is abundant in so many foods—the problem is not that you aren't getting enough calcium in your bones, but *keeping* it in your bones. To do that you need other nutrients, particularly magnesium, otherwise all the calcium you eat will end up in your tissues and will then be excreted. This is why, rather than loading up on dairy foods (which are acid forming and thus deplete minerals from your body), women would be better advised to eat far more magnesium- rich foods, such as green leafy vegetables, to buffer excess acidity."

Foods to Avoid

- Generally cut down on caffeine. More than three cups of strong coffee a day can increase your risk of developing osteoporosis by as much as 80%.
- Our Western diets tend to be very high in acid-forming foods, which cause calcium to leach from the bones. These include all "white" foods: breads, cakes, croissants, cookies, refined sugars, white pasta and rice and so on. (See *Acid–Alkaline Balance*.)
- Gluten sensitivity can be an issue (see under *Allergies*) as celiacs, for instance, are more likely to suffer from osteoporosis due to poor calcium absorption.
- Some people eat too much animal protein, which increases acidity of the blood and promotes calcium loss from the bones.

- Avoid carbonated drinks because the artificial carbonation creates carbonic acid, which dissolves bone, and the excess phosphates force more calcium to be excreted.
- Avoid excess alcohol. Consuming more than two alcoholic drinks daily decreases calcium absorption from your diet. It also interferes with the synthesis of vitamin D, which helps the bones absorb calcium.
- All dairy foods from animal sources increase calcium loss, but also provide calcium. Eating 4oz (100g) of kale or spring greens will have at least as much of a beneficial effect on calcium balance as 8oz (200g) of milk or 4oz (100g) of cheddar cheese.
- Avoid fluoride as much as you can, which is also linked to bone loss. (See *Fluoride*.)

Friendly Foods
- Fewer vegetarians tend to suffer from osteoporosis because their diet usually contains far more vegetables, pulses, grains, and fruits.
- Foods that are high in calcium and magnesium will help reduce calcium loss from bones, so eat more green leafy vegetables, such as kale, alfalfa, watercress, kelp, broccoli, cabbage, and spring greens.
- Fish and sesame seeds contain as much calcium as many animal- source milks.
- Eat more fermented soy-based foods, such as tempeh and natto, which are high in phyto-estrogens (isoflavones). (See this section under *Menopause*.)
- Magnesium is found in brown rice, buckwheat, lentils, peas, corn, almonds, cashews, and Brazil nuts, as well as sunflower, sesame, and pumpkin seeds, wheat germ, and wholegrain cereals.
- Vitamin D is found in egg yolks, oily fish, organ meats, and milk. It allows the body to absorb the calcium and phosphorous needed for healthy bones.
- Vitamin K is vital for healthy bones, as it keeps calcium in the bones and out of the arteries, where calcium deposits add to arterial plaque. Vitamin K is found in broccoli, green cabbage, lettuce, and especially kale.
- As low stomach acid is often a factor in osteoporosis, eat more pineapple or papaya before meals to aid absorption. (See *Low Stomach Acid*.)
- Silica is another important mineral for healthy bones and is found in lettuce, celery, cucumber, green and red peppers, bean sprouts, asparagus, millet, oats, and parsnips.
- Boron is a trace mineral needed for healthy bones. It is found in raisins, prunes, nuts, non-citrus fruits, and vegetables.
- Add 1 tablespoon of organic cider vinegar and honey to a glass of warm water daily. Sip throughout the day. This helps the body assimilate more calcium.
- Drink mineral waters in place of tap water. Fiji water is rich in silica.
- Otherwise, try Kangen Water—a water system unit that ionizes and greatly alkalizes water, thus supporting your bones. It has been used in Japanese hospitals with highly beneficial health results. For full details, visit www.kangenwaterusa.com

Useful Remedies
- Natural plant phyto-estrogens and soy-based estrogen supplements (isoflavones) promote a positive calcium balance. They also help make bone more resistant to releasing calcium and reduce urinary calcium loss. Estrogen levels decline with age in both men and women, with a particularly dramatic drop in women during menopause. **VC**
- Natural phyto-estrogen creams contain bio-identical (meaning the exact molecule that is found in the human body) progesterone made from wild yam. When used in tandem with estrogen from soybeans and proper nutrition, this combination can help increase bone density. To find out if you are at risk of osteoporosis, have a bone-density scan via your doctor and also ask for a urine DPD test to show if you are currently losing bone. If the bone scan is

OK and the urine test shows no bone loss, then you don't need extra hormones. But if your density is low and the urine test shows excessive bone breakdown, then natural hormones, the right diet, supplements, and exercise can be very useful. For a free information sheet on phyto-estrogen cream, call 1-310-301-4015 or visit www.pharmwest.com (Also see under *Menopause* for a full list of bio-identical hormones and where to source them.)

- As mentioned before, magnesium and calcium are also an important part of an overall supplement program. An optimum dose **for anyone with osteoporosis** would be 600mg of magnesium and 500mg of calcium daily taken in a chelated (or citrate) form, as they are more easily utilized by the body. They should be taken in divided doses throughout the day, with the final dose taken just before bedtime, as these minerals are known as nature's tranquillizers.

- To **prevent** osteoporosis, start taking around 300mg of calcium citrate and 400mg of magnesium citrate daily from your early 40s.

- Vitamin K2 (100mcg daily) is very important for gluing calcium into your bone matrix. Research has shown that vitamin K2 can reduce fracture risk by 65%. Most bone multi formulas contain some vitamin K2. **NB: If you are taking blood-thinning drugs, check with your doctor before taking any vitamin K.**

- Vitamin C (1–2g taken daily with meals in an ascorbate form) promotes the formation of proteins required in bone and is also involved in the synthesis and repair of all collagen, including cartilage and matrix of bone.

- Collagen is a vital component of healthy joints, cartilage, ligaments, and tendons and also improves bone strength. It is the most widely distributed protein in the body, and we lose about 1.5% annually after the age of 30. Take daily in a glass of water or diluted juice 30 minutes before a main meal to support your bones. Super Collagen drink from NeoCell. **VC**

- Zinc (15mg per day) is necessary for bone building. This should be in any multi-vitamin/mineral.

- Vitamin D3 (1,000IU daily) is **essential** for calcium and phosphorus absorption. Lack of vitamin D is now linked to more than 17 major diseases associated with aging.

- Boron (3mg per day) is necessary for the conversion of vitamin D into its active forms. It also helps the body produce natural estrogen. This mineral is vital for healthy bones.

- Vitamin B6 (100mg per day) is a necessary co-factor for many enzyme reactions involved in bone building.

- All the companies listed on pages 15–16 make multi-vitamin/mineral and bone formulas that contain a balanced supply of most of these nutrients and hydrochloric acid (stomach acid) to aid absorption. Don't be afraid to call and ask a nutritionist for help.

- The mineral strontium (citrate) has the unique ability to bind calcium into the bone and thus increase bone density. Take 200mg a day; however, it must be taken 12 hours away from calcium supplements. **VC**

Helpful Hints

- Because of our fast-paced lifestyles, our tissues tend to be more acid, causing calcium to be leached from our bones and magnesium from the muscles (these are the minerals that help re-alkalize our bodies). Therefore, learn to deal with stress in your life and your reaction to it. Basically, the more stressed you become, the more damage you are doing to your bones in the long run.

- After the age of 50, or before if you have surgery or go through early menopause, have a bone scan every two years and have all hormone levels checked.

- Do not smoke. Women who smoke generally experience menopause up to a year and a half earlier than non-smokers, and thus face a longer period of estrogen deficiency and accompanying bone loss. Smoking also hampers efficient processing of calcium. Smokers have a higher rate of spinal fractures than non-smokers.

- Osteoporosis is a largely preventable disease, and there are some commonsense things you can do to reduce your risk. As well as keeping your hormones balanced, another important preventative action is doing weight-bearing exercise. Swimming and cycling are great exercises, but they don't increase bone density because they are not weight bearing. Skipping, jogging, walking, using weights, aerobics, and rebounding (mini-trampolines) are great exercises to beat osteoporosis. Tennis players have a 30% higher bone density in their serving arm compared to their non-serving arm. For anyone already suffering from osteoporosis, join a local gym and begin exercising with a professional. In an ideal world begin weight training in your 20s and 30s before your bones start to thin, but it is never too late.
- Sunlight is needed to make active vitamin D in the body, so even if you are not an avid sunbather, expose your skin to at least 15 minutes of sun regularly—but not between 11am and 3pm.
- Dr Marilyn Glenville is one of the UK's leading experts on natural ways to cope with the menopause and osteoporosis. She has also written an excellent book: *Osteoporosis, The Silent Epidemic* (Kyle Cathie). For more information, visit www.marilynglenville.com

P

PALPITATIONS

(see also Adrenal Exhaustion, Heart Disease, Low Blood Sugar, Stress, and Tachycardia)

This is a fairly common problem that just about everyone experiences at one time or another. If you are under stress, have suffered a shock, are anxious or even over excited, then as the stress hormones adrenalin and cortisol are released, your heart automatically responds by beating faster. Once the anxiety has passed, your heart rate should calm down, but if it doesn't, then you have a problem. Palpitations occur when the heart beats irregularly; it can skip a beat or feel like a fluttering in the chest. If you find that you regularly suffer from any of these symptoms, that they do not recede when you are calm, or if you are regularly short of breath, then you definitely need to see your doctor. Palpitations can also indicate that there is a problem with the electrical circuitry in the heart.

Not only does over-production of the stress "fight-or-flight" hormones adrenaline and cortisol trigger palpitations, but food sensitivities can also be a factor. Low blood sugar can also contribute to palpitations and panic attacks. (See *Low Blood Sugar.*)

A lack of iron or imbalanced hormone levels, especially thyroid hormone and/or progesterone levels, can also be potential factors. A blood or saliva test administered by your doctor should indicate if hormonal imbalances are to blame.

Also, in highly sensitive individuals, electro-pollution from cellular phones, digital cordless phones, and WIFI is known to trigger palpitations. (See under *Electrical Pollution.*)

Foods to Avoid
- Avoid heavy alcohol intake, which can damage the heart muscle.

- Caffeine found in teas, coffee, all chocolates (pure dark chocolate has the highest concentration of caffeine), soft drinks, etc. stimulates the release of adrenaline into the bloodstream. I know of several people, including relatives of mine, who suffered from this problem if they touched **any** caffeine. Once caffeine was eliminated, their palpitations disappeared.
- Too much refined sugar, stress, and caffeine deplete magnesium from the body —the very mineral the body needs to stay calm.
- Food additives can trigger an attack in sensitive individuals.
- Generally don't eat large, heavy meals, which place an additional strain on the body.
- Avoid any energy drinks that contain the plant extract guarana, which is basically neat caffeine. Same for drinks like Red Bull.
- Any foods that you are intolerant to may also cause palpitations. The most common are wheat, eggs, dairy products from cows, and citrus fruits.
- Avoid eating large meals if you are anxious.

Friendly Foods.

- See *Angina, Atherosclerosis, Stress*, and *General Health Hints*.
- Drink more passiflora or chamomile tea to help calm yourself down.
- Use small amounts of brown rice syrup, organic agave syrup, stevia, or xylitol instead of refined sugar. Available from all health stores.
- Make sure you drink plenty of water, as dehydration can also be a contributing factor in palpitations.

Useful Remedies

- A pinch of cayenne pepper swallowed with a little water in most cases helps regulate the heartbeat very quickly.
- An irregular heartbeat is also linked to electrolyte imbalances, including calcium, magnesium, potassium, and even sodium. Take 99mg of potassium daily for one month. **SVHC** Also take a calcium/magnesium formula that contains 100–400mg of magnesium and 200mg of calcium twice daily in divided doses, taking the final dose at bedtime. (Your doctor can do a blood test to see if you are lacking potassium, sodium, or calcium.)
- Folic acid (600 mcg daily) helps stabilize the heartbeat. Sometimes a high homocysteine level can contribute to this problem. (See *High Blood Pressure*.)
- Vitamin B5 (pantothenic acid) helps combat feelings of stress; take 100–500mg daily. Also take a B-complex, as all the B-group vitamins work together to calm the nerves.
- Take a good-quality multi-vitamin/mineral that contains 400IU of natural-source vitamin E. This helps the heart muscle receive more oxygen.
- Co-enzyme Q10 is a vitamin-like substance made in the body that helps regulate heartbeat. As we age we manufacture less, so try taking 60mg daily, and then increase to 100mg daily. **VC**
- Vitamin D3 has been shown to help alleviate arrhythmia; take 1,000IU daily.
- Cortisol Manager tablets contain ashwagandha, phosphatdlyserine, and L-theanine (an extract of green tea). This combination is excellent for reducing cortisol production and calming you down. If you are a Type A person who rushes around all day, feels stressed, and needs to "slow down," then try taking one of these tablets when the adrenaline starts "pumping," thus triggering palpitations, plus take one or two before bed. I have found that they are wonderful for reducing "fight-or-flight"-type symptoms, and they help me get a better night's sleep. However, if you are at the point of total and utter exhaustion, then read the *Adrenal Exhaustion* section, because if your body is not producing sufficient cortisol you will get no benefit from taking this formula. Available from Integrative Therapeutics, Inc. Tel: 1-800-931-1709. Website: www.integrativeinc.com

- Otherwise try plain L-theanine capsules. Take 100mg three times daily spread throughout the day. If you would rather drink green tea, look for decaffeinated brands.

Helpful Hints
- As palpitations can be linked to an over-active thyroid, ask your doctor to do a blood test to check for thyroid and other hormone imbalances.
- Learn to meditate to reduce stress, as worrying about this condition can precipitate an attack. (See *Adrenal Exhaustion* and *Stress*.)
- To combat worrying, which only exacerbates the condition, learn how to breathe properly by taking yoga classes.
- Take a calm, deep breath every 20 minutes.
- Essential oils of lavender and ylang ylang have a calming effect. Try a few drops in your bath. You can also inhale the ylang ylang directly from the bottle to help slow your breathing. Try regular aromatherapy massage, which is very relaxing.
- Go for leisurely walks, breathing slowly and deeply.

PANIC ATTACKS

(see also Adrenal Exhaustion, Low Blood Sugar, Palpitations, Phobias, and Stress)

Panic attacks occur during periods of acute anxiety, and about one in three Americans has a panic attack during any given year. Feelings of intense panic induce hyperventilating (breathing too fast), which can cause light-headedness and tingling in the fingers and toes because of reduced carbon dioxide concentrations in the blood. Panic attacks have a huge variety of causes, most of them based on fears or phobias. Obviously, if a loved one dies suddenly—in a car accident, for example—and you are with them, a panic attack would be triggered by acute shock. Some people have panic attacks if they see spiders; or, if they have had a heart attack or stroke before, the least sensation of pain may induce panic out of the fear that another attack is imminent. During 1998 following a near-death experience, I suffered panic attacks for almost two months—and believe me, if someone tells you to pull yourself together, they are wasting their time. Reassurance and patience are what's needed. Panic attacks are hugely linked to adrenal exhaustion and low blood sugar. (See these sections.)

Foods to Avoid
- Avoid stimulants (especially caffeine), refined sugar, and alcohol, which can all trigger severe mood swings and disrupt blood sugar levels.
- Sugar substitutes such as aspartame should also be avoided.
- Canned and pre-packaged foods are high in salt. Combine this with a panic attack and your blood pressure can rise.
- People who tend to eat too many starchy foods, such as breads, potatoes, croissants, bananas, and so on, are more likely to suffer from panic attacks, as blood sugar is greatly affected by these types of foods.

Friendly Foods
- Protein, fiber, and healthier fats like eggs, fish, quinoa, amaranth, sunflower, pumpkin, flax or hemp seeds, plus protein powders, will help balance blood sugar levels and reduce the likelihood of a panic attack. Eat small amounts of protein, fiber, and fats with every meal.
- Eat more calming foods (with some added protein) that will also help to balance your blood sugar, such as brown rice, buckwheat, couscous, sweet potatoes, oatmeal, quinoa, whole-

wheat bread and pastas, lentils, beans, and rice and corn pastas. These slower-release carbohydrates are essential for stabilizing blood-sugar levels, which are often a factor in panic attacks.

- Eat small meals regularly. Don't skip meals.
- Snack on organic nuts, seeds, and low-fat yogurts. Health stores now sell numerous low-sugar seed/protein bars.
- Cut down on sodium-based salts; use a magnesium- or potassium-based salt. Try seasoning food with Himalayan Crystal Salt or nori flakes instead, as they are high in minerals.
- Generally include more beans, pulses, fruits, and vegetables in your diet.
- Eat more oily fish rich in omega-3 fats, and seeds such as sunflower, sesame, and pumpkin, as well as walnuts, almonds and Brazil nuts, flaxseeds and hemp seeds, which are all rich in omega-6 essential fats. (See *Fats You Need To Eat*.)
- Low levels of serotonin are linked to feelings of depression. Serotonin is made from a constituent of protein called tryptophan. Fish, turkey, chicken, cottage cheese, beans, wheat germ, avocados, and bananas are all rich in tryptophan, which helps keep you calm. If you tend to eat lots of bananas, then try eating them with a few sunflower seeds or an oatcake to slow the fast-releasing sugars.
- Sprinkle wheat germ over a low-sugar breakfast cereal. Nature's Path makes cereals from spelt, quinoa, and kamut, which are sweetened with apple juice. Cereals are rich in B vitamins, which help keep you calm.
- Oatmeal is a very calming food. Use a few raisins or xylitol to sweeten. Add fresh fruit for added fiber.
- Eat more lettuce, mushrooms, peppers, and root vegetables, which are also calming foods.
- Use small amounts of brown rice syrup, organic agave syrup, stevia, or xylitol instead of refined sugars, as they have a much lower glycemic index. Available online and from health stores.

Useful Remedies

- Homeopathic argent nit, gelsemium and aconite taken in combination help reduce anxiety. These are very potent. King Bio has these and more in an Anxiety and Nervousness oral spray. Take as soon as you feel onset of symptoms. **VC**
- Take a high-strength B-complex daily to help support your nerves.
- Inositol, one of the B-group vitamins, has been shown to reduce panic attacks. A good source is lecithin granules. Sprinkle liberally over yogurts, fruit, and so on.
- Take up to 2g of vitamin C daily with meals. Mild to moderate vitamin C deficiency is associated with nervousness.
- Take 400mg of calcium and 600mg of magnesium daily. Many people who suffer from panic attacks are lacking these minerals. Take in divided doses throughout the day.
- Take 99mg of potassium per day. Low levels can increase susceptibility to anxiety. **SVHC**
- Tryptophan is the precursor to serotonin, which is called the "happy brain neurotransmitter." Panic attacks can be reduced by increasing serotonin levels in the brain. Take 250–500mg per day. Take one tablet in the morning and one in the evening if needed. **VC**

Helpful Hints

- Bach Flower Remedies are generally known to be helpful for reducing panic attacks. Try Star of Bethlehem, Rescue Remedy, or Jan de Vries Emergency Essence. If you feel an attack coming on, treat the flower remedy as your medicine. Say to yourself as you place it under your tongue, "This will calm me down in under 3 minutes." Keep repeating this phrase, and it will help.
- Regular exercise reduces stress and builds confidence. A regular aromatherapy massage with

lavender oil helps you stay calm and balances the emotions. A warm, relaxing bath and sound, restful sleep do wonders to ease stress.

■ Learn how to control the attacks; fighting them will just make them worse. Tell yourself that this is the body's way of getting you to take care of yourself. Speak to yourself gently, as you would to comfort a child.

■ Hypnotherapy and self-hypnosis called Neuro-Linguistic Programming have proven very successful for reducing panic attacks and phobias. (See *Useful Information*.)

■ If you regularly suffer from panic attacks, carry a large paper bag with you, and immediately blow into it, slowly and calmly, if you begin hyperventilating. This should help calm you down and stop you from fainting.

■ Carry homeopathic Aconite 200c, and take it at the onset of an attack. This is a great remedy if you have intense fear.

■ Daily Strength is an online support group and community for people with anxiety, panic, and phobias. For more information, visit www.dailystrength.org

PARASITES
(see Irritable Bowel Syndrome)

PARKINSON'S DISEASE *(see also Leaky Gut and Mercury Fillings)*

Parkinson's Disease (PD) is a degenerative disorder of the central nervous system that becomes more common with increasing age. Men tend to be more affected than women. Around one in every 272 people in the US has Parkinson's, and an estimated one in 90 people has the disease but doesn't know it. Although Parkinson's tends to mainly affect people over the age of 50, it sometimes occurs in younger people if they have suffered any type of brain inflammation, carbon monoxide poisoning, long-term over-exposure to toxic metals and pesticides, or certain drugs. People who use a cocktail of pesticides in their homes have been found to be at twice the risk of Parkinson's.

This condition triggers deterioration of the nerve centers in a small part of the brain called the substantia nigra, which is responsible for sending messages down the nerves in the spinal cord to control muscles in the body. These messages are passed between brain cells, nerves, and muscles by neurotransmitters, with dopamine being the main neurotransmitter produced within the substantia nigra. In PD patients, a number of these cells die, and the amount of dopamine produced is therefore reduced.

As these events occur, a PD sufferer will generally find walking or getting out of a chair more of an effort. Muscles can stiffen and generally feel tenser. It's common for patients to experience tremors, rigidity, and muscular spasms in different limbs to varying degrees. Other symptoms can include unsteadiness, chronic constipation, bladder problems, insomnia, difficulty swallowing, depression, weight loss, impulsive behavior, impaired speech, a fixed facial expression, and a shuffling gait. The person knows what they want the muscle to do, but the messages received by the muscle group are not properly coordinated to allow for smooth movement.

People with PD also tend to suffer from more melanoma skin cancer, which is why any PD sufferer should always use organic, high-factor sunscreens and wear a hat.

No single cause has yet been proven, but nutrient deficiencies, heavy metal toxicity (especially from mercury and aluminum), exposure to pesticides, over-consumption of the artificial sweetener aspartame, viruses, and carbon monoxide poisoning are all linked to neurological conditions.

Children and adults should keep away from anything containing aluminum and mercury if they have had a recent vaccination, because many vaccinations contain heavy metals that could potentially trigger neurological and other disorders later in life. (See *Mercury Fillings*.)

Some prescription drugs can cause Parkinson-like symptoms. In addition, patients with Parkinson's have been found to have high levels of iron in the substantia nigra area of the brain, which can react to destroy dopamine-producing cells.

To replace dopamine most patients take a synthetic form of the amino acid L-dopa, which the body then makes into dopamine, helping to restore brain function. Nutritional physician Dr Shamin Daya, based at the Wholistic Medical Centre in Harley Street, London, UK, says: "The main problem for these people is that they often lack the important co-factors of nutrients such as zinc, magnesium, sometimes B1 or/and a type of activated vitamin B6 known as Pyridoxal 5 Phosphate, which are required to convert L-dopa to dopamine."

Many of the drugs used to treat Parkinson's can cause lethargy and extreme mental confusion or completely uncontrolled jerky movements if there is too much L-dopa in the body. As every case is unique, I strongly recommend that anyone with Parkinson's consults a nutritional physician, as this condition needs specialized care.

Anyone with PD also needs to take care of their liver function and make sure that they do not have a leaky gut. The gut is known by nutritional physicians as our "second brain"—and if it is not working properly, then you may not be absorbing sufficient nutrients from your diet and also suffer from food intolerances. (See *Leaky Gut* and *Liver Problems*.)

P

Foods to Avoid

- As much as possible, only eat organic-source foods and never use chemical-based pesticide sprays in or near your home.
- Avoid foods cooked in aluminum or iron pots.
- Reduce stimulants, such as coffee, soft drinks, tea, and alcohol, as these foods can affect tremors.
- Cut down on animal fats, especially red meat, cow's milk, and cheese, which impair the metabolism of essential fats. (See *Fats You Need To Eat*.)
- Avoid processed foods that are filled with refined sugar, such as mass-produced cakes, sugary drinks, refined breakfast cereals and bars, cookies, pies, and pre-packaged meals.
- Especially avoid additives and preservatives, such as monosodium glutamate (MSG) and aspartame, because of their negative effects on the brain.
- With professional guidance you may also need to eliminate gluten, which is found in grains such as wheat, rye, oats, and barley, as gluten can prevent the absorption of nutrients and medication in some people.
- Don't fry food and avoid all hydrogenated and trans-fats, like those found in margarines and pre-prepared foods. Frying foods causes more oxidation in the brain, which basically means more damage. These fats are also found in most mass-produced cakes, cookies, pies, and so on. Always check labels. Avoid all mass-produced vegetable oils.
- Protein foods can interfere with the absorption of L-dopa; therefore, only eat protein such as fish, organic chicken, or lean meats in the evening after the final dose of L-dopa has been taken.

Friendly Foods

- Ensure an adequate dietary intake. Because chewing can become difficult, loss of appetite is common, and nutrient deficiencies can speed the progression of the disease. Foods can be liquefied or use meal replacements instead.
- As much as possible, only eat organic foods since they contain fewer pesticides and

herbicides. A University of Miami post-mortem study in 1994 found pesticides more commonly in those who had died of Parkinson's disease.

- Research has shown that restricting protein intake is helpful and that 90% of the daily intake should be eaten with the evening meal, when you are not having your L-dopa medication. This is extremely important advice that is not always given to patients on L-dopa. Protein competes for absorption with the L-dopa, so eating protein during the day, when most sufferers take their medication, can block its efficacy.

- Protein can be found in organic lean meats such as turkey, plus fresh fish, eggs, beans, quinoa, lentils, nuts and seeds, fermented soy foods, and whole grains. The best sources of protein for Parkinson's sufferers are small amounts of soy, egg yolks, oily and white fish, and poultry. You can also add organic hemp seed protein or whey protein to breakfast smoothies. (See *General Health Hints* for a great smoothie recipe.)

- Generally, eat more beans and pulses rather than gluten-based foods such as breads. You can buy gluten- and wheat-free breads in most supermarkets and health stores.

- Include apples, pears, papaya, pumpkin, mangoes, cabbage, kale, watercress, cauliflower, carrots, and broccoli in your diet.

- Root vegetables tend to be sprayed with pesticides less, so eat more red beets and their tops, green beans, turnips, spinach, and pumpkins.

- Use unrefined, organic sunflower, sesame seed and olive oils for salad dressings and to drizzle over cooked foods such as brown rice or quinoa. These oils are rich in essential fats, which are vital for healthy brain function, as they enhance brain cell wall stability. (See *Fats You Need To Eat*.)

- Get into the habit of juicing. Use organic carrots, beets, and artichokes, which are high in vitamins and minerals and help cleanse the liver. (See *Liver Problems*.)

- If you have mercury fillings in your teeth, eat more nori seaweed flakes, chlorella, apples, and cilantro, which detoxify metals from the body. (See *Mercury Fillings*.)

- Dried or ready-to-eat organic fruits such as prunes, figs, and apricots help ease or prevent constipation, as does drinking at least 6 glasses of water daily.

- Black and purple grapes, blackberries, and blueberries are high in antioxidants that help support the brain.

- Flaxseeds are high in omega-6 and -3 fats and really help ease constipation. Soak a tablespoon of flaxseeds in cold water overnight, drain the next morning, and eat sprinkled over low-sugar cereals, oatmeal, or in smoothies.

- Begin drinking green or white teas, which are rich in antioxidants.

- Eat low-fat, live probiotic yogurts to ensure there are plenty of friendly bacteria in the bowel.

Useful Remedies

- The specific nutrients and amounts you need to take will be different for each individual case. Supplements will also depend on what medication you are taking and the time of day you take it. Again, I strongly recommend that you see a qualified nutritionist or nutritional physician who can devise a program specifically for you.

- Studies from the Birkmayer Institute for Parkinson's in Vienna, Austria, have shown that NADH, a co-enzyme form of vitamin B3, can help increase energy levels, reduce depression, and stimulate the body's production of more L-dopa. 5mg should be taken on an empty stomach at least 40 minutes before food. Professor Birkmayer's highly absorbable NADH is called Enada. VC. **NB: Anyone who is very stressed and suffers from palpitations should avoid this supplement. However, in some cases the intravenous form of this nutrient is more effective in Parkinson's—speak to your doctor about the IV form.**

- L-methionine, an essential sulfur amino acid, readily crosses the blood-brain barrier where it can be converted into the vital nutrient S-adenosylmethionine (SAM-e). L-dopa supplementation reduces the brain's SAM-e levels. Try 500mg of methionine twice daily, taken 30 minutes before meals. **VC**

- Take a full-spectrum antioxidant formula since vitamin C, in combination with other antioxidants such as vitamin E, helps counteract the negative side effects of L-dopa. **VC**
- The amino acids tyrosine and phenylalanine help ensure that the brain has sufficient raw materials for the synthesis of dopamine. Dosages need to be set by a qualified doctor or nutritionist.
- The amino acid acetyl L-carnitine is very important because it helps protect the brain and improves memory. Take 1–1.5g daily in divided doses 30 minutes before meals.
- Lipoic acid is a powerful antioxidant that supports brain function and removes heavy metals. Take 200mg three times daily.
- When we are young the body makes a vitamin-like substance called Co-enzyme Q10, but as we age levels fall. Parkinson's patients have been found to have 35% less CoQ10 than healthy people, which is an issue as CoQ10 is needed to protect neurons in the brain. Under medical supervision take around 200–400mg daily with a small amount of fat (such as olive oil or butter). **VC**

- Chlorella helps rid the body of unwanted heavy metals; take 500mg twice daily. Otherwise use Greens Plus in smoothies or simply drink with a little water. This powder contains Hawaiian spirulina, chlorella, lecithin, barley, pectin apple fiber, soy and barley sprouts, and lactobacillus acidophilus. It is a great all-around way to ingest good nutrients, encourage healthy bacteria, keep the body more alkaline, and help keep you regular. **GP**
- Melatonin, produced by the pineal gland at night, is a very important antioxidant for the brain as it induces natural sleep. Many PD patients have issues sleeping, and bioelectromagnetics scientist Roger Coghill says, "When you take melatonin supplements that you can buy online…, most synthetic tablets contain thousands of times the natural dose that your pineal gland normally produces." Therefore, Roger has developed a supplement called Asphalia, which contains natural melatonin extracted from certain grasses that mimics the normal dose made by your pineal gland at night, rather than the larger doses you get in mass-produced tablets. Take 1–2 capsules 30 minutes before bed. Roger's exclusive distributor in the US is Diva Marketing, Don't Disturb Me!, 2612 Sleepy Hollow, Pearland, TX 77581; Tel: 1-713-221-1873 or 1-866-692-8037; website: www.dontdisturbmesite.com **NB: Asphalia should not be taken by severe asthmatics, children under the age of one, and pregnant women in their third trimester.**
- If you have mercury fillings, see this section under *Mercury Fillings*.

Helpful Hints

- Because mercury fillings are linked to Parkinson's, have them checked by a holistic dentist and removed if necessary (with all of the necessary protection during removal—otherwise you can become even more contaminated). See *Mercury Fillings*.
- Since many of the world's oceans are heavily polluted, high levels of mercury are also being reported in some coastal fish. (See *Mercury Fillings*.)
- There is a strong link between aluminum/mercury toxicity and PD; therefore, avoid all aluminum cookware and aluminum foil. Read labels carefully as cake mixes, antacids, buffered aspirin, self-raising flour, pickles, processed cheeses, and most deodorants and toothpastes contain aluminum.
- Both the food additive monosodium glutamate (MSG) and the artificial sweetener aspartame have been linked to Parkinson's; therefore, avoid all additives and preservatives whenever possible. More than 3,000 foods and drinks contain artificial sweeteners.

- Also avoid using "air fresheners" in your home, because many of them contain a cocktail of chemicals.
- The anti-aging hormone DHEA is well known for supporting brain function and can be used as a supplement. Ask your doctor to test your hormone levels with a blood or saliva test. Never self-medicate with hormones.
- See the *Allergies* section for details of the York and Genova Tests for food intolerances.
- Reduce stress. At times of stress the body uses dopamine to make the stress hormones noradrenaline and adrenaline, using up your already short supply. Tools for reducing stress include exercise, massage, relaxation techniques, meditation, or enjoyable hobbies. (See *Stress*).
- If tremors are worse at or after meals, avoid eating protein (meat, fish, beans, nuts, and seeds) at meals where you take your medication, as protein competes with the L-dopa for absorption.
- Constipation is a major symptom that must be dealt with to ensure the proper elimination of toxins. In addition to dried fruits, flaxseeds, and water, try massaging your stomach in a clockwise circular motion to stimulate the bowel. Take walks after meals or use magnesium supplements (150mg three times a day) to relax the bowel. (See *Constipation*.)
- Because organophosphates (OPs) from pesticides and herbicides are now found in our drinking water, use a good-quality water filter such as Kangen Water. This ionized, antioxidant water system helps alkalize, rehydrate, and re-balance the body. It has been used in Japanese hospitals with highly beneficial health results. For more details, visit www.kangenwaterusa.com
- Read *Parkinson's Disease, The Way Forward* by Dr Geoffrey Leader and Lucille Leader (Bath Press). This user-friendly book presents an integrated approach to the management of Parkinson's disease.
- Dr David Perlmutter, a neurologist in Naples, Florida, has pioneered the use of intravenous glutathione, which has had a dramatic effect on most of his Parkinson's patients. His book, *The Better Brain Book* (River Head Books) makes for a fascinating read. Available from Dr Perlmutter's website: www.perlhealth.com
- Stem-cell therapy holds great promise for Parkinson's patients. For more details about where you can find cutting-edge treatments, see the *Multiple Sclerosis* section.
- For further help, contact the National Parkinson Foundation by calling 1-800-327-4545 or visiting www.parkinson.org You can also contact American Parkinson Disease Association. Tel: 1-800-223-2732. Website: www.apdaparkinson.org

P

PCOS (polycystic ovarian syndrome)

(see also Infertility, Low Blood Sugar, and Liver Problems)

Between one in 10 and one in 20 women of childbearing age has polycystic ovarian syndrome (although they may or may not have "polycystic ovaries"). This means that as many as 5 million women in the US alone suffer from irregular or no periods, erratic or no ovulation, sub-fertility, recurrent miscarriages, excess facial and body hair, fatigue, acne, weight gain that is hard to shift, hair loss, mood swings, abdominal pain, aching joints, and dizziness. In the long term, there is a sevenfold increase in the risk of cardiovascular problems and diabetes. Depression, anxiety, low self-esteem, and possibly low iodine levels are also factors with this condition.

The job of the ovaries is to produce hormones, ripen and release eggs ready for fertilization, and prepare the lining of the womb for pregnancy. If no fertilization occurs, then the lining is shed, leading to a period. This whole process is governed by sex hormones. Follicle-stimulating hormone (FSH) and luteinizing hormone (LH) are made by the pituitary gland in the brain. These hormones then stimulate the ovaries to produce progesterone, testosterone, and estrogen. PCOS occurs when there is an imbalance in these hormones, namely high estrogen, testosterone, and LH. High levels of the hormone insulin, which is needed to balance blood sugar levels, are also produced. The body's insulin receptors on the surface of cells seem to switch off and stop listening to the signal from insulin, and so to compensate, the body overproduces insulin, which further disrupts the sex hormones. Research has shown that by enhancing the body's ability to register insulin signaling, all hormone levels can be normalized.

Foods to Avoid

- Also see this section under *Low Blood Sugar*.
- Nutritionist Gareth Zeal says, "Most women with this problem tend to be eating too many animal-based products including milk, cheese, and meat, plus excessive amounts of starchy refined carbohydrate foods, such as cakes, cookies, bread, white potatoes, and so on."
- Eat less red meat, pork, animal-source dairy products, and fried foods. Excess consumption of the wrong kinds of fat can lead to weight gain and cardiovascular problems. (Women with PCOS have a higher risk of developing cardiovascular problems.) When preparing foods grill, bake, or stir-fry with olive oil. (See *Fats You Need To Eat*.)

- Stay away from refined sugar in all forms, as sugar affects hormone levels in the body. Avoid it in mass-produced breakfast cereals and bars, cakes, cookies, sweets, soft drinks, store-bought juices, and chocolate.
- Alcohol exerts an estrogen-like action in the body, so it is best avoided. If you must indulge, keep it to a minimum and drink red wine, as this helps protect against cardiovascular disease.
- Keep caffeine to a minimum because it can disrupt hormone levels. This means very little to no coffee, tea, soft drinks, chocolate, energy drinks, and some painkillers.

Friendly Foods

- Eat small regular meals that contain complex carbohydrates, such as brown rice, pasta, rye bread, millet, sweet potatoes, and quinoa, as these foods help keep blood sugar levels in the body more even, reducing the release of insulin levels and stabilizing hormone levels. (See *Low Blood Sugar*.)
- Eating small amounts of protein with all meals and snacks helps make insulin more effective by slowing the relase of sugars into the blood. Lentils, beans, eggs, fish, lean chicken and turkey, nuts, and seeds are ideal sources of protein.
- Foods from the brassica family (cauliflower, broccoli, watercress, cabbage, and Brussels sprouts) help encourage excretion of excess hormones.
- Omega-3 essential fatty acids found in flaxseeds, hemp seeds, and oily fish (salmon, mackerel, sardines, pilchards, herring, and anchovies) have an important role to play in helping control insulin resistance and hormone disruption.
- Go organic, as many of the pesticides liberally sprayed onto foods can have hormone-disrupting actions.
- Fiber is known to bind to excess hormones and help remove them from the body. Eat more whole grains, brown rice, millet, beans, lentils, oats, and lots of fresh fruit and vegetables.
- Eat live, sugar-free yogurt daily to feed the good bacteria in the gut, as this helps break down excess hormones.
- Phyto-estrogens help reduce high estrogen levels. Therefore, eat foods such as miso and tempeh (a fermented form of soy), as well as flaxseeds, beans, and lentils.

- Use organic rice/agave syrup or xylitol instead of refined sugars, because they have a much lower glycemic index.
- As PCOS can be related to low iodine levels, use nori seaweed or kelp flakes as a salt substitute. You can also increase your intake of sea vegetables such as samphire or kelp.

Useful Remedies

- Ask at your health store for a multi-vitamin/mineral for your age. Take daily.
- B vitamins are essential for balancing sugar levels in the body and helping with estrogen-related hormonal problems. Most multi-vitamin/mineral formulas contain plenty of B vitamins, so there's no need to take an additional supplement.
- The combination of agnus castus (1ml twice daily) and saw palmetto (1ml twice daily) has been used for centuries to balance female hormones and is also great for reducing PCOS symptoms.
- Methionine is an amino acid that helps support liver function. Take 500mg twice daily 30 minutes before main meals. (See *Liver Problems*.)
- The mineral chromium helps balance blood sugar, which is a major factor in PCOS. Take 100–200mcg twice daily.
- Most of the companies featured on pages 15–16 offer vegetable extract capsules that contain cabbage and mustard greens, which help balance hormones. The Life Extension Foundation makes a Triple Action Cruciferous Vegetable Extract with resveratrol (from red grapes). **LEF**

Helpful Hints

- If you are overweight, lose weight. Studies at St Mary's Hospital in London, UK, found that moderate weight loss helped correct hormonal abnormalities, reduced body hair, and improved a woman's chances of conception.
- Exercise not only helps with weight loss and strengthening the heart, but also releases feel-good hormones in the body. Aim for at least three 20-minute sessions per week. Start with a brisk walk outside, as daylight is also known to lift low moods and prevent depression.
- Use a water filter. Millions of women currently take the contraceptive pill and excrete it in their urine, whence residues find their way into the water supply. Drinking unfiltered tap water is known to have an effect on hormone levels.
- Food wrapped or cooked in plastic containers or plastic wrap will have a negative effect on hormone balance. The risk is increased when these plastics are heated. If you do have to buy food that is wrapped in plastic, transfer it to a glass container as soon as you get home. Above all, never microwave food covered in plastic wrap or in plastic containers.
- Women with PCOS have found acupuncture to be useful in helping kick start non-existent cycles and regulating cycle length.
- Learn to relax and tackle your stresses, both physical and emotional. Stress contributes to high insulin levels and hormonal imbalances.
- Essential oils of agnus castus, geranium, and rose may be beneficial for balancing hormones, while sandalwood, neroli, ylang ylang, and mandarin are good for relaxation. Add to a relaxing bath or use in an oil burner.
- www.pcosupport.org is a great, informative website with lots of practical information and fact sheets. They also produce a free monthly newsletter.

P

PHLEBITIS

(see also Atherosclerosis, Circulation, and Leg Ulcers)

Phlebitis is caused by inflammation of the walls of the veins, usually near the surface of the skin. It is often combined with the formation of small blood clots on the area of the inflammation. It may be triggered by a sensitivity to external irritants, such as laundry detergents, or by food intolerances. The condition can occur after injections or intravenous infusions and is common in intravenous drug abusers. It is more common in people who have varicose veins or blood vessel disorders such as Buerger's disease. Symptoms include swelling and redness along and around the affected segment of the vein, which can become very tender when touched. The best way to prevent this condition is to keep your circulation in good condition by eating more of the right foods.

Foods to Avoid

- Identify and avoid foods that you have a sensitivity to. The most common culprits are wheat and dairy products from animal sources (especially cows). See under *Allergies* for details about the York, Genova, and Bio Meridian Tests for food intolerances.
- You may also be sensitive to gluten.
- Cut down on all saturated fats, which are found in animal products, sausages, full-fat cheese, milk, chocolate, and hard margarines.
- Don't fry food and never use mass-produced, refined, hydrogenated oils. (See *Fats You Need To Eat*.)
- Reduce your intake of cakes, burgers, cookies, highly refined breakfast cereals, and mass-produced white breads and pastas. Many of these foods are packed with fats, salt, and refined sugar. Refined sugars convert into fat in the body if not used up during exercise. (See *General Health Hints*.)

Friendly Foods

- Increase your intake of oily fish, which are rich in the omega-3 essential fats that help thin the blood naturally.
- Sprinkle wheat germ and/or lecithin granules over low-sugar cereals and desserts. They help emulsify the bad fats and aid circulation.
- Buy a packet each of organic, unsalted walnuts, Brazil nuts, almonds, sunflower and pumpkin seeds, sesame seeds, and flaxseeds, which are high in omega-6 essential fats. Grind them all in a blender and keep in an airtight jar in the fridge. Sprinkle over any foods you like. These will add healthy fats, fiber, and minerals such as zinc to your diet, which are vital for skin and wound healing.
- Eat more stone-ground whole-wheat bread, pasta, and noodles. Also try lentil-, corn-, and rice pastas, which are available in most supermarkets and health stores.
- Use skimmed milk or try non-dairy alternatives, such as rice or almond milks.
- Include garlic in your diet because it thins the blood naturally.
- Olive oil and avocados are rich in mono-unsaturated fats, which are healthy and aid healing.
- Eat more fresh fruits and vegetables, especially pineapple and papaya, which are rich in digestive enzymes that aid healing. They are also anti-inflammatory.
- Eat more curries because they are rich in turmeric, which also has anti-inflammatory properties.

Useful Remedies

- Take 400IU daily of natural-source vitamin E to help thin the blood naturally and ease discomfort. **VC**
- Take a high-strength multi-vitamin/mineral made specifically for men and/or women over 50.

- Some people find relief by placing raw papaya on the affected area for an hour each day.
- Bromelain, extracted from pineapple, has potent anti-inflammatory effects. Take 500mg daily.
- Use Vari-Vein capsules, which contain witch hazel, horse chestnut, ginger, bilberry, and more. All of these ingredients help increase circulation and reduce the swelling associated with this condition. Available online from Amazon and other retailers.
- Pycnogenol, pine bark extract, has been shown to reduce inflammation, ease pain, improve blood flow, and help make veins more elastic Start with 80mg twice daily, and then reduce to 40mg daily after a month.

Helpful Hints
- Basically you need to get moving. Begin by walking for 15 minutes daily and gradually increase over a one-month period to 1 hour a day.
- When applicable, use stairs instead of elevators.
- An extremely gentle and easy exercise regime, such as swimming, yoga, qigong, or tai chi, would also be helpful; as would reflexology and acupuncture. (See *Useful Information*.) Tai chi can be practiced by people of any age—even if you are in your 80s or 90s.

PHOBIAS *(see also Adrenal Exhaustion, Low Blood Sugar, and Panic Attacks)*

A phobia is an extreme or irrational fear attached to a specific object or situation that is not life threatening. However, for the person with the phobia, the fear is often overwhelming and their lives can become a nightmare. The most common phobias are a fear of confined spaces or of various animals and insects, such as birds or spiders. Certain social situations provoke anxiety in some people who fear they will become trapped or embarrassed. As adrenal exhaustion and low blood sugar can contribute to this problem, please also read these sections.

Foods to Avoid
- Also see *Low Blood Sugar* and *Insulin Resistance*.
- As much as possible, avoid stimulants such as coffee, tea, and refined sugars. Also cut down or eliminate alcohol and foods or drinks that contain caffeine or sugar.
- Also see *Panic Attacks* and *General Health Hints*.

Friendly Foods
- Low levels of serotonin are linked to feelings of depression. Serotonin is made from a constituent of protein called tryptophan; therefore, include more foods such as fish, turkey, chicken, cottage cheese, beans, avocados, bananas, and wheat germ in your diet to help raise your mood and keep you calmer.
- Calming foods also include brown rice, pastas, noodles, couscous, sweet potatoes, lettuce, mushrooms, peppers, and root vegetables.
- Oats are a great food for helping rebuild nervous system tissue. Have oatmeal with a protein shake for breakfast daily.
- Sprinkle wheat germ over breakfast cereals or fruit whips. There are plenty of cereals available made from amaranth, quinoa, and kamut that are sweetened with a little apple juice. Cereals, including oatmeal, are rich in B vitamins, which help keep you calm.
- Drink more decaffeinated green tea and licorice tea.

Useful Remedies
- The amino acid L-theanine, found in green tea, really helps keep you calm without making you feel tired in any way. Take 100mg four times throughout the day. **VC, VS**

- The herbs ashwagandha, Siberian ginseng, and gotu kola are adaptogenic herbs that help normalize the adrenal system. These are all included in the Jarrow advanced stress formula called Adrenal Optimizer. **JF, VC**
- Take a high-strength vitamin B complex daily to help support your nerves.
- 5-Hydroxytryptophan (5-HTP) is a supplement that naturally raises serotonin levels in the brain, helping to improve mood and calm you down. Start with 25mg and increase over 10–14 days to 75mg three times daily. **VC, VS**

Helpful Hints

- Learn to meditate. People who practice this skill regularly have lower blood pressure than they would have otherwise, are less anxious, and are more able to cope with stressful situations.
- Daily Strength has an online support group and community for people with phobias. For more information, visit www.dailystrength.org
- Hypnotherapy is an excellent way to find the root cause of your problem and learn how to let it go so you can lead a normal life. (See *Useful Information*.)
- Celebrity hypnotherapist Paul McKenna, has made some great self-hypnosis CDs that help to remove phobias. Website: www.paulmckenna.com
- Homeopathic Aconite 200c is a good remedy when you are experiencing intense fear or terror.
- Take more exercise to stimulate the production of more mood-boosting chemicals in the brain.

P

PILES (Hemorrhoids)   *(see also Constipation and Varicose Veins)*

Piles are basically enlarged varicose veins that form inside the anus. If you suffer from chronic long-term constipation, then the veins can break through the anus and protrude externally. If you feel this happening and the vein is still soft and pliable, you can carefully ease the swollen vein back inside the anus. But if the pile becomes hardened and forms a clot and remains outside the anus, this calls for immediate medical attention. When you go to the bathroom, if you have piles or an anal fissure, you can often see blood in the stools and experience extreme discomfort and itching in that area. Also, if your liver is congested, which is common with this problem, it can place more pressure on your back, which in turn adds pressure to your venous system, making piles worse.

Other factors involved in the formation of piles are persistent coughing, pregnancy and childbirth, standing and/or sitting for long periods, overuse of laxatives, and traveling long distances while in a seated position for hours on end—all of which raise pressure in rectal veins. If you bleed from the anus at any time, you should seek medical attention immediately.

The secret to avoiding piles is to avoid constipation in the first place.

Foods to Avoid

- Generally, you need to avoid eating too many flour-based foods such as cakes, mass-produced white breads, refined cookies, pies, and desserts, as flour and refined sugars plug up the bowel. If you mix flour and water together you get a very sticky paste, and this does not change consistency in the bowel!
- Melted cheese and full-fat cheeses can also cause constipation.
- Red meat takes a long time to digest. If you must eat meat, only have a small portion no more than twice a week.

- Coffee, soft drinks, and alcohol all dehydrate the bowel.
- Avoid mass-produced foods, such as burgers and high-fat fast food.
- Reduce your intake of full-fat dairy products from cows.
- Avoid sodium-based salt.
- For some people, eating citrus fruit and tomatoes makes the situation worse.

Friendly Foods

- Drink at least 6–8 glasses of water daily, even if you are not thirsty.
- Eat far more fresh, lightly cooked vegetables and salads, especially green leafy vegetables such as celery, spinach, kale, watercress, bean sprouts, spring greens, and cabbage.
- Figs, prunes, apples, pineapples, apricots, bananas, mangoes, papaya, avocados, grapes, and melons will all help reduce constipation. Strawberries, raspberries, peaches, sultanas, raisins, and dates can be eaten regularly (unless you have blood sugar, candida or another fungal-type problem).
- Flaxseeds are really helpful for keeping the bowels more regular. Soak one tablespoon of flaxseeds in cold water overnight, drain, and then add to low-sugar breakfast cereals, oatmeal, or smoothies. Adjust the amount to suit your individual needs.
- Eat high-quality protein, such as skinless chicken, fish, tempeh, beans, peas, and pulses.
- Eat more whole-wheat bread, pastas, and noodles.
- Enjoy low-sugar, high-fiber cereals for breakfast. Try cereals made from quinoa, amaranth, rice, or millet, which are less likely to irritate the gut than wheat bran and other cereals.
- Use oat and rice brans over cereals and in smoothies.
- Try blackstrap molasses, unsweetened jams, organic agave syrup, or xylitol instead of refined sugars.
- Replace cow's milk with low-fat goat's milk and organic rice, almond, quinoa, or coconut milks.
- Almonds, sunflower, pumpkin, and sesame seeds are all rich sources of fiber.
- Experiment with coffees made from rye and chicory or herb teas, such as rose hip, and unsweetened fruit juices.
- Use more unrefined organic olive, sunflower, and walnut oils for salad dressings.
- Eat more live, low-fat yogurt, which is rich in friendly bacteria that encourage healthy bowels.

Useful Supplements

- A pine bark extract known as pycnogenol is a powerful antioxidant that has been shown in studies conducted at the University of Munster in Germany to help stop bleeding and significantly reduce pain from hemorrhoids. Take 300mg daily while symptoms are acute, then after four days, reduce to 150mg daily for a further four days. You can also use pycnogenol-based creams. **VC**
- The herb butcher's broom helps improve circulation in the lower body and helps tone the veins. Take 500mg twice daily.
- Horse chestnut capsules help strengthen the capillaries. Take 50–75 mg of standardized escin (the active ingredient) twice daily.
- Take 2g of vitamin C spread throughout the day with meals plus 1g of bioflavonoids and 400IU of full-spectrum, natural-source vitamin E daily to strengthen blood vessel walls.
- Taking 20,000IU of vitamin A per day for a month will help repair tissue damage. **NB: Only take this dose for 1 month, and take no more than 3,000IU daily if you are pregnant or planning to become pregnant.** Also, note that liver is very rich in vitamin A; if you eat a lot of liver, you do not need to take extra vitamin A as a supplement. After one month, switch to a natural-source carotene complex (7mg daily), which naturally converts to vitamin A in the body and is very safe. **SVHC**

- Take a vitamin B complex to aid digestion, which in turn will aid bowel function.
- Zinc is vital for soft tissue healing; take 30mg daily with 1–2mg of copper.
- After 3 months on this regimen, switch to a good-quality multi-vitamin/mineral.
- Rutin (found in buckwheat) helps strengthen vein walls. Take 300mg daily.
- Prebiotic fiber from agave and other plant sources helps encourage the colonization of friendly bacteria in the bowel, which in turn aids more efficient bowel function. Try Agave Digestive Immune Support powder from The Life Extension Foundation (**LEF**) or call any of the companies mentioned on pages 15–16 to ask for their prebiotic formulas.

Helpful Hints

- Insert pilewort suppositories, which are best used before going to bed. They are made from olive oil, beeswax, and pilewort and help soften the pile and reduce any swelling. **OP**
- After you have opened your bowels, squeeze the cheeks of the bottom together several times. This action will encourage blood flow into that area, which helps stop piles from forming.
- Take one or two cayenne pepper capsules with main meals to increase circulation and help reduce any bleeding. **VC, VS**
- Apply combinations of zinc oxide, vitamin E, and aloe vera gel or olive oil to the affected area. This should help soften the piles and make them less painful.
- Apply cold witch hazel lotion frequently to hemorrhoids to shrink the swollen blood vessel. Derma E supplies a witch hazel, bilberry, and horse chestnut cream called Clear Vein Crème, available online.
- In an acute situation, or if you cannot see your doctor immediately, try dissolving 1 tablespoon of Epsom salts into 6 tablespoons of lukewarm water and then carefully applying it to the affected area with a cotton ball. This helps reduce the swelling until you can see your doctor.
- Nelson's Homeopathic Pharmacy makes a natural hemorrhoid relief cream called H+care, which is very useful. Visit www.nelsonsnaturalworld.com/en-us/us/ to order online or to find a store near you.
- Homeopathic remedies, such as staphysagria or aesculus (horse chestnut) can also help. See a qualified homeopath for individual remedies.
- Bathing the anus in cold water every morning can help prevent the recurrence of piles.
- Bowel function can be affected by drugs such as antacids, anti-depressants, excessive iron tablets, and laxative abuse. If you think these may be a factor, talk to your doctor.
- Long-term laxatives use can make the bowel lazy and can increase the need to strain.
- Instead of sitting, squat to open your bowels. This will take pressure off the lower part of the bowel.

PILL, CONTRACEPTIVE

The progestogen- (synthetic progesterone) only, or mini-pill, provides contraception by thickening the mucus in the cervix, making it impenetrable to sperm. The combined pill, which contains both estrogen and progestogen, prevents pregnancy by thickening the mucus and suppressing ovulation. Potential side effects from taking the pill are an increased risk of cancers of the breast and cervix, blood clotting in the legs, high blood pressure, increased risk of heart disease and stroke, weight gain, fluid retention, and migraines. Women who took the pill for ten years or more back in the 1960s have a much higher risk of developing breast cancer. The pill depletes the body of vital nutrients, such as vitamins B and C, plus the minerals magnesium, calcium, and zinc. I took the pill for more than 10 years from the late 1960s to the early 1970s, which I believe was the root cause of my continual heavy bleeding, so that at 31 I needed an emergency hysterectomy. If you must take the pill, then have regular breaks of several months at a time. Taking the pill over long periods can increase the risk of developing candida. (See *Candida*.)

Foods to Avoid
- Greatly reduce your intake of refined sugars, animal protein, dairy products from cows and the saturated fats found in dairy, hard margarines, cakes, pastries, burgers, sausages, and so on.
- Reduce your intake of sodium-based salt, caffeine, and tobacco.
- Reduce your alcohol intake.
- Also see *General Health Hints*.

Friendly Foods
- Include organic raw wheat germ in your diet, as it is rich in vitamins B and E.
- Eat far more whole grains, including brown rice, millet, quinoa, couscous, whole-wheat breads and pastas, fruits, and vegetables.
- Cereals and oats are also rich in B vitamins.
- Cherries, papaya, mango, cantaloupe melons, apricots, and most other fruit and vegetables are rich sources of vitamin C.
- Eat more fish, plus sunflower, pumpkin, and sesame seeds, which are high in zinc, as the pill raises copper levels, which lowers zinc levels.
- Eat more live, low-fat yogurt that contains healthy bacteria, which are depleted by the pill.
- Eat more cabbage, watercress, broccoli, and cauliflower, which contain a hormone-regulating substance called indole-3-carbinole.
- Also see *General Health Hints*.

Useful Supplements
- Take a multi-vitamin/mineral such as Synergy by NSI. **VC**
- Make sure any multi you take contains at least 30mg of zinc.
- Take a B-complex, as the pill depletes all of the B vitamins.
- Take 250mg–500mg of vitamin C a day in an ascorbate form with food to help prevent any deficiency caused by the pill.
- Indole-3-carbinol is an important nutrient extracted from broccoli, watercress, and cabbage that helps regulate hormones. Take 200mg daily. Available from all good health stores.
- Support your liver by taking supplements that aid detoxification of excess hormones from the liver, such as NSI's Liver Detox. Three capsules daily with meals. **VC**
- Also see *Liver Problems*.

Helpful Hints
- Studies conducted since the 1960s have consistently shown that women are at a greater risk of a pulmonary embolism when taking the pill, even the lower estrogen-containing pills. If you are on the pill you should not smoke, as this considerably increases the risk of some hazards, such as blood clots and heart disease. For more information, call the National Women's Health Resource Center at 1-877-986-9472 or visit www.healthywomen.org

PLANTAR WARTS
(see also Immune Function)

Plantar warts are non-cancerous skin growths that occur on the soles of the feet. They are extremely common, highly contagious, and can be very painful. Plantar warts are essentially a viral infection, and you are more likely to contract them if you are really run down.

Foods to Avoid
- Reduce your intake of all foods and drinks that contain refined sugar, which lowers immune function.
- Reduce caffeine, alcohol, and all highly processed white-flour-based foods.
- Also see dietary advice under *Immune Function*.

Friendly Foods
- Eat lots of garlic, asparagus, parsley, avocados, sea vegetables (such as kelp and samphire), apples, cucumbers, millet, rice bran, sprouts, and whey, hemp, pea or soy protein powders,
- Also see *Immune Function* and *General Health Hints*.

Useful Remedies
- If you regularly get plantar warts, start taking a high-strength bee propolis tincture or capsules, which are highly anti-viral and greatly boost your immune system.
- To fight off the virus, take 20,000IU of vitamin A daily for 1 month only and then reduce to 5,000IU daily in a multi-vitamin/mineral complex. You could also eat organic liver once a week. **NB: If you are pregnant or planning to become pregnant, take no more than 3,000IU of vitamin A daily.**
- After 1 month of vitamin A supplementation, begin taking a natural-source carotene complex. It will naturally convert to vitamin A in the body and is totally non-toxic. **SVHC**
- Take a garlic capsule daily for its anti-viral properties.
- Vitamin C is vital for boosting your immune system; take 2g daily with food in divided doses.
- Take 30mg of zinc daily for its immune-enhancing properties. This is found in most multi-vitamin/mineral complexes.
- See this section under *Immune Function*.

Helpful Hints
- Apply a tiny amount of crushed garlic or tea tree oil onto the affected area twice a day. **NB: Garlic oil can cause burning, so make sure it is placed only directly on the wart for several minutes at a time.**
- There is an enzyme in banana skin that can attack the wart. Many people have written to say that, although it sounds somewhat bizarre, this remedy really does work! Apply the inside of the banana skin to the plantar wart and tape on. Change every two days until the wart disappears.
- Homeopathic Thuja 6C and Thuja Mother tincture can be applied directly onto the warts and covered with a bandage.
- Place a tiny amount of fresh urine on a small cotton ball and attach it to the wart with a bandage. Change the dressing twice daily. Urine is a sterile liquid that contains anti-viral and antibacterial components and also softens the skin.

POLYCYSTIC OVARIAN SYNDROME

(see PCOS—Polycystic Ovarian Syndrome)

POLYMYALGIA RHEUMATICA *(see Fibromyalgia)*

POSTPARTUM DEPRESSION (postnatal depression) *(see also Adrenal Exhaustion and Low Blood Sugar)*

Although the birth of a child is, for most women, a time of great joy, up to 80% of women feel extremely low immediately after giving birth, which in itself can be incredibly exhausting. This 1–2-week period of "postpartum blues" usually goes away on its own; however, for about 12–15% of women, this will develop into postpartum depression. This can be due to hormonal changes, fluctuating blood sugar levels and/or nutrient deficiencies. In naturopathic terms postpartum depression is linked to adrenal exhaustion, as the hormones produced during pregnancy and the birth, such as cortisol and adrenaline, sap the adrenal glands, which can leave you feeling totally exhausted and emotionally drained. (See *Adrenal Exhaustion*.)

In addition, anxiety about coping with a new baby, lack of sleep, perhaps financial problems, and, of course, the realization that life has changed for good, can all add to this condition. For a few women, the feeling of depression lasts for months, which can seriously undermine their ability to cope.

Firstly ask your doctor to test for low iron levels—an obvious factor if there was heavy blood loss during or after the birth. This condition can be greatly alleviated by taking the right supplements for a few weeks. Symptoms vary from increased or decreased appetite, a feeling that one is a failure, depression, an inability to cope, feelings of panic, and sometimes aggressive feelings toward the baby. (See also *Low Blood Sugar* and *Depression*).

Nutritional physician Dr Shamin Daya says, "Depression basically denotes an imbalance in the brain chemistry. Once the right nutrients are given in the right amounts, especially B vitamins, then the depression can easily be alleviated."

Nutritionist Gareth Zeal adds: "Women who take 3–4g of omega-3 fish oils, plus 1000IU of vitamin D3, during and after pregnancy are dramatically less likely to suffer postnatal depression. Their children are also less likely to suffer many childhood conditions such as ADD or to have poor eyesight and will be far less likely to develop depressive-type conditions in later life."

P

Foods to Avoid
- Reduce stimulating foods, such as refined sugar and caffeine, as well as alcohol, as they all trigger the release of more cortisol.
- Also see *Adrenal Exhaustion* and *Low Blood Sugar*.

Friendly Foods
- See this section under *Adrenal Exhaustion, Depression*, and *Low Blood Sugar*.

Useful Remedies
- As low levels of B vitamins are associated with this condition, take a high-strength vitamin B complex daily for at least 2 months.
- You can take the herb agnus castus to help re-balance your hormones, even if you are breast-feeding. Take 5ml of the tincture daily.
- Magnesium helps induce feelings of calm. Take 1000mg daily in divided doses with food, plus 30mg of zinc (which supports brain chemistry) and iron (in a formula such as Spatone or take

iron phosphate in doses based on blood tests via your doctor). Taking these minerals will greatly ease symptoms after a few days.

- Take a multi-vitamin/mineral that contains at least 500mg of vitamin C and 150mcg of selenium.
- Try Christopher's Female Reproductive Formula, an herbal formula that contains raspberry leaf, squaw vine, and uva ursi, which all help balance hormones following childbirth. **VC**
- Taking 4g of omega-3 fish oils daily can really help both mother and baby (via breast milk).
- Take homeopathic caullophylum, cimicifuga pulsatilla, and sepia—one pill, four times a day. This blend helps balance hormones and reduces feelings of doom and hopelessness, tears, and so on. These are all in the King Bio Menopause Spray. **VS**
- Taking 1,000IU of vitamin D3 daily can also help both mother and baby (via breast milk).

Helpful Hints

- Postpartum depression is often caused by the sudden drop in progesterone levels that occurs just before birth, especially in women whose bodies are slow to begin making progesterone again. You can use a natural progesterone cream, which is easily absorbed, to bring your progesterone levels up again until your body takes over. Your doctor can tell you if your progesterone levels need to be topped off by doing a simple blood or saliva test. For more information about natural progesterone or help finding a doctor who uses it, visit www.natural-progesterone-advisory-network.com

- In the US, natural progesterone cream is available over the counter and can be ordered for your own use. For an information sheet call PharmWest at 1-310-301-4015 or visit www.pharmwest.com
- Homeopathic Ignatia 30c, taken twice daily for up to a week, is particularly good for mothers who thought that having a baby was going to be all roses.
- And for those who feel enveloped by a black cloud, try homeopathic Cimicifuga 30c twice daily for up to a week.
- Because many cases of depression are linked to the liver, see also *Liver Problems* and *Depression*.
- Getting more sleep and getting out of the house and away from the baby for brief periods can greatly help mild postpartum depression. Don't bottle up your feelings; talk things over with a friend or relative. Releasing your feelings really helps put things in perspective and will make you realize just how many women are in a similar situation.
- For more help and advice, call Postpartum Support International at 1-800-944-4773 or visit www.postpartum.net

PRE-MENSTRUAL TENSION and PRE-MENSTRUAL SYNDROME (PMT/PMS)

(see also Low Blood Sugar and Liver Problems)

PMS causes a variety of physical and emotional symptoms in the days prior to menstruation. They vary from mood swings, food cravings, and depression to breast tenderness and enlargement, fluid retentionm and bloating. Changes in hormone levels also cause some women to experience migraine-type symptoms. For 8% of women, though, pre-menstrual mood changes are extreme, causing premenstrual dysphoric disorder (PMDD).

PMS is associated with imbalanced levels of progesterone and estrogen (see *Menopause* for details about natural progesterone and estrogen creams). Low blood sugar is common prior to a period, and once blood sugar is balanced symptoms often disappear (see *Low Blood Sugar*). Many women with PMS also have candida (see also *Candida*) and food intolerances mainly to wheat, caffeine, gluten, and sometimes animal-source dairy products. Congestion of the liver is also linked to PMS. (See *Liver Problems*.)

Foods to Avoid
- Generally you need to cut down on animal fats, burgers, sausages, and heavy, rich, meat-based meals that usually contain high levels of saturated fat and salt.
- All high-salt foods, such as potato chips and salted peanuts, and highly processed meat, such as salami, should be avoided, as salt will add to the water-retention problem.
- Stimulants, such as tea, coffee, caffeine in any form, sodas, energy drinks, and chocolate, as well as snacks like cakes, cookies, croissants, and Danish pastries, will all play havoc with your blood sugar.

Friendly Foods
- Starting the day with an oat-based cereal, such as oatmeal, mixed with a chopped apple and a few sunflower seeds and raisins will help balance blood sugar until lunchtime.
- It would also be wise to eat some protein with breakfast, because it helps balance blood sugar for longer (proteins take longer to digest). An omelet, or poached or boiled eggs would be good choices, or make a smoothie with nuts and seeds with added whey or hemp seed protein powders. (See *General Health Hints* for a delicious smoothie recipe.)
- Drink more water, and try calming herbal teas such as chamomile.
- Include small amounts of quality protein with each meal. Fresh fish, eggs, chicken and turkey without the skin, cottage cheese, cooked tofu, lentils, quinoa, peas, and sunflower, pumpkin, and sesame seeds, plus all dried beans and pulses, are rich in fiber, protein, and essential fats.

- Foods such as tempeh or miso, sweet potatoes, pumpkin, broccoli, cauliflower, and Brussels sprouts all help balance your hormones naturally.
- Add organic sunflower and/or walnut oil to salad dressings.
- Snack on apples, pears, and bananas. Also try spreading low-fat humus, tahini, or goat's cheese on rice/oatcakes, spelt/amaranth crackers or whole-wheat bread. If you tend to eat too many bananas this can affect blood sugar, so always eat a few pumpkin or sunflower seeds at the same time to slow the sugar release.
- Many health food stores now sell low-sugar snacks. Eating these with a piece of fruit will help reduce any cravings.

Useful Remedies (to be taken all the time, not just during a period)
- Taking a B complex that contains at least 50mg of B6 per day will help the liver process estrogens.
- Gamma-linolenic acid (GLA) is the main ingredient in evening primrose oil and helps reduce breast pain. Take 100–500mg of GLA daily. **VC**
- Take 1g of omega-3 fish oils daily to help reduce tender breasts and help raise your mood.
- Take 400mg of calcium and 600mg of magnesium per day in divided doses to reduce the symptoms of PMS. Both of these minerals help keep you calm. Most companies make a two-in-one formula.
- Also take a multi-vitamin/mineral for women that contains a further 50mg of B6 to make your total daily intake 100–150mg per day.
- If your sugar/carbohydrate cravings are acute, take 150mcg of chromium daily. It will take a few days for the chromium to kick in, but it will really help reduce sugar cravings.
- The amino acid L-glutamine also helps reduce sugar/starch cravings and will heal any leaky gut. Take 500mg twice daily 30 minutes before food.

- Try the herbal menstrual formula Christopher's Female Reproductive Formula, which contains blessed thistle, squaw vine, barberry, and cramp bark, to cleanse the reproductive organs and balance hormones. **VC**

Helpful Hints

- When you are stressed, you produce too much adrenaline, which eventually exhausts your endocrine (hormone) system and depletes calcium from your bones. (See *Osteoporosis* and *Stress*.)
- To reduce stress, start exercising more regularly or learn to meditate. Find some time each day to call your own, even if it's only a relaxing bath for 30 minutes.
- Treat yourself to an aromatherapy massage each month, or add essential oils of rose, ylang ylang, neroli, jasmine, or geranium to your bath. Clary sage is great for reducing cramping period pains.
- If you smoke, give it up.

PRICKLY HEAT

Basically, prickly heat arises because the skin cannot release perspiration adequately. This irritating and unsightly condition usually affects fair-skinned people, such as myself, in tropical or sub-tropical climates. It initially appears as an itchy red, raised rash of hundreds of tiny bumps anywhere on the body. It has been linked to food intolerances (see *Allergies*) and chemical levels in drinking water, but can just as easily be triggered by sunscreen, shower gels, and soaps to which the individual becomes more sensitive in the heat and sun. I tend to suffer from prickly heat on my shins if I stand for too long in tropical temperatures, which causes blood to "pool" in my legs. Alcohol, antibiotics, and aspirin can also trigger prickly heat. Many people who suffer from these types of reactions have a leaky gut (see *Leaky Gut*).

Foods to Avoid

- Try cutting out cow's milk and dairy products, as well as wheat, peanuts, tea, and coffee. However, the culprits could be something unusual such as radishes or orange juice. (See *Allergies*.)
- Avoid really hot drinks and highly spiced foods.

Friendly Foods

- Eat more foods that nourish the skin from the inside out, such as apples, carrots, spinach (best raw), watercress, broccoli, pumpkin, cantaloupe melons, apricots, mango, papaya, and figs.
- Artichokes, beets, and asparagus cleanse the liver, which in turn aids skin healing.
- Onion and garlic are rich sources of quercetin, which is a natural anti-histamine.
- Avocados and oily fish are fabulous for the skin.
- Include more organic sunflower and pumpkin seeds, flaxseeds, almonds, and Brazil nuts in your diet; these are are rich in essential fats.
- Use more organic, unrefined extra-virgin olive, walnut, or sunflower oils in salad dressings.
- Drink bottled or pure filtered water.
- Muesli and most cereals are high in B vitamins, which help prevent dry skin.
- Nettle tea will help reduce the inflammation.

Useful Remedies

- Take 2–3g of vitamin C in an ascorbate form with meals, as vitamin C acts like a natural anti-histamine.

- Take a natural-source carotene complex for 14 days before you travel and throughout your vacation.
- Take a high-strength B complex daily.
- Take a multi-vitamin/mineral formula for your age and gender daily.
- Omega-3 fish oils help protect against free radical damage in the skin from the sun, and if you are taking sufficient amounts, these fats can help reduce your risk of sunburn. However, you still need to apply organic sunscreens! Take 2g daily for the long term.
- Take 1000IU of vitamin D3 daily throughout the year.

Helpful Hints

- If at all possible, expose your skin to sensible amounts of full- spectrum light prior to going into intense sunshine, as this helps build more pigment in the skin. Buy Full Spectrum Real Sunlight Lamps in which the harmful UVA and UVB rays have been greatly reduced, which enables you to make more vitamin D, while encouraging production of the natural pigment. Available in many stores like Target, Walmart, Kmart, and online from Amazon and other retailers.
- In most cases, prickly heat will clear up on its own in a few days if the affected area is kept cool and dry. Take regular cool showers and allow the skin to dry naturally.
- Use a skin brush regularly to help remove dead skin cells and allow the pores to work correctly.
- Avoid using any insect repellent on the affected areas.
- Once your skin is dry, apply aloe vera gel.
- Don't use any type of oil-based product, which can block your sweat glands.
- If the prickly heat does not clear up within 4–5 days and/or gets infected, you must see a doctor.
- To prevent prickly heat, avoid situations that can lead to excessive sweating, such as hot, humid environments and strenuous physical activity.
- Wear loose-fitting cotton clothes.
- Buy products in their most natural and unadulterated state. For anyone who suffers from dermatitis or skin allergies, Burt's Bees makes natural skin and hair products, body lotions, sunscreens, and toothpaste, and they also have an advice line. Visit www.burtsbees.com for more information.
- Many strong antibiotics and drugs make the skin very sensitive to the sun. If you are taking antibiotics, stay out of the sun.
- The herb St John's wort can also make the skin sensitive.
- Essential oils, such as lemon oil, can make your skin hyper- sensitive when exposed to sunlight. Do not use such oils if you are going out into the sun.
- Stay out of the midday sun and never allow your skin to go red.
- Take the homeopathic remedy Urtica 6c three times daily in between meals to reduce the redness. Discontinue use once the rash begins to fade. Or try homeopathic Sol/Urtica 30c, which helps prevents prickly heat. You can also use an Urtica Cream such as Weleda Burn Care. **VC, VS**
- Avoid hot baths and showers.

P

PROSTATE PROBLEMS *(see also Cholesterol)*

The prostate is a walnut-sized gland that sits below a man's bladder. Its job is to secrete seminal fluids and to contract strongly during orgasm to cause ejaculation. As men get older it is common for the prostate gland to gradually enlarge, up to 2–4 times its normal size, to about the size of a lemon. About half of all men over the age of 50 will have some degree of prostate enlargement at some point in their lives. This is largely attributable to the hormonal changes associated with ageing. After the age of 50 or so, a man's levels of testosterone decrease, while his levels of other hormones, including estrogen, increase. Despite decreasing testosterone levels, some of it is converted into a far more potent form—dihydrotestosterone (DHT)—and the normal process that breaks it down is inhibited by the excess estrogens. The potent DHT collects in the prostate and causes the overproduction of prostate cells, which ultimately results in prostate enlargement.

Other common factors affecting the prostate are heavy metal toxicity (mercury and aluminum), over-proliferation of fungus in the gut that spills over into the prostate, and long-term exposure to plastics, petrochemicals, and pesticides, which all have hormone-disrupting, estrogenic-like effects in the body.

The tube that takes urine from the bladder to the outside (the urethra) passes through the prostate, so the enlarged gland places pressure on the urethra, impeding the flow of urine and triggering the need to urinate more often. Many men get up three or four times during the course of the night. Other symptoms include difficulty in beginning urination, poor stream, dribbling at the end of urination, and sometimes pain. An enlarged prostate can also trigger urinary infections, bladder stones, and kidney damage.

In younger men these symptoms, as well as blood in the sperm, are usually linked to prostatitis, which is an inflammation of the prostate gland. Treatment of this condition is generally by antibiotics. The majority of prostate problems, though, are a result of the gradual enlargement that comes with age, termed benign prostatic hypertrophy (BPH). Still, the prostate can be affected by cancer. Prostate cancer is the most common cancer in men (after skin cancer), and one in every six American men will be diagnosed with it during their lifetime. If you have blood in your urine, difficulty in passing urine, or any swelling in your testicle area, please, please go see your doctor.

Lifestyle factors may play a role in prostate cancer prevention. A study involving 5,000 men conducted at the Johns Hopkins Bloomberg School of Public Health found that those with lower LDL cholesterol levels can potentially reduce their risk of developing high-grade prostate cancer by as much as 60%. (See dietary guidelines under *Cholesterol*.)

Foods to Avoid
- Because pesticide and herbicide residues are linked to prostate cancer, avoid non-organic foods as much as possible.
- Reduce your intake of animal fats found in meat, full-fat milks and cheeses, chocolate, hard margarines, and fatty fast food. Consuming too much animal-source dairy products and non-organic red meat (usually high in chemical and hormone residues) increase the risk of prostate cancer.
- Don't eat processed pies and pastries.
- Avoid fried and barbecued foods.
- Reduce your intake of caffeine, alcohol, and refined sugars.
- Also see *General Health Hints*.

Friendly Foods

- The carotene lycopene is the most abundant nutrient stored in the prostate, and studies have shown that men who eat 10 or more cooked tomatoes weekly are 45% less likely to develop prostate cancer. The lycopene in tomatoes is released when they are heated in a small amount of oil. A great way to do this is to cut tomatoes in half, brush them with a little olive oil, and add chopped garlic and basil. Grill or bake for a few minutes and serve. Lycopene is also found in guava, pink grapefruit, and watermelon.

- Eat organic foods as much as you can to avoid pesticide residues on fresh produce and hormones used in animal production. Additionally, locally grown seasonal fruits and vegetables contain more nutrients than those transported over thousands of miles.

- Sprinkle flaxseeds, soaked overnight and drained (or use ready-cracked flaxseeds) over cereals and yogurt or add to soups and smoothies. They are rich in essential fats and zinc. (See *General Health Hints* for a delicious smoothie recipe.)

- Pumpkin seeds are rich in zinc, magnesium (a muscle relaxer), and essential fats, helping reduce the conversion of testosterone to the potent DHT. Eat them raw or try lightly toasting them in a little soy sauce and sprinkling them over a salad to make a delicious, and very prostate-friendly, snack. Alternatively, grind 2 tablespoons each of hemp, sunflower and flaxseeds (use ready-cracked flaxseeds) and keep them in an airtight jar in the fridge. Sprinkle daily over cereals, salads, fruits, and yogurts.

- Eat more oily fish, which are rich in omega-3 essential fats, and use unrefined organic walnut, sesame, sunflower, and olive oils for salad dressings or drizzle over cooked foods. (See *Fats You Need To Eat*.)

- Include plenty of fiber in your diet from fruits and vegetables, especially broccoli, kale, cauliflower, and Brussels sprouts, which help balance hormones naturally.

- Lentils, alfalfa, tomatoes, salad leaves, yellow peppers, organic carrots, watercress, and pumpkin will help protect against cancers.

- Eat more brown rice, quinoa, millet, oats, cereals, and oat and rice bran. The fiber helps remove excess hormones from the body.

- Eat more pulses, such as barley, kidney beans, soybeans, and lentils, as well as corn, rice and lentil pastas.

- Have one serving of cooked tempeh (a fermented form of soy), miso, or soy sauce daily.

- There is currently a lot of discussion about soy-based foods, such as tofu and soy milk. While this argument is ongoing, it is generally accepted that fermented soy in the form of miso or tempeh is beneficial if taken in moderation. Cooked tofu is OK, but if in any doubt, avoid unfermented soy products, such as soy yogurt and soy milk, or check with your health professional.

Useful Remedies

- The mineral zinc is more abundant in the prostate than in any other organ in the body, and supplementation has been shown to reduce prostate overgrowth and symptoms of BPH. Zinc inhibits the conversion of testosterone to DHT, the primary hormonal trigger for prostate enlargement. Zinc deficiency is common in those with prostate problems. Take 20mg of zinc 2–3 times per day. As zinc depletes copper levels, take a proportionate amount of copper— approximately 1mg of copper for every 15mg of zinc.

- The herb saw palmetto has been proven to effectively reduce enlargement of the prostate gland and dramatically improve the symptoms of BPH. Its active components reduce the production and activity of DHT. Take 150–350mg of standardized extract twice a day as capsules. Or try Prostaguard from Kordel, which contains saw palmetto, horsetail, couchgrass, and hydrangea, which all help normalize prostate function. Available from lifepluspharmacy.com

- Another good herb for an enlarged prostate is pygeum. It is particularly good for relieving symptoms such as frequent or difficult urination and associated sexual dysfunction. Take 50–100mg of standardized extract twice daily.
- One of the oldest remedies for enlarged prostate is nettle, taken either as a tincture or as tablets. Take 5ml of tincture or 200–300mg of standardized extract capsules 2–3 times per day. You can also try nettle tea with a little honey.
- Prosta DHT by Apex Energetics is a multi-formula that contains most of the supplements mentioned above. Take two daily. Visit www.naturalhealthyconcepts.com or call 1-866-505-7501 for more information or to order.
- Otherwise, most of the companies featured on pages 15–16 have multiple prostate formulas for men.
- The mineral selenium has been found to help prevent prostate enlargement, and there is a significant inverse relationship between selenium levels in the body and prostate cancer. Taking 200mcg per day can significantly reduce your risk of both. Check your multi before adding extra selenium.
- Essential fats, especially omega-3 fish oils, can also help prevent prostate enlargement. Take 1g of fish oil with 4g of flaxseed oil daily. **VC NB: Diets that are too high in omega-6 fats (from refined margarines, pies, etc) and saturated fats (from animal products) are linked to an increased risk of prostate problems (see under *Fats You Need To Eat*), whereas omega-3 fats from oily fish, flaxseeds, and hemp seeds can help reduce the risk.**

- Include a natural carotene-source supplement that is rich in lycopene. Take 20–40mg daily.
- Because a deficiency of vitamin D3 is linked to prostate, colon, breast, and many other cancers, take 1000IU every day.
- Take 2g of vitamin C with added bioflavonoids daily with food because seminal fluid, which the prostate produces, requires large amounts of vitamin C.

Helpful Hints

- Filter your main tap water supply before drinking. This is because hormone residues from the pill and HRT are found in most water supplies, and they have an estrogen-like "building" effect in the body, which in the long term can trigger hormonal cancers. Kangen Water is an ionized, antioxidant water system that helps re-alkalize the body, thereby killing fungus and other pathogens. It has been used in Japanese hospitals with highly beneficial health results. For full details, visit www.kangenwaterusa.com
- A doctor usually discovers an enlarged prostate during a rectal examination. Therefore, all men over 40 should have an annual rectal examination. Early detection greatly increases your chances of a complete cure.
- Ask your partner to see if they can feel any abnormalities. Make this a fun thing, but try doing it once a month.
- Regular exercise is vital as it boosts immune function and also naturally reduces stress hormone levels. However, do not cycle, as this will put pressure on the prostate. Swimming and walking are great exercises.
- To help improve circulation to the area and reduce inflammation, lie on your back, bend your knees, bring the soles of your feet together, and then bring your feet as close to your buttocks as possible. Relax your legs, letting your knees fall outwards toward the ground. Hold this position for 5 minutes. Attempt this exercise only if you are fit and have no joint problems in your hips and legs.
- Massage essential oils of cypress, tea tree, and juniper berry mixed with a little jojoba carrier oil into your lower back and groin areas to help strengthen the prostate.

- See an osteopath or chiropractor to check that your pelvis and spine are not misaligned. In certain cases a major nerve connection from the lower part of the spine to the prostate becomes trapped, and once this is released water can be passed normally. (See *Useful Information*.)
- If you have prostate cancer, see *Useful Remedies* under *Cancer*.
- There is a test for prostate health called a PSA, or Prostate-Specific Antigen, test. If your levels of PSA are elevated, it can mean that your prostate is becoming enlarged, or it may possibly be an indication of prostate cancer. This is not a test for cancer *per se*, but it indicates prostate-cell activity. Another good test is the PCA3, Which is short for prostate cancer gene 3. This test uses a urine sample to see if you are over-expressing the PCA3 gene. Because this gene is over-expressed in 90% of prostate cancer cases and not expressed in BPH or prostatitis, it is much more specific than a PSA test. Both these tests can be administered by your doctor.
- Other factors can raise the PSA levels. For example, ejaculation can raise levels for 2 days, although in general, the higher the level, the more likely it is to be a sign of cancer. Biopsies are needed to confirm this.
- Men who self-medicate with the anti-aging hormone DHEA should take care, since DHEA can convert into testosterone and then into estrogen, which can trigger hormonal cancers. Always have blood and saliva tests to monitor your hormone levels before taking any hormone supplements, creams, pills, or patches.
- Harvard University has published a book entitled *Testosterone for Life,* showing research that men with low testosterone levels are at a higher risk of prostate cancer. Again, have your hormone levels checked.
- For further help and advice, contact the American Prostate Society by calling 1-877-859-3735 or visiting www.americanprostatesociety.com If you are interested in learning more about on-going prostate cancer research, visit www.pcf.org or call 1-800-757-2873.
- If your prostate is enlarged, be cautious about using over-the-counter cold or allergy remedies. Many of these products contain ingredients that can inflame the condition and cause urinary retention.
- Read *Prostate Health in 90 Days* by Larry Clapp (Hay House) or *Prostate Cancer* by Philip Dunn (Ostrich Publishing).

PSORIASIS   *(see also Candida, Leaky Gut, and SAD Syndrome)*

This is a chronic skin condition that can occur at any age. It is characterized by patches of red, raised, and scaly skin. Once it begins scaling, the skin can take on a silvery, fish-like look. It does seem to have some hereditary links, but symptoms often don't appear until adulthood. It usually does not itch but can cause discomfort and embarrassment. Areas most commonly affected are the arms, elbows, behind the ears, scalp, back, legs, and knees. Psoriasis may also be triggered by prolonged stress, a traumatic event, food intolerances, essential-fatty-acid deficiencies, low levels of stomach acid, constipation, liver congestion, and vitamin B deficiency. It is also linked to a leaky gut, food intolerances, and a yeast fungal overgrowth such as candida. Many people with psoriasis may have poor liver function, as skin problems can be a sign that the liver is under stress, in which case you need to see a qualified nutritionist who can modify your diet to help detoxify the liver. (See Liver Problems.) Lack of vitamin D and a lack of exposure to full-spectrum sunlight also factor in this condition.

Foods to Avoid
- Eliminate wheat and any wheat-containing foods for one month and see if this helps. Some people also have an intolerance to gluten. (See *Allergies* for useful tests to identify food sensitivities).
- Dairy from animal sources can be a problem, but skimmed milk should be OK.
- Citrus fruits and tomatoes aggravate the problem in some sufferers.
- Cut down on saturated and hydrogenated fats, especially red meat, mass-produced vegetable oils, fast food, cakes, pastries, pies, and full-fat dairy products. All of these foods are acid forming in the body. (See *Acid–Alkaline Balance*.)
- Keep a food diary and note when symptoms become worse. It's often the foods you eat and/or crave the most, such as starchy, sugary foods, that are the underlying trigger for this condition.
- As much as possible, eliminate alcohol, as it makes the liver work harder and thus affects the skin. In some people, the single biggest trigger for psoriasis is alcohol consumption.

Friendly Foods
- Most people with psoriasis are deficient in essential fats. Therefore, eat salmon, sardines, mackerel, herring, pilchards, or anchovies at least twice a week. (See *Fats You Need To Eat*.)
- Eat as wide a variety of fresh foods as possible.
- Eat more brown rice, millet, and buckwheat, which are gluten-free.
- Eat more pectin-rich foods, such as apples and carrots. Greatly increase your intake of whole fruits and vegetables.
- Figs, prunes, kiwi, spinach, watercress, and papaya are all great for the skin. (See *Candida*, as high-sugar fruits can exacerbate fungal conditions such this.)
- Add unrefined, organic walnut, sunflower, sesame, and olive oils to salad dressings or drizzle over cooked foods.
- Use organic rice or low-fat goat's milks instead of cow's milk. Otherwise try almond milk.
- Pumpkin seeds, flaxseeds, and sunflower seeds are all high in zinc and essential fats.
- Begin making fresh vegetable juices with raw beets, artichokes, carrots, and apples or any vegetables you have on hand. Add a teaspoon of green food powder (see details under *Acid–Alkaline Balance*), 20 drops of dandelion and milk thistle tincture and half a cup of organic aloe vera juice to help cleanse the liver. Drink immediately after juicing.
- Another good green food powder is Greens Plus, which contains Hawaiian spirulina, chlorella, lecithin, barley, pectin apple fiber, soy and barley sprouts, and lactobacillus acidophilus. It is a great all-around way to ingest good nutrients, encourage healthy bacteria, keep the body more alkaline, and make the skin healthier. Details onwww.greensplus.com
- Celeriac, artichoke, and kale are also great for the liver.
- Stay hydrated by drinking plenty of water and other fluids.

Useful Remedies.
- Taking 5–6g of evening primrose oil daily will help reduce the inflammation associated with psoriasis. Evening primrose oil is high in gamma-linolenic acid (GLA), so if you don't want to swallow high doses of evening primrose oil, take 1–2g of pure GLA daily instead. **VC**
- Omega-3 fish oils are highly anti-inflammatory and help nourish and lubricate the skin from the inside out. Taking at least 3–5g daily is highly effective for this condition.
- Take a B-complex that contains 400mcg of folic acid and 100mg of B6, which are often low in people with this condition.
- Vitamin B12 injections have helped many people who have low stomach acid (see *Low Stomach Acid*).
- Take vitamin C with bioflavonoids (2g daily in divided doses with meals) to help reduce the inflammation.

- Take a multi-vitamin/mineral that contains at least 30–40mg of zinc. A good multi-vitamin should also contain a full spectrum of the B vitamins. If it does, there is no need to take an additional B-complex.
- Betaine hydrochloride (stomach acid) is often useful. One capsule taken with main meals aids digestion and the absorption of nutrients. If you have active stomach ulcers, take a digestive enzyme that is free of betaine hydrochloride instead.
- Most psoriasis sufferers are very deficient in vitamin A. For one month take 25,000IU of vitamin A daily and then reduce to 5,000IU daily (this amount should be in your multi). **NB: If you are pregnant or planning to become pregnant, do not take more than 3,000IU of vitamin A daily.** Liver is very high in vitamin A, so if you eat a lot if it, you may not need to take a supplement—but I don't know anyone who eats liver every day!
- After supplementing vitamin A for a month, switch to a daily intake of natural-source carotenes, which naturally convert to vitamin A in the body and are non-toxic.
- There has been extensive research into the healing properties of the plant *Mahonia aquifolium* for psoriasis sufferers. It is available as a liquid, cream, or ointment from many online retailers, including Amazon.
- Take at least 1000IU of vitamin D3 daily, as a lack of D3 is linked to many skin conditions and a host of other diseases.
- A highly concentrated form of whey called DermaWhey has been shown to soothe skin conditions such as psoriasis. **LEF**

Helpful Hints

- Regular colonic irrigation therapies help detox the bowel. (See *Useful Information*.)
- Sea bathing is beneficial for psoriasis. Many sufferers find relief after bathing in Dead Sea salt because of its high mineral contents. Add 2.25lb (1kg) to your bath and soak for 10 minutes.
- Homeopathic Ars-iod 6x, taken twice daily for a few weeks, is particularly good for dry, scaly, itchy skin.
- Moderate sun exposure also helps psoriasis, but remember to wear a hypoallergenic sunscreen.
- Smokers run a greater risk of developing psoriasis.
- Many people with this skin condition tend to be holding on to emotional issues, such as resentment, anger, and bitterness. If emotions are repressed, the liver is affected and skin problems can result.
- For more help, read *Healing Psoriasis: the Natural Alternative* by Dr John Pagano (Pagano Organization).

R

RAYNAUD'S DISEASE

(see also Circulation, Sjogren's Syndrome, and Stress)

Raynaud's is five times more common in women than in men and commonly begins between the ages of 18 and 30, although it can occur later. This condition develops when small blood vessels that supply blood to the skin constrict, triggering intermittent spasms—usually in the fingers and toes, but occasionally in the nose and tongue. If Raynaud's-type symptoms appear alone, without any other condition being present, it's known as Raynaud's disease, but if other symptoms are apparent such as a dry mouth, eyes and nose, aching joints, and/or osteoporosis, then you may have Sjogren's syndrome, an autoimmune condition. (See *Sjogren's Syndrome*.

Initially symptoms occur when the extremities are exposed to cold temperatures, especially if the person is stressed. The nerve receptors in these areas become particularly sensitive to the slightest chill, and fingers and/or toes can become white, bluish or red; tingling and numbness are also common. This condition is linked to poor circulation and a diet low in essential fats and other nutrients, including iron. Another trigger for Raynaud's is smoking, which greatly affects microcirculation. In rare cases the skin can ulcerate if it is starved of blood for too long. (See *Circulation, Fats You Need to Eat*, and *Leg Ulcers*.) Other factors include repetitive activities using the hands, such as typing or using vibrating tools.

Sometimes Raynaud's remains dormant for years, but can re-surface under conditions of extreme stress, exhaustion, or after an infection. Raynaud's can also affect the tissue in the lungs, in which case cold air can trigger coughing attacks.

If Raynaud's is allowed to worsen, or if the skin ulcerates, it can become serious, and in rare cases it can lead to gangrene severe enough to require amputation. Therefore, it needs to be taken very seriously from the outset. People who tend to be stressed much of the time, are highly strung, and have poor circulation are at greater risk. Rheumatoid arthritis, lupus, and some thyroid conditions may also be linked to Raynaud's-type symptoms, as may scleroderma, a chronic connective tissue autoimmune condition in which the body accumulates too much collagen, resulting in hardening of the skin and various internal tissues. Other symptoms of scleroderma include joint pain or puffy hands and feet, gut problems, dry mucous membranes, dental and jaw problems, and sometimes, as it progresses, fatigue. The earlier you can recognize such symptoms and seek medical advice and specialist help, the better. People who suffer from scleroderma are likely to also have Sjogren's syndrome. Anyone with autoimmune disease should read the section on *Leaky Gut*, which is often a major contributing factor in all autoimmune conditions.

People suffering from Raynaud's are also at a much greater risk of heart disease and stroke, another reason to take this condition seriously. As people with A and AB blood types have a propensity to clot more readily than other blood types, they are more likely to suffer from conditions relating to circulation, such as Raynaud's.

Foods to Avoid

- Cut down on saturated fats found in hard margarines, fatty meats, full-fat milk, and animal-source dairy products.
- Avoid the caffeine found in coffee, energy drinks, and chocolate (the darker the chocolate, the more caffeine), which constricts blood vessels.
- Also see this section under *Atherosclerosis* and *Circulation*.

Friendly Foods

- You need to eat more foods that are high in natural-source vitamin E, such as wheat germ, avocados, nuts, and seeds.
- Rutin-rich foods help strengthen small blood vessels. These include buckwheat, the peel of citrus fruits, rose hips, apple peel, and cabbage.
- Make stews, soups, and casseroles that are full of root vegetables (sweet potatoes, carrots, pumpkin, and so on) as these types of foods warm you from the inside out and are rich in minerals.
- Eat iron-rich foods: lean red meat, liver, poultry, eggs, blackstrap molasses, fish, broccoli, kale, and leafy green vegetables such as spinach and watercress.
- Magnesium is a nutritional vasodilator, so be sure to include more low-sugar cereals, oats, honey, whole-wheat bread and pastas, almonds, Brazil nuts, walnuts, mustard, and curry powder in your diet. All leafy green foods are rich in magnesium, and foods like chlorella and green food powders are also high in iron.
- Cook with garlic and onions, which help thin the blood naturally. Also use plenty of fresh root ginger and cayenne pepper, which warm the body.
- Eat plenty of fruit high in vitamin C, such as cherries, kiwi, and blueberries. In winter, make berry-and-fruit compotes, or lightly glaze fresh fruit with a little honey and grill on kebab sticks. Serve with low-fat, live yogurt and sprinkle with lecithin granules (which lower LDL-cholesterol levels).
- Eat more oily fish, which are rich in omega-3 essential fats
- Flaxseeds are also rich in omega-3 and -6 fats. Soak them overnight in cold water, drain, and then eat sprinkled over cereals or oatmeal or mixed in fruit smoothies daily.

Useful Remedies

- If you are not on blood-thinning drugs, take 400–600IU of natural-source full-spectrum vitamin E daily.
- Take 1–3g of vitamin C with bioflavonoids a day with food. These play a vital role in the synthesis of collagen, which is the key component in the walls of blood vessels. Vitamin C is also essential for protecting the small arteries that supply the fingers from damage during attacks.
- Take niacin (vitamin B3) in a formula that creates a flushing sensation. Start by taking around 30–50mg, two or three times daily, and gradually increase to 100–1000mg or more per day (in divided doses) under medical supervision. **Be aware, this vitamin really boosts circulation and for about 30–45 minutes after swallowing, it can cause a pronounced red flushing effect on the skin. Anyone suffering from liver disease should not take high doses of niacin.**
- If you take the flavonoid quercetin earlier in the day, before taking the niacin, this reduces flushing and suppresses inflammatory responses. Take 500mg daily.
- Otherwise take a high-strength vitamin B complex daily, and if symptoms are severe ask your doctor for a vitamin B12 injection.
- Take a high-strength multi-mineral that contains 500mg of magnesium, 500mg of calcium, and 20mg of potassium, plus a trace amount of manganese.

- Gamma-linolenic acid (GLA) is an essential fatty acid found in evening primrose, borage, and blackcurrant oils, and is important for relaxing muscles. A recent study found that 12 capsules a day of evening primrose oil dramatically decreased the number of Raynaud's attacks. But as most people don't want to swallow 12 pills a day and the ingredient they really need is the GLA, take 2–4 Mega GLA capsules daily. **VC**
- Essential polyunsaturated fatty acids, known as omega-3 and omega-6 fatty acids, have been shown to lower "unhealthier" LDL fats and thin the blood naturally. Therefore, you can either take 8g of flaxseed oil capsules *or* 4g of pure omega-3 fish oils daily. Fish oils also improve your tolerance to cold, which is why the Inuits rarely feel the cold! (See *Fats You Need To Eat*.)
- The herb gotu kola really helps increase circulation. Take 500mg twice daily during the winter or while symptoms are acute.
- Cayenne pepper capsules help improve circulation. Start by taking one capsule three times daily with food and increase if desired. You should see the benefits after a month.
- If the cayenne pepper causes too much warmth in the stomach, then try Christopher's Blood Circulation Formula, which contains a small amount of cayenne as well as ginger, hawthorn, low-odor garlic, ginseng, and parsley. **VC**
- Add a few drops of a liquid ginger product to water and sip throughout the day. This really helps warm you right though. **VC**

Helpful Hints

- If you suffer from Raynaud's-type symptoms year round, have a blood test to determine what's going on and to get a proper diagnosis.
- Wear mittens, which are more effective at keeping you warm than gloves. At all costs, keep your hands and feet warm. Many stores now sell cashmere or wool hand/wrist covers, which leave fingers free to work.
- Avoid handling cold items from the fridge. Wear gloves in cool supermarkets.
- Do not clap hands together and rub them too hard, as this can damage blood vessels.
- Run hands under warm (NOT hot) water. Moist heat is preferable to dry heat sources.
- Otherwise place your hands under your armpits to warm them up gently.
- Exercise regularly to improve your circulation. Swimming, walking while swinging your arms in circles, skipping, and rebounding on a mini-trampoline are all wonderful ways to improve circulation.
- If your feet are affected, then wear warm socks to bed at night and avoid tight-fitting shoes that restrict circulation.
- Learn to control your stress levels, as stress has a huge impact on Raynaud's. (See *Stress*.)
- Make tea infusions with fresh root ginger, cinnamon twigs, or angelica root.
- Try massaging your hands and toes regularly with **diluted** essential oils of black pepper, rosemary, lavender, or geranium, or add a few drops of each of these oils to your bath.
- Use good-quality, rich hand cream, preferably organic, to help soften the skin.
- Use only pH-balanced cleansing bars rather than mass-produced soaps.
- Avoid damaging the affected fingers, especially if they are ulcerated. Wear gloves.
- Reflexology and acupuncture have helped many sufferers. (See *Useful Information*.)
- For further information, contact the Raynaud's Association by calling 1-800-280-8055 or visiting www.raynauds.org

REPETITIVE STRAIN INJURY (RSI)

(see also Carpel Tunnel Syndrome)

According to U.S. Department of Labor, Occupational Safety and Health Administration, hundreds of thousands of American workers suffer from chronic pain in their wrists, elbows, shoulders, or necks due to RSI, making it the most common occupational health issue. And thanks to the huge numbers of us that work on computers, these statistics are on the rise. In typing this book I, too, have succumbed to RSI, but I keep it under control by wearing a wristband that goes through my thumb and around my wrist, which contains magnets. It has certainly helped me. You can find these bands in all good sporting goods stores.

Meanwhile, employers spend more than $7 billion in workers' compensation claims, which obviously needs to be taken seriously. Common symptoms include numbness, tingling pains, loss of grip, and restricted movement. Anyone who has a job or plays a sport regularly that involves repetitive movements is at risk of developing RSI. The condition is basically caused by inflammation of the tendons, known as tendonitis. Tendonitis usually heals within a few weeks, but if it becomes chronic, calcium salts can deposit along the tendon fibers. The tendons most commonly affected are the Achilles, biceps, elbow, thumb, knee, inside of the foot, or shoulder joint.

Foods to Avoid
- Caffeine reduces the body's ability to cope with pain.
- Cut down on refined sugars and junk foods, which trigger inflammation in the body.

R

Friendly Foods
- Eat more oily fish, which are rich in vitamin A, to aid tissue healing and reduce inflammation.
- Eat plenty of foods that are high in natural carotenes for their anti-inflammatory properties. These include asparagus, French beans, broccoli, carrots, papaya, raw parsley, red peppers, spring greens, sweet potatoes, watercress, spinach, apricots, pumpkin, tomatoes, and cantaloupe melon.
- Nuts (unsalted) and seeds, especially pumpkin, sesame, sunflower, and flaxseeds, plus fish, are all high in zinc.
- Include more turmeric in food, because it has highly anti-inflammatory properties.
- Pineapple, cherries, and ginger all have anti-inflammatory properties.

Useful Supplements
- Take 2g of vitamin C in an ascorbate form daily in divided doses with food, as vitamin C plays a major role in the prevention and repair of injuries. **VC**
- Natural-source beta-carotenes will help reduce inflammation and maintain tissue integrity. Take 30mg daily.
- Zinc (30mg per day) functions alongside vitamin A. An increased copper-to-zinc ratio is often found in individuals with chronic inflammatory conditions.
- Bioflavonoids are extremely effective at reducing inflammation. Take 1g of a bioflavonoid complex daily.
- Include a multi-vitamin/mineral in your regimen that includes 400IU of natural-source, full-spectrum vitamin E, 200mcg of selenium, and 100–150mg of vitamin B6.
- Take glucosamine (1000mg daily in divided doses) and MSM (1000mg) daily. MSM is an organic form of sulfur and has proved useful for alleviating this problem. Most glucosamine supplements are derived from crab shells. If you are allergic to shellfish, ask for the vegetarian version made from corn. Available at health stores.
- Omega-3 fats have an anti-inflammatory effect on the body; take 2–4g daily.

- Take 600mg of magnesium daily in divided doses to help soothe nerve endings and repair muscles.
- Collagen is a vital component of healthy joints, cartilage, ligaments, and tendons. It is the most widely distributed protein in the body, but we lose about 1.5% annually after the age of 30. Take daily in a glass of water or diluted juice 30 minutes before a main meal to support your tendons. Super Collagen drink from NeoCell. **VC**

Helpful Hints

- Magnets help increase circulation, which brings more oxygenated blood to the problem area. Take a look at www.magnetsandhealth.com or www.therionmagnetics.com for more information.
- A proper warm-up and stretching before exercise are important to prevent injury.
- Rest the injured area as soon as it hurts to avoid further damage.
- Wrap some ice or a bag of frozen peas in a towel and apply to the painful area for 10 minutes every hour while symptoms are acute. Do not wrap so tightly that circulation is impaired.
- Compress the area with an elastic bandage to limit swelling.
- Elevate the injured body part above the level of the heart to increase drainage of fluids out of the injured area.
- You can also massage the affected areas with essential oil of wintergreen, which has anti-inflammatory properties. This really helps.
- If you sit for long hours at a desk, take regular breaks and really stretch out.
- Life-Flo makes an organic sulfur (MSM) muscle balm that really helps ease pain. **VC**
- The Alexander Technique helps individuals learn about healthy posture and, therefore, how to reduce or even eliminate RSI problems. Acute problems may benefit from treatment with osteopathy, chiropractic, or acupuncture. (See *Useful Information*.)
- If after trying all these suggestions for 6 weeks you are no better, consult a specialist in sports injuries or at least have an x-ray or scan.

RESTLESS LEGS
(see also Circulation)

This is a very distressing yet very common condition, which causes tickling, burning, or pricking sensations or an irresistible urge to kick your legs, combined with involuntary twitching in the muscles of the lower legs. Between 5 and 15% of adults are affected—more than 12 million in the US alone! It can occur sporadically during the day, usually if you sit for long periods, but it's more likely to occur when you are resting, which is why this condition can greatly affect sleep patterns. Also known as Ekbom's syndrome, restless legs is more common in pregnant and middle-aged women, smokers, diabetics, people with low blood sugar (see *Low Blood Sugar*), and those who drink too much coffee. It could also be partly hereditary. Common factors are a lack of iron, full-spectrum vitamin E, and the mineral magnesium. (See also *Circulation*.)

Foods to Avoid

- Cut down on your alcohol intake.
- The biggest trigger is caffeine in any form, so avoid coffee, tea, and soft drinks. Also eliminate any foods that contain caffeine, including chocolate.
- Avoid foods that contain too much sugar, which can cause your blood sugar to fluctuate and make symptoms worse.

- Reduce refined pastries, cakes, mass-produced pies, and cookies.
- Also see *General Health Hints*.

Friendly Foods

- You need to eat quality protein from chicken, fish, eggs, low-fat cheeses, pulses, beans, peas, cooked tofu, and so on at least once a day.
- Eat more brown rice, quinoa, and couscous. For snacks, eat rye crisp breads or amaranth/rice crackers, which are delicious spread with a little low-fat humus or tahini.
- Eat more leafy green vegetables, especially kale and watercress, as well as fruit and honey, which are all rich in magnesium.
- Iron-rich foods include liver, lean red meat (such as venison), rabbit, free-range chicken, eggs, cereals, and blackstrap molasses.
- Essential fats are vital; therefore, include oily fish in your diet at least twice a week and sprinkle organic unsalted sunflower and pumpkin seeds over cereals and salads.
- Eat raw wheat germ and avocados, which are rich in vitamin E and healthier monounsaturated fats.
- Eat more blueberries and bilberries when they are in season.
- Drink calming herbal teas, such as chamomile, lemon balm, or vervain.
- As you need plenty of B vitamins with this condition, eat more oatmeal, low-sugar oat-based cereals, and oat bran.
- Invest in a low glycemic index (GI) cookbook.

Useful Supplements

- If you are deficient in iron, take a liquid formula such as Spatone that is easily absorbed and does not cause constipation. Available from health stores worldwide.
- Take a high-strength B complex to calm the nerve endings. Folic acid (5mg) and B6 (100mg) are the most important. Take these with breakfast or lunch.
- Natural-source, full-spectrum vitamin E (400IU daily) can be extremely effective at alleviating this condition. **NB: If you are on blood-thinning drugs, vitamin E thins the blood naturally, so tell your doctor and have regular blood tests so that you can reduce your prescription dosages.**
- The mineral magnesium is very important for relaxing muscles, so take a good-quality multi-vitamin/mineral that contains 500mg of magnesium and 400mg of calcium. Take with your evening meal.
- Cayenne pepper capsules really rev up the circulation and have an anti-cramping affect. Take three a day in divided doses with meals.
- Also see *Useful Supplements* under *Circulation* and *Raynaud's Disease*.

Helpful Hints

- A simple blood test will tell you if you are anemic and actually need to take extra iron. (See *Anemia*.)
- Get plenty of exercise.
- Massage your legs and feet (especially before bed) with essential oil of rosemary in a carrier of almond or olive oil, using kneading movements from the ankle upwards toward the knee. The legs can be bathed in alternate hot and cold water to improve circulation.
- Use cramp bark cream before going to bed. **VC**
- Try reflexology, acupuncture, or regular aromatherapy massage to rev up the circulation.
- Take all the suggested supplements for at least 3 months.
- Wearing magnets in your shoes or in bed socks greatly aids circulation, which can considerably reduce symptoms at night. Magnets are available from all large pharmacies.
- If it's practical, go for a walk for at least 30 minutes in the evenings.

RHEUMATOID ARTHRITIS

(see Arthritis)

ROSACEA

(see also Candida, Leaky Gut, Low Stomach Acid, Lupus, and Sjogren's Syndrome)

This is a common skin disorder in adults between the ages of 30 and 50, and women are three times more likely to be affected than men. It's thought that hormones play a role in this condition, and naturopaths state that lymphatic congestion is often a factor. Symptoms are a chronic acne-like eruption or flushing of the face, which usually affects the area around the nose and chin. Sometimes the tiny pustules are filled with sebum, while others are just filled with fluid.

Rosacea can be inherited, but it is more commonly associated with drinking too much alcohol, prolonged stress, coffee, tea, spicy foods, menopause, and a lack of stomach acid and/or B-vitamins. It can also be triggered by food intolerances, the most common triggers being wheat, cow's milk, and oranges. Many people who suffer from rosacea also suffer from migraines (see *Migraine*). A leaky gut is also highly implicated in rosacea (see *Leaky Gut*), and you may be intolerant to the gluten found in wheat and grains as well. You also need to take care of your liver (see *Liver Problems*). Generally, the worse your digestion (usually linked to food intolerances in combination with stress), the worse your symptoms are likely to become.

Facial butterfly-type rashes are linked to autoimmune conditions such as lupus. (See *Lupus*.)

R

Foods to Avoid
- Generally cut down on coffee, tea, alcohol, hot drinks, and hot spicy foods, which increase blood flow and hence flushing.
- Minimize your caffeine intake by cutting down on coffee, chocolate, energy drinks, sodas, and so on.
- Keep a food diary and note what you were eating, drinking, or feeling prior to the onset of symptoms.
- Avoid heavy, rich or fried foods, which place a strain on digestion and the liver.
- Avoid eating too many foods made with flour (pies, cakes, and so on), as they are often high in refined sodium-based salt, refined sugar, and saturated fats.
- Avoid oily, spicy foods.

Friendly Foods
- Bitter foods, such as radicchio, fennel, chicory, celeriac, and young green celery, stimulate stomach acid.
- Take a teaspoon of apple cider vinegar or lemon juice in warm water before a meal.
- Drink plenty of water, even if you are not thirsty.
- Eat more pineapple and papaya to improve your digestion.
- Eat plenty of leafy green vegetables, especially spinach, watercress, kale, cauliflower, broccoli, cabbage, and celery.
- Eat more beets and artichokes to help cleanse your liver.
- Include plenty of live, low-fat yogurt in your diet to help replenish healthy bacteria in the gut.

Useful Remedies
- Prebiotics feed the healthy bacteria in your gut. They usually contain inulin, a compound

found in chicory and artichokes. Take daily as recommended. Most of the vitamin companies featured on pages 15–16 produce prebiotic capsules and powders.

- Probiotics, healthy bacteria, can also be helpful if taken for a month. They help restore healthy levels of bacteria in the gut, which in turn can reduce the facial rashes. Jarro-Dophilus EPS, made by Jarrow, will help replenish gut flora; take one daily after food. They are enteric-coated, which means they can pass through stomach lining and there's no need to keep them refrigerated. **JF**
- If you are not suffering from active stomach ulcers, take one betaine hydrochloride (stomach acid) capsule with main meals. If this causes a slight burning sensation, switch to a pancreatic digestive enzyme capsule that is free from betaine hydrochloride. **VC**
- Rosacea sufferers often don't secrete enough of the pancreatic enzyme, lipase. Take one Source Naturals Pancreatin capsule with main meals. **VC**
- As B-group vitamins are often depleted, also take a B complex.
- There is a skin regime called Your Skincare Solution Rosacea Skin Kit by Pevonia that has helped many sufferers. For full details, contact Pevonia. Tel: 1-800-446-3751. Website: www.shoppevonia.com
- Applying a cream containing pine bark and blackcurrant leaf helps reduce redness and inflammation and has potent anti-inflammatory properties. One such cream is Decleor NutriDivine Nutriboost Ultra Cocooning Cream, available from Nordstrom and online from Amazon and other retailers.
- People who take pycnogenol, pine bark extract, regularly report great improvement after 3 months. Take 80mg twice daily. **VC**
- Try an herbal tincture made specifically for rosacea that includes milk thistle, red clover, bilberry, and gingko. **OP** Alternatively, take a product containing all these ingredients such as Udo's Choice Wholesome Fast Food. **VC**
- Mix 1 teaspoon of fenugreek seeds in a cup of boiling water, allow to cool, strain, and then drink twice daily. This really helps clear lymphatic congestion.

Helpful Hints

- Sipping diluted lemon juice with main meals can help treat low stomach acid, which is a factor in this condition.
- Homeopathic Arsenicum Brom 6c taken twice daily for 2 weeks helps reduce symptoms.
- Exposure to heat and cold can trigger an attack.
- Try regular rebounding (buy a mini-trampoline) to help clear any lymphatic congestion.
- Some women who take the hormone DHEA are affected by pimples appearing on their faces and foreheads, which can mimic rosacea-type symptoms. Check with your health professional in case you are taking too high a dose of DHEA.

R

S

SAD SYNDROME (seasonal affective disorder)

(see also Depression)

Approximately 10 million people are affected by this problem in the US, and at least 20 million more are affected by a milder form known simply as the "winter blues." It's far more common in women (75% of sufferers) than men, and symptoms include low moods, increased appetite and food cravings (usually for starchy, sugary, fatty foods), PMS-type symptoms, weight gain, depression, loss of libido, irritability, difficulty concentrating, an increased feeling of being of "no use" to anyone, lack of energy, and an increased desire to sleep during the winter months. Many people report that they feel sleepy during the day, yet cannot sleep well at night.

Symptoms usually begin in late autumn or early winter and tend to disappear by late spring or early summer. Due to a lack of full-spectrum light in northern latitudes during the winter months, our pineal gland, which is situated in our brain, produces more melatonin, the hormone that regulates glandular function and makes us feel more sleepy.

Melatonin is crucial for controlling our biological rhythms and is secreted mainly at night, while its counterpart serotonin, the "feel-good chemical," is secreted on exposure to bright daylight. Melatonin helps you sleep, while serotonin raises mood and makes you feel positive. Therefore, when there is a lack of natural sunlight, you make more melatonin and less serotonin. This is why suicide rates increase in countries where sunshine is rare during the winter months.

Foods to Avoid

- When there is insufficient light, the body naturally craves sugary carbohydrates to increase its serotonin levels, which is why many women put on weight in the winter. Do your best to reduce your intake of stimulants, such as coffee, mass-produced chocolate, caffeine, and refined sugary, starchy-based foods and drinks.
- Alcohol lowers brain levels of the neurotransmitter serotonin, which helps keep us positive.
- Reduce your intake of refined, sugary, starchy foods. If you crave sugar, use a little brown rice syrup, organic agave (plant-based) syrup and/or xylitol as a sweetener. **VC, VS**
- See section on *Low Blood Sugar*, as it usually goes hand in hand with SAD Syndrome.

Friendly Foods

- Eat foods that help the body produce more serotonin, such as fish, turkey, chicken, cottage cheese, beans, avocados, bananas, whey protein, and wheat germ.
- Sixty percent of the brain is made up of fat, so eat plenty of oily fish, which is rich in omega-3 fats. Add flaxseeds to your breakfast cereal, as they are also rich in essential fats.
- Organic milk is also a good source of the amino acid tryptophan, which helps raise serotonin levels.
- Include more organic tempeh, miso soup, and beans in your diet. Kidney, cannellini, and black-eyed beans are rich sources of fiber and proteins that will help raise your mood.

- During the winter, make rich stews with plenty of green and root vegetables, and add brown rice and pastas.
- Low-sugar, oat-based muesli and cereals are rich in B vitamins, which are great mood foods. Eat oatmeal for breakfast that is sweetened with a chopped apple and a few raisins.
- Try dairy- and sugar-free organic chocolate made with agave syrup, goji and acai berries with blueberry and coconut oil. Glamour Food is available from the Organic Pharmacy in Beverly Hills. Tel: 1-310-272-7275.

Useful Remedies

- First, take a good-quality multi-vitamin/mineral supplement that contains at least 200mg of magnesium and 30mg of zinc.
- Add a high-strength B complex, as a lack of vitamins B3, B6, B12, and folic acid are all linked to depression. Vitamins B6, B3, and inositol are necessary to convert tryptophan into serotonin.
- Lack of vitamin D (especially D3) is closely associated with SAD syndrome. During the winter months, take a minimum of 1000IU daily, and if symptoms are acute take 2000–4000IU daily for a couple of weeks. During a day in the sun, you can naturally produce as much as 20,000IU of vitamin D!
- Tryptophan, an amino acid, helps boost serotonin levels. This supplement has been shown to be as effective as orthodox antidepressants, without the negative side effects. 250mg can be taken twice daily. **VC, VS**
- St John's wort has proven very effective for this condition; take 500–1000mg a day. **NB: Do not take if you are already on blood-thinning drugs. If you are taking any prescription drugs, ask your doctor about any contraindications.**

- Take 2g of omega-3 fish oil capsules daily, as a lack of essential fats can contribute to feelings of depression.

Helpful Hints

- Make an effort to walk in natural daylight for at least 15 minutes a day, especially when the sun is out. We need around 10,000 lux of full-spectrum light daily to maintain serotonin levels. One lux is equal to the light of one small candle!
- Try using Real Sunlight lamps, available at major retailers such as Target, Wal-Mart, and Kmart. The harmful frequencies of UVA and UVB have been filtered out, making this sunlight safe. Developed in Sweden, they are now used in many nursing homes to boost immune function and relieve the depression associated with SAD Syndrome. They have been so successful that the Swedish Government is installing them in nursing homes in which residents are rarely exposed to natural sunlight. These lamps increase levels of vitamin D3 naturally, boost immune function, and reduce depression.
- Tanning beds should not be used to treat SAD. The light sources in tanning beds are high in ultraviolet (UV) rays, which harm both your eyes and your skin. Light boxes emit full-spectrum light. Use Biolight's full-spectrum light bulbs, available at health and specialty stores across the US. For more information, visit www.sunlifelighting.com
- Exercise as much as possible during daylight hours to increase the production of serotonin, the "feel-good" hormone.
- Take a winter vacation to someplace sunny.
- Mental Health America has an informative factsheet available on its website: www.nmha.org as well as a crisis hotline: 1-800-273-8255. You may also want to visit the SAD Association (UK)'s website, www.sada.org.uk, for advice about buying a SAD light.
- Otherwise, you can learn more through the Society for Light Treatment and Biological Rhythms' website: www.sltbr.org

■ A number of manufacturers make light boxes used specifically for SAD Syndrome. Search online and on Amazon.

SCALP PROBLEMS

Dry, flaking, itching scalp or dandruff

This condition occurs when the tiny cells that make up the outer layer of skin are shed at a faster rate than normal. Dandruff usually results from a malfunction of the sebaceous glands that affects the amount of sebum or oils they produce. If too little sebum is secreted, the hair becomes brittle and dandruff appears. Dry skin on the scalp is also linked to eczema and psoriasis. An itchy scalp can also be associated with candida. (See *Candida*.) Dandruff is connected with food intolerances as well.

Foods to Avoid
■ I'm afraid it's the usual culprits of highly refined, starchy foods that are high in animal fats, full-fat dairy products, and refined sugars.
■ Also see *General Health Hints*.

Friendly Foods
■ You need to increase your intake of essential fats found in oily fish, as well as sunflower, pumpkin, hemp, flax, and sesame seeds.
■ Use organic walnut and olive oils, not only for salad dressings, but also drizzled over cooked dishes. Udo's Choice Oil is a balanced blend of omega-3 and -6 fats, which will help feed the skin from the inside out. (See *Fats You Need To Eat.*)
■ Eat more whole foods, brown rice, and stone-ground whole-wheat bread, barley, quinoa, amaranth, buckwheat, millet, and pasta.
■ Greatly increase your intake of fresh fruits and vegetables, especially organic carrots, spinach, watercress, papaya, apricots, cantaloupe melon, guava, mango, pumpkin, sweet potato, and squash, which are all rich in natural-source carotenes.
■ Eat pineapple and papaya with main meals to aid digestion.
■ Include more low-fat, live yogurt in your diet to aid digestion.
■ Eat more wheat germ and avocados, which are rich in vitamin E.
■ Dry skin is also a sign of dehydration so drink at least 6–8 glasses of water daily.
■ Use nori seaweed flakes instead of salt, as they are a rich source of minerals that help nourish the scalp. Available at all health stores.

Useful Remedies
■ Take a good-quality multi-vitamin/mineral that contains 30mg of zinc, which is vital for skin healing.
■ Take a B complex (usually included in any multi).
■ You will need an extra 2.5–4mg of biotin (a B vitamin) daily, as it is excellent for scalp problems.
■ Your multi should contain some vitamin A, but take an additional supplement for up to 2 months to raise your intake to 10,000IU per day. **NB: If you are pregnant or planning to become pregnant, take no more than 3,000IU of vitamin A a day. Also avoid taking extra vitamin A if you eat a lot of liver.** After 2 months, start taking a natural-source carotene complex that naturally converts to vitamin A in the body. **SVHC**

- Most people with dry skin or scalp are lacking essential fats, usually omega-3 fish oils. These fats that help nourish your skin from the inside out. Take 2g daily.
- A cream made from the plant/herbal extract *Mahonia aquafolium* can really help moisturize the scalp. For more information about PsoEcze products, visit www.goapharma.com or call 011-1-905-480-0409.

Helpful Hints

- Use natural-based shampoos that contain no chemicals or colorings. Weleda and Burt's Bees both make great ranges. All health stores also sell ranges of other organic products.
- Massage your scalp with pure rosemary oil mixed with jojoba or olive oil and leave on overnight.
- Homeopathic Arsenicum album 6x can be taken once or twice daily for a week.
- You can loosen dandruff, which sticks to the hair and scalp, by rinsing the hair with sour milk or a mild solution of lemon juice. Use 2 tablespoons of lemon juice mixed in a pint (a little less than 0.5 liters) of cooled boiled water.
- For more help, see *Hair Problems*.

Greasy scalp

Greasy hair and scalps are usually caused by overactive sebaceous glands, which produce a waxy, natural oil known as sebum that keeps hair supple. This problem is more common during the teenage years because, as most of us age, our scalps will gradually become drier. It is far more common in men and teenagers and is linked to acne and hormonal changes. (See also *Acne*.) A greasy scalp can be aggravated by frequent washing with strong shampoos, which destroy the acid balance of the scalp. Always use a pH-balanced shampoo or add a little vinegar or lemon juice to your final rinse.

Foods to Avoid

- Cutting down on refined carbohydrates, especially sweets, chocolates, and soft drinks, often helps.
- Reduce your intake of red meat, which takes a long time to digest and can putrefy in the gut.
- Cut down on alcohol, caffeine, and saturated fats, which place an extra burden on the liver. (See *Liver Problems*.)
- Avoid melted cheese, which is very difficult to digest.

Friendly Foods

- Eat more organic tofu, broccoli, watercress, cauliflower, Brussels sprouts, lentils, and beans, which help regulate hormone levels.
- Drink at least 6–8 glasses of water every day.
- Drink organic beet juice to help cleanse the liver. (See *Liver Problems*.)
- Eat more fish, especially oily fish, plus avocados, sunflower, pumpkin, hemp, and sesame seeds and flaxseeds. Also use their unrefined oils for salad dressings. See *General Health Hints* for a great breakfast smoothie recipe that includes plenty of seeds.

Useful Remedies

- Vitamin A helps balance oil production. Take 5000IU daily for 2 months and then switch to a natural-source carotenoid complex, which naturally converts to vitamin A in the body and is completely non-toxic. **NB: If you are pregnant or planning to become pregnant, do not take more than 3000IU of vitamin A a day. Natural-source carotenes are safe to use.**
- Take an essential fatty acid formula. (See *Fats You Need To Eat*.)
- Take a multi-vitamin/mineral plus 2–3mg biotin, a B vitamin that is often deficient in people with this problem. (Good multis should contain biotin.)

Helpful Hints

- Wash your hair regularly with mild or very dilute shampoo. Try using herbal shampoos, such as seaweed or rosemary.
- Do plenty of exercise, which will help reduce over-production of sebum.
- Massage your scalp regularly.
- Homeopathic Nat Mur 6x can be taken once daily for 7–10 days.
- Apply chickweed ointment to itchy areas.
- Consult a qualified nutritionist who can help you rebalance your diet. For details of good trichologists, see *Hair Loss*.
- Avoid hair products that contain sodium lauryl sulfate, which is used for cleaning concrete!

Head lice

This is a common problem, especially in school-age children. The most obvious symptoms are a constantly itching scalp and gray-colored insects in the hair upon examination. These are the adult lice. The lice eggs (nits) are white and stick to the hair. As the eggs have a 7–14-day incubation period, patience and regular daily treatments are necessary to get rid of them. Many orthodox treatments contain organophosphates (pesticides), which are now linked to cancers. Head lice are attracted to clean and dirty hair alike.

Foods to Avoid
- See *General Health Hints*.

Friendly Foods
- See *General Health Hints*.

Useful Remedies
- Licenex contains a blend of homeopathic ingredients in a base of aloe vera and essential oils to naturally kill lice and nits and relieve the itching and irritation. For more information, visit www.licenex.com or call 1-800-875-0850.
- Chinese Whispers is an herbal, non-chemical-based formula that has been shown in medical trials to kill head lice. Sold at www.lifepluspharmacy.com
- There are several body oils, sprays, and essential oils containing neem, from the Indian neem tree, which is a great insect repellent. Available online from Amazon,

Helpful Hints
- Comb hair daily with a fine-toothed comb to remove the lice.
- Check the head daily, as close personal head-to-head contact with someone who is infested can spread lice.
- Wash all clothing in really hot water and then leave in the freezer for 2–3 days to kill any remaining lice.
- Combine one part lavender oil and one part tea tree oil to three parts olive oil. Massage into the head and then rinse with vinegar.

SCIATICA

Sciatica is usually a symptom of a structural problem in the lower back, where the sciatic nerve becomes trapped or pinched. The pain tends to affect the buttocks and backs of the thighs, but it can travel down the back of the leg as far as the feet in some cases. It may also cause numbness, pins and needles, and/or weakness in those areas. The most common cause is a trapped nerve, but a slipped or bulging disc in the lower back that puts pressure on the sciatic nerve can also be a trigger. Other causes include an abscess and inflammation of the sciatic nerve. Sciatica may also result from a minor injury to the back, for example, from lifting a weight that is too heavy at the gym or sitting in an awkward position. If you suffer from shingles in that area, then you may experience post-herpetic neuralgia pain.

Foods to Avoid
- Avoid consuming excessive amounts of foods that drain the body of thiamine (vitamin B1) and magnesium. These include coffee, tea, soft drinks, chocolate, and refined sugars, which all reduce the body's ability to cope with any kind of pain. Sugar also triggers inflammation in the body.
- Lack of magnesium and thiamine can also contribute to muscular pain and spasms.
- Red meats, full-fat dairy products, and cheeses are high in arachidonic acid, which exacerbates inflammation.

Friendly Foods
- Cereals, wheat germ, meats, fresh peanuts, brewer's yeast, and Brazil nuts are all rich in thiamine.
- Magnesium-rich foods are cereals, honey, wheat germ, almonds, Brazil nuts, mustard, and curry powder.
- Eat plenty of green leafy vegetables, yellow peppers, and fresh fruits, which are all nutrient rich, to support your nerves.
- Add more turmeric and cayenne pepper to foods because they act like powerful anti-inflammatories.
- Ginger helps reduce pain; add to cooking or make fresh ginger tea.
- Eating oatmeal for breakfast helps support the nerves. Sweeten with a chopped apple and a few organic raisins or chopped dried apricots (which are also rich in magnesium).

Useful Remedies
- Take a B vitamin complex supplement and passion flower capsules, to help calm the nerves. **VC**
- Also try magnesium malate (500mg twice daily) to help relax the nerve endings.
- Calcium has anti-spasmodic properties; take 400–600mg daily in divided doses.
- Take thiamine (vitamin B1) to nourish the nervous system. This should be in any good high-strength vitamin B complex. Take 100mg daily with meals.
- Vitamin B12 injections may be helpful in some cases.
- Take 200IU of natural-source, full-spectrum vitamin E twice daily, which helps reduce any inflammation.
- Organic sulfur (MSM) plus the amino sugar glucosamine, has shown great results in reducing this type of pain. Take 1000mg of MSM daily, plus 500mg of glucosamine twice daily until symptoms ease. If you are highly sensitive to shellfish, ask for the Health Perception Glucosamine, which is derived from corn.
- DLPA, an amino acid, encourages the production of the body's own pain-killing chemicals. Take 400mg three times daily until symptoms ease. It also helps lift your mood. **SVHC**
- Take 1–3g of vitamin C with bioflavonoids to aid tissue healing.

Helpful Hints
- To reduce pain and discomfort, use an ice pack plus a hot water bottle wrapped in towels. Place each alternately on the site of the pain for 10 minutes; try this twice daily.
- To relieve sciatica, lie down on your back with your knees bent, feet flat on the floor. Place your hands underneath your buttocks (palms down) beside the base of your spine. Close your

eyes and, while taking long, deep breaths, rock your knees from side to side for two minutes. Reposition your hands every few minutes to enable different parts of the buttocks' muscles to be pressed against your hands. Then gently move your legs from side to side with your knees pulled in to your abdomen and your feet off the floor. Support your legs by holding them with your palms just behind your upper legs.

■ See a qualified osteopath or chiropractor as soon as possible and then try acupuncture, which is excellent for pain relief. (See *Useful Information*.)

■ Many alternative practitioners have found that regular deep tissue massage gives enormous relief to sciatica sufferers, as muscular spasms in this area can be mistaken for sciatica.

■ Essential oils of wintergreen and peppermint are nature's painkillers.

■ Homeopathic Lachesis is good for left-sided sciatica. Take 30c, 3–4 times daily, for up to 4 days. For right-sided sciatica, try Lycopodeum 30c.

■ Join a local yoga or tai chi class, which helps keep you supple but is very gentle exercise.

■ When sleeping or resting, lie on your side with a pillow between your knees to minimize pelvic strain. If you sleep on your back, put a soft pillow under your knees.

SHINGLES (herpes zoster)

(see also Immune Function and Stress)

S

Shingles is caused by the same virus as chickenpox. The basic rule is that you cannot contract (or have a very low risk of contracting) shingles if you have never had the chickenpox, as the virus lies dormant for many years in a nerve root in the spine. There is anecdotal evidence that a person suffering from shingles can pass the virus on, especially to young children, and give them chickenpox. Also, if a child who has chickenpox comes in contact with an elderly relative who has once suffered from chickenpox, the contact may reactivate the virus in the form of shingles. All people who have had the chickenpox are at risk of contracting shingles.

Shingles is common after the age of 50, but younger people are beginning to suffer from it, too. People infected with HIV are at a greater risk of developing shingles. It is unusual to have more than one attack, but if you do then you need to boost your immune function. The virus can be activated by shock, stress, or lowered immune function. As the virus multiplies and attacks the nerve, it can cause searing pains along the nerve pathways. After a few days, the skin erupts with itchy blisters. These generally heal within two to four weeks, but nerve pains may last for several weeks, causing what is known as postherpetic neuralgia (PHN). If the facial nerves are affected (known as trigeminal neuralgia), there may be temporary paralysis, and if the optic nerve is affected, the cornea may also be damaged. Shingles most commonly appears on the trunk but can also appear on the palms, inner areas of the arms, legs, or feet. (See also *Herpes* and *Cold Sores* since shingles is caused by a form of herpes virus.) If the blisters for any reason become infected, seek immediate medical attention.

In rarer cases, the person may experience middle ear and throat problems and/or a loss of taste and smell. See under *Taste and Smell (Loss of)*.

The secret to preventing shingles is to keep your immune system in good shape. (See *Immune Function*.)

Foods to Avoid

■ Foods that are rich in arginine, an amino acid commonly found in chocolate, carob, lentils, beans, and nuts, feeds the virus and can make symptoms worse.

■ Avoid refined sugary foods made with white flour, as well as foods high in saturated fat.

SHINGLES (HERPES ZOSTER) 361

These foods have a negative effect on the immune system, and sugar increases inflammation in the body.

Friendly Foods

- Eat high-quality protein at least once a day—for example, lean meats (such as turkey and lean pork), fish, corn, and tempeh, all of which are rich in lysine, an amino acid that has been shown to interfere with the replication of the virus.
- Most people feel very ill when they have shingles; therefore, eating homemade vegetable soups that are easy to digest and rich in nutrients is very beneficial.
- Add whey protein to smoothies to aid skin healing. (See *General Health Hints* for a great smoothie recipe.)
- Live, low-fat yogurts aid digestion and replenish healthy bacteria in the bowel.
- See *General Health Hints*.
- Garlic and rosemary are highly anti-viral. Use them in your cooking daily.
- Drink plenty of organic green tea, which is rich in compounds that help kill the virus.

Useful Remedies

- At the onset of symptoms, begin taking 500–1000mg of lysine daily. If you already have symptoms, take up to 4g daily.
- While symptoms are acute, take up to 5g of vitamin C daily in an ascorbate form spread throughout the day with meals. This may trigger loose bowels, in which case reduce the dose by 1g at a time until this stops.
- Beta Glucans 1–3, 1–6, which are derived from yeast cell walls, are proven to strengthen the body's innate immune system (the immune system you were born with). Take 250–500mg daily while symptoms last and also take it whenever you feel "run down". Dr Paul Clayton is a medical pharmacologist based in the US and UK. His website (www.healthdefence.com) contains a wealth of research about Beta Glucans and is well worth a look. **VC**
- Try Peaceful Mountain Natural Shinglederm Rescue cream containing St John's wort and lemon balm. Both are anti-viral, and regular applications can help reduce pain and speed healing. From www.peacefulmountain.com
- Oregano capsules have highly anti-viral properties. Take two daily in divided doses with meals while symptoms last. If you have problems taking or swallowing the capsules, reduce to just one daily. **VC**
- Apply zinc cream regularly to fight the virus. Also take 30mg of zinc daily internally in the form of a multi-vitamin/mineral.
- Licorice can also help kill the virus.
- Omega-3 fish oils are highly anti-inflammatory. Take 3g with meals while the condition lasts.
- Use coconut oil for cooking, as it reduces replication of the virus.
- During an attack, take 30,000IU of vitamin A daily for 2 weeks only, as this will aid skin healing and boost immune function. **NB: If you are pregnant or planning to become pregnant, do not take more than 3000IU of vitamin A daily**. After the 2 weeks, switch to a natural-source carotene complex that will naturally convert to vitamin A in the body and is non-toxic.
- Olive leaf extract acts as an anti-viral. (See *Antibiotics*.)
- The herb St John's wort is very useful for relieving the depression and nerve pain associated with shingles. Take 500mg three times daily. **NB: This herb should not be taken by anyone already on blood-thinning drugs such as Warfarin. You may also become sensitive to the sun while taking this herb.**

Helpful Hints

- Rest as much as possible when the attack starts, and make sure you see your doctor in case of complications such as infection.

- Make sure you change your toothbrush and face towels regularly, as these can harbor the virus.
- Calendula or melissa (lemon balm) cream or oil can be applied to the sores to help calm them down. **VC**
- Taking homeopathic Rhus Tox 6x 3–4 times daily for three days will help reduce the pain.
- Applying a mixture of plain yogurt and a little zinc oxide cream along the path of the affected nerve 2–3 times daily can clear herpes zoster in 24–48 hours if you start the regimen at the first sign of an outbreak.
- Hot and cold compresses help relieve nerve pain.
- Essential oils of wintergreen and peppermint are nature's painkillers.

SINUS PROBLEMS *(see also Allergies, Allergic Rhinitis, and Catarrh)*

Sinusitis is an inflammation of the mucous membranes in the sinuses. It usually occurs after a viral or bacterial infection, such as a cold or the flu, has affected another part of the respiratory system. It can also be caused by injury to the nose, dental treatment, or swimming. Common symptoms are a blocked nose and nasal-sounding speech, often accompanied by facial pain and headaches, which can be made worse by bending forward. If you suffer from chronic sinus problems, they are more than likely linked to food intolerances (see *Allergies* and *Leaky Gut*) and/or stress. Some people also have deviated septa or polyps in the nasal cavity, which can increase the likelihood of suffering from chronic sinus problems.

Foods to Avoid
- If symptoms are acute, avoid mucus-producing foods at all costs, including full-fat animal-source milks, cheese, chocolate, white bread, croissants, pastries, cakes, and anything else containing refined white flour, fat, sugar, and/or milk.
- At the onset of an acute sinusitis attack, try eating very light meals. This helps to clear the body of toxins and gives the digestive system and liver a rest, which in turn boosts immune function.
- Avoid refined sugar in any form for at least 6 days, as sugar greatly impairs your immune system and encourages bacterial growth.
- Basically avoid any foods that you are intolerant to, the most common being wheat, dairy products from animal sources, oranges, and eggs. I have also met people who develop sinus symptoms after eating foods as diverse as garlic, kiwi fruit, and even bananas. You need to be tested for food intolerances before cutting any large food groups from your diet. Find details of the York and Genova Tests in the *Allergies* section.

Friendly Foods
- For 3 or 4 days, live on really thick soups that are full of fresh vegetables and a little bit of chicken, lentils, brown rice, or barley.
- Eat more garlic (if you are not sensitive to garlic) and onions.
- Hot curries with cayenne pepper also help clear the sinuses, because the spices dilate blood vessels, increase blood flow to the area, and help clear any mucus.
- Drink plenty of freshly blended vegetable juices, especially cucumber, carrot, parsley, beets, kale, and apple, which are very cleansing.
- Snack on fenugreek seeds and add fresh root ginger to meals.
- Drink plenty of water and elderflower tea to help reduce congestion.
- Salads are great with some added protein, such as fresh fish or lean meats.

Useful Remedies

- The amino acid N-acetyl-cysteine (NAC) really helps support the liver and breaks down mucus, enabling it to be expelled. Take 500mg before meals twice daily.
- B-group vitamins are often lacking in people with this condition; take a high-strength vitamin B complex daily with food.
- Take up to 3g of vitamin C a day in divided doses with meals to reduce allergic responses to foods and external allergens, since vitamin C acts like a natural antihistamine.
- Take a multi-mineral that contains 400mg of magnesium and 30mg of zinc to boost immune function.
- The bioflavonoid quercetin (400mg 1–3 times daily) acts as a highly effective natural antihistamine.
- Echinacea and golden rod also help reduce mucus. They are both available in liquid drops. **VC**
- Try Sinus Take Care by New Chapter, which contains eucalyptus and golden seal, to help balance and tone the mucous membranes. Power Garlic and eyebright (if the eyes are affected) are also good herbs to use for this condition. **VC**
- Try the homeopathic remedy Kali Bich 6c three times a day between meals until symptoms are relieved.

Helpful Hints

- Inhaling steam is another useful treatment. Add a few drops of mint or eucalyptus oil to boiling water, place a towel over your head, and inhale for 5 minutes daily.
- The NeilMed Sinus rinse is a godsend for people with sinus problems. It's a very simple "wash out" for the nose that takes less than two minutes to use. Use once or twice daily. They also make a spray gel that helps soothe and hydrate irritated nasal passages. I was told about this range by an ear, nose and throat specialist, and it really does help when used daily. Available from most major pharmacies. For more information, visit www.neilmed.com/usa/index.php

- Add some sea salt to tepid water and place a small amount in the palm of your hand, then inhale this mixture up each nostril to help clear the nasal passages. You could also buy a sea salt nose spray instead. Available from most pharmacies.
- Avoid dry conditions. When the heating is on, make sure there is a bowl of water near the vents to keep the air moist.
- Blow your nose very gently, as some people can suffer nosebleeds when the nasal cavity becomes infected or very dry.

SJOGREN'S SYNDROME

(see also Raynaud's Disease, Rheumatoid Arthritis, Leaky Gut, Lupus, Osteoporosis, and Stress)

Sjogren's Syndrome is named after Henrik Sjogren, a Swedish ophthalmologist who, in 1933, noted that many of his female patients with various forms of arthritis also suffered from dry mucous membranes. Sjogren's is an autoimmune condition, in which the body's immune system turns on itself and starts attacking the moisture-producing glands, such as the eyes, nose, skin, throat, mouth, and vagina, which can all become chronically dry. Ninety percent of sufferers are women, and this condition can cause further health complications. Chronic dry mouth can trigger an increase in dental problems. The skin may also become so dry that highly irritating skin rashes appear along with thread veins close to the skin's surface. The skin may darken and become infected if scratched intensely.

There are two types of Sjogren's: Primary and Secondary. Primary Sjogren's patients are likely to have different antibodies circulating in their blood than those who have the secondary form, which is linked to other autoimmune conditions such as rheumatoid arthritis and lupus.

This condition often goes undiagnosed for several years, as the symptoms are so varied. As well as inflammation in the body and the dryness of mucous membranes, other symptoms can include Raynaud's Syndrome, osteoporosis, joint and muscle pains, chronic low white blood cell counts, fatigue, a propensity for lung problems such as bronchitis, high cortisol levels, hormone imbalances (especially around the menopause), low thyroid function and sleep problems, low levels of the hormone DHEA, and/or excess acidity in the body. Some sufferers, especially those who have previously been diagnosed with lupus or rheumatoid arthritis, may also be highly sensitive to sun exposure and suffer from rosacea-type facial rashes around the nose and chin.

Other important causative factors often overlooked by the orthodox medical establishment include leaky gut syndrome, in which the gut wall becomes permeable and food particles leach into the blood stream, thus triggering an autoimmune-type response. Multiple food intolerances (usually to refined sugars, wheat and/or gluten, and animal-source dairy products), in conjunction with a highly strung personality or a highly stressed lifestyle, can also play a part in this condition. Therefore, it's very important that you read the *Acid–Alkaline Balance, Candida, Leaky Gut, Lupus, Raynaud's Disease, Rheumatoid Arthritis*, and *Stress* sections before reading on.

It's usually a rheumatologist who eventually diagnoses Sjogren's by taking a full medical history and doing blood tests. The Epstein-Barr Virus is also linked to this condition.

The main point to stress with Sjogren's and other autoimmune conditions is that it has probably taken years for your symptoms to develop, and while you may feel, or be told, that such conditions are "incurable," there is a huge amount you can do to help yourself—but it will take time. The first step is to start thinking positively and be kind to yourself. Then you need to find a good nutritionist who can organize the appropriate tests to discover the root factors that have contributed or triggered your condition. (See *Useful Information* at the back of this book to source a qualified nutritionist.)

It's also important to note that several prescription drugs have side effects that mimic some Sjogren's Syndrome symptoms, which is another reason to investigate all of your symptoms thoroughly.

Foods to Avoid

- See this section under *Acid–Alkaline Balance, Leaky Gut*, and *Rheumatoid Arthritis*. Also keep in mind that it can take several months to re-alkalize your body, which has probably been too acid for many years.
- Avoid tomato juice and acid fruits (in the mouth), such as oranges and grapefruits.
- Avoid all soft drinks and other beverages high in refined sugars.
- Cut down on diuretics, such as alcohol, coffee, and excess black tea, as these can contribute to dryness in the body.
- Cut down on all flour-based foods, because flour and water make a sticky paste when combined. In the bowel these types of foods also draw fluids from the body to aid excretion and thus add to dryness.
- Generally cut down on refined, starchy, sugary foods because they can affect immune function and trigger tooth decay.
- Once you have been tested for food intolerances (see *Allergies*), avoid the offending foods. In the meantime, greatly reduce your intake of wheat, gluten, refined sugars, and animal-source dairy products.

Friendly Foods

- When the body is dry it requires far more essential fats; therefore, eat more oily fish, organic nuts, and seeds and use walnut, olive, sesame, and flax seed oils for salad dressings.
- Drink alkalizing water such as Kangen Water, a water system that attaches to your kitchen faucet to ionize and greatly alkalize water. This water aids healing, as tissues heal more quickly when they are more alkaline. It has been used in Japanese hospitals with highly beneficial health results. For full details visit www.kangenwaterusa.com
- Green tea has antioxidant and anti-inflammatory properties. Drink regularly, but only the organic decaffeinated versions. Steep for at least 5 minutes before drinking. Sweeten with a small amount of xylitol, organic agave syrup, or stevia, which have a low impact on blood sugar levels.
- Instead of wheat-based breads, try amaranth crackers or oatcakes (but avoid these if you are chronically constipated).
- Use almond, quinoa, or rice milks instead of animal-source milks.
- Eat far more pulses, lentils, barley, quinoa, brown rice, plus any fresh vegetables and fruits. However, please read the *Leaky Gut* and *Candida* sections before you start to eat huge amounts of fruit!
- Increase your intake of foods that are high in carotenes, such as watercress, pumpkin, papaya, carrots, all green leafy foods, apricots, and cantaloupe melons.

Useful Remedies.

- This list could go on almost into infinity, which is why it's vital for you to consult a nutritionist who can pinpoint your main triggers and then deal with the problems in order of urgency!

- Gamma -inolenic acid (GLA), the main ingredient in evening primrose oil, is very important for this condition as it helps reduce inflammation. Take 2g daily in divided doses with meals. **VC**
- Omega-3 fish oils or flaxseed oil capsules (if you are a vegetarian) are important for nourishing the mucous membranes and help alleviate dryness. Take at least 2g daily.
- Co-enzyme Q10 helps protect teeth and gums and also increases energy levels. Take 100mg daily with breakfast or lunch.
- Find a good-quality multi-vitamin/mineral for your age and gender that contains at least 30mg of zinc per day, as many people with this condition are often low in zinc. Try Zinc by Twinlab, which contains three types of zinc (picolinate, gluconate, and dihydrate). These are easy to absorb and improve zinc levels quickly. Initially take two capsules daily for 6 weeks, then one a day for 6 weeks, and then just one capsule per week.
- Healthy bacteria are important for gut health, which is almost always an issue in autoimmune conditions. Take a probiotics supplement daily after main meals—they are available from all health stores.
- Use liquid hyalauronic acid (HA), a naturally occurring protein found in all bone and cartilage structures in the body. HA helps cushion the joints and is what keeps young people's joints so supple. HA also helps relieve the dryness in tissues due to its ability to maintain hydration. Take one dose daily in water on an empty stomach before breakfast. **VC**
- Omega-7, extracted from the sea buckthorn, is an essential fatty acid useful for reducing dryness in the eyes, nose, vagina, etc, by helping the body retain moisture. Take four capsules daily for the first month and then two daily after that. **VC**
- Lack of vitamin A is very much linked to dryness. Therefore, take a natural-source carotene complex daily, as this naturally converts to vitamin A in the body and is totally non-toxic.
- A fermented wheat germ extract known as AWGE has demonstrated remarkable immune-modulating effects and helps normalize over-stimulate immune systems. AWGE has been shown to reduce the symptoms of autoimmune disease in numerous trials. Take one sachet

daily in water at least one hour before breakfast. Also available in capsules. Must be kept refrigerated. For more details, visit www.avemarwge.com

Helpful Hints

■ As long-term stress of any kind is very much linked to this condition, do all you can to control your reactions to stressful situations. Regular meditation and tai chi are both proven ways to reduce the "fight-or-flight" stress responses that can do so much damage to the body. (See *Stress*.) Don't worry if there are no classes in your area, there are plenty of at-home DVDs available from Amazon, such as *Tai Chi Exercises for Lifelong Health and Well-Being*, starring Tricia Yu.

■ Some sufferers have very dry mucous membranes in their noses, so try using Naso Gel from NeilMed to keep it moist. Otherwise, you may suffer from nosebleeds. For more information call 1-877-477-8633 (toll free) or visit www.neilmed.com/usa/index.php

■ Use sterile "natural tears"-type eye drops if and when your eyes become very dry. Always use these natural tears during flights.

■ Practice good dental hygiene and see an oral hygienist at least twice a year. Dry mouth can cause gums to recede more quickly and trigger dental issues.

■ The Biotène range of products, including toothpaste, mouthwash , liquids, and gels, are especially formulated for people with dry mouth problems. They are based on a unique LP3 salivary enzyme-protein system. For more information, visit www.biotene.com

■ As lack of the hormone DHEA is linked to Sjogren's, have a blood test and supplement as needed under medical supervision.

■ Have your thyroid function tested.

■ Warm, moist atmospheres are preferable to dry "desert-like" conditions.

■ Use a high-quality body-butter-type body cream to keep your skin moisturized.

■ Use pH-balanced moisturizing soaps based on ingredients such as olive oil.

■ Be sensible with sun exposure, as it can add to skin dryness.

SKIN CANCERS
(see Sunburn)

SMOKING
(see also Bronchitis)

Smoking and exposure to cigarette smoke is the leading cause of premature, preventable death in the United States, causing 438,000 premature deaths on average every year. Of these deaths, 40% are from cancer, 35% are from heart disease and stroke, and 25% are from lung disease like Chronic Obstructive Pulmonary Disease (COPD). More than 44 million Americans are smokers, and every day about 3,000 kids under the age of 18 start smoking.

If you smoke, the best favor you can do for yourself and for those around you is to give it up. Smoking a pack a day equates to losing a month of life each year. Smoking a pack of cigarettes a day depletes 500mg of vitamin C from your body yet, the average daily intake is 60–100mg. Cigarettes increase carbon monoxide levels in the blood, and it takes the circulatory system six hours to return to normal after you have smoked a cigarette. This is because one cigarette can increase your heart rate by 20 beats a minute and can also increase your blood pressure.

Perhaps now you understand why heart disease, cancer, and strokes, as well as high blood pressure and numerous other chronic diseases, are linked to smoking. (People with A or AB blood types tend to have stickier blood; therefore, smoking would increase their risk for heart disease and strokes even more.) It's also worth noting that smoking ages your skin, and tests have shown that the skin of a 40-year-old smoker is comparable to that of a 65-year-old non-smoker.

The more you can control your blood sugar, the easier it will be to avoid the mood swings associated with withdrawal and give up smoking for good. (See *Low Blood Sugar*.)

Foods to Avoid
- Cut down on foods that you have just prior to enjoying a cigarette, such as wine, beer, or coffee.
- Cut down on saturated animal fats, which will harden your arteries over time.
- Cut down on caffeine, sodas, refined sugary and starchy foods, tea, and other stimulants.
- Also see *Heart Disease*.

Friendly Foods
- As smoking makes your body far more acid, eat plenty of foods that will help re-alkalize your system, such as fruits, vegetables, millet, buckwheat, and wheat germ. (See *Acid–Alkaline Balance* for a longer list.)
- Oats are a nerve tonic that should help reduce addictions. Have organic oatmeal every morning.
- Begin using unrefined walnut, sunflower, and olive oils for salad dressings, and sprinkle sunflower, pumpkin, and flaxseeds over breakfast cereals and salads.
- Eating more leafy greens, such as cabbage, watercress, spring greens, spinach, and kale, reduces your risk of lung cancer.
- Drink organic green and white teas, which are high in antioxidants. Some researchers believe that Japanese men who smoke have a lower risk of cancer and other lung diseases thanks to the protective effects of green tea.
- Cantaloupe melons, pumpkin, apricots, carrots, papaya, French beans, mangoes, raw parsley, and watercress are all high in natural-source carotenes, which help protect lung tissue.
- Eat more oily fish, which is rich in vitamin A.
- Generally eat small meals regularly to control blood sugar. (See *Friendly Foods* under *Low Blood Sugar*.)
- If you eat meat, then have one portion of organic liver once a week, as it is rich in lung-protective vitamin A.

Useful Supplements
- Taking a high-strength multi-vitamin/mineral formula that includes essential fats and antioxidants provides some protection.
- Make sure that any multi-formula you take contains a full spectrum of B vitamins.
- Take 2g of vitamin C daily in divided doses with meals.
- Natural-source beta-carotenes (30mg daily) will help prevent some of the damage done in the lungs by smoking. However, it is still far better to stop smoking ASAP.
- Taking 500mg of magnesium daily before bed helps ease difficulties with breathing.
- The amino acid N-acetyl-cysteine (500mg twice daily before meals) helps bronchial conditions, as it loosens mucus and strengthens tissue.
- 200mcg per day of the mineral chromium helps keep your blood sugar level, as many people who stop smoking struggle to balance their blood sugar. Take between meals.
- Try taking an herbal extract tincture made from crushed lobelia leaves, ginger, oats, licorice, and thyme twice daily. It will help reduce cravings and support the lungs. Take with homeopathic remedies Staphysagria, Tabacum, and Nux Vomica, which all really help reduce withdrawal symptoms and cravings.

Helpful Hints

- Soak in an Epsom-salt or sea-salt bath, which helps remove nicotine through the pores. Accompanying this with skin brushing would be even better.
- For more help and information, contact the American Lung Association's helpline: 1-800-548-8252 or visit www.lungusa.org
- smokefree.gov is a national initiative to help people stop smoking. It provides an online, step-by-step stop smoking guide and a number of other resources. You can also talk to a cessation counselor by calling 1-877-448-7848.

SORE THROATS   *(see also Colds and Flu and Immune Function)*

If you tend to suffer from a persistent sore throat, it is usually a sign that your immune system is struggling to cope. When I become overtired and my throat becomes sore, I know that if I eat any foods high in refined sugars, it could send my immune system off the deep end and trigger a cold or infection. I now know my limits and listen to my body. If you are at this point, never underestimate how the things you eat during the subsequent 48 hours can be the deciding factor in whether you become ill or not. Also make sure that you are getting sufficient rest, which is one of the easiest ways to help boost immune function.

Regular bouts of tonsillitis (see *Tonsillitis*) mean that your lymphatic system is under stress and your body is telling you to detoxify. Regular sore throats are also associated with the yeast fungal overgrowth candida. (See *Candida*.)

Inflammation and pain in the throat can trigger symptoms such as pain upon swallowing or speaking, a dry tickling feeling, build-up of mucus in the nose and sinuses, and occasionally a husky voice or losing your voice. These types of infections are caused by bacteria or viruses. A sore throat caused by a streptococcal infection (often called strep throat) needs to be identified and treated or it could trigger rheumatic fever in some cases. If symptoms are severe, please see your doctor.

If I start feeling a sore throat coming on, I take homeopathic Streptococcus 10M immediately along with the Wellness Formula (see *Useful Remedies*, below), and the soreness almost always disappears within a day.

Foods to Avoid

- Eliminate refined sugar in any form for 4 days to give your immune system a chance to fight off any infection.
- Greatly cut down or avoid all white flour-based products, snacks, and burger-type meals. Avoid all "white" foods.
- Coffee, sugary drinks, and alcohol dehydrate the body and are stimulants. If your adrenal glands are exhausted, these foods will add to the problem.
- Cut down on all full-fat animal-source dairy products, especially chocolate and full-fat milks.

Friendly Foods

- Increase fluid intake. Include lots of filtered water, herbal teas (especially green and white tea), diluted fruit juices, and broths.
- Sip warm water mixed with powdered vitamin C, plus lemon juice, ginger and/or garlic with a little honey.
- Also see *Friendly Foods* under *Colds and Flu*.

Useful Remedies

- One of the best remedies I have found for alleviating a sore throat, which usually heralds the start of a cold, is the Wellness Formula made by Source Naturals Inc. It contains garlic, propolis, elderberry extract, olive leaf extract, vitamin C, astragalus, zinc, and grape seed extract. This is an excellent combination of nutrients needed to boost immunity, as they are anti-viral and antibacterial. At the first sign of a sore throat or that feeling that you are "coming down with something," take one or two tablets three times daily. See www.sourcenaturals.com for more information.

- At the same time take homeopathic Streptococcus 10M as directed for 3 days; it really helps eliminate a sore throat. Available from specialist homeopathic pharmacies.
- Ask at your health store for either a bee propolis (avoid if you are highly sensitive to bee stings) or an echinacea throat spray and use as directed.
- Alternatively, try Echinacea, Astralagus & Reishi by Nature's Way, which also contains astragalus (which boosts the immune system). VC
- Natural-source beta-carotene will naturally convert to vitamin A in the body, which hugely supports a healthy immune system. Take up to 30mg daily when you feel sick.
- Take at least 2–3g of vitamin C daily in divided doses with meals.
- Take a vitamin B complex to support your adrenal glands along with an extra 500mg of vitamin B5.
- Low levels of selenium are linked to viral infections. Take a multi-vitamin/mineral that includes 200mcg of selenium and 30mg of zinc.
- Zinc gluconate lozenges really help reduce a sore throat; take 3–4 daily. Available online and at health stores.
- If you end up taking antibiotics, make sure you replenish the healthy bacteria in your gut by taking acidophilus/bifidus capsules twice daily for 6 weeks. (See *Antibiotics*.)

S

Helpful Hints
- Crush some fresh sage and make it into a tea by steeping it in boiling water. After letting the tea cool, gargle it for a few minutes. Sage is antiseptic and will ease the soreness. If your throat is really sore, soak a cloth in the sage mix and apply it to the throat area.
- You can also crush an onion, wrap it in a cloth, and place it on the throat.
- Propolis tincture can be diluted in water and used to gargle.
- Change your toothbrush regularly.
- At the onset of a sore throat, use homeopathic Aconite or Belladonna 30c if the throat is red and worse on the right-hand side. For children's sore throats, a hacking cough, and swollen tonsils, try Chamomila 30c, three times daily for two days.
- The herb thyme is also a natural antiseptic. It can be made into a solution and used to gargle with for sore throats or sipped as a tea mixture to help relieve sore throats and coughs. You can also mix oregano, thyme, and basil essential oils and massage onto the throat area.
- Tea tree oil is a natural antiseptic; use diluted with a little sea salt as a gargle but do not swallow. You can also gargle with a mixture of warm water, a quarter of a teaspoon of turmeric powder, and a pinch of salt.

SPIRITUAL EMERGENCY

(see also Adrenal Exhaustion, Depression, Low Blood Sugar, and Panic Attacks)

This title may appear out of place in a health book, but believe me, a spiritual emergency (when a spiritual awakening becomes a physical and sometimes mental crisis) is a well-known phenomena in the East. And as our interest in spiritual subjects gains pace, it is becoming far more common in the West. I have yet to meet an orthodox doctor (apart from a handful, including my own) who has heard of this condition or recognizes any of its specific symptoms; however, it definitely exists.

Most psychiatrists tend to diagnose a spiritual emergency as psychosis, depression, schizophrenia, or a total nervous breakdown (which it may well be), but if this subject could receive wider attention, many people could avoid being sent to mental care facilities, given strong prescription drugs, and labeled as being "mentally ill."

Of course, mental illness can have a huge range of causes, including the overuse of social drugs (such as crack, LSD, or cannabis), extreme and prolonged stress that severely alters brain chemistry, and a poor diet lacking in essential brain nutrients—but it can also be linked to a spiritual-type breakthrough.

Back in 1998 I experienced a huge spiritual emergency in which I began affecting electrical equipment, could clearly see people's energy or auric fields, became super-psychic, telepathic and could clearly "hear" people in the spirit world. I received huge amounts of information, which placed an enormous strain on my brain and nervous system. The full story is told in my book *Divine Intervention* (CICO Books).

Symptoms of intense breakthroughs are diverse and wide-ranging; this is an abbreviated version. The body may experience muscle tremors, fever, or cold. Some people hear voices or, depending on their culture and beliefs, see visions of angels, demons, or archetypal animals. The person may undergo a physical near-death experience or a symbolic feeling of death and rebirth. There may also be a sense of having "married God" or even that you are the reincarnation of Jesus, Buddha, or another important spiritual figure. You may manifest objects such as holy ash or phenomena such as stigmata. Can you imagine an orthodox doctor's reaction to such a list of symptoms?

And whatever your personality is at the time of a spiritual breakthrough, it becomes hugely amplified. Feelings of humility alternate with a belief that you are a super-being; you may wonder, "Why doesn't everyone want to listen to *me?*" You may believe that you can fly, have a sense that you have become indestructible, or feel unconditional love interspersed with episodes of panic.

At such times people often experience various phenomena, such as seeing auras and hearing other realms, either spontaneously as in my case, or during spiritual development courses. Also, growing numbers of people who regularly use social drugs, such as cannabis, crack, or ecstasy, are suffering from similar mental-health-type symptoms.

While researching my spiritual/science books *The Evidence For the Sixth Sense* (CICO Books) and *Countdown to Coherence* (Watkins Publishing) in which I deal in depth with these types of issues, I spoke at length to Professor Frederick Travis, head of the Center for Brain, Consciousness, and Cognition at the Maharishi University in Iowa, who has studied brain function for more than 30 years.

When I asked him about the effects of dangerous social drugs, he told me: "These types of drugs block the uptake of neurotransmitters. Within the brain you have 'pleasure circuits,' which fire when you eat a favorite food such as chocolate, or you see a fabulous sunset. The neurotransmitter dopamine is released and travels to the receiving part of a cell, where it is held for a moment, then 'let go' and recycled and taken back up by the neuron that fired it. But if you take a drug like cocaine, it fills up the re-uptake receptors, and the dopamine just sits in the space between the two cells, so the receptors just keep firing. That is the basis of the 'rush' that users experience."

"Which causes what to happen in the long term?" I asked. "The dopamine circuits can eventually be destroyed," Travis told me. "Users no longer enjoy such intense highs on a single dose, so they take more and more drugs to feel that rush again. This spiral takes them ever further away from living a stable life, as their brains suffer more and more damage which can trigger psychosis, depression, suicidal tendencies, sometimes multiple-personality disorders, and schizophrenia."

With regard to schizophrenics, Travis and others have found that they have a thinning of the brain cortex, which means they have less gray matter and fewer cortical connections. Therefore, they find it difficult to maintain a coherent sense of individualized "self," as they cannot integrate thinking, feeling, and a sense of self at the same time. This means they can easily become disoriented into other levels of feeling and of reality. A shaman might term such events as a spirit "walk-in," but Travis says that such people are "picking up" energetic aspects of the Whole Consciousness and therefore are becoming confused in their everyday reality, as their brains are flooded with information. This also helps explain phenomena such as speaking in tongues, as at times of intense religious experiences, people may link to the universal field of consciousness that contains all knowledge, and since their brains cannot process so much information, it comes out as a garbled mess!

Studies have demonstrated that if schizophrenics learn to meditate and also have counseling, over time, in conjunction with a good diet, their condition can improve.

There is not sufficient space in this type of book to deal with the huge panoply of mental health conditions, but it's important to realize that in some cases people can be helped via diet, supplements, and the right specialist support. Nevertheless these types of conditions/symptoms are in many cases linked to adrenal exhaustion and low blood sugar (see these sections before continuing).

We all have psychic abilities and are capable of miracles, but most of us don't truly comprehend this ultimate truth. When you undergo this type of experience, you need to find professional help to determine the most appropriate course of action.

If, during your spiritual growth, you begin to feel ultra-special and your ego comes into play, you need to ground yourself (see below). Find your nearest spiritualist church, which will undoubtedly know of someone who can help you. Hands-on healing would definitely be of benefit during a spiritual-type emergency (see *Healing*).

But if anyone starts to self-harm, threatens others, thinks they can fly, and generally becomes a danger to themselves or others, medical help is needed immediately.

Foods to Avoid
- Sometimes during this type of situation you don't want food, but it is imperative that you eat to help ground yourself.
- The last thing you need is stimulants so avoid caffeine, refined sugars (although, see below), and alcohol.

Friendly Foods
- If your brain is in absolute overdrive and feels as though it's on fire, then eat some sugary food quickly. The brain uses pure glucose as a fuel, and as you may be processing huge amounts of information, your brain will need an energy supply. It is always preferable if you can eat small healthy meals regularly, but if the situation is acute, then eat sugar or a banana. Controlling your blood sugar helps control the events and your ability to cope with them. (See *Adrenal Exhaustion* and *Low Blood Sugar*.)
- Generally eat far more "earthy" grounding foods, such as oatmeal made with organic rice milk, stews, and thick vegetable or grain-based soups.
- You may not want it, but you need protein, which helps balance your blood sugar levels for longer periods of time. Fish and animal products might repulse you, in which case eat some beans, pulses, cooked tofu, and brown rice with plenty of fruits and vegetables. Otherwise,

make smoothies with fruits, sunflower and pumpkin seeds, and add a tablespoon of whey, hemp seed or rice-based protein powder, which is easy for the body to utilize. (See *General Health Hints* for a great smoothie recipe.)

- Drink plenty of water and calming herbal teas such as vervain, licorice, or chamomile.
- Your digestion may be upset so include fresh ginger in soups and drink ginger teas. (See *Leaky Gut* and *Stress*.)

Useful Remedies

- Begin taking Bach Rescue Remedy and Star of Bethlehem immediately and then every 2 or 3 hours after that.
- Also begin taking homeopathic Arnica 200c every few hours to help reduce feelings of shock.
- For anyone who is quite psychic, intuitive, and has a very open personality, try homeopathic Phosphorous 30c three times daily, which will help balance the energies.
- Take one homeopathic Aconite 200c daily. Taken at the onset of any symptoms, this can help to relieve some of the stress and reduce fear.
- Take a high-strength B complex to support your nerves. Try an extra 1000mg of pantothenic acid (vitamin B5) daily to support your adrenal glands, which are most likely working overtime.
- Take a multi-vitamin/mineral formula daily.
- The brain is made up of 60% fats so take 3–4g of fish oil daily. If you are vegan or vegetarian, take flaxseed oil instead.

Helpful Hints

- Contact the Spiritual Crisis Network, a charity formed by clinical psychologist Isabel Clarke and her colleagues, plus Catherine Lucas (www.breathworks-mindfullness.co.uk) who went through a profound spiritual emergency. You can e-mail them at info@SpiritualCrisisNetwork.org.uk; website: www.SpiritualCrisisNetwork.org.uk
- You could also contact the Spiritual Emergency Resource Center by calling 1-415-648-2610 or visiting www.spiritualcompetency.com/se/resources/senciis.html
- Ask your health professional to read *Madness, Mystery and the Survival of God* or *Psychosis and Spirituality* by Dr Isabel Clarke (available from www.o-books.net). Her latest book is *Psychosis and Spirituality: Consolidating the new paradigm* (Wiley-Blackwell).
- In London, the College of Psychic Studies takes students from all over the world and helps them integrate their newly found gifts and knowledge in a balanced and safe environment. Tel: 011-44-20-7589-3292. Website: www.collegeofpsychicstudies.co.uk
- At this time you need all of the support and patience friends and family can provide, as you may say and do many things (such as levitate or produce ash) that can initially be very frightening. You may also experience periods of complete and utter bliss. I beg of you to write any insights or channeling down, but don't try sharing them with everyone you know, as this can elicit negative responses. At such times a person can also easily be persuaded to join cults.
- Avoid negative thoughts as much as you can. For every negative thought, try to replace it with a positive one.
- Try not to panic—the experience will pass; it just takes time. (See *Panic Attacks* and *Stress*.)
- Read *Spiritual Emergency* by Stanislav and Christina Grof, MD. This book really helps when personal transformation becomes a crisis (available from www.holotropic.com). So would my books *The Evidence For The Sixth Sense* (CICO Books) and *Countdown to Coherence* (Watkins Publishing).

STITCH

This is a sudden, sharp pain in the side or abdomen, triggered by exercise, which usually wears off after a few minutes of rest. A stitch is the body's way of telling you that it needs more oxygen, so stand still and breathe deeply.

The pain is almost certainly caused by a spasm in the gut wall. It can also be triggered by too much exercise after a heavy meal. This is because, after eating a large meal, blood is diverted from the muscles momentarily to aid digestion. So, if we do some type of physical exercise at this time, a stitch will occur. Therefore, it makes sense not to exercise until at least an hour after eating.

People who tend to be sedentary and eat insufficient fresh fruit and vegetables as well as too much sugar, caffeine and animal protein are often lacking in calcium and magnesium, which causes a build-up of lactic acid, resulting in regular attacks of muscle cramps or a stitch. Basically, a stitch is triggered by an over-acidic environment. (See *Acid–Alkaline Balance.*)

Foods to Avoid
- Generally, cut down on refined sugar/starchy foods, such as croissants, cookies, cakes, pizza, and white-flour-based foods.
- Avoid any foods that remove the mineral magnesium from the body, which is needed to alleviate a stitch. Magnesium is particularly depleted by too much alcohol and caffeine.

Friendly Foods
- Magnesium-rich foods, such as green leafy vegetables, fruits, brown rice, barley, lentils, and whole grains rich in fiber, will give you more protection in the long term. Blackstrap molasses are rich in magnesium and calcium.
- Honey and dried apricots are also high in magnesium.
- Eat good-quality protein, such as fresh fish, eggs, cooked tofu, and lean meats, at least once a day.

Useful Remedies
- Take a high-strength vitamin B complex daily.
- Take 400mg of calcium and 600mg of magnesium to help reduce spasms and relax the muscles. Take in divided doses with food.
- Take Emergen-C or electrolyte sachets, which are high in vitamin C and minerals. Take one sachet before exercising to help reduce any chance of a stitch. Available from most pharmacies.

Helpful Hints
- If you can, bend down and touch your toes to relieve a stitch. Or take a deep breath and stretch really well.
- A stitch is more likely to occur if you exercise while food is still digesting in the gut. Avoid strenuous exercise for an hour after a substantial amount of food.
- Generally, do regular exercise to avoid lactic acid accumulation in the body.
- Before doing heavy exercise, especially jogging/running, drink a small glass of diluted fruit juice with a quarter of a teaspoon of baking soda mixed in. This will help delay the onset of lactic acid build-up and should help you avoid developing a stitch.
- A stitch generally occurs when you have not warmed up properly before exercise.
- Do not sit for long periods without going for a walk or stretching.
- Breathe deeply more often.

S

STOMACH AND DUODENAL ULCERS

(see also Acid–Alkaline Balance, Acid Stomach, Low Stomach Acid, and Stress)

Stomach ulcers are small raw areas on the walls of the stomach where the protective mucous coating has worn away. This may be due to the mucous lining being insufficient to start with and so being affected by factors such as stress, smoking, alcohol, excess caffeine intake, erratic eating habits, over-consumption of refined starchy foods, and so on.

Duodenal ulcers are also small raw spots, but they appear in the lining of the duodenum (the first section of the small intestine) and tend to be smaller than stomach ulcers. Duodenal ulcers are predominantly caused by stomach acid infiltrating the sphincter muscle and flowing into the small intestine. This is why having too much stomach acid (which tends to affect Type O blood types) can be a problem. This condition is also exacerbated by smoking and alcohol, as both relax the pyloric sphincter muscle, thereby allowing acids to escape onto the walls of the small intestine, which lacks the same protection as the stomach.

A bacterium called *Helicobacter pylori* has been found in more than 90% of duodenal ulcers and 80% of gastric ulcers. This bacterium is also linked to stomach cancers, low energy levels, and skin conditions such as rosacea and urticaria. Inflammatory conditions such as migraines are also linked to *Helicobacter pylori*. Treatment with high-dose antibiotics usually kills the bacterium; however, it commonly re-occurs.

Stomach ulcers are more common in Type A blood types and tend to affect older people whose protective stomach lining has been eroded. There is a link between stomach ulcers and cancer. The pain of a stomach ulcer is often made worse after eating. Duodenal ulcers are more common in Type O blood types and tend to affect younger people. They generally do not progress to cancers, and the pain of duodenal ulcers is usually relieved by food.

Stress is a major factor in any type of ulcers, because when you are stressed the body produces more stomach acid. Intolerances to foods such as wheat, cow's milk (animal dairy in general), and prescription drugs, plus long-term use of aspirin, steroids, and non-steroidal anti-inflammatory drugs (NSAIDs) such as ibuprofen, can also be contributory factors in ulcer development. (See *Leaky Gut*.

Nutritionist Gareth Zeal says, "In clinical practice I have found that if people take an omega-7 essential fat known as sea buckthorn with a meal at the same time as using aspirin (if this has been prescribed), the omega-7 helps to reduce the risk of internal bleeds."

Foods to Avoid

- There is a proven link between over-consumption of caffeine and ulcers, so avoid or greatly reduce coffee and sodas. Organic decaffeinated coffee is usually tolerated in small amounts.
- Eliminate all animal-source dairy products for at least one month.
- Alcohol irritates the gut wall, so keep it to a minimum or eliminate it completely for a while.
- Don't eat too much refined sugar and too many rich fatty foods, which tend to severely irritate the gut.
- Avoid spicy foods, which can aggravate the gut lining.
- Avoid eating late at night, which places a great strain on your digestive system and liver.
- Avoid citrus fruits (especially oranges and grapefruit), raw tomatoes, rhubarb, plums, and pineapple. The concentrated juices seem to cause the most problems.
- Avoid all refined white-flour-based foods.
- Avoid thermally hot or cold foods and drinks.
- Reduce your consumption of animal proteins, such as beef and pork, as these increase stomach acid production.

- Eliminate soft drinks, which play havoc with gut lining.

Friendly Foods

- Eat lots more fresh cabbage, which is rich in the amino acid L-glutamine, known to heal the gut. Eat it raw or add to fresh vegetable juices. If you cook the cabbage, use the water it cooked in for gravy or drink it once it has cooled.
- Replace cow's milk with organic rice or almond milk.
- Eat plenty of vegetables and fruits, such as bananas, figs, lychees, or pears. Before eating lots of fruit, though, read the *Candida* section, as ulcers are often linked to fungal overgrowth.
- Include barley, brown rice and whole-wheat bread, pastas and noodles, as well as lentils, millet, amaranth, quinoa, and couscous in your diet.
- Eat more baked potatoes, sweet potatoes, peas, corn, and apples, which are high in fiber.
- Mashed pumpkin is great for healing the gut, as is papaya.
- Add seaweed, such as kombu, to your bean dishes. Seaweed aids ulcer healing.
- Use nori flakes instead of salt, as they are high in minerals and are delicious.
- Fish, nuts and seeds (flaxseeds and sunflower, pumpkin, and sesame seeds) are high in zinc, which aids tissue healing. See *General Health Hints* for a delicious smoothie recipe that includes hemp seed protein.
- Eat more live, low-fat yogurt, manuka honey, and licorice, which will help heal the gut and kill *Helicobacter pylori*.
- Add cinnamon to fruit dishes.
- Slippery elm (preferably in a tea) helps soothe and heal the whole digestive tract, including the stomach and duodenum. Sip throughout the day in between meals. **VC**
- Drink more organic green and white teas.

Useful Remedies

- The herbs marshmallow, barberry, pau d'arco, and poke root help promote gut healing.
- Chew 1–2 tablets of deglycyrrhized licorice 20 minutes before food. This encourages healing of the stomach lining and helps eradicate *Helicobacter* if it is present.
- Take Gastro ULC, a formula designed to help heal gastric ulcers and leaky gut. Take one with each main meal. To order contact Apex Energetics, 16592 Hale Ave., Irvine, CA 92606. Tel: 1-800-736-4381. Website: www.apexenergetics.com
- Vitamin A is vital for the stomach lining to be able to heal. Take 20,000IU daily for the first month and then reduce to 10,000IU for another month. **NB: If you are pregnant or planning to become pregnant, do not exceed 3000IU of vitamin A daily.**
- After two months take a carotene complex daily for ongoing maintenance, as it naturally converts to vitamin A in the body and is completely non-toxic.
- B vitamins aid digestion and reduce the risk of ulcers. Take a B complex daily.
- Take 500mg of vitamin C in an ascorbate form before meals and at bedtime, as most ulcer patients are lacking this vital vitamin. **VC**
- Mastica is a resin from a plant found in the Greek Aegean Sea. Taking 500–1000mg per day for two weeks has been shown to rapidly heal gastric ulcers. It also helps remove any *Helicobacter*.
- Taking L-glutamine (2–4g twice daily) 30 minutes before meals (for one month, then half dose) really helps heal the gut. **VC**
- Omega-7 essential fats from sea buckthorn help rebuild mucosal tissue. Take 2g daily for 3 months, then reduce this to 1g daily with meals. **PN**
- N-acetyl cysteine (NAC) is an amino acid derivative that can inhibit the growth of *Helicobacter* if taken regularly. Take 600mg twice daily in between meals. This is also a great supplement to support liver function.

Helpful Hints

- Chew food thoroughly. Never rush a meal, because digestion becomes difficult when you are stressed or in a hurry.
- Don't drink too much liquid with meals, as this dilutes digestive juices.
- Ulcers can be encouraged to heal by eating small quantities of food at a time.
- Avoid stress and rushing as much as possible, as stress over a prolonged period can cause great harm to our digestive systems.
- Smoking greatly increases the risk of ulcers.
- Drinking 75ml of concentrated aloe vera juice 20 minutes before meals also helps soothe the digestive tract. Lakewood Organic Juices make a good pure aloe juice, which greatly soothes the stomach lining. Available from some supermarkets and health stores. www.lakewoodjuices.com
- Homeopathic Mercurius Corrosivus or Argentum Nitricum 6c can be taken three times daily for a week.

STRESS

(see also Adrenal Exhaustion, Depression, and Immune Function)

More than half of the estimated 550 million lost working days in the US every year are due to stress-related conditions, and stress is a major contributing factor for a host of health problems. Not all stress is bad; it can help keep you sharp and alert. But in the longer term, how your body copes depends on your *reaction* to the stress.

Eons ago when our ancestors were faced with life-and-death situations, the hormones adrenaline and cortisol were released from the endocrine system, which includes the pancreas, thyroid, and pituitary, plus the adrenal glands which are situated just above the kidneys. These hormones made the heart pump faster, giving an instant energy boost to the body and brain. Muscles tensed, cholesterol production increased, and enzymes caused the blood to thicken so that if our ancestors were injured, their blood would clot more easily. Blood vessels would constrict; endorphins, the body's own painkillers, would be released; and oxygen consumption increased. Known as the "fight-or-flight" reaction, these responses saved many lives back when our ancestors fought off marauding animals and invaders.

Today, our automatic physical response to stress remains the same, but unfortunately these days it tends to trigger heart attacks, strokes, cancers, stomach ulcers, and even Alzheimer's disease. Why? Because if we don't disperse this constant stream of stress hormone production through regular exercise and relaxation, then, in the longer term, excess fight-or-flight hormones become highly toxic to every major organ and set up inflammatory responses in the body. It's like putting rocket fuel in a scooter: you eventually burn out the engine.

For the most part these days, instead of going for a walk, breathing deeply, and calming down, we tend to head for the coffee/soda machine or eat another refined sugary "treat" to keep us going, which triggers even more adrenaline to be released, thus exacerbating the situation. Make no mistake—prolonged, chronic, relentless stress can kill you.

The first signs of stress usually show up as behavioral and/or emotional changes, such as feeling constantly irritable, a sense-of-humor failure, suppressed anger, feeling like you cannot cope, breaking down in tears, and/or feeling tired yet "wired."

Then come the physical symptoms: palpitations and headaches, lack of appetite or cravings for refined sugary/starchy foods, insomnia, poor digestion, muscle cramps, frequent urination, constipation and/or diarrhea, a dry mouth, constant thirst, feeling clammy and cold or too hot.

Also, your brain doesn't work properly and you forget simple words or names. That's because stress creates more free radicals, and research at Stanford University has shown that raised cortisol levels damage the connections between brain cells, affecting brain functions. Luckily, if you stop the stress, the connections can grow back. Long-term stress also makes the body far more acid, and vital minerals are then leached from the bones and muscles to re-alkalize the body. (See *Acid–Alkaline Balance*.) Long-term stress and the over-acidity it triggers can be an important factor in the development of leaky gut syndrome and all of its consequences, such as autoimmune conditions, skin conditions (like eczema and psoriasis), and eventually osteoporosis.

If any or all of these symptoms sound familiar, you need to **stop and rest** because the next stage could be a total burn-out, possible mental health problems, a heart attack, or a stroke. Whether your stress comes from a bad relationship, work, children, illness, lack of money – whatever it is, if possible make space and time between what is stressing you out and your reactions to it. Talk to someone and tell him or her how you are feeling. Start going for counseling. If more people could do this, thousands of lives could be saved.

Additionally, research from Glostrup University Hospital in Denmark showed that women who have high-stress jobs are more than twice as likely to develop heart disease later in life—you have been warned.

Research has also demonstrated that if you think negatively, tend to be angry a lot of the time, and are under long-term negative stress, especially after age 50, then you are more likely to suffer from heart and arterial disease. This is because so many of us hold in emotions that we should literally "get off our chests." Remember, the more indirect you are, the more stressed you become. Emotions held in for long periods of time will eventually cause a fuse to blow.

There are also those infuriating (but wise) souls who are always positive; they love stress and positively thrive on it. However, we are all unique, and you need to learn your limits and listen to your body. There are many things you can do to reduce the negative effects of stress on your body, which can help you stay healthier.

Foods to Avoid
- Never underestimate just how much your diet can affect your stress levels and your ability to cope with it. Avoid any foods and drinks that contain alcohol, caffeine, refined sugar, and artificial sweeteners, especially aspartame, which all stimulate the adrenal glands to work harder.
- Reduce refined (white) and processed foods. They are high in additives/preservatives and sugar, and usually low in nutrients. The more refined and processed food you eat, the more stress you place on your liver, digestive system, and ultimately your adrenal glands.
- Cut down on heavy meals, especially red meat, which is hard to digest, because digestion is one of the first things to be affected when you are stressed.
- Don't eat in a rush.

Friendly Foods
- When you are stressed, it is vital to eat small, balanced meals regularly to help control your blood sugar and thus support your adrenal glands. (See *Low Blood Sugar*.)
- Stress breaks down protein in the body very quickly. This is why most people who are very stressed tend to lose weight. Make sure that you eat around 4–6oz (100–175g) of quality protein daily, preferably at breakfast and lunch, as it helps balance blood sugar levels. Eat protein such as eggs, fish, lean organic meats, tofu, cheese, amaranth, quinoa, peas, lentils, beans, and pulses.

- Whey is an easily absorbed form of protein. If you don't have a problem with cow's milk, then try Solgar's Whey to Go, otherwise use organic-sourced hemp seed, pea, rice, or soy protein powders. (See *General Health Hints* for a great smoothie recipe.)
- Eat oily fish and unrefined sunflower, pumpkin, and hemp seeds. They are all rich in essential fats that reduce the inflammation triggered by stress hormones. (See *Fats You Need To Eat*.)
- Licorice tea helps support adrenal function, and echinacea tea will help support your immune system, which is greatly affected by stress. Valerian and chamomile teas with a little honey will help calm you down.
- Green tea contains L-theanine, an amino acid that encourages the production of alpha waves, the brainwaves you produce during relaxation. Drink a decaffeinated green tea.
- Make sure to eat breakfast. Low-sugar muesli, eggs, protein powder, or whole-wheat toast would be fine. Try oats, especially oatmeal made with rice milk, as oats are a rich source of B vitamins, which help you stay calm.
- Whole-wheat pasta, noodles and breads, couscous, quinoa, amaranth/oat crackers, lentils, brown rice, and barley are all calming foods.
- Avocados, turkey, cottage cheese, bananas, potatoes, ginger, yogurt, leafy green vegetables, lettuce, and low-fat milks will also help you de-stress.
- Increase your intake of easy-to-digest foods, such as homemade vegetable soups, mashed sweet potatoes, poached fish, stewed fruits, and so on to help take some of the burden off of your digestive system.
- Also see *General Health Hints*.

Useful Remedies

- If the stress has been induced by shock or trauma, use homeopathic Aconite 30c, and take it every hour in between meals for a few days. Give the traumatized person some sweet tea, as the brain uses more glucose during times of shock.
- Take a high-strength multi-nutrient formula that contains vitamins, minerals, antioxidants, and essential fats because your body needs more nutrients when it is under stress. Ask any of the companies listed on pages 15–16 to recommend a formula that will suit your age and gender.
- If you are not taking a high-strength multi-vitamin/mineral, then begin taking at least a high-strength B complex daily with breakfast to support your nerves.
- Urinary excretion of vitamin C increases with stress so take 1–2g of vitamin C in divided doses with meals. Also take 400IU of natural-source, full-spectrum vitamin E to thin your blood, as stress also thickens the blood. **NB: Avoid vitamin E supplements if you are on blood-thinning drugs such as Warfarin.**
- Jarrow's Adrenal Optimizer contains vitamins C and B5, as well as Siberian ginseng and other nutrients involved in the support of the adrenals. Take one capsule three times per day. It will also calm anxiety. **JF**
- You will need additional calming minerals so take 400mg of calcium and 600mg of magnesium, which are known as nature's tranquillizers. Take in divided doses with the last dose at bedtime. (Both of these minerals should be part of any good multi formula.)
- Take a high-strength fish oil (1g daily) that contains both EPA and DHA essential fats. These fats thin the blood naturally and help keep blood pressure down.
- L-theanine is an amino acid found in green tea that helps increase alpha wave production, the brain waves you produce when you are calm. It is available in capsules and will help you feel more relaxed without inducing drowsiness. Take as needed. **SVHC**
- If you are a Type-A person who rushes around all day and feels very stressed, try taking Cortisol Manager tablets, which contain ashwagandha, phosphatidyl serine and L-theanine.

Take one of these tablets when the adrenaline starts "pumping" and a further one or two before bed. They are excellent for reducing cortisol production and calming you down. I have found them wonderful for reducing "fight-or-flight"-type symptoms, and they really help me to get to sleep. However, if you are at the point of total and utter exhaustion, then your body may not be producing sufficient cortisol, in which case there would be no benefit in taking this formula. (See *Adrenal Exhaustion* and *Low Blood Sugar*.) Available from www.amazon.com and Natural Healthy Concepts. **NHC**

Helpful Hints

- Do all you can to change your reaction to stressful situations. Long-term chronic stress makes your whole body **far** too acidic, which can trigger or exacerbate a huge range of conditions, from eczema and arthritis to cancers and heart disease. The easiest way to do this is to practice regular meditation or tai chi, which are proven to reduce the release of stress hormones over time and help you cope more positively in stressful situations.
- Learn how to relax! Have a weekly massage, play soothing music, walk in the park breathing deeply and slowly, have a long bath... anything that gives your body space and time to relax.
- Make sure you get sufficient sleep (about 6–8 hours). Sleep deprivation is a major stress on the body in itself and lowers your tolerance to other stresses.
- Numerous validated studies carried out at the Institute of HeartMath in Boulder Creek, California, have demonstrated that once you learn how to entrain your heart and mind as one, then production of the anti-aging hormone DHEA is increased, while cortisol production linked to stress decreases. You can literally entrain your alpha brain activity, produced during relaxation, to synchronize with your heart rate. Your heart can influence your brain and thus reduce your stress levels. By attaching a small sensor to a fingertip, you can watch your heart rhythms in real time on your computer screen and then experience how your thoughts can change its beating. The Institute of HeartMath offers software, devices and downloadable books that can help you develop heart-brain coherence. Find them at www.heartmath.org
- Apply pure rosemary, nutmeg, and clove oils directly to the adrenal area (on your back near your waist area) to support adrenal function and help you feel more positive.
- If you tend to regularly wake up between 3am and 5am, this is a sign that your adrenal glands are struggling. (See *Adrenal Exhaustion*.)
- Take stock of your life. An important first step is to identify the sources of your stress. Keep a diary and write down the things that are winding you up. After a month you will see it's most probably the same things over and over again. Take steps (if possible or practical) to remove what stresses you can from your life. Change your attitude from being negative to positive.
- Laughter releases stress. Learn to lighten up and don't take life so seriously.
- I know it's hard but, as much as you can, stop worrying so much. Dale Carnegie once said that 85% of the things we worry about never actually happen. Trust that things will turn out for the best.
- Keep a pet. Studies of cat and dog owners have shown the considerable stress-reducing abilities of furry companions. When cats purr they produce calming alpha waves, so stroke your cat and de-stress!
- Concentrate on what you can change in your life, and let go of the things you have no control over.
- Doctors agree that if we could all practice a pleasurable hobby that requires a fair amount of concentration, it would take our minds off what is stressing us, reduce the release of stress hormones, and help calm us down. At the very least, watch a movie that makes you laugh.
- Avoid obvious pressures, such as taking on too many commitments and deadlines. Learn to see when a problem is someone else's responsibility, and refuse to take it on.

S

- Learn to say no and mean it; stop feeling guilty.
- If you are in a very stressful situation, walk away (if possible). Go for a walk, take some slow deep breaths, calm down, and then go back. If you do this, you will feel better able to cope.
- Get plenty of exercise, as relaxed muscles mean relaxed nerves that reduce stress. A brisk walk or vigorous exercise session is instant first aid for feelings of stress. If this is impossible, you will still benefit from regular exercise.
- Take a deeper breath every 20 minutes. This helps to re-alkalize the body and slows the release of stress hormones.
- Try a simple progressive muscle relaxation exercise to free the body of physical tensions and distract the mind. Lie down flat on the floor with your palms up and breathe into your tummy. Then, beginning with your feet and calves, tense the muscles as hard as you can, and then relax. Work your way up your body, tensing and releasing each muscle group in turn, finishing with your head and face. Then just relax and stay there for 5 minutes, imagining that you are simply in empty space; and just let go.
- Have a regular massage using essential oils of lavender, valerian, frankincense, neroli, jasmine, or ylang ylang, which will help calm you down. Your body will absorb these oils, so leave them on overnight to increase their effectiveness.
- Hypnotherapy on a weekly basis will really help calm you down. (See *Useful Information*.)
- If you have an emotional problem that you cannot solve or if you can't handle the stress in your life, seek outside help and advice. Simply talking with a trusted friend can be very beneficial, although it is often better to find a professional counselor who can help you handle your problems and teach you effective stress-reduction techniques.

Cortisol and Stress

Cortisol is a steroid hormone made by the adrenal glands in response to any stressful "fight-or-flight" situation. Eons ago, this perfectly normal and natural response gave us the extra energy boost and mental sharpness to either run from our attacker or stand and fight. Either way, our bodies would utilize the cortisol and then levels would return to normal.

Cortisol is both good and bad. It is needed to help regulate blood pressure and cardio-vascular function, as well as to regulate the body's use of proteins, carbohydrates, and fats. It is also released during times of infections, trauma, fatigue, temperature extremes, and crucially when you worry too much. Basically, cortisol signals the liver to release stored sugars (glycogen) to fuel the brain and muscles. However, if this continues unabated it can lead to insulin resistance. (See *Insulin Resistance*.) In the short term cortisol is a good guy, but if levels circulating in your body become, and remain, too high—that is, chronically elevated—then cortisol damages tissues and organs, and greatly affects memory and brain function. High levels of stress hormones also deplete bone in the long term.

Other common symptoms of chronically high stress levels include palpitations, depression, sleep disorders, high blood pressure, anorexia, low blood sugar, insulin resistance, thyroid problems, menstrual disorders, osteoporosis, and obesity (when combined with high insulin levels). You get the picture. Too much stress and cortisol can kill you. Think of the Pacific salmon: after spawning, it undergoes rapid cortisol-induced aging, and death follows in a matter of days. You should also be aware that estrogen replacement from orthodox HRT can increase cortisol levels.

One of the best methods for measuring cortisol levels is an adrenal stress index saliva test. This test measures cortisol levels from early morning to midnight. The results are plotted on a graph and compared with a normal daily output of cortisol. This test is available via

Genova Diagnostics (Tel: 1- 800-522-4762; www.genovadiagnostics.com) or contact your health care practitioner.

STROKE

(see also Angina, Atherosclerosis, Heart Disease, High Blood Pressure, and Stress)

Strokes are the third most common cause of death in the United States and are a major cause of disability and dementia in older adults. Every year between 700,000 and 750,000 Americans have a stroke, and about 275,000 of them die as a result. Nine out of every ten cases occurs in someone over the age of 55, but children and young people can also suffer a stroke. Still, the risk of having a stroke increases with age.

Other significant risk factors are: Raynaud's disease, an overactive thyroid (especially before the age of 45), and Asian or African-American ethnicity.

A stroke occurs when there is a loss of blood supply to the brain that damages or destroys an area of brain tissue. Arterial blockages cause nine out of ten strokes (called ischemic strokes). These blockages may be the result of the gradual build-up of sticky cholesterol-like substances in the arteries that leads to arterial thickening (see *Atherosclerosis*). Sometimes blood clots travel from another part of the body, such as the heart or neck, to the brain, causing a cerebral embolism. The other 10% of strokes (called hemorrhagic strokes) are caused by bleeding into the brain from a ruptured blood vessel, which is most commonly caused by high blood pressure.

Depending on the part of the brain affected, there may be sudden loss of speech or movement, heaviness in the limbs, numbness, blurred vision, confusion, dizziness, loss of consciousness, or coma. Strokes often cause weakness and paralysis on one side of the body, involving the arm and/or leg and face. Symptoms can last for several hours or the rest of a person's life, depending on the severity of the stroke. "Mini" strokes may even go unnoticed and can contribute to subtle reductions in mental function. Many people who have a stroke go on to make a partial or even complete recovery. In fact, an estimated 5.4 million stroke survivors live in the US today.

The risk of having a stroke is higher among people with an unhealthy lifestyle. Smoking, eating too much salt and saturated fat, high estrogen levels, prolonged stress, high LDL (bad cholesterol) levels, and being overweight all contribute. People who tend to be angry or aggressive a lot of the time are also at a far higher risk, as stress and anger raise LDL cholesterol levels, which thickens the blood. People with Type A or AB blood are also at a higher risk, as they tend to have stickier blood.

A lack of vitamin C weakens the matrix of the artery wall, making it more prone to damage and plaque build-up. Free radicals from smoking, prolonged stress, and eating excessive amounts of fried and high-fat foods can lead to increased arterial damage, especially if the person is deficient in antioxidants, such as vitamins C and E.

But there is another factor produced by the body that many nutritional doctors believe is equally as dangerous as having high cholesterol; it's called homocysteine. High levels of homocysteine, which is a toxic by-product of the metabolism of proteins, are known to cause damage to arteries. Researchers have discovered that high homocysteine levels in the blood are as big of a risk factor for cardiovascular disease as factors such as smoking or having high cholesterol.

The good news is that if you have sufficient vitamin B6, B12, and folic acid intake, your body will convert homocysteine into less toxic substances. Studies have confirmed that the

S

less vitamin B6 and folic acid in your blood, the higher your levels of homocysteine. This is why taking a high-strength vitamin B complex daily could save your life.

At times, the symptoms of stroke are not obvious. If you suspect that someone may have recently had a stroke, ask him or her to do **all** of the following ASAP. It could save the person's life:

- Ask the person to smile.
- Ask the person to raise both arms at the same time.
- Ask the person to speak a simple sentence, such as: "It's sunny outside today."
- Ask the person to stick out their tongue.

If the person has trouble with any of these four tasks, take them to hospital or call for **immediate** medical assistance. The faster anyone who has suffered a stroke can be treated, the less damage that will be done to his or her brain. Stroke victims **need urgent medical attention within 3 hours.**

As an over-acid system is also linked to strokes, see *Acid–Alkaline Balance*.

Foods to Avoid

- Avoid mass-produced, refined white foods. Replace refined grains (white bread, pasta, rice, cakes, and cookies) with whole grains, such as brown rice, wholegrain breads and pastas, quinoa, and oats. Whole grains contain more vitamin B, which has often been removed in processed "white" products.
- Reduce your intake of saturated fats from red meats, full-fat dairy products, cheese, and mass-produced chocolate.
- Avoid fried foods or hydrogenated margarines. Those most at risk of having high homocysteine levels are high-protein (meat) eaters with a poor dietary intake of vitamin B6, B12, and folic acid. (See *Fats You Need To Eat*.)
- Reduce your intake of animal-based dairy products. They are associated with an increased risk of cardiovascular disease, especially strokes. There are two possible reasons for this. First, while high in calcium (which is often poorly absorbed), dairy foods are relatively low in magnesium. Calcium requires adequate magnesium to be deposited in the bones; otherwise, it is usually deposited in soft tissues, including joints and arteries. Second, dairy foods are often high in fat and protein, which can raise homocysteine levels, and lack adequate levels of the B vitamins needed to process it into less toxic substances.
- Avoid all soft drinks, because the sugar content causes damage to the circulatory system and leads to an increased risk of strokes.
- Caffeine can drive up blood pressure. Cut down on coffee, tea, soda, and other caffeine-based energy-type drinks and foods. Good alternatives include green or white tea, peppermint tea, fruit teas, or diluted fruit juices.
- Cut down on wines and beer, but an occasional small whisky at night is fine.
- Eliminate sodium-based salts from your diet because of their effects on blood pressure. Replace them with magnesium- or potassium-based salt, such as Solo Sea Salt, or sprinkle powdered kelp or nori seaweed flakes (available from all health stores) onto food.
- Avoid all highly preserved meats (such as bacon and salami), salted nuts, and smoked foods.

Friendly Foods

- Eat plenty of fresh fruits and vegetables and drink freshly made juices for the vitamin C and the other protective antioxidants they contain.
- Eat more beta-carotene-rich foods, such as carrots, sweet potatoes, papaya, spinach, watercress, spring greens, mangoes, cabbage, broccoli, cantaloupe melon, pumpkin, and

tomatoes. In the Nurses' Health Study, which monitored 121,000 US female nurses aged 30–55 over a 20-year period beginning in 1988, those who consumed more than 15–20mg of beta-carotene a day had a 40% lower risk of stroke than women who reported eating less than 6mg a day.

- Potassium-rich foods help prevent strokes, and a recent study showed that low potassium intake can increase the risk of stroke by 50% in the over-65s. Therefore, eat more potassium-rich foods. Bananas, low-fat yogurt, baked potatoes with the skin, prune juice, tomato juice, Swiss chard, spinach and all leafy greens, squash, asparagus, dried apricots, oranges, kidney beans, and lentils are all rich in potassium. **NB: If you have kidney disease or take a diuretic medication to lower your blood pressure, check with your doctor before taking any extra potassium.**

- Vitamin B6 and folic acid are found in oranges, lemons, bananas, tomatoes, green leafy vegetables, beans, nuts, seeds, and wholegrain products. Many breakfast cereals are fortified with additional folic acid. Enjoy organic oatmeal for breakfast made with half skimmed milk and half water; add a chopped apple and a few raisins for sweetness, plus some wheat germ for its vitamin E.

- Make sure to eat a serving of green vegetables, especially dark green leafy vegetables, every day. Spinach, cabbage, lettuce, spring greens, kale, chard, broccoli, peas, and watercress are all good.

- Eat more foods rich in essential fats, such as oily fish, and use unrefined olive, walnut, and sunflower oil for salad dressings. Include more raw, unsalted nuts and seeds, especially flaxseeds, pumpkin, and sunflower seeds, in your diet. The easiest way to get seeds in your diet is to sprinkle them whole or freshly ground on your breakfast every morning. (See *Fats You Need To Eat*.)

- Trials at the Johns Hopkins University School of Medicine in Baltimore have found that resveratrol, a phytopolyphenol compound found in red wine, red grapes, raspberries, blueberries, and cranberries, contains a protective enzyme that helps protect oxygen-starved cells from death in the event of a stroke. Therefore, it makes sense to increase your intake of these foods.

- Garlic and onions help thin the blood naturally.

- People who drink at least three cups of green or black tea daily can reduce their risk of having a stroke.

- Dark chocolate contains a compound called epicatechin that was found in research from Johns Hopkins University to help protect the brain from damage done by strokes by "shielding" brain cells. One or two squares of organic dark chocolate a day should be fine. Otherwise, try small amounts of dairy- and sugar-free organic chocolate made with agave syrup, goji and acai berries with blueberry and coconut oil. Glamour Food is made by the Organic Pharmacy and is only available at their Beverly Hills store, 453 North Beverly Drive, Beverly Hills, CA 90210. Tel: 1-310-272-7275. Epicatechin nutrients can also be found in green tea.

- Magnesium-rich foods include honey, kelp, raw wheat germ, dates, almonds, Brazil nuts, and curry powder.

- Cayenne pepper is a powerful heart and circulation tonic and has been known to reverse arterial plaque formation.

Useful Remedies
- Magnesium relaxes constricted arteries and reduces the risk of a blockage. Take 400–600mg a day in divided doses. Many doctors have found that anyone who has suffered a stroke caused by a clot in the brain should be given intravenous magnesium as soon as possible after

the stroke. Magnesium has a powerful dilatory action on the arteries and helps restore blood flow to the damaged tissue.

■ Take a high-strength vitamin B complex to help lower homocysteine levels.

■ Fish oils (1–3g daily) thin the blood naturally. If you're a vegetarian, then take flaxseed oil capsules instead.

■ Take 1g of vitamin C plus 400IU of natural-source vitamin E to protect against clotting. **NB: If you are on blood-thinning medication, check with your doctor before taking vitamin E as it naturally thins the blood.**

■ Co-enzyme Q10 (100mg per day) helps strengthen the heart muscle. People who have adequate levels of CoQ10 are less prone to strokes.

■ Taking 1g of bioflavonoids daily helps strengthen capillaries.

■ Take a good-quality antioxidant formula that contains at least 200mcg of selenium.

Helpful Hints

■ Research has shown that people living in soft-water areas are more prone to high blood pressure, which can lead to strokes, as soft water is low in minerals, including magnesium. Therefore, if you live in a soft water area, supplement around 400–600mg of magnesium daily (taken in divided doses). Avoid drinking artificially softened water, which uses sodium.

■ Stop smoking, because it doubles your risk of having a stroke.

■ Certain types of combined oral contraceptives can make the blood stickier, which increases the risk of clotting. Orthodox HRT is also linked to an increased stroke risk. (See *Menopause*.)

■ Control your blood pressure. (See *High Blood Pressure*.)

■ Exercise regularly to make your heart stronger and improve circulation. Exercise also helps control weight. Being overweight increases the likelihood of high blood pressure, atherosclerosis, heart disease, and adult-onset (Type II) diabetes. (See *Weight Problems*.) Just walking briskly for a total of 2–3 hours a week has been shown to reduce the risk of strokes in women by up to a third. Also, cycling and swimming lower the risk of both stroke and heart disease. Remember to start gently if you have not exercised for a while, and if you have heart or circulation problems, consult your doctor before starting any exercise program.

■ Homeopathic Aconite 30c (taken three times daily between meals for 3 weeks) helps reduce the effects of shock on the body.

■ Read *Put Your Heart In Your Mouth* by Natasha Campbell-McBride.

■ Another helpful resource is *Heart and Blood Circulatory Problems* by Jan de Vries (Mainstream Publishing).

■ For more help and information, visit the American Stroke Association's website: www.strokeassociation.org

SUNBURN

(see also Age Spots and Aging)

Because the sun has gotten such a bad press over the years and skin cancer rates are rising, we are all supposed to have become more sensible about the sun. However, most people haven't changed a bit. No matter where I am in the world, I see pale North Americans of all ages literally cooking their skin, as I once did. A few wise people stay out of the midday sun, but I still see far too many young children with no hats, sunglasses, or T-shirts out during the brightest parts of the day. Their parents are often nearby, doing the same thing.

At the opposite end of the spectrum you have people such as the actress Nicole Kidman, who never sunbathes—so I hope she takes plenty of vitamin D3!

Sunshine gives off a cocktail of light frequencies, but principally the sun produces ultra violet (UV) radiation. The UVA rays are the aging rays; UVB are the burning rays; and UVC are the most dangerous. Both UVB and UVC are mostly absorbed by the ozone layer (or what's left of it), so it's mostly UVA that reaches us. UVA can penetrate deeper into the skin than both UVB and UVC, and UVA causes damage down into the fat layer of your skin—0.25in (2.5mm) into the dermis. To try to protect itself, your skin begins to thicken and turns brown. We all know that too much sun accelerates aging. In fact, 80% of age-related skin damage comes from too much sun exposure.

Yet, the slower you can tan, the more you reduce the sun's aging effects on your skin. When the skin turns red in the sun, it is the red blood cells' response to the heat that is being generated on the skin. Your blood is basically trying to cool your skin.

African-Americans' and Asians' skin contains more melanin, the thick treacle-like substance that resides in your epidermis. The darker the skin, the more melanin it contains and the more easily it can reflect UV rays. Also, darker skin is able to resist the penetration of the sun's rays down to the dermis—five 5 times more effectively than white skin. People with greasy skin make more sebum, which helps block UV rays, hence people with dark and oilier skins are able to tan better and suffer less wrinkling. Basically, the fairer you are the more easily you will burn, the faster your skin will age, and the greater your risk of developing skin cancers.

But sunshine on your skin makes you feel so good. If you don't expose your skin to sufficient sunlight, then you can become depleted in vitamin D, especially vitamin D3, which is vital for healthy bones, teeth, and immune function. Lack of sunshine and full-spectrum light can also trigger SAD Syndrome (see that section), as the body produces less serotonin, the "feel-good" hormone. Therefore it should be no great surprise that getting enough full-spectrum light is vital for good health and your state of mind. Modest sunbathing helps lower cholesterol and increases hair and nail growth, but too much will lower your immune function. People who live in colder climates and have little sun tend to suffer a higher incidence of internal cancers. What we need to do, as always, is to find a healthy balance. For example, if you expose your skin to just 15 minutes of sun a day, then you can produce several days' supply of vitamin D.

(See *Helpful Hints* for details of how to recognize various types of skin cancer.)

S

Foods to Avoid
- Avoid foods and drinks that will trigger dehydration, such as alcohol, caffeine, and too many soft drinks.

Friendly Foods
- If you are out in the hot sun, you will obviously sweat more. However, this can quickly dehydrate you, which can lead to low blood pressure, which in turn can trigger a fainting episode. Drink plenty of water, and if it's really hot, add a little extra sea salt to your food. You can also use an electrolyte mixture (available from all pharmacies) to replenish lost minerals.
- The most important foods you need to eat more of to help protect your skin from the inside out (at any age) contain essential fats and carotenes. Carotenes are found in carrots, sweet potatoes, tomatoes and tomato paste, asparagus, mustard and cress, raw parsley, red peppers, steamed spinach, apricots, pumpkin, papaya, spring greens, watercress, mangoes, and cantaloupe melon.
- Essential fats are found in sunflower, pumpkin, sesame, hemp, and flaxseeds. Use their unrefined oils in salad dressings and drizzle over cooked foods. (See *Fats You Need To Eat*.)
- When you are in the sun, eat plenty of grilled oily fish and enjoy avocado and olive salads.

Useful Remedies

- Take a high-strength multi-vitamin/mineral and an antioxidant formula that contains at least 100mcg of selenium (known to reduce the incidence of skin cancer).
- Taking 3000–5000IU of vitamin D3 daily for 2 months prior to a vacation should help reduce your risk of burning. But still be sensible in the sun.
- Take 30mg of natural-source carotene complex for 6 weeks before and a month after your vacation in the sun, as research in Germany has found that taking carotenes for around 10 weeks or more helps protect your skin from the ravages of sunburn.
- Take 2g of omega-3 fish oils daily, as essential fats nourish your skin from the inside out. Vegetarians can use flaxseed oil capsules.
- People who take 2g of vitamin C daily along with 400IU of full-spectrum, natural-source vitamin E, appear to have added sun protection. But obviously also with a sunscreen!
- Melanin is made from the amino acid L-tyrosine. Try taking 1000mg daily 30 minutes before meals to help the body tan naturally. You should also start taking it a week or so before you go on vacation.
- Pine bark extract, known as pycnogenol, has been proven to reduce skin inflammation triggered by UV radiation and reduces the likelihood of cell abnormalities. Once again, though, continue to be sensible in the sun. Take one or two capsules daily. **VC**
- Try an Urtica cream such as Weleda Burn Care, which reduces the stinging and inflammation of sunburn. **VC, VS**

Helpful Hints

- The incidence of skin cancer is on the rise, especially in countries and latitudes that enjoy hot sunshine all year round. And as the holes in the ozone layer become larger and more widespread, skin cancers are increasing proportionately, especially after the age of 50. The most dangerous type of skin cancer is malignant melanoma, which is a tumor of the melanocyte (the melanin-producing cells). They are usually either black or brown in color and can develop from an existing mole or just simply appear. It begins to itch, grows larger, and the skin can break down around the "mole." The secret to surviving melanoma is to consult a doctor, dermatologist, or oncologist as fast as you can. If caught before the cancer spreads internally, it can be treated successfully. The good news is that if you have reached your 60s and have no skin cancer, the incidence of melanoma reduces. Taking 200mcg of selenium daily plus natural-source carotenes can help reduce the likelihood of developing malignant skin cancers. If you have a malignant cancer, see the *Cancer* section.
- You may see small skin ulcers, tiny flaking patches or small areas of skin that start to bleed, keep scaling and won't heal. This could be a squamous or basal cell carcinoma. These are not as dangerous as melanoma, but they still need prompt attention and treatment.
- If you are using rejuvenating creams based on Retin A, glycolic acids, AHAs, etc, then wear a higher SPF sunscreen and be really careful not to let your skin go red. Use these types of creams in the winter months. (See *Aging*.)
- Don't allow your skin to go really red. This can trigger skin cancers and cause broken and unsightly capillaries.
- If you suffer from skin conditions such as eczema or psoriasis, moderate sunbathing and seawater will help your skin.
- No matter how much people tell you that tanning beds are safe, they are not. Continued use greatly increases the risk of skin and other cancers.
- Real Sunlight lamps, available at several retailers such as Target, Wal-Mart, and Kmart, are safer than sunlight as the harmful UVA and UVB frequencies have been filtered out. Developed in Sweden, and now used in many nursing homes to boost immune function, they

can relieve the depression associated with conditions such as SAD syndrome. They have been so successful that the Swedish Government is installing them in nursing homes in which residents are rarely exposed to natural sunlight. These lamps increase levels of vitamin D3 naturally, boost immune function, and reduce depression.

- If you carry the herpes simplex virus, too much sun can trigger an attack of cold sores. (See *Cold Sores*.)
- Anyone with lupus must be careful in the sun. (See *Lupus*.)
- Many scientists now believe that chemical-based sunscreens (containing ingredients such as sodium lauryl/laureth sulfate, octylmethoxycinnamate (OMC), benzophenones, synthetic fragrances and colorants) may do more harm than good. Certain preservatives in sunscreens, such as parabens, mimic the affect of estrogens, which can disrupt hormones and are linked to hormonal cancers. If you develop a rash after sun exposure, check out the ingredient list in the cream. PABA (a constituent of folic acid and a member of the B-vitamin family) can trigger skin reactions in some people.
- Try Kimberly Sayer's organic family sunblock. The UV protection comes from zinc oxide and titanium dioxide. It also contains green tea extract, buckthorn, chamomile, aloe vera gel, grape seed oil, avocado oil, and organic echinacea. It is available in SPF 25. Available from www.kimberlysayer.com and a number of other online retailers.
- Other good makes are Curasol by Curaderm (www.antiaging-systems.com/PRG-71/curasol.htm) and Caudalíe (www.caudalie.com).
- During tests it was found that the amount of sunblock you put on your body can be crucial in protecting your skin. Most people only apply enough to achieve 20% of the sun protection factor advertised on the bottle. Apply protection regularly.
- To help avoid cataracts and aging eyes, wear good wrap-around sunglasses that block 99–100% of UVA rays.
- Wear a hat, which greatly reduces UV radiation exposure to the eyes.
- Avoid the sun between 11am and 3pm in northern states and make that 11am and 4pm in hotter climates.
- Please try to be sensible. Wear a light wrap or T-shirt in the heat of the day and always re-apply sunscreen after swimming.
- Certain antibiotics, arthritis drugs, diuretic drugs, and antihistamines (such as Benadryl) can trigger extreme reactions. If you are taking any of these drugs and you are going to be in the sun, check with your doctor.
- The herb St John's wort is also known to trigger sun sensitivity in some people. Large amounts of the herb gotu kola can do the same.

SUPERBUGS *(see MRSA)*

SWOLLEN FEET AND ANKLES *(see Foot Problems and Water Retention)*

T

TACHYCARDIA (rapid heart beat)

(see also Adrenal Exhaustion, Palpitations, Panic Attacks, and Stress)

Tachycardia is a sudden increase in heart rate to over 100 beats per minute in an adult. It occurs in healthy people during exercise, but if tachycardia occurs when you are resting, then you should urgently consult a doctor. Symptoms may include palpitations, breathlessness, light-headedness, sweating and/or dizziness. These types of symptoms may also denote extremes in blood sugar or blood pressure levels. Low or especially high (hyperthyroidism) thyroid function can also be a factor in some people. Low iron levels or low levels of the hormone progesterone may also need to be considered. Food intolerances are well known to trigger tachycardia and should be investigated. (See *Allergies*.) For example, some people develop a rapid heartbeat within 10 minutes of eating wheat. Keep a food diary and note which foods trigger the symptoms. Whatever the trigger, this condition needs thorough investigation by your healthcare professional or doctor.

Foods to Avoid
- Don't drink too much alcohol, which can damage the heart muscle.
- Caffeine triggers the release of adrenaline into the bloodstream and therefore can precipitate an attack.
- Avoid high-energy drinks that are full of refined sugars and caffeine at all costs.

Friendly Foods
- As dehydration can also be a factor in these types of symptoms, make sure you are drinking sufficient fluids.
- Eat more potassium-rich foods. These include all leafy green vegetables, bananas, fresh and dried fruits, nuts, fish, and sunflower seeds.
- See *Friendly Foods* under Heart Disease.
- Eat more garlic, onions, and pomegranate, which are heart-healthy foods.

Useful Remedies
- Take a high-strength multi-vitamin/mineral for your age and gender that contains a full spectrum of B vitamins. See pages 15–16 for a list of companies that would be happy to help you.
- Co-enzyme Q10 is a vitamin-like substance manufactured by the body; however, production slows as we age. Taking 100mg daily helps strengthen the heart muscle and increases energy levels.
- Natural-source, full-spectrum vitamin E helps the heart muscle receive more oxygen and naturally thins the blood. Take 400IU daily. **NB: If you are on blood-thinning medication such as Warfarin, avoid taking vitamin E supplements until you have spoken to your doctor.**
- The mineral magnesium, which helps regulate the heartbeat, is often deficient in people with tachycardia. Take 300–600mg daily in divided doses with meals.
- L-theanine (extracted from green tea) helps keep you calm. Try taking 50–100mg two or three times a day. **VC**

■ Putting a pinch of cayenne pepper under your tongue can help normalize your heartbeat.

Helpful Hints

■ Because palpitations may be linked to an overactive thyroid or low iron levels, ask your doctor to do a blood test.

■ To combat worrying, which only exacerbates this condition, learn how to breathe properly by taking yoga, tai chi, or relaxation lessons.

■ Practice meditation regularly, as this helps you cope with stressful situations in a calmer way. If you feel an attack coming on, splash your face with cold water, then lie down, close your eyes, and breathe slowly and deeply for a few minutes until the attack passes.

■ Essential oil of lavender or ylang ylang has a calming effect, so add a few drops to your bath. Try regular aromatherapy massage, which is very calming.

■ Go for leisurely walks, breathing deeply.

TASTE AND SMELL, LOSS OF

In young people this condition can occur after a cold or with blocked sinuses, but as we get older and our immune system weakens, loss of taste and smell is very common. If the nose becomes too dry and "stuffed up", then the sense of smell can quickly be impaired. When you have a cold your ability to taste and smell can be reduced by as much as 80%. Hay fever, allergic rhinitis, nasal polyps, and smoking can all interfere with taste and smell. A lack of zinc is often the culprit, as many people do not absorb sufficient zinc from their diets. Certain heart and prescription drugs can also cause a loss of taste and smell. It is generally easier to smell and taste in warm, moist atmospheres than in cold, dry ones.

Babies have many taste buds in their mouths, including the cheeks, but once we become adults the sensitivity of all of our taste buds is diminished and is greatly diminished by old age.

Your tongue is covered with tiny projections called papillae, inside which are the sensory nerves that enable you to taste. Saliva is needed for taste and without it our diet would be virtually tasteless.

The average nose can detect approximately 4,000 different odors, while an especially sensitive one can recognize around 10,000. Inside the nose we have two small receptor sites, which are yellow-brown patches of mucus-covered membrane, found in the roof of the nasal cavities. They are covered in millions of hair-like antennae. As we age, these antennae become less effective.

Foods to Avoid

■ Generally you need to avoid mucus-forming foods, such as full-fat milk, chocolate, cheese, and other animal-source dairy products. Soy milk can also be a problem for some people.

■ Sugary, fatty, starchy white foods will also make the situation worse.

■ Also see *Foods to Avoid* under *Colds and Flu*.

Friendly Foods

■ Keep your diet clean with plenty of fresh fruits and vegetables.

■ Eat more brown rice, quinoa, barley, lentils, cereals, oats, and whole-wheat bread and pastas.

■ Increase your consumption of zinc-rich foods, including lean steak, lamb, beef, calves' liver, raw oysters, fresh (preferably organic) peanuts, hazelnuts, Brazil nuts, ground ginger, and dry mustard.

■ Sunflower, pumpkin, sesame, and flaxseeds all contain fair amounts of zinc.

■ Try organic-source rice, almond, or coconut milk as non-dairy substitutes.

■ Eat more garlic and onions, which are antibacterial and anti-viral.

Useful Remedies

■ Take 15–30mg of chelated zinc or zinc picolinate, which can be useful for helping restore the sense of smell. For best results, take on its own at night before bed. Otherwise take Zinc by Twinlab, which contains three types of zinc (picolinate, gluconate, and dihydrate). These are easy to absorb and improve zinc levels quickly. Taking 1–3 capsules daily for 6 weeks should be fine, then reduce to one capsule daily for a further 6 weeks, and then just one capsule a week.

■ If an infection triggers a loss of taste and smell, take 10,000IU of vitamin A for a month, which helps support the upper respiratory tract. After the month, switch to a natural-source beta-carotene supplement, such as Solgar, which naturally converts to vitamin A in the body and is non-toxic. **NB: If you are pregnant or planning to become pregnant, you should take no more than 3000IU of pure vitamin A daily. Carotenes are safe and non-toxic.**

■ Include a high-strength multi-vitamin/mineral and an extra 1g of vitamin C daily in your regimen.

■ If the problem is linked to a cold or sinus infection, then see *Colds and Flu, Sinus Problems,* and *Immune Function*.

Helpful Hints

■ Homeopathic Nat Mur, Silica, and Pulsatilla are very useful for loss of taste. Belladonna or Hyos are useful for loss of smell.

■ Tap water is often contaminated by chemicals that can exacerbate this problem. Invest in a reverse-osmosis water filter system, which is more effective than over-the-counter carbon filters. Visit www.freedrinkingwater.com

■ See a qualified nutritionist who can help rebalance and detoxify your system.

TENNIS ELBOW
(see Bursitis and Carpal Tunnel Syndrome)

THROAT PROBLEMS
(see Sore Throat)

THRUSH
(see also Candida and Cystitis)

Vaginal thrush is caused by the same fungus, *Candida albicans*, that causes oral thrush. Infections develop when the good bacteria in the vagina are destroyed. This happens if we take too many antibiotics, eat too much refined sugar or starchy mass-produced junk foods, become very run down, or use highly perfumed soaps and deodorants. Symptoms can include itchiness or general soreness of the vagina, and sometimes the vulva swells and is accompanied by a thick, whitish discharge that smells rather yeasty. You may feel the need to urinate more frequently, and there could be some slight stinging when you pass urine. If the infection takes hold, the lymph glands in the groin can swell. If this happens, you must see a doctor (*see Candida*). If you suffer from cystitis (bladder infections) regularly, then you may be very run down, and this can lead to thrush. If this is the case, then avoid sexual intercourse for at least a week to help ease symptoms.

As chronic thrush is also linked to diabetes, see your doctor.

Foods to Avoid

- See *Foods to Avoid* under *Candida*.
- Because the body needs to be kept more alkaline, see the dietary advice in *Acid–Alkaline Balance*.
- Completely avoid pistachio nuts and peanuts, which harbor molds that can add to the problem.
- Avoid all blue cheeses.
- Avoid all refined sugary foods, since the fungus feeds off sugar.

Friendly Foods

- Eating 250ml of plain, live yogurt daily helps clear thrush.
- See *Friendly Foods* under *Acid–Alkaline Balance* and *Candida*.

Useful Remedies

- Take 1000mg twice daily of the herb pau d'arco, which has anti-fungal properties.
- Grapefruit seed extract (800–1200mg daily) is anti-fungal. It also acts like a natural antibiotic.
- Take a course of acidophilus/bifidus. These healthy bacteria will help kill the yeast overgrowth. **VC, VS**
- Dilute a few drops of thyme and rose essential oils in a douche of lukewarm water twice daily to help kill the bacteria.
- Douche with yogurt (one pot of natural live yogurt to 3 pints/1.75 liters of cooled boiled water). Or douche in lukewarm water with a few drops of tea tree oil, a crushed garlic clove, and a little organic cider vinegar. Or use apple cider vinegar diluted into water (4 tablespoons of vinegar to 0.75 pint/1 liter of cooled boiled water). This helps re-acidify the vaginal area, as the good bacteria prefer a slightly acid environment.
- Include a high-strength multi-vitamin/mineral in your regimen.
- Eat more garlic, which is highly anti-fungal.

Helpful Hints

- Avoid sexual intercourse while an attack lasts, because it could be extremely painful. Your partner will also need to be treated for candida, as you are more than likely passing the problem back and forth.
- Try lavender and tea tree pessaries until symptoms ease. Never use tea tree oil directly on any affected area. Always dilute in lukewarm water.
- In conjunction with the above, you can also take pau d'arco and powdered or garlic oil capsules orally as directed until the condition eases, as they are highly anti-fungal.
- Wear cotton underwear and change it every day.
- Avoid vaginal deodorants, perfumed bath salts, and talcum powder.
- Only use pH-balanced soaps.
- Vitamin E or calendula cream may relieve itching.
- Take homeopathic Lycopodium 6c or Kali Mur 6c 2–3 times daily for up to a week to help reduce symptoms.
- For oral thrush, use Borax 6c twice daily for up to a week.

THYROID, UNDERACTIVE AND OVERACTIVE

(see also Adrenal Exhaustion and Fluoride)

Undiagnosed thyroid problems have reached epidemic proportions, mostly because the symptoms can vary so hugely. Your thyroid is often the most ignored gland in your body. It is situated in your neck, just below the Adam's apple, and produces hormones that affect every major organ and the metabolism and repair of every single cell in your body. Every drop of our approximately 8–10 pints (4.5–5.5 liters) of blood circulates through the thyroid every hour, bringing with it the substances the thyroid needs to do its work.

Thyroxine (also known as T4) is the main hormone produced by the thyroid gland and is converted by the liver into T3 (tri-iodothyronine), which is the active form of the hormone. Basically, the more T3 you produce, the faster your metabolism. If you don't produce sufficient thyroid (T3) hormones, many systems in your body begin to slow down—heartbeat, circulation, blood pressure, energy levels, metabolism, and temperature. Slower metabolism will mean that you don't burn calories as efficiently as you could, so you gain weight more easily. Also when the body slows down, its ability to detoxify harmful substances is greatly impaired.

Up to 20% of the population is probably suffering from some degree of hypothyroidism (underactive thyroid), and the older you get the more prone you are to this condition. But it doesn't have to be that way. Symptoms that should make you investigate whether your thyroid may be underactive include persistent low energy levels, mental "fogginess," depression, cold hands and feet, weight gain (even with a poor appetite), high cholesterol even if you eat sensibly, a slow pulse, low blood sugar (see *Low Blood Sugar*), headaches, infertility, dry and sometimes puffy skin, brittle nails, poor vision and memory, constipation, sore throat, nasal congestion, thinning hair, low libido, and heavy periods.

Your ability to metabolize beta-carotene (from foods such as sweet potatoes, papaya, and carrots) can be decreased if you have an underactive thyroid. This can case further problems, as beta-carotene is needed for optimum immune function and tissue repair.

An underactive thyroid is seven times more common in women than in men, especially in women with low levels of the hormone DHEA. Unfortunately, because some of the symptoms associated with an underactive thyroid are often attributed to menopause, thousands of women go undiagnosed or are offered orthodox HRT as a one-stop cure-all. Yet there is much you can do to help yourself.

If you have your thyroid tested, make sure they test your TSH, T4, T3, and thyroid antibodies. Ask your health professional to organize a Total Thyroid Profile (a blood test) by Genova Diagnostics. Tel: 1-800-522-4762. Website: www.genovadiagnostics.com

Otherwise you can try a temperature test developed by Broda Barnes that is used by some nutritionists. Here's how it works. Shake out a thermometer and keep it by your bed. When you wake up in the morning (before getting out of bed), put the thermometer under your arm and lie there for 10 minutes. Your temperature should be 97.7–98°F (36.5–36.7°C). Do this for at least 2 days. (Women should do this test on days 2 and 3 of their period, as body temperature fluctuates during the cycle.) If either of your temperature readings is below 97.7°F (36.5°C), take it again over a longer period of time, say a week, to see if it is low on a fairly regular basis. If it is, you probably have an underactive thyroid. For more help, visit www.brodabarnes.org

In many cases a low temperature will not necessarily indicate a condition that would be medically diagnosed as an underactive thyroid (and treated with synthetic thyroid hormones), but nevertheless you could benefit from the following guidelines. If you do decide to take steps to improve your thyroid efficiency, check your early-morning temperature again for a couple of mornings every month or so. As it starts to increase, you should find that some of your symptoms also start to improve.

An overactive thyroid (excess T3 production) is known as hyperthyroidism and is relatively rare. In this condition the thyroid produces too many hormones, which can trigger symptoms such as goiter (when the thyroid becomes more prominent and the eyes bulge). Other common symptoms are anxiety, insomnia, an inability to relax, shakiness, excessive sweating, feeling warm even on cold days, rapid heartbeat, palpitations, breathlessness, and weight loss even with a hearty appetite. If you are diagnosed with an overactive thyroid, you need the help of a competent physician or nutritional practitioner.

Long-term adrenal exhaustion can disrupt many processes in the body, including the thyroid (see *Adrenal Exhaustion*).

Foods to Avoid—for an underactive thyroid

- Certain foods are known to inhibit thyroid function. These include soy (soy milk, tofu and so on), apples, pine nuts, cruciferous vegetables (such as cabbage, broccoli, mustard, and kale), spinach, peaches, pears, and turnips. Also avoid walnuts, pine nuts, peanuts, mustard, and millet. These foods are generally good for you, but avoid them until your thyroid has stabilized. This is more of a problem if you aim to eat these foods raw; once cooked, they can be eaten in moderation.
- Avoid all caffeine-containing foods and drinks because they will stimulate the release of adrenaline, which can affect the thyroid.
- Avoid fluoride, as it interferes with thyroid function. (See *Fluoride*.)

T

Friendly Foods—for an underactive thyroid

- Iodine and the amino acid tyrosine are the two nutrients the body uses to make thyroid hormones. Iodine can be found in seafood and seaweed (for example, kelp, nori, and arame), mushrooms, Swiss chard, butter beans, pumpkin seeds, sesame seeds (tahini), egg yolk, lecithin, ground beef, artichokes, onions, leeks, and garlic. **NB: Those suffering from autoimmune thyroid disease such as Hashimoto's or Graves disease would not be helped by extra iodine.**
- Use organic sea salt or sprinkle powdered kelp or nori flakes over meals.
- The amino acid tyrosine is in all protein-rich foods, especially fish, butter beans, pumpkin seeds, bananas, and avocados. If you have adequate protein in your diet, you should be getting enough tyrosine.
- Essential fatty acids are vital for proper thyroid function so include plenty of oily fish, seeds, and cold-pressed oils in your diet. (See *Fats You Need To Eat*.)
- Eat more radishes, watercress, wheat germ, brewer's yeast, mushrooms, tropical fruits, watermelon, seeds, and sprouted foods such as alfalfa. Make your own watermelon juice and then add aloe vera juice for a great thyroid blend.
- Use organic-source coconut oil for cooking, as it helps stimulate the thyroid. Available in most supermarkets and health stores.
- The trace mineral manganese is also important for thyroid function; therefore, eat more pecans, almonds, Brazil nuts, rye, barley, and buckwheat.
- Since low selenium is also linked to low thyroid function, eat more asparagus and garlic.

Useful Remedies—for an underactive thyroid

- Taking a high-strength multi-vitamin/mineral complex every day provides a foundation of nutrients for the body to work with.
- Inflammation and oxidation within the body can trigger problems with manufacturing certain

enzymes that are necessary for proper thyroid function. Therefore, take a broad-spectrum antioxidant formula.

- Selenium is needed for the manufacture of thyroid hormones. Selenium levels are low in the soil of many countries, and if the minerals are not in the soil, they won't be in your food! Take 200mcg daily.

- Kelp tablets contain iodine, which is vital for manufacturing thyroid hormones. Follow the directions on the label, aiming for around 150mcg of iodine a day. **NB: Don't take more than 500mcg of iodine a day unless it is under your doctor's instruction, as too much iodine can upset thyroid balance. Do not take iodine if you have Graves or Hashimoto's disease.**

- The body makes thyroxine from the amino acid L-tyrosine, so take 500mg twice daily on an empty stomach (plus 50mg of vitamin B6 and 100mg of vitamin C to aid absorption).

- Take 1–3g of Korean ginseng (or 2–6ml of tincture) daily for a month, then stop and start taking it again a month later. This can help reduce the effects of stress on your adrenal glands, your thyroid and your health in general. **NB: Avoid Korean ginseng if you suffer from high blood pressure.**

- Take 1g of vitamin C with food, as well as 100mg of CoQ10, early in the day to help raise energy levels.

- Essential fats are crucial for helping normalize thyroid function. Take 4–6g of fish oil daily with food until you note an improvement. If you are vegetarian, take 40–60ml (just over a tablespoon) of flaxseed oil per day stirred into vegetable juices until your condition improves. Then reduce to 2g of omega-3 a day, or 2 teaspoons of flaxseed oil.

Helpful Hints

- As well as checking your thyroid hormone levels, ask your doctor to check levels of DHEA, which can easily be supplemented if low.

- Stop smoking. Smoking is known to make an underactive thyroid worse. Cigarettes aren't an easy addiction to give up, but it is definitely worth the effort. For smokers, the number one thing you can do to improve your health and have a healthy lifespan is to quit smoking.

- Managing stress is often the key. Learn to relax, ensure you have regular "down time," try yoga, tai chi, massage, or meditation, and exercise regularly. (See *Stress*.)

- Support your digestion. It is well established that our digestive capacity declines with age or when you are under stress at any age. Tyrosine, needed to make thyroid hormones, is a component of protein. Protein is relatively difficult to digest, so less digestion means less tyrosine and therefore less thyroid hormones. The answer is to chew well, relax during meals, and ensure you have an optimum level of nutrients in your diet to support digestion. If you have low stomach acid (needed to digest protein), you'll find that eating beets gives you pink urine, which doesn't normally happen, so this can be used as a simple at-home test. Both digestive enzymes and betaine hydrochloride (stomach acid) capsules may be needed in the short term until your digestion becomes more efficient. (See *Low Stomach Acid*.)

- Consider food intolerances. Dr James Braly reports in his book *Dangerous Grains* (Avery Publishing) that there is a correlation between wheat (gluten) intolerances and thyroid problems. You can check for food intolerances with an at-home blood test from YorkTest Laboratories (www.yorktest.com).

- Exercise regularly. Exercise stimulates thyroid function, so aim for 30 minutes of aerobic exercise at least three times per week. If you are just starting an exercise program, start gently and build up.

- Avoid fluoride (in toothpaste) and chlorine (in tap water), as they are both chemically similar to iodine and block iodine receptors in the thyroid. Consider installing a good water filter.

- If an underactive thyroid is diagnosed early enough and the patient is otherwise energetic, homeopathic thyroid treatment can be very useful. Thyroidea Compositum, made by the German company HEEL, is one of the most useful non-drug substances. Available from homeopathic pharmacies with a prescription from a licensed practitioner, as well as from www.smallflower.com
- Read *Hypothyroidism, the Unsuspected Illness* by Broda O. Barnes and Lawrence Galton (Harper and Row) or *Why Am I So Tired— Is Your Thyroid Making You Ill* by Martin Budd (Thorsons).
- For further information or to order Broda's book, log on to www.brodabarnes.org

TINNITUS

Tinnitus is a chronic and distressing condition in which the patient suffers from a ringing, buzzing, or humming noise in one or both ears. This condition can have a variety of causes, which include high blood pressure, exposure to loud noises or an explosion, long-term use of aspirin, use of beta blockers and antibiotics, compacted ear wax, spinal or cranial misalignment (which can reduce circulation to the ears), or food intolerances. Low zinc levels can also be a major contributing factor in this condition. Tinnitus is more common in older people, but is appearing in younger people who are exposed to excessively loud music. Aging rock stars who were exposed to loud music over many years often suffer from tinnitus. In Chinese medicine, adrenal and kidney function are linked to ear problems; therefore, if you are totally exhausted and/or stressed, this could also trigger tinnitus or make any existing problem worse. This condition can also be linked to a congested liver. (See *Liver Problems*.)

Foods to Avoid
- Avoid alcohol, smoking, and caffeine, all of which may aggravate the condition.
- Cut down on sodium-based salt, which can trigger a build-up of fluid in the ear or raise blood pressure.
- Avoid all full-fat cow's milk and dairy products for 2 weeks, because they are mucus-forming, which can block the ears and sinuses. (See *Sinus Problems*.)
- Generally cut down on saturated fats, such as red meat, cheese, chocolate, highly refined white-flour-based foods, pies, pastries, cookies, and so on.
- Yeasty breads and other yeast-based foods can also make this problem worse.
- Don't use hard margarines or highly refined cooking oils, and eliminate fried foods.
- Read labels carefully to avoid any foods that contain hydrogenated or trans-fats. (See *Fats You Need To Eat*.)

Friendly Foods
- Eat plenty of garlic and onions, which are very cleansing.
- Choose low-fat dairy options such as fully skimmed milk or cottage cheese.
- Use organic rice milk for making oatmeal and on cereals. Also try live, low-fat yogurts in desserts instead of creams.
- Try organic-source almond or coconut milks.
- Generally increase your consumption of fruits and fresh vegetables, and include more nutritious foods, such as lentils, barley, and corn-, rice- and spinach-based pastas, in your diet.
- Baked potatoes are a wonderful food; add a little yogurt or use a non-hydrogenated spread such as Biona or Olivia. Also try organic walnut, pumpkin seed, hemp seed, or coconut butters, available from most health food stores.

■ Add more cayenne pepper to foods to help increase circulation.

Useful Remedies

■ For 1 month take 25,000IU of vitamin A to nourish inner ear nerve cells. (If you are pregnant or eat lots of liver, which is high in vitamin A, then limit your intake to 3000IU a day.) After the month, switch to natural-source carotenes daily, which naturally convert to vitamin A in the body. These are safe and non-toxic. Take 1–2 capsules daily. **SVHC**

■ Take 30mg of zinc in a multi-vitamin/mineral supplement, as a lack of zinc is greatly associated with tinnitus. For the first month take an extra 30mg of zinc three times daily before bed to aid absorption until symptoms ease. Otherwise take Zinc by Twinlab, which contains three types of zinc (picolinate, gluconate, and dihydrate). These are easy to absorb and improve zinc levels quickly. Taking 1–3 capsules daily for 6 weeks should be fine; then take just one a day for 6 weeks followed by just one capsule a week.

■ Taking vitamin B12 (1000mcg a day) helps reduce noise-induced tinnitus, as it nourishes nerve endings.

■ As all of the B vitamins work together, also take a high-strength B complex.

■ Taking ginkgo biloba (120–240mg of standardized extract daily) helps increase circulation to the ear, which should help people if poor circulation is the underlying cause.

■ Try garlic and horseradish tablets or tincture, which act as decongestants.

■ Herbs such as gotu kola, cayenne pepper, and prickly ash will all help increase circulation to the head. Also have a word with an herbalist to find out which herb may help you most effectively.

Helpful Hints

■ Recordings of soothing music or sounds help mask the unwanted noise, especially when you are trying to get to sleep.

■ Regular exercise may provide relief by increasing blood circulation to the head.

■ Practice relaxation techniques, such as Mindful Meditation, which has been proven to help tinnitus sufferers.

■ Cranial osteopathy or chiropractic treatment can release built-up tensions in the head and neck, which can trigger tinnitus.

■ Acupuncture has proved very beneficial for some sufferers. (See *Useful Information*.)

■ For up-to-date research and news about tinnitus, visit the American Tinnitus Association's website: www.ata.org

■ Impacted wisdom teeth and tooth decay can cause this problem. When we grind our teeth over many years, the jaw can become misaligned; this is known as TMJD (Temporomandibular joint disorder). Dentists who specialize in treating TMJ problems (or any good dentist) can make a small brace to be worn at night that holds the jaw in its correct position, which often alleviates tinnitus. There is a craniofacial pain center at Tufts University in Boston, Massachusetts, that specializes a multidisciplinary approach to treating head, neck, and facial pain. Tel: 1-617-636-6828. Website: http://dental.tufts.edu/1176988224004/TUSDM-Page-dental2ws_1262786838313.html There are also a number of other craniofacial pain clinics based at other universities and hospitals around the country.

TONGUE PROBLEMS

The tongue is a great indicator of your overall health and mirrors the levels of toxicity in the body. A healthy tongue should be pink, moist, and clean, with little to no coating. A white coating is usually a sign that the digestive system is not working as it should, that your liver and bowels are sluggish, and that you are eating too many mucus-forming foods (such as full-fat, animal dairy-based foods, refined sugary/starchy foods, and red meat). Smokers are more likely to have a coated tongue. Candida, the yeast overgrowth, can cause a thick white coating on the tongue (see *Candida*). If you have a heavily coated tongue, this can also contribute to bad breath so buy a tongue scraper from any pharmacy and use daily.

A swollen tongue can denote dehydration; therefore, drink plenty of fluids. It may also be linked to an iron deficiency so have a blood test to check. If your tongue swells suddenly, this can be an acute allergic reaction, which can be triggered by nuts, shellfish, or anything to which you have a severe intolerance, and you need to seek immediate medical attention.

Naturopath and Chinese doctor Stephen Langley says: "By looking at a person's tongue, I can easily determine the overall state of that person's health. For example, if the coating is yellow, this indicates excessive heat in the body associated with constipation, over-acidity or pain, and inflammation. If the tongue is 'scalloped' looking, as though it is indented with teeth marks along the sides (which is very common), this can indicate either poor absorption and assimilation in the gut or exhaustion of the adrenal glands."

Foods to Avoid
- Red meat, full-fat animal-source dairy products, and most starchy foods made with mass-produced, highly refined white flour can add to the mucus load in the body and slow digestion.
- Reduce your intake of alcohol, caffeine, fried foods, and junk/fast food, which place a strain on the liver. (See *Liver Problems*.)
- Also see *General Health Hints*.

Friendly Foods
- To clear the coating, you need to keep your diet really clean for 7–10 days.
- During any detoxification process the tongue is likely to become even more furred as the body begins eliminating acidity.
- Drink plenty of fresh vegetable juices made with garlic, ginger, and any fresh vegetables you have on hand. Celery, artichoke, chicory, celeriac, kale, and beets are great liver cleansers.
- See *Friendly Foods* under *Constipation*.
- Eat more pineapple and papaya, which greatly aid digestion.

Useful Remedies
- Take a probiotic that contains acidophilus/bifidus daily for 6 weeks to replenish healthy bacteria in the bowel. **VC, VS**
- Prebiotics are plant compounds that encourage the growth of healthy bacteria in the bowel. Try Agave Digestive Immune Support. One scoop daily with breakfast really helps keep you regular. **LEF**
- Take a digestive enzyme with main meals.
- The herb milk thistle (500mg three times daily) will help improve liver function.
- The celloid mineral sodium phosphate (600mg daily) will help reduce the creamy coating. NuAge Nat Phos is a good product. **VC**

Geographical tongue

In this condition, discolorations form irregular shapes on the surface of the tongue, often making it look like a map. Usually it disappears on its own, but sensitivity to certain foods can exacerbate the problem. (See *Allergies*.) I have had letters from pregnant women whose geographical tongues disappeared once the baby was born. This problem is also linked to iron and/or vitamin B deficiencies. The patches can also be caused by an infection or irritants such as vinegar.

Foods to Avoid
- Cut down on caffeine, highly spiced foods, vinegar, pickles, pineapple, and plums.
- Refined orange juice may also be a problem for some people.
- Alcohol will also irritate the delicate tissues of the mouth.

Friendly Foods
- Include more ginger and live, low-fat yogurt in your diet, which are very soothing.
- Garlic and onions are very cleansing.
- Drink plenty of water.
- Eat more foods that contain B vitamins, such as whole grains, oat bran, wheat germ, quinoa, amaranth, brown rice, organic muesli, oats, lecithin granules, and brewer's yeast. Liver is also high in vitamins A and B, but only eat it once a week and make it organic.
- Eat plenty of fresh fruits and vegetables.
- Also see *General Health Hints*.

Useful Remedies
- Greens Today Joint Formula is a combination formula that brings together horsetail, silica, kelp, vitamin C, boron, and digestive enzymes to improve absorption of nutrients from food and encourage soft tissue healing. **VC**
- Take a high-strength B complex daily with breakfast or lunch.
- Take a multi-vitamin/mineral suitable for your age and gender that contains around 30mg of zinc, as low zinc levels are linked to this problem.
- Ask your doctor to check if you are low in iron, in which case take a liquid formula, such as Spatone, which will not cause constipation. Available worldwide from health stores.
- Take NuAge Calc Fluor (calcium fluoride) tissue salts four times a day. **VC**

Helpful Hints
- Tea tree oil can be diluted in warm water and used as a mouthwash, as can 1% hydrogen peroxide.
- Some sufferers report an improvement after taking a garlic capsule daily.

TONSILLITIS
(see also Immune Function and Sore Throat)

A nasty sore throat accompanied by difficulty swallowing and ear pain are the most common symptoms of tonsillitis. It makes you feel horribly tired, and symptoms may also include fever, nausea, headache, and swollen, painful lymph glands in the neck. Tonsillitis is especially common among children. Antibiotics are not necessarily needed as more often than not tonsillitis is caused by a virus, which is not killed off by antibiotics. It is only if a secondary bacterial infection occurs that antibiotics are warranted. Recurrent infections indicate that the immune system is struggling or that food intolerances, especially to animal-source dairy, are involved. (See *Immune Function*.)

Foods to Avoid
- While an infection is present, anything that increases mucus production needs to be avoided. This includes dairy products (most especially from cows)—cheese, milk, full-fat yogurts, chocolates, cream, and butter—along with eggs, soy milk, and nut butters.
- Foods such as toast, potato chips, and spicy foods can cause discomfort to an inflamed throat.

- Soft drinks and other refined sugary/fatty foods and drinks will greatly lower immune function.
- Caffeine, found in tea, coffee, chocolate, and sodas, adds stress to the immune system and is best avoided.
- Once the infection is over, if you suspect that dairy foods are causing a problem, continue to keep them out of the diet. Keep calcium levels high by eating lots of sesame seeds or tahini (ground sesame seeds), almonds, Brazil nuts, bony fish such as sardines and pilchards, plus dark green leafy vegetables, including kelp, broccoli, cabbage, and watercress.
- Reduce packaged and processed foods that are high in hydrogenated and trans-fats, artificial flavorings, colorings, preservatives, and sweeteners.

Friendly Foods

- Make low-sugar, diluted fruit juices into popsicles by freezing them. This is a great way to help soothe a sore throat while an infection is present. Blackcurrant and apple are particularly good.
- Vegetable soups and chicken broths are full of healing nutrients that will boost the immune system and are easier to swallow than regular food. Use plenty of sweet potatoes, cabbage, squash, pumpkin, carrots, and broccoli, plus lentils or brown rice, with a little chicken or lamb.
- To tempt a child with a low appetite, put lots of different colors on the plate—oranges, reds, purples, blues, yellows, and greens. Colorful foods contain bioflavonoids, which have many immune-boosting and protective properties. A bowl full of blueberries, blackberries, cherries, plums, apricots, papaya, and oranges will give any child lots of nutrients. Or blend these fruits with a small amount of rice milk to make a nutritious smoothie. For a recipe, see *General Health Hints*.

- When your child is ready to return to solid foods, begin with light, easily digested meals, as the digestive system has been taxed during the infection. Go for thicker stews or lightly steamed vegetables with chicken or fish.
- Eat more fresh fruits and vegetables and whole grains, as these will help supply the immune system with the raw ingredients it needs to function well.
- Include more foods rich in vitamin C, such as strawberries, kiwi, sweet potatoes, blackberries, red and yellow peppers, broccoli, and peas.

Useful Remedies

- Try Sambucol, an extract of elderberries, which has proven anti-viral action and tastes great, too. Children can have 2 teaspoons twice a day, and adults can have 2 teaspoons four times a day. It also comes as a lozenge. Adults should have one lozenge four times a day.
- Vitamin A is known to help heal inflamed mucous membranes and boost immune function. During an infection, children over the age of 5 can have 10,000IU for 2 days before reducing the dose to 2,500IU daily. Seven- to 10-year-olds should take 10,000IU for just 2 days before reducing the dose to 3,500IU daily until symptoms ease. After this time, you can switch the child to a beta-carotene capsule daily, which is completely safe. Watercress, pumpkin, papaya, carrots, and watermelon are all rich in carotenes. **NB: If you are pregnant or planning to become pregnant, you cannot take more than 3000IU of vitamin A daily, but carotenes, which naturally convert to vitamin A in the body, are fine.**
- Take phytolacca, an herb that specifically helps alleviate the symptoms of tonsillitis. Also take a complex such as Wellness Formula by Source Naturals that contains echinacea, goldenseal, and astragalus—all known to boost immune function. **VC, VS**
- Applying a little neat tea tree oil externally to the painful area on the throat should help ease the pain.

- Suck zinc lozenges three times a day, as zinc aids the immune system and has been shown to reduce the duration of a sore throat.
- During an infection, add 4g of powdered vitamin C to water and sip throughout the day. This will keep levels boosted and help the immune system fight the infection. Source Naturals makes a good non-acidic one called magnesium ascorbate. **VC**
- Beta Glucans 1–3, 1–6, which are derived from yeast cell walls, are proven to strengthen the body's innate immune system (the immune system you are born with), making it more resistant to pathogens from food and air. Take 250–500mg daily. It can also be taken by children and reduces the likelihood of food intolerances that are triggered by a weakened immune system. Dr Paul Clayton is a medical pharmacologist based in the US and UK. His website (www.healthdefence.com) contains a lot of research about Beta Glucans and is well worth a look. **VC**

Helpful Hints

- Add manuka honey and root ginger to hot water for a soothing drink. The ginger is full of zinc, which is healing, and the manuka honey has strong antibacterial action.
- Gargling with salty water or red sage and echinacea four times a day really helps.
- Slice an onion, wrap it in an old cloth, and wrap the cloth around the throat. Replenish every 3 hours. This can really help clear congestion from the lymph glands in the neck.
- Get lots of rest and maintain a high fluid intake.
- Humidifiers can help keep a dry throat moist and ease discomfort.

- If the tonsils become infected and antibiotics are necessary, then follow them up with a probiotic supplement. Probiotics are healthy bacteria needed by the gut that are killed along with the infection by the antibiotics. (See *Antibiotics*.)

TRAVEL SICKNESS

This is an extremely common condition, especially in children and older people. Just worrying about a journey can be enough to trigger symptoms in a sensitive individual. Eating a large meal prior to traveling and stuffy atmospheres can also make symptoms worse. Some people can read while moving, but for others trying to focus on something stationary while in a moving vehicle can disturb the balance in the inner ear, resulting in nausea. Also, if anyone who suffers from travel sickness looks out the window and notices the scenery flashing by, this often makes symptoms worse because the balance of the inner ears is linked to receptors in the eyes. Symptoms include looking pale, feeling clammy and sometimes nausea, vomiting, and in extreme cases, fainting.

Food to Avoid

- On short trips, avoid eating and drinking anything immediately prior to your journey.

Friendly Foods

- On the day prior to travel, eat lighter foods, salads, fish, tofu, and fresh fruit compotes; or grilled fruits, soups, and low-fat yogurt.
- If you are on a long trip and can face food, eat really light, low-fat foods such as rice or oatcakes. Otherwise, try dry toast or a cheese biscuit.
- Sip small amounts of fresh lemon or lime juice in warm water.
- Peppermint and ginger herbal teas can also be sipped to calm the digestive tract and stomach.
- Recently on a cruise I suffered from seasickness and was told that if I ate a green apple very slowly it would help—and it did.

Useful Remedies

- Magnesium is nature's tranquillizer. If you tend to start feeling nervous the day before a trip, begin taking 200mg of magnesium three times a day for a couple of days prior to traveling.
- Ginger is really successful at reducing feelings of nausea, and you can take four ginger capsules 2 hours prior to travel. However, it is often more effective when you can taste the ginger.
- Make tea with a small piece of fresh root ginger and a little honey and take in a flask or thermos to sip during your trip. You could also take 1–2ml of the tincture in a little water.
- Take a high-strength vitamin B complex daily with meals to support your nerves.

Helpful Hints

- Stay fairly still and breathe calmly. Look ahead to the horizon and not downward to help keep the fluid in the ears balanced.
- Try to sit at the front of any vehicle.
- If possible, open a window.
- Avoid the company of people eating strong-smelling foods.
- A drop of peppermint oil on the tongue helps reduce feelings of nausea.
- You can even simply inhale the aroma of peppermint oil, as it has been shown to reduce feelings of nausea and subsequent vomiting.
- Acupressure can help control motion sickness. Press the point that is approximately 2 in. (5 cm) up from the center of your wrist on the underside of your arm (it's the point between two tendons). Press for 20 seconds every half hour or so to reduce symptoms. You can also wear Sea Bands, which work on a similar principle. Available from most large pharmacies.
- Try homeopathic Cocculus 30c. Take one pilule before traveling and one every few hours during the trip.

T

TREMORS   *(see also Alzheimer's Disease and Parkinson's Disease)*

This problem can be triggered by a huge variety of causes, such as extreme nervousness, excessive consumption of caffeine or alcohol, and/or an overactive thyroid gland. Recovering alcoholics and drug addicts often suffer tremors. If the tremors occur when resting or you suffer involuntary jerking, this may be associated with conditions such as Parkinson's disease or rheumatic fever. On rare occasions, tremors can be inherited. Mercury and heavy-metal toxicity are linked to tremors (if you have mercury amalgam fillings, see *Mercury Fillings*). Cigarettes are high in cadmium and nickel, so stop smoking. If you suffer from blood sugar problems, this could make symptoms worse (see *Low Blood Sugar*).

As certain prescription drugs are also known to have tremors as a side effect, check with your doctor. If your adrenal glands are totally exhausted, then tremors may result (see *Adrenal Exhaustion*).

Foods to Avoid

- Avoid any foods or drinks that contain aluminum at all costs (see *Alzheimer's Disease*).
- Greatly reduce any foods or drinks containing caffeine. This includes chocolate, soft drinks, guarana, coffee, and strong tea.
- Avoid alcohol and spicy foods, which are stimulants.
- Don't eat too many sugary, starchy foods, which can make you feel even more nervous.
- Avoid preservatives and additives.

Friendly Foods

- Generally you need calming foods, such as sweet potatoes, pasta, whole-wheat bread, brown rice, lentils, barley, cereals, and oats.
- Oatmeal made with organic rice milk, with a chopped raw apple or banana plus a little manuka honey to sweeten, makes a very calming breakfast or supper.
- Turkey, chicken, cooked tofu, bananas, wheat germ, avocados, sunflower seeds, pumpkin seeds, flaxseeds, and oily fish are all calming foods because they nourish the nerves.
- Almonds, dates, Brazil nuts, mustard, curry powder, and all green leafy vegetables are good sources of magnesium, which calms the muscles.
- Drink more water.
- Drink more green or white tea, which contains L-theanine, an amino acid that helps calm you down. Avoid drinking these teas at night, as they contain some caffeine, or ask for decaffeinated versions. Otherwise, you can take 100mg of L-theanine twice daily in between meals.

Useful Remedies

- Include a multi-vitamin/mineral supplement that contains a full spectrum of B vitamins to nourish your nerves and also contains at least 30mg of zinc. (Often when we are falling off to sleep our bodies jerk; this is usually due to a lack of zinc.)
- Calcium and magnesium help reduce muscle spasms. Take 400mg of calcium with 600mg of magnesium in divided doses, with the final dose being taken before going to bed.
- Either take four evening primrose oil capsules daily or 400mg of gamma-linolenic acid (GLA)—a fatty acid found in evening primrose oil that helps reduce tremors). **VC**

ULCERS, DUODENAL AND STOMACH   *(see Stomach Ulcers)*

VARICOSE VEINS   *(see also Circulation, Constipation, and Piles)*

Varicose veins are caused by long-term poor circulation and weakened valves in the veins, which allow blood to accumulate, thus stretching the vein walls. The most commonly affected areas are the legs, where the veins eventually can be clearly seen on the skin's surface. Over time they bulge, become bluish and lumpy looking, and can become painful.

If they are not treated, they can also ulcerate, especially in older people. Anything that slows the return of the blood from the legs to the heart will aggravate varicose veins.

This condition is closely linked to constipation because, if you strain when you go to the bathroom, blood is forced into your lower body, which makes the problem worse. Vein problems are also linked to standing or sitting for long hours, being overweight, pregnancy, and crossing your legs too much. Perhaps most frightening of all, vascular surgeons are seeing children as young as 11 with this problem, because they are "couch potatoes" who sit at computers or watch TV all day. (See also *Diabetes* and *Deep Vein Thrombosis*.)

Another common condition, known as thread or spider veins, involves chronically dilated and overly permeable capillaries near the surface of the skin. While they are harmless and rarely cause any problems, they can be distressing for cosmetic reasons. You can prevent them from developing or worsening by following much of the advice below. (See also *Helpful Hints*.)

When I became pregnant at 18, after working long hours standing in a supermarket, I developed varicose veins. In my 20s these were made worse when I worked for 9 years as an air stewardess and often had to be on my feet for 15 hours at a time. Today, I tend to sit at a desk for lengthy spans, which greatly restricts my circulation. My mother and father both had vein problems. Yes, you can inherit a tendency for veins—but if I had known then what I know now, I could definitely have prevented their onset. In my 40s I had some veins stripped, but the problem has returned. However, today, thanks to more efficient diagnostic techniques and improved surgical procedures, you can in many cases eliminate varicose veins, but it is much better to prevent them in the first place.

Foods to Avoid
- Cut down on heavy meals, red meat, and cheeses, as they're low in fiber and take a long time to pass through the bowel, potentially contributing to constipation. Furthermore, saturated, fried, and hydrogenated fats thicken the blood, which makes it travel more slowly through your veins and arteries, increasing the risk of vascular problems.
- Foods made with flour from any source tend to block the bowels; therefore, reduce your intake of flour-based foods, especially croissants, pies, pizzas, cakes, cookies, and so on. Choose grains that are easier to digest, meaning ones that are low in gluten, such as wholegrain spelt breads or 100% rye breads. Also eat more brown rice, rolled oats, quinoa, and barley.
- Coffee, tea, sodas, and especially alcohol will dehydrate the bowel.
- Also see *Constipation* and *Circulation*.

Friendly Foods
- Eat more bilberries, blueberries, blackberries, sweet potatoes, pumpkin, squash, cherries, apricots, spinach, spring greens, and cabbage. In addition, eat more citrus fruits, broccoli, red grapes, papaya, tomatoes, tea, and red wine, which are all rich sources of flavonoids and vitamin C—powerful antioxidants that help strengthen capillaries and reduce the risk of hemorrhoids, thrombosis, and bruises.
- Rose hips (try rose hip tea), buckwheat, and apple peels contain the bioflavonoid rutin, which also helps strengthen your veins. Buckwheat makes great pancakes and can also be added to breads and biscuits. You can buy organic buckwheat pancake mixes from most health stores.
- Avocados, sprouted seeds (such as alfalfa), eggs, raw wheat germ, and unprocessed nuts are rich in vitamin E, which reduces stickiness in the blood.
- Garlic, onions, ginger, and cayenne pepper all aid circulation.
- Eat plenty of fish, especially oily fish. The essential fatty acids (EFAs) they contain reduce pain and keep blood vessels soft and pliable. Aim for 2–3 portions per week. Eat more unrefined, preferably organic, sunflower, hemp, pumpkin, sesame, and flaxseeds, which are all high in essential fats and fiber. (See *Fats You Need To Eat*.)
- Drink more water; aim for 6–8 glasses a day of bottled or filtered water. Water maintains blood pressure and helps reduce constipation.

- Make sure that your diet contains plenty of fiber to prevent constipation. Fruits, vegetables, whole grains (such as brown rice and quinoa), beans, and lentils are your best sources. If you feel you need more than you're getting in your diet, skip the bran (a harsh, insoluble fiber) and use soluble fiber-rich cracked flaxseeds, such as Arrowhead Mills, or psyllium husks, instead. Both are available from your local health food store.
- Sprinkle oat bran over cereals and into smoothies. (See *General Health Hints* for a good basic smoothie recipe.)
- If constipation is a real problem for you, in addition to the fiber, water, and exercise recommended above and below, eat four prunes prior to each meal.

Useful Remedies

- For centuries plant extracts such as butcher's broom and horse chestnut seeds (commonly known as buckeyes) have been used to reduce the inflammation and swelling associated with leg problems, and science has now validated these age-old remedies. Dr John Wilkinson, a scientist who specializes in plant research, says: "We have found that saponins, a group of active agents found in the roots and seeds of these plants, constrict and strengthen veins, have anti-inflammatory properties, and reduce swelling, thus making venous return to the heart more efficient. The compounds in these plants are safe and can be taken internally in capsule form daily (but not during the first three months of pregnancy, or by people on blood-thinning drugs). Plant extracts can also be used topically in a cream or gel. We have found that butcher's broom is highly effective when taken in isolation, but its effects appear to be amplified when combined with horse chestnut, vitamin C, and the flavonoid rutin."

- Most health stores sell butcher's broom, which also reduces the heaviness, tingling, and cramping associated with varicose veins. Take 100–300mg of standardized extract 2–3 times daily, or try Ultra Vein-Gard Leg Therapy Cream, available from most online retailers.
- Horse chestnut seed extract can also be taken either in combination or on its own. Clinical trials have confirmed its ability to aid vein contraction, reduce vein fragility and permeability, and significantly reduce lower-limb swelling. You need 50–75mg of escin twice daily (escin is the active ingredient in horse chestnut). If you prefer a liquid, take 1–4ml twice a day.
- Another herb, gotu kola, has also shown impressive clinical results in treating both varicose veins and varicose ulcers by improving circulation in the lower limbs and stimulating connective tissue repair. Try taking 500mg twice daily with meals.
- Pycnogenol, pine bark extract, improves the elasticity of vein walls and reduces inflammation. Initially take 80mg twice daily for a month and then reduce to 80mg daily. **PN**
- Silica is an excellent mineral for toughening up veins. Take 200mg of silica compound daily. Try Cellfood Essential Liquid Silica **VC**
- An antioxidant complex containing vitamins A, C, and E, selenium, and Co-enzyme Q10 helps prevent free-radical damage to the blood vessels as well as aiding in connective tissue repair. Take 1–2g of vitamin C daily with meals and 400IU of natural-source, full-spectrum vitamin E, which also enhances circulation through its anti-clotting effects.
- If veins are sore and swollen, buy some witch hazel in tincture or cream form and apply directly to the veins. Witch hazel in capsules and tincture can also be taken internally to reduce the swelling. **VC**
- Apply a little vitamin E cream mixed with two drops of juniper oil topically where the skin is sore.
- If you have facial thread veins, try Jason Vitamin K Cream for the face, which contains bioflavonoids, ginkgo biloba, and calendula. It is available online and from most natural/health food stores. For a list of stores in your area, visit www.jason-natural.com or call 1-877-527-6601.

Helpful Hints

- If the veins are swollen, itchy, and painful, soak a bandage in cold witch hazel, apply it to the affected area, and wrap firmly for 30 minutes with the leg elevated. This should help reduce the swelling.

- For those who are on their feet all day, physiotherapist Geraldine Watkins recommends lying on the floor, bending the knees, and placing the lower legs on a chair or bed for 15 minutes daily to give the leg valves a rest and encourage excess fluid to be absorbed back into the system. If the legs are swollen, then a cold compress should be applied.

- It's vital for your overall health that you stay active. Even walking briskly for 45 minutes to an hour a day will help. Otherwise rebounding on a mini-trampoline, skipping, playing tennis, jogging, and dancing are all wonderful exercises for supporting veins. And if your legs ache, no matter what your job, swimming is the best all-around exercise for keeping legs healthy.

- Also, if you stand a lot, wear insoles to support your arches. They are available from any good pharmacy or back store. Also avoid heels over 2 in. (5 cm) and start wearing support tights or socks at the first sign of vein problems.

- If you are at a desk for much of the day, take regular breaks, look for some stairs, and climb them! Make sure you move for at least 30 minutes a day. While sitting, use a rocking footrest, available from office stores and online, as bending and circling the feet keeps circulation moving. When at your desk make sure your knees are lower than your hips, which reduces compression in the arteries and veins in the groin area. Also avoid wearing tight-fitting pants, which add to compression in the groin and the back-of-knee areas when seated for long periods.

- Avoid crossing your legs, doing heavy lifting, or putting any unnecessary pressure on your legs.

- Reflexology, acupuncture, and a firm massage can all help increase circulation. (See *Useful Information* at the back of this book.)

- If the veins are sore and throbbing, make a warm-water compress with added cypress and geranium essential oils. Use cold compresses to reduce any swelling.

- To prevent varicose veins, avoid constipation and/or straining to pass stools. Continually straining to go to the bathroom forces blood into your lower body, which makes the problem worse. Hemorrhoids are similar to varicose veins of the anus (see also *Constipation* and *Piles*).

- Facial thread veins can be treated using a fine needle, often called red vein treatment. The needle is quickly inserted into each end of the vein and a current passes through the needle, which cauterizes the tiny capillary. Then the needle is quickly injected down the length of the vein, which makes the vein disappear. Available at most electrolysis or laser hair removal centers. You then need to keep the treated areas dry for several days.

- You can also have spider veins lasered, which I found more effective. The laser literally "smashes" the spider vein and, although you may have some bruising for a few days, it works very well. To find a vein center near you, visit www.veindirectory.org

- To avoid facial thread veins in the first place, don't use very hot or very cold water on your face, as any extremes in temperature can cause delicate veins to rupture.

- Avoid strong winds, and if you are out on a boat or skiing, wear really thick protective creams.

- Avoid too much sunbathing.

- Finally, get a proper diagnosis, says John Scurr, a consultant vascular surgeon based at the Middlesex Hospital in London, UK. "Many people believe there is little point in having veins, hemorrhoids, and so on treated, thinking they will return. But these days newer diagnostic and treatment techniques are giving good long-term, and in many cases permanent, relief." For any further information about all aspects of vein problems, visit Dr Scurr's website: www.jscurr.com

VEGETARIANISM

This subject is obviously not a health condition, but as I receive numerous letters from parents who are concerned that their children are not getting sufficient nutrients from their diet, I thought I should include a few guidelines. Because of increasing awareness about the hormones given to livestock in this country and the living conditions for animals on commercial farms, more and more people are turning to a vegetarian diet, which basically means not eating any foods or products derived from the slaughter of animals. Generally a vegetarian diet is a healthy diet, and vegetarians tend to have fewer cases of arthritis and inflammatory conditions than meat eaters. But many people, especially teenagers who call themselves vegetarians, often have a pretty unhealthy diet that includes lots of dairy foods, especially melted cheese, plus refined sugar and white-flour-based foods. These people are at a higher risk of increased homocysteine levels, because they are more likely to have fewer B vitamins and zinc in their diet. (For full details about homocysteine, see *High Blood Pressure*.)

Vegetarians generally suffer less ill health, heart disease, and cancer than meat-eaters, mainly because vegetarian diets tend to be higher in fiber and lower in saturated fats. Many parents worry that their children will become deficient in nutrients, especially vitamin B12, iron, zinc, and vitamin D, but this tends to be more of a problem for vegans. Dr Shamin Daya, a nutritional physician based at the Wholistic Medical Centre in London, UK, says: "In clinical practice we often find that many people, including vegetarians and vegans who eat a highly refined diet, suffer from leaky gut syndrome. They should definitely investigate this possibility and take plenty of hemp seed protein-type powders. They should also make sure that they and their children eat as great a variety of foods as possible." (See *Leaky Gut*.)

Foods to Avoid
- Don't go overboard on full-fat cheeses, which are high in saturated fats.
- Products that are high in processed palm oil should be kept to a minimum, as they are also very high in saturated fats.
- Avoid too many starchy foods that are high in white flour, refined sugar, and unsaturated fats. (See *Fats You Need To Eat*.)

Friendly Foods
- Green leafy vegetables, sesame seeds, low-fat yogurts (organic soy), and Parmesan cheese are all high in calcium.
- For protein, eat lentils, quinoa, beans (especially soybeans), tempeh, miso, brown rice, peas, cereals, corn, organic almonds, Brazil nuts, peanuts, sunflower seeds, and sesame seeds, which also contain good levels of zinc.
- For non-vegans, mozzarella, goat's or sheep's cheese (such as feta) are better absorbed by the body than cow's products.
- Eggs and dried skimmed milk are rich sources of vitamin B12. Alfalfa sprouts and spirulina also contain small amounts.
- For carbohydrates, eat low-sugar cereals, oats, whole-wheat bread, brown rice and pasta, barley, amaranth, millet, buckwheat, and rye. Quinoa is an excellent source of protein.
- Potatoes, sweet potatoes, parsnips, pumpkin, turnips, and rutabaga are also good sources of carbohydrates.
- Red or yellow vegetables, carrots, tomatoes, pumpkin, sweet potatoes, dried apricots, and leafy green vegetables are all rich in vitamin A.
- Nuts and seeds are high in essential fats.
- Wheat germ can be sprinkled on cereals and desserts as a rich source of B vitamins.

- Mushrooms and peas also contain B-group vitamins.
- Use unrefined walnut, sunflower, and olive oils for salad dressings.
- Iron is found in leafy green vegetables, whole-wheat bread, blackstrap molasses, eggs, dried fruits (especially apricots), beans, seeds, pulses (peas and chickpeas), nuts, chocolate, and cocoa.
- Eat plenty of fruits that are rich in vitamin C, such as kiwi and cherries, as vitamin C aids absorption of iron from foods.
- Use organic soy-, rice-, hemp-, or pea-based protein powders in smoothies. (See *General Health Hints* for a basic smoothie recipe.)
- Instead of sugar use xylitol, stevia, or organic agave syrup, which have minimal impact on blood sugar levels.

Useful Remedies
- Take a high-strength vitamin B complex daily with breakfast or lunch.
- Take a multi-vitamin/mineral that contains a full spectrum of B vitamins, plus zinc (30mg) and selenium (100mcg) and that is suitable for vegetarians. If your multi has good amounts of B vitamins, then you do not need to take them separately.
- If you have been found to be low in iron, take a formula such as Spatone. Available worldwide from health stores.

Helpful Hints
- Most bookstores now sell a huge range of healthy vegetarian cookbooks. Treat yourself to a couple, and remember that the greater the variety of foods you eat, the more nutrients you will be ingesting.

VERTIGO
(see also Adrenal Exhaustion, Ménière's Syndrome, and Stress)

Around three in every ten adults over 65 suffer from vertigo—a very unpleasant sensation of moving or spinning or a feeling that you are losing your balance, even when you are standing or sitting still. It can also be accompanied by nausea. Symptoms usually last for a few minutes but can continue for hours, days or, in extreme cases, much longer.

Such symptoms may be triggered by impacted earwax, blockage of the eustachian tube, or a viral infection in the balancing mechanism of the inner ear (see *Catarrh* and *Sinus Problems*). High blood pressure can also be a factor, as can iron deficiency (see *Anemia*).

Vertigo is also linked to blood sugar problems (see *Adrenal Exhaustion* and *Low and High Blood Sugar*) and poor circulation. It is also a symptom of Ménière's syndrome and may also be triggered by an injury to the head or neck. Beta blockers and some prescription drugs can trigger an attack, so make sure to carefully note any contraindications with drugs. Nutritional physician Dr Shamin Daya adds, "In practice, we have also found that some patients with vertigo are deficient in zinc."

Extreme exhaustion and an overgrowth of the yeast candida may also be contributing factors in vertigo (see also *Candida*), as can a misalignment of the neck and skull. If you suspect this is the cause, consult a cranial osteopath or chiropractor as soon as possible.

Dutch researchers found that as many as 50% of people with chronic dizziness are actually suffering from some type of cardiovascular disease (see *Heart Disease*), and more than 60% of patients have two or more causes for their problem. Therefore, if you suffer from vertigo that continues for more than a couple of weeks, consult your doctor for a thorough check-up and possibly X-rays.

Nutritionist Gareth Zeal says: "We often see patients with this problem who may be low in iron, so this should also be tested, and if people are extremely stressed it can trigger vertigo. Once they reduce their stress levels, symptoms can disappear."

Naturopath Stephen Langley adds: "Many people who are chronically stressed will not have been absorbing nutrients such as zinc or iron from their diet, possibly for quite some time. And once stress levels are reduced and the gut is working properly, then as absorption is restored, symptoms are often alleviated." (See *Adrenal Exhaustion* and *Stress*.)

Foods to Avoid

- Generally you need to cut down on saturated fats found in full-fat animal-sourced milk and dairy products, meat, mass-produced high-fat chocolates, cakes, cookies, pies, sausages, and so on.
- Avoid caffeine (especially in cappuccinos, chocolates, and soft drinks), fried foods, alcohol, and aspartame.
- Cut down on your intake of sodium-based salts; there are now plenty of magnesium- and potassium-based salts available from health stores.

Friendly Foods

- If you have a specific ear problem, vitamin A and carotene-rich foods are needed for sensory cells in the inner ear to function normally. Eat more oily fish and fish oils, sweet potatoes, pumpkin, papaya, watercress, apricots, and sweet potatoes.
- Liver is very high in vitamin A, but only eat it once a week.
- Eat more garlic, onions, and ginger.
- Calf's or lamb's liver, eggs, and leafy green vegetables are also a rich source of iron and vitamin A.
- Use organic rice, oat, or almond milk instead of cow's milk.
- Eat more sunflower, pumpkin, and flaxseeds, which are rich in essential fats and zinc. Also use their unrefined oils for salad dressings.
- Eat more bananas, dried fruit, fish, and sunflower seeds, which are rich in potassium.
- See *General Health Hints*.

Useful Remedies

- Take 25,000IU of vitamin A per day for one week. The inner ear needs a high concentration of vitamin A, and sensory cells are dependent upon vitamin A. NB: If you are pregnant or planning to become pregnant, only take 3000IU of vitamin A daily.
- A full-spectrum B complex helps nourish the nerve endings in the inner ear.
- Take a multi-mineral that contains at least 100mg of calcium and 99mg of potassium. The potassium reduces sodium (salt) levels in the body. High levels of sodium in the blood can make symptoms worse.
- Try Zinc by Twinlab, which contains three types of zinc (picolinate, gluconate, and dihydrate). These are easy to absorb and improve zinc levels quickly. Initially take two capsules daily for 6 weeks, then reduce to one a day for 6 weeks, and then take just one capsule per week.
- The herb ginkgo biloba helps improve circulation to the inner ear. Take 120–150mg of standardized extract twice daily until symptoms ease. NB: People taking anticoagulant drugs need to check with their doctor before taking any ginkgo. Take no more than 120mg daily.
- Take up to 2000mg of a vitamin C and bioflavonoid complex daily in divided doses with meals.
- Ginger capsules can be taken 4–6 times a day during an attack to help reduce feelings of nausea.

- Co-enzyme Q10, a vitamin-like substance, helps improve cellular function in the brain and may help alleviate vertigo. Take 100mg daily with either breakfast or lunch.
- As low vitamin D levels are associated with an increased risk of falling, take 1000IU of D3 daily. This also greatly boosts the immune system.

Helpful Hints
- If you smoke, stop. Smoking thickens your blood and slows circulation to the head.
- Avoid rapid body movements, especially of the head. Avoid standing up quickly after lying down, especially first thing in the morning.
- Use two pillows at night and avoid sleeping on the affected side as much as possible.
- Reduce stress levels and make sure you are getting sufficient sleep.
- See a chiropractor or cranial osteopath to make sure your neck and spine are not misaligned, which can trigger problems in the ear. Hypnotherapy and acupuncture have also helped in some cases. (See *Useful Information*.)
- If you have been taking prescription drugs for a long period of time, check with your doctor, as high blood pressure and beta blockers are known to cause this problem.
- Ask your doctor to check if you have impacted earwax, which can trigger vertigo-like symptoms. (See *Glue Ear*.)

VIRAL INFECTIONS
(see Immune Function)

VITILIGO

This is a difficult multi-factorial condition that causes natural pigment production to stop and white patches to appear on the skin. The darker your skin color, the more obvious and distressing the appearance of your skin can become. This condition has been linked to low stomach acid levels, stress, low levels of B vitamins, pernicious anemia, and an overactive thyroid gland. It could also be triggered by nutritional deficiencies or a fungal overgrowth. Dr Shamin Daya, a nutritional physician based at the Wholistic Medical Centre in Harley Street, London, says: "In patients with this autoimmune condition, we have found in clinical practice that certain parasites in the gut produce chemical toxins, which can have a "bleaching" effect on the skin; therefore, it's well worth patients have a Genova Test to find out if parasites are indeed a contributing factor." (See *Allergies*.)

Foods to Avoid
- Alcohol, caffeine, processed foods, and refined sugar deplete the body of B vitamins.
- See *General Health Hints*.

Friendly Foods
- Papaya and pineapple contain enzymes that aid digestion and improve the absorption of nutrients.
- Foods rich in B vitamins include wheat germ, brewer's yeast, calf's liver, eggs, whole grains (such as brown rice and quinoa), nuts, fish, chicken, turkey, dates, oats, cereals, mushrooms, green vegetables (especially kale, watercress, broccoli, and spinach), black strap molasses, fruits, and apricots.
- As low zinc levels are linked to vitiligo, eat more fresh fish, nuts, and sunflower and pumpkin seeds.
- Live, low-fat yogurt also aids digestion.

- Drink plenty of water; aim for at least 6–8 glasses daily.
- Eat more foods high in natural carotenes, such as apricots, cantaloupe melon, pumpkin, carrots, tomatoes, sweet potatoes, papaya, red and yellow peppers, and mangoes.

Useful Remedies

- As lack of stomach acid is also linked to this problem, take betaine hydrochloride (HCl) for up to 2 years with main meals. If you have active stomach ulcers, take a digestive enzyme without HCl with main meals instead. **VC**
- Take a high-strength B complex, plus 400mcg of folic acid and 500mcg of vitamin B12.
- PABA is a B-vitamin; take 100mg three times daily to help to re-pigment the skin.
- Include 1–2g of vitamin C daily, as it is vital for collagen production. Take in divided doses with food.
- Take 2mg of copper per day. Copper makes up a number of enzymes that are required for skin pigmentation. Take 30–40mg of zinc at the same time. Both of these are usually found in most multi-vitamin/mineral formulas.
- Take 22.72mg per pound of body weight of the amino acid phenylalanine on an empty stomach in divided doses daily. Combining this supplement with careful sun bathing should help to re-pigment the skin. Take this suggested dose for one month and then reduce to half the dose until desired effects are achieved. If no positive results are noted after 3 months, discontinue. Use a high SPF sunscreen and don't sit in the midday sun. Just take 15 minutes twice daily for a few days and gradually the skin should re-pigment.
- Natural-source carotenes are great for the skin. Take daily.

- The herb ashwagandha has been found to help prevent abnormalities in skin pigmentation if 1–2g is taken daily. Again, try this dose for 2 months, and then reduce to 1g daily until it is no longer needed.

Helpful Hints

- Some people believe that small amounts of sun are beneficial for vitiligo. However, I believe that you should keep areas of vitiligo out of the sun or at the very least use a strong sunscreen (see *Sunburn*). Never allow these areas to burn, as your skin has no natural protection against the sun.

VOMITING

(see also Food Poisoning)

Vomiting can have many causes, the most obvious being food poisoning, food intolerances, and binge drinking, but it could also be caused by prescription drugs that disagree with you. Morning sickness, migraines, bulimia, drinking too much alcohol, and eating a really high-fat, rich meal can all trigger nausea. If an infant vomits violently within a few minutes of being fed, you need to seek medical attention. Urgent medical attention is also needed if a child begins vomiting after drinking a poison such as bleach, or swallowing an object.

Dehydration is the biggest concern with vomiting. If the person is small, also has diarrhea, and cannot keep down any fluids, obviously the rate of dehydration will be much faster than in a tall, weighty person. If a baby or small child suffers frequent vomiting and diarrhea, they are at a greater risk of dehydration and need immediate medical attention.

When some people vomit, low blood pressure can kick in, thus triggering loss of consciousness, in which case a saline IV is needed to bring the person around; seek urgent medical attention. If you suffer from low blood pressure and begin vomiting frequently, call a doctor. If you have severe abdominal pain or begin vomiting any blood, have a fever, and the vomiting has continued for more than 24 hours, seek urgent medical help. Nausea after fatty foods can be related to liver congestion, in which case you need to greatly reduce your intake of fats, coffee and alcohol. (See *Liver Problems.*)

Foods to Avoid
- See all dietary advice under *Food Poisoning*.

Friendly Foods
- Sip clear fluids, such as boiled water, fruit juices, or a powdered electrolyte drink such as Pedialyte (available from all pharmacies).
- If you can tolerate it, sip a little ginger ale or ginger tea.
- Don't drink more than a couple of tablespoons of liquid at any one time until the nausea has stopped.
- Once vomiting has stopped, gently increase your fluid intake. Drink no coffee or black tea for 24 hours.
- Slowly begin eating again. Dry toast, dry crackers, arrowroot, tapioca or semolina, fresh soups, a little poached fish with mashed potatoes, low-fat yogurts, or brown rice should be fine.
- Once you feel you are able to eat, start replacing lost potassium by eating high-potassium foods such as bananas and most fresh fruits.

Useful Remedies
- (Don't take these supplements until at least 24 hours after the vomiting has stopped.)
- Drinking a small capful of pure aloe vera juice before eating will help soothe the gut. Lakewood Organic Juices make an excellent pure aloe juice. Available from many supermarkets and health stores. www.lakewoodjuices.com
- Fifteen drops of deglycerrhized licorice twice daily will help soothe the digestive tract.
- Take two capsules of a probiotic that contains acidophilus/bifidus daily for a couple of weeks. This will help replenish healthy bacteria in the bowel. **VC**

Helpful Hints
- Place some essential oils of ginger and peppermint under your nose; this greatly helps reduce the dreadful feeling of nausea.
- Take one dose of homeopathic Nux Vomica 6x or Arsenicum Album 6x every 30 minutes (up to 10 doses daily) until symptoms ease.

WARTS

(see also Immune Function)

Warts are caused by a varied assortment of viruses that invade the skin, causing cells to multiply rapidly and form raised lumps. When your immune system is weak, you are more likely to pick up one of these viruses. Warts are contagious, and touching warts can transfer viruses to new sites and encourage new warts to develop. They are commonly found on the soles of the feet (see *Plantar Warts*) and on the hands or arms. They can also occur if your tissues become too acid. (See *Acid–Alkaline Balance.*)

Foods to Avoid
- See *Foods to Avoid* under *Acid–Alkaline Balance* and *Immune Function*.

Friendly Foods
- Since vitamin A and carotenes are vital for healing the skin, eat more leafy greens—especially spinach, watercress, cabbage, broccoli, and kale—pumpkin, papaya, apricots, sweet potatoes, tomatoes, cantaloupe melon, oily fish, and liver.
- Eat more sulfur-containing foods, such as onions, leeks, garlic, Brussels sprouts, cabbage, and broccoli.
- Eat more low-fat, bio yogurt.
- See *Friendly Foods* under *Immune Function*.

Useful Remedies
- If you are not pregnant take 20,000IU of vitamin A daily for 1 month to help fight the virus. **NB: If you are pregnant or planning to become pregnant, take no more than 3000IU of pure vitamin A daily.** After a month, switch to natural-source carotene complex capsules, which are safe and non-toxic. Take 1 or 2 capsules daily. **SVHC**
- Take 2g of vitamin C twice daily in divided doses with food to boost your immune system.
- Take a high-strength multi-vitamin/mineral that contains 200mcg of selenium and 30mg of zinc.
- Olive leaf extract is highly anti-viral; take 500mg twice daily for a month.

Helpful Hints

- Oregano or thyme therapeutic grade essential oils are very powerful. Dab a small amount of neat oil onto the wart twice daily until it disappears. It will take about 2–3 weeks.
- Dissolve a little baking soda in a drop or two of water in the palm of your hand. Apply the resulting paste to the wart, cover with a bandage, and change daily. The wart should be gone within a week.
- You could also crush half an aspirin, place this on a bandage, and immediately place it over the wart. Change the bandage daily. It's the salicylic acid that helps get rid of the wart. It should disappear within 2 weeks.
- Dandelion tincture can be added to the wart through a small piece of card in which you have cut a small hole. Dab on the tincture for 3 days.
- Apply the following mixture twice daily for up to 10 days: add a little freshly crushed garlic to the contents of one vitamin E and one vitamin A capsule and mix with some zinc cream. Apply only to the site of the wart, and cover it with a bandage. If the skin surrounding the wart becomes inflamed, eliminate the garlic.
- Homeopathic Thuja 6c or Causticum 6c can be taken twice daily, but you must stop this remedy as soon as you see an improvement.

WATER ON THE KNEE *(see also Water Retention)*

This condition is triggered when the little fluid-filled sacks that surround the knee joint become inflamed. The problem is usually caused by a knock or a fall, or by a chronic condition such as arthritis.

Foods to Avoid
- Reduce or avoid red meat, salt, caffeine, black tea, and all highly processed sugary, starchy foods. All of these can exacerbate inflammation in the body.

- Any foods that are high in salt, such as potato chips, olives, and preserved meats, will make the body retain more water.
- Avoid foods from the nightshade family (tomatoes, potatoes, eggplant, and sweet peppers), especially if you suffer from any arthritis-type conditions.
- See *Foods to Avoid* under *Bursitis*.

Friendly Foods
- Since an over-acid system can make this condition worse, eat more dark leafy greens, especially watercress, kale, spinach, cabbage, broccoli, and bok choy, as they are rich in magnesium, which helps alkalize the body. (See *Acid–Alkaline Balance*.)
- Squash, fruits, vegetables, and organic raw honey also help alkalize the body.
- Add a teaspoon of apple cider vinegar and a touch of raw, organic honey to boiled water that has cooled and sip throughout the day to help re-alkalize the body.
- Eat plenty of potassium-rich foods: bananas, papaya, celery, most fruits, flaxseeds, sunflower seeds, pumpkin seeds, and nuts.
- Eat more avocado and raw wheat germ, which are rich in vitamin E.
- Pineapple is a rich source of bromelain, which has anti-inflammatory properties. Cherries are also anti-inflammatory.
- Eat oily fish, such as mackerel, pilchards, salmon, and sardines, twice a week.
- Drink plenty of water. For details as to why, see *Water Retention*.
- Use nori seaweed flakes or kelp flakes instead of sodium-based salts.
- Instead of sugar, use small amounts of xylitol, stevia, or organic agave syrup, which have a less of an effect on blood sugar.

Useful Remedies
- Silica helps strengthen tissues in the knees. Take 200mg daily or drink more Fiji water, which is high in silica.
- Take 1g of vitamin C with bioflavonoids twice daily to help reduce swelling.
- Bromelain from pineapples is highly anti-inflammatory; take 500mg twice daily while symptoms last.
- Take 30mg of zinc per day, as it helps the body fight inflammation.
- Take 2g of omega-3 fish oils daily, which are highly anti-inflammatory.
- MSM is an organic form of sulfur that counteracts inflammation and pain. Start by taking 1g a day and then increase to 2g daily. It is great for your skin, too.
- Celery seed extract acts as a mild diuretic, which helps flush excess fluid from the body. Take 200mg twice daily with food.

Helpful Hints
- At the onset of inflammation, rest the affected area and avoid putting pressure on the joint for a few days. Keep your leg raised as much as possible.
- Alternating hot and cold compresses can help disperse the swelling.
- Homeopathic Ruta 6c, taken twice daily for 3–5 days, really helps reduce knee problems. Also Apis 6c, taken three times daily between meals, helps reduce the swelling.
- Perseverance with this regime is important, as knee problems can take some time to heal.
- Regular acupuncture not only greatly reduces the pain, but also has a major impact on the swelling. (See *Useful Information* at the back of this book.)
- Ask at your local health or sports store for a knee brace that contains magnets, as magnets help increase blood flow to the area, thereby boosting the amount of oxygenated blood in the knee and speeding healing.

WATER RETENTION (edema)

(see also Allergies and Rheumatoid Arthritis)

Water retention can be seen throughout the body; however, unlike water on the knee, general water retention is not caused by an injury. It can usually be seen in the hands, legs, ankles, feet, or around the eyes. The most common cause is excess sodium-based salt in the body, but it can also be triggered by food intolerances (the usual culprits being wheat and dairy products from cows—see *Allergies*). It can also occur during pregnancy or when taking the contraceptive pill or HRT. It is very common in women, especially those over the age of 60.

Another trigger can be standing for too long in hot weather. Occasionally, fluid retention can denote more serious problems that affect the heart, kidneys, or liver. Therefore, if these suggestions do not work after 2–3 weeks, please have a thorough check-up by your doctor. Some people mistakenly think that if they cut back on their fluid intake, their water retention will disappear—but in fact, the opposite is true. The problem is that, as we get older, water finds it harder to penetrate your cells; therefore, a person can be suffering from water retention but technically be dehydrated. The secret is getting the water into the cells that need it.

Foods to Avoid

- Cut down on high-salt foods and pre-packaged meals, and don't add salt to meals.
- Hot dogs, cheese, sauces, pizza, olives, potato chips, preserved meats, and pickles can all be high in sodium.
- Some breakfast cereals contain more salt than the average bag of potato chips.
- Don't add salt while cooking unless it's a potassium- or magnesium-based salt. Powdered kelp and nori seaweed flakes are two other good salt alternatives.
- Even some chocolate drinks can be very high in salt.
- Alcoholic and caffeinated foods and drinks act as diuretics. They cause water to be leached out of the cells where it is needed, which increases dehydration.

Friendly Foods

- Eat lots of fresh fruit and vegetables, as they are very rich in potassium.
- Include more spinach, celery, kale, watercress, cabbage, bananas, almonds, sunflower seeds, apricots, sweet potatoes, raisins, blackberries, cherries, bilberries, and blueberries in your diet.
- Drink at least 6–8 glasses of pure filtered water daily.
- Eat good-quality protein, such as fish, eggs, quinoa, chicken, turkey, or tempeh, at least once a day.
- Otherwise, try a protein powder drink for breakfast. You can find a great smoothie recipe under *General Health Hints*.
- Ask at your health store for various seaweeds, such as kombu, arame, nori, or kelp. Soak them for 5 minutes, chop, and then sprinkle over meals. Seaweeds are high in potassium and really help remove excess fluid from the body. They are also high in organic sodium, but this does not cause the body to hold water to the same extent as normal table salt.
- Drink more green or white tea, which acts as a natural diuretic.

Useful Remedies

- Dandelion leaf tea or tincture is a gentle diuretic that puts more potassium into the body than it takes out. 1ml can be taken three times a day. **VC**
- Take 1–2g of vitamin C in an ascorbate form with meals in divided doses, which can help lymph drainage. **VC**
- Take a vitamin B complex that contains 100mg of B6, which is a natural diuretic.

- Take one 200mg celery seed extract capsule twice daily. Celery is a natural liver and kidney cleanser and helps neutralize excess acid in tissues. **VC**
- The herb gotu kola stimulates circulation in the lower limbs and improves lymph drainage. Take up to 500mg twice daily when symptoms are acute.
- Celloid sodium sulfate is known as the problem-fluid remover. Take 200mg three times daily. Try NuAge Nat Sulph. **VC**

Helpful Hints

- Try to elevate your feet for at least 15 minutes every day. Lie on the floor and place your lower limbs higher than your waist. This really helps excess fluids drain via the lymphatic system.
- Rebounding on a mini-trampoline is particularly good for enhancing lymph drainage. Have regular lymph-drainage massages. (See *Useful Information* at the back of this book.)
- The homeopathic drops Lymphomyosot, made by Heel, can be used to help lymph drainage. For more information, visit www.heelusa.com
- Do regular exercise, such as swimming, walking, skipping, or jogging.
- Skin brushing is a great way to remove excess fluids from the body. Start at the feet and work toward the heart. Then brush your chest and shoulders, once again working toward the heart area. When you brush your arms, work from the hands up toward the shoulders and throat area.
- If you are overweight, try to lose weight.

WEIGHT PROBLEMS

(see also Allergies, Candida, Insulin Resistance, Low Blood Sugar, Stress, and Thyroid)

In 1991 only 12.2% of women and 11.7% of men were obese, whereas now about 34% of the adult US population is clinically obese. Childhood obesity has more than tripled over the past 30 years and now affects at least one in every five children. If this growth in obesity continues unabated, then children and young people will undoubtedly have a shorter life expectancy than their parents.

This is shocking if you also consider that obesity contributes to more than 300,000 premature deaths, which could have been prevented, a year in the US alone. It's time for us all to take greater responsibility for our health.

Research has shown that women who gain more than 44 pounds after the age of 18 (above the weight they should be for their height and age) are 2.5 times more likely eventually to suffer a stroke. People who are significantly overweight are five times more likely to develop late-onset (type II) diabetes. More than 80% of people with type II diabetes are overweight when first diagnosed. Obese men are 33% more likely to die of cancer and this figure rises to 55% in women.

The basics of finding your perfect weight and then maintaining it are: controlling your blood sugar levels, eating a varied diet that contains plenty of fiber, and doing sufficient exercise. If you feel that you have truly tried every diet and you are still finding it hard to lose weight, then you may have an underactive thyroid, a chronic food intolerance that is causing water retention, or insulin resistance. Steroids are also a well-known trigger of weight gain.

The human body contains 30–40 million fat cells, and any extra calories we eat are stored as fat. A lot of people now do regular exercise, but the majority still do not. Lack of regular exercise slows down our metabolic rate and toxins begin to accumulate. The net result is "middle-age spread," which is happening to young and old alike.

How many overweight people do you know who regularly say: "I really cannot imagine why I'm overweight, I hardly ever touch bread, cakes, chocolate and so on,"—but when they think no one is looking, they eat a chocolate croissant followed by a cappuccino? I realize that weight gain can have a multitude of causes, **but 98% of people who are overweight are simply eating too much and doing insufficient exercise.** After all, if we are truly honest about obesity, I have yet to see anyone leave a prison-type camp looking overweight. This book is about living consciously—you can choose. Choose what you put in your mouth, and you can choose your weight. And if you choose to lose weight, then do it for yourself; if you are happy being "overweight," then so be it.

Meanwhile, I believe it is important to stop thinking about the word "diet' and start thinking about "eating more healthily for the rest of our lives." There are cabbage diets, protein-only diets, carbohydrate-free diets, eat-a-Twinkie-only-at-night diets, and so on. Almost half of women between the ages of 25 and 35 are on a diet, but in the long term **they don't work.**

Naturopath Stephen Langley says: "The major problem today is blood sugar problems; basically, thanks to our increased love of refined sugary, starchy foods, our bodies are over-producing insulin to try to balance loss of sensitivity in our cells. Insulin causes excess sugar to be converted into fat and excess insulin then prevents that fat from being released by the body."

If this is allowed to continue, not only does the person pile on weight, but also the insidious insulin resistance can eventually lead to full-blown diabetes.

If you are 20% or more over your ideal weight, you are technically obese. This extra weight puts undue stress on your back, legs, joints, circulation, and internal organs. Obesity increases the body's susceptibility to infection, the risk of heart disease, high blood pressure, arthritis, late- onset (type II) diabetes, stroke, and other serious health problems that can result in premature death.

So how do you know if, for your height, build, age, and sex, you're "normal," overweight or obese? There have been numerous charts produced, but the most recognized method that's easy to do is the Body Mass Index (BMI). Your BMI is simply the ratio of your weight in kilograms to your height in meters squared; it's a good rough guide and is widely used. The "normal" range is 18.5–24.9, over 25 is considered overweight, over 30 is moderately obese, and over 40 is very obese. For example, a man of 1.83 m (6ft) who weighs 80 kg (176lb) has a BMI of 24. This means he falls in the normal weight category. However, a man who is 1.52 m (5ft) tall and weighs 80 kg (176lb) has a BMI of 34, which is considered obese. This man's "normal" weight should be no more than 127.6lbs.

The math is a little more complicated using US measurements, but not impossible. Divide your weight in pounds by your height in inches squared, and then multiply that number by 703. Let's take the example above: a man who is 6ft tall and weighs 176lb. (Remember that there are 12 inches in a foot.) To calculate his BMI:

> 176lb divided by (72 in. x 72 in.) = 0.03395
> Then multiply this number by 703 (0.03395 x 703)
> BMI = 24

Now you can calculate your BMI and use it to determine what your target weight should be. (Visit www.cdc.gov/healthyweight/index.html for an easy-to-use BMI calculator that will do all of the math for you.)

Many fad diets suggest consuming lots of protein and few to no carbohydrates, such as rice or potatoes, as protein can be harder to digest and metabolize and therefore releases its energy more slowly. People do experience initial weight loss on this diet, perhaps due in large part to the exclusion of wheat and refined sugars (most people's main carbohydrate). However, this diet isn't a good long-term weight-loss strategy, as too much protein makes the blood and tissues too acid, which can become a high-risk factor for osteoporosis in later life. Excess protein also places a great burden on the kidneys and unbalances metabolism. The saturated fat that accompanies animal protein can increase the risk of heart disease. A far better approach is to eat as great a variety of foods as possible and to make life-long changes to your diet, while cutting down on wheat-based, white starchy foods.

Many people find that they lose weight easily on a trial "exclusion diet" for food intolerances, while still eating heartily. The most common food intolerances are usually starchy or sugary in nature (wheat, corn, milk from cows, refined sugar, and potatoes), and this is not unlike the low-carbohydrate diet mentioned above. But avoiding any food that is badly tolerated, whether it is "fattening" or not, usually enables rapid weight loss. Also, naturopath Stephen Langley says: "If people can eat according to their blood type, they will naturally lose weight. For example, people with Type A blood will tend to put on weight if they eat meat and dairy products, whereas those with Type O will increase their weight by eating gluten and corn. Therefore, I suggest that people read Peter J D'Adamo's books such as *Fatigue: Fight It with The Blood Type Diet* (Berkley Trade) or *Eat Right For Your Type* (Putnam Adult)."

Finally, don't be tempted to cut corners and use weight-loss pills that claim to be fat blockers. These types of products encourage you to eat a cheeseburger, and then take a pill so you won't gain weight. This is definitely not the way to try to improve your health. Like low-fat diets, they can stop you from absorbing essential fats (the healthy fats), as well as other fat-soluble nutrients that depend on fats for transportation into the body, such as vitamins A, D, E, and K. Weight loss is best done slowly and for the long haul if you want to improve not just your weight but also your health.

At the end of the day you need to ask yourself honestly:
1. Am I exercising enough?
2. What foods do I tend to eat and crave the most? If the answer to this is wheat, flour, breads, pies, cookies, sodas, coffee, etc., then you may well have a leaky hut and fungal overgrowth problems, such as candida, as well as food intolerances (commonly to refined carbohydrates, wheat, and possibly gluten, caffeine, sugar, or alcohol). All of these are huge factors in people who cannot lose weight. (See under *Allergies* to organize a test.)
3. Could my thyroid be underactive? This is incredibly common; to answer this question see the *Thyroid* section.
4. Am I drinking 6–8 glasses of water a day?
Be honest with your answers. Face the truth!

Meanwhile, a research study from The University of Buffalo in New York found that 40% of obese men had low testosterone levels. Therefore, both men and women should have their hormone levels checked by a doctor. If testosterone and other hormones such as DHEA and estrogen are too low, you can easily supplement them as needed. (See *Menopause*.)

Foods to Avoid
- Cut down on refined carbohydrates: white breads and rice, croissants, Danish pastries, pies, desserts, anything with pastry, burgers, pizzas, and melted-cheese-type snacks. By all means have a treat once a week or so, but once you start losing weight and stop eating these foods all the time, your need for them will gradually disappear.
- Gluten, found in grains, is very hard for the body to digest. Eating gluten-containing foods

can trigger overeating, because you are not absorbing the nutrients that you should be from the grains (such as zinc, magnesium, selenium, vitamin C, and B vitamins). As a result, you are getting the calories but not the corresponding energy, which makes you crave these foods even more. Try eliminating any foods that contain gluten for a few weeks; all supermarkets sell alternatives.

- Artificial sweeteners are found in more than 3,000 foods and low-calorie drinks, but they place a strain on the liver and can slow weight loss. The worst offender is aspartame. Manufactured fructose, maltose, dextrose, etc. should also be avoided.
- Cut down on fried, processed, and fast foods. Indian foods in sauces are among the worst offenders.
- Research has shown that many adults are consuming up to 46 teaspoons of sugar a day. Keep in mind that many foods that are labeled as being "low-fat" may be high in sugar or sweeteners; always check the labels. Reduce all foods high in refined and artificial sugars, which will convert to fat inside the body if not used up during exercise. Remember, though, we all need a certain amount of fat, and fat-free diets are dangerous. (See *Fats You Need To Eat*,)
- Chocolates are highly acid forming and, although dark chocolate is high in antioxidants and can often contain fewer calories than potato chips, please remember that it may still be high in saturated fats and sugar. The occasional piece of dark chocolate is fine, but keep in mind the word "occasional." You could also look for sugar- and dairy-free chocolates such as Glamour Food, which is made with coconut oil, goji and acai berries. Glamour Food is only available from the Organic Pharmacy, 453 North Beverly Drive, Beverly Hills, CA 90210. Tel: 1-310-272-7275.

- Avoid salted nuts, chips, and preserved meats.
- Reduce sodium-based table salt.
- Avoid all hard margarines, full-fat milk, and full-fat cheeses.
- Stop ordering desserts or try eating the fruit salad or a low-fat yogurt instead.
- In most cases, the weight is coming from foods that you tend to eat every day or crave the most. Start keeping a food diary and note down what you eat and when—you will soon know the culprits!

Friendly Foods

- Eat more organic foods, which contain fewer pesticides. Pesticides live in your fat tissue and are really hard to eliminate.
- In the summer, eat nothing but fruit before noon. This is a great way to kick start a sluggish metabolism. (See *General Health Hints* for a great smoothie recipe with added protein powder that keeps you well satisfied until lunchtime.)
- In the winter, try eating gluten-free oatmeal with a grated raw apple and a few raisins for breakfast. This should help reduce mid-morning cravings.
- Instead of white-flour-based foods, use whole-wheat, stone-ground bread and experiment with various pastas and meals made from corn, rice, spelt, quinoa, buckwheat, millet, lentil, amaranth, and potato flour.
- Instead of wheat-based breads, try amaranth or rice crackers or oatcakes. Spread a little humus or cottage cheese on them or add a tomato and a cucumber for a quick healthy snack.
- Eat far more brown rice, lentils, chickpeas, barley, and dried (or canned) beans.
- Eat plenty of fresh fruits and vegetables—the more fiber the better. Cabbage, broccoli and cauliflower are great healthy foods, but avoid cabbage and cauliflower if you have an underactive thyroid or have Type O blood. (See *Thyroid*.)

- Onions, ginger, spring greens, spinach, bok choy, celery, pineapple, and apples are all great foods for assisting weight loss. Radicchio, chicory, fennel, celeriac, and bitter foods help cleanse the liver, which also aids weight loss. (See *Liver Problems*.)
- Use organic rice milk, skimmed milk, or skimmed goat's milk instead of full-fat milk. Experiment with almond or coconut milks.
- Eat one portion of quality protein a day, such as fish, eggs, chicken, or cooked tofu, as protein balances blood sugar for a longer period of time. Try to eat this protein at breakfast and/or lunchtime.
- A small baked potato is fine (sweet potato would be even better), but fill it with low-fat bio yogurt and chives instead of butter. Or use a spread such as Olivio, or hemp- or pumpkin-seed butters. Available from good health stores.
- Always eat breakfast. There are dozens of organic low-sugar cereals now available, and another great breakfast is organic oatmeal made with half water and half rice milk. Use a few raisins and a chopped apple to sweeten.
- If you are desperate for sugar, try xylitol, stevia, or organic agave syrup, which are plant-based natural sugars that do not greatly impact your blood sugar levels. For a longer list see *Low Blood Sugar* and *Insulin Resistance*.
- Drink lots of herbal teas and at least 6–8 glasses of water a day. Water suppresses appetite and helps prevent fat from depositing in the body; it reduces water retention and encourages toxins to be flushed out of the body. Researchers from Virginia have found that drinking two glasses of water before every meal can help you lose an average of 5lbs more.
- Essential fats are vital if you want to lose weight. (See *Fats You Need To Eat*.)

- Use rice or oat bran for extra fiber.
- Ask at your health store for a magnesium- and/or potassium-based salt such as Himalayan Crystal Salt, or use powdered kelp or nori seaweed flakes as a salt substitute.
- In general, fewer vegetarians suffer from obesity, heart disease and cancer. (See *Vegetarianism*.)
- Caffeine is an appetite suppressant, although a fairly toxic one.
- Use organic coffee.

Useful Remedies

- Refined foods deplete the body of many vital minerals, and virtually everyone who eats them to excess is lacking in the mineral chromium. Begin taking 200mcg daily in between meals to help reduce your chance of developing late-onset diabetes and to reduce cravings for sweet and refined foods. It takes a while to kick in, but it really does help reduce sugar cravings. Furthermore, scientific investigations have shown that it can help reduce body fat and increase muscle concentration during exercise.
- Take a high-strength B complex to support your nerves and aid digestion.
- Include a good-quality multi-vitamin/mineral for your age and gender in your regimen. The vitamin companies listed on pages 15–16 would be happy to help you choose the right supplement.
- Co-enzyme Q10, a vitamin-like substance, is needed for the conversion of fat into energy within body cells. Research shows that as many as half of all obese people are deficient in CoQ10. Take 100mg per day with breakfast or lunch.
- The amino acid L-carnitine helps the body produce energy from fat; take 500mg twice daily 30 minutes before food.
- Soluble fiber, such as ready-cracked flaxseeds, aids fat elimination from the intestines and helps prevent the re-absorption of toxins by keeping you regular. Soak a tablespoon of flaxseeds overnight in cold water, drain, and add to smoothies or oatmeal daily.

- The amino acid tyrosine helps you maintain your chosen weight once you have reached it. Take 500mg twice daily before meals.
- Try a carb blocker with Phase 2, made from white kidney bean extract, which helps prevent the digestion and absorption of approximately 60% of starches (such as pasta, rice, cereals, potatoes, and bread) that you may consume. However, if you continue to eat lots of white-flour-based cakes, cookies, and desserts, this supplement would be less effective. **VC**

Helpful Hints

- Some people find it easier to lose weight by "grazing" all day on healthy snacks, which helps balance their blood sugar. So regular nibbling is one of the simplest, but most effective, ways to start losing weight. Others say that if they eat three sensible meals a day, which includes an oatmeal-type breakfast, a good lunch (without dessert), and a light supper, with no snacks in between, they also lose weight. Listen to your body.
- Many people now consider food combining as being out of date, but naturopath Stephen Langley says: "There is no doubt that food combining aids better digestion and encourages weight loss. The basic rule is, if you are eating a protein food such as meat, eggs, cheese, fish or chicken, then avoid the major starches such as bread, pasta, rice or potatoes in the same meal. And if you are eating starches, then eat them without any of the major proteins."

- Regular exercise increases your metabolic rate, decreases fat deposits, and helps reduce food cravings. Regular exercise also increases muscle mass, which burns more energy just to keep the muscles functioning properly. The most important part of regular exercise is that it needs to be **regular**, and burning yourself out in the first week is the easiest way to ensure you won't continue. Aim for 30 minutes of exercise at least five times a week. The best way is simply to walk for 30 minutes or more every single day. I have a girlfriend who was 224lbs and would not diet at all, but she agreed to start walking daily. At first she hated it, but as the pounds fell away over several months, she was delighted and now feels irritable if she does not get her daily walk. She is 69 years old, so it's never too late to start!
- Gradually build the intensity and vary the style of your exercise. Consider joining a local dance, aerobic exercise, or swimming club. It really helps if you work out with people who have the same goal in mind. For this reason, join Weight Watchers. To find a meeting near you, visit www.weightwatchers.com
- Eat the majority of your food before 7:30pm if possible and try to make breakfast and lunch your larger meals of the day.
- An excess of estrogen can cause weight gain and water retention if your body is low in progesterone. (For details of natural progesterone cream, see *Menopause*.)
- Try reading *Eat More, Weigh Less* by Dr Dean Ornish (Quill Press) or the *End of Overeating* by David A Kessler (Penguin).
- If you think you might suffer from an eating disorder, get professional help. Call the National Eating Disorders Association's information and referral helpline: 1-800-931-2237 or visit www.nationaleatingdisorders.org

Author's note

After six months of intense research, hundreds of hours of typing, plus phone calls and interviews that I thought would never end, I am delighted to have reached the end of the Hints Section!

In updating this book I have learned huge amounts, and I hope you will, too. I have added several new headings, but if your specific condition is not mentioned I apologize. If I had tried to feature every illness, this book would be thousands of pages thick rather than an easy-to-read health reference guide. But without a doubt Steve, Gareth, and I have endeavored in our own ways to give you a good foundation to enable you to become your own health detective.

Due to my work schedule I can no longer answer individual letters, but there are plenty of names and addresses to turn to for more help. Or you can find more on my website: www.hazelcourteney.com

Remember, you can still enjoy treats, but simply balance them with plenty of healthy foods. It's never too late, and always keep in mind that the right food is the best medicine! Your body is perfectly capable of healing itself if it's given the right tools for the job. Above all, reduce the stress in your life, exercise regularly if you can, and as much as possible, enjoy your journey.

Good luck and good health.

Hazel Courteney, Stephen Langley, and Gareth Zeal

USEFUL INFORMATION

ACUPUNCTURE

This practice goes back more than 3,000 years. Basically, an acupuncturist inserts fine sterile needles into specific meridian energy points in the body, which encourage energy and blood to flow more freely. Specialist scanners can now clearly see blocked energies within the human body (see *Electrical Pollution* and *Healing*). And when these blockages are released, the body's self-healing mechanisms become more effective. Acupuncture is medically and scientifically proven to reduce pain and can also help alleviate inflammation, water retention, balance hormones and emotions, help infertility and pregnancy problems, nausea, sciatica, back and neck pain, migraines and so on. To find your nearest nationally certified practitioner, contact:
National Certification Commission for Acupuncture and Oriental Medicine
76 South Laura Street, Suite 1290,
Jacksonville, FL 32202
Tel: 1-904-598-1005
Fax: 1-904-598-5001
Website: www.nccaom.org

Stephen Langley, MBAc, my co-author, specializes in facial acupuncture at the Hale Clinic, 7, Park Crescent London, UK W1B 1PF.
Tel: 011-44-20-7631-0156

ADVANCED REFLEXOLOGY

Anthony Porter has been a reflexologist since 1972. During the 80s he went to China and the Far East to teach reflexology and found that their methods, when combined with his own, gave even better results. He has taught his advanced techniques to thousands of reflexologists internationally and says: "With ART we can not only balance various parts of the body (which is what happens with normal reflexology), but we can also feel more subtle changes within the 7000 nerve endings or reflex areas of the feet, and, after working on them, this has a profound therapeutic effect." Medical research with a leading gynecologist has shown huge success with easing the pain and distress of many gynecological conditions that might have otherwise needed surgery. Anthony has also had had great success with infertility, stress, and a host of health problems. To find more details about ART or Anthony's practice in Central London, visit www.artreflex.com or call 011-44-20-8920-9555.

In the US, you can contact Lil M. Mueller, Wisconsin (www.rayofhopereflexology.com); Pauline S. Uri, California (www.mtshastareflexology.com); or Guadalup Verhaeghe, Michigan (Manual Therapeutics, Tel: 1-989-631-0088).

ALEXANDER TECHNIQUE

This technique teaches you how to use your body more efficiently, as well as how to have balance and poise with minimum tension in order to avoid pain, strain, and injury. To find your nearest practitioner, contact:

American Society for the Alexander Technique
P.O. Box 2307, Dayton, OH 45401-2307
Tel: 1-800-473-0620 or 1-937-586-3732
Fax: 1-937-586-3699
Website: www.alexandertech.org
E-mail: info@amsat.ws

AROMATHERAPY

Aromatherapy is the use of essential oils to improve health and well being through massage, inhalation, compresses, and baths. It is excellent for reducing muscle spasm, stress, and anxiety.
For a register of practitioners, contact:

Aromatherapy Registration Council
5940 SW Hood Ave., Portland, OR 97039
Tel: 1-503-244-0726
Fax: 1-503-244-0727
Website: www.aromatherapycouncil.org
E-mail: info@aromatherapycouncil.org

National Association for Holistic Aromatherapy
P.O. Box 1868, Banner Elk, NC 28604
Tel: 1-828-898-6161
Fax: 1-828-898-1965
Website: www.naha.org
E-mail: info@naha.org

The International Society of Professional Aromatherapists (IFPA)
82 Ashby Road, Hinckley, Leicestershire, UK LE10 1SN
Tel: 011-44-1455-637987
Fax: 011-44-1455-890956
Website: www.ifparoma.org
E-mail: admin@ifparoma.org

BACH FLOWER REMEDIES

This is a healing system used to treat emotional problems, such as fear and hopelessness. The

liquid remedies are made from the flowers of wild plants, bushes, and trees.
For further information contact:

The Bach Centre
Mount Vernon, Bakers Lane, Sotwell,
Oxfordshire, UK OX10 0PZ
Tel: 011-44-1491-834678
Fax: 011-44-1491-825022
Website: www.bachcentre.com

Flower Essence Society
P.O. Box 459, Nevada City, CA 95959
Tel: 1-800-736-9222 or 1-530-265-9163
Fax: 1-530-265-0584
Website: www.flowersociety.org
E-mail: mail@flowersociety.org

BOOKS
If you have difficulty finding any of the recommended books, or simply want to find a book on your condition, search online at Amazon.
Website: www.amazon.com

CHELATION
Chelation, an intravenous treatment using the synthetic amino acid EDTA, has been proven to improve blood flow in blocked arteries in heart, diabetic, and stroke patients by removing toxic metals from the body. When combined with antioxidants and other substances, the healing and anti-aging effects are amplified. It is very useful if you have any of the above conditions, plus senile dementia, Alzheimer's disease, Parkinson's disease, ME, chronic fatigue, arthritis or multiple sclerosis, or if you want to prevent cancers. It is also known as IVAT—Intravenous Antioxidant Therapy.

For further details read *Detox With Oral Chelation* by David Jay Brown (Smart Publications) or *Everything You Should Know About Chelation Therapy* by Dr Morton Walker (McGraw Hill).

In the US there are a number of chelation clinics. Search Google for your area or check the following websites:
www.holisticnetworker.com
www.worldwidehealthcenter.net
www.alternativesforhealing.com

CHIROPRACTIC
This is a manipulation treatment for disorders of the joints and muscles and their effects on the nervous system. Chiropractors treat the entire body to bring it back into balance and restore health. Once a month I visit my chiropractor, who keeps my spine and neck mobile after an injury several years ago. To find a practitioner in your local area, contact:

The American Chiropractic Association,
1701 Clarendon Blvd., Arlington, VA 22209
Tel: 1-703-276-8800
Fax: 1-703-243-2593
Website: www.acatoday.org
E-mail: memberinfo@acatoday.org

COLONIC HYDROTHERAPY
Colonic hydrotherapy is a method of cleansing the colon that flushes away toxic waste, gas, accumulated feces, and mucus deposits. This is a safe treatment when given by a qualified professional. Check with your doctor before undertaking this therapy. Colonics are very useful if you are chronically constipated or have taken antibiotics or painkillers, which can cause constipation. For a list of practitioners, contact:

International Association for Colon Hydrotherapy
11103 San Pedro, Suite 117,
San Antonio, TX 78216
Tel: 1-210-366-2888
Fax: 1-210-366-2999
Website: www.i-act.org
E-mail: homeoffice@i-act.org

COUNSELING
If you, or a member of your family, is in need of professional counseling, contact:

American Counseling Association
5999 Stevenson Ave., Alexandria, VA 22304
Tel: 1-800-347-6647
Fax: 1-800-473-2329
Website: www.counseling.org

American Association of State Counseling Boards
3-A Terrace Way, Greensboro, NC 27403
Tel: 1-703-212-2239
Fax: 1-703-212-4884
Website: www.aascb.org
E-mail: aascbinfo@counseling.org

American Psychological Association
750 First Street, NE, Washington, DC 20002
Tel: 1-800-964-2000
Website: www.apa.org

CRANIAL OSTEOPATHY
This is a gentle method of osteopathy that concentrates on the nerves and bones in the head, neck, and shoulders. Many readers have reported relief from ME (chronic fatigue syndrome), facial pain, jaw pain, and arthritis

after having this therapy. It is also excellent for draining lymph from the head and neck area. To find your nearest practitioner, contact:

The Cranial Academy
8202 Clearvista Parkway #9-D,
Indianapolis, IN 46256
Tel: 1-317-594-0411
Fax: 1-317-594-9299
Website: www.cranialacademy.org
E-mail: info@cranialacademy.org

GENERAL ORGANIZATIONS

If you want to know more about specific alternative therapies, the following organizations will be happy to give you advice and put you in touch with the practitioners and societies that meet their high standards of practice and therapy:

Alternative Medicine Foundation
PO Box 60016, Potomac,
MD 20859
Fax: 1-301-340-1936
Website: www.amfoundation.org

Hipocrates Health Institute
1443 Palmdale Court, West Palm Beach,
FL 33411
Tel: 1-800-842-2125
Fax: 1-561-471-9464
Website: www.hippocratesinst.org
E-mail: it@hippocratesinst.org
(This clinic is a leader in natural and complementary health care in the US, offering in- and out-patient services utilizing multiple ways of restoring or preserving health, plus educational programs.)

HEALING

Healers channel healing energies through their bodies and out through their hands into the patient's energy field, which encourages the body to heal itself. Healing is especially good for chronic fatigue and for raising energy levels when you are under the weather or suffering from any illness.

Although there are hundreds of good healers in the US alone, there is one I will mention—William Rand, who is a well-known Reiki healer, teacher, and author. Tel: 1-800-332-8112. Website: www.reiki.org.

There is now a wealth of scientific research to show how healing works. See under the *Healing* section.

To find your nearest practitioner, contact:

American Association of Healers
Tel: 1-970-586-3565
Website:
www.americanassociationofhealers.com

HEALING, REIKI

This is a very popular form of hands-on healing. For general enquiries or to find a Reiki Master, contact:

The Reiki Alliance
204 N. Chestnut Street, Kellogg, ID 83837
Tel: 1-208-783-3535
Website: www.reikialliance.com
E-mail: info@reikialliance.com

International Association of Reiki Professionals
P.O. Box 104, Harrisville, NH 03450
Tel: 1-603-881-8838
Website: www.iarpreiki.org
E-mail: info@iarp.org

HERBALISM

This is the practice of using plants to treat disease. Treatment may be given in the form of fluid extracts, tinctures, tablets, or teas. For further details or to locate a qualified practitioner, contact:

American Botanical Council
P.O. Box 144345, Austin, TX 78714
Tel: 1-800-373-7105 or 1-512-926-4900
Fax: 1-512-926-2345
Website: http://abc.herbalgram.org

American Herbalist Guild
P.O. Box 230741, Boston, MA 02123
Tel: 1-857-350-3128
Website: www.americanherbalistsguild.com
E-mail: ahgoffice@earthlink.net

American Herbal Products Association
8484 Georgia Ave., Suite 370,
Silver Springs, MD 20910
Tel: 1-301-588-1171
Website: www.ahpa.org

HOMEOPATHY

Homeopathy works in harmony with the body to stimulate the body's natural healing mechanisms. It uses minute amounts of a particular substance (made from animal, vegetable, or mineral matter), working under the concept that if you are exposed to minute amounts of the same bacteria or virus, or whatever ails you, this stimulates the body's natural defense mechanisms. It treats like with like. For example, a large amount of the "poison nut" found in nature (which becomes homeopathic nux vomica) would make you feel very ill indeed; however, a minute amount in homeopathic form can alleviate symptoms of vomiting and nausea in most cases very quickly.

For a register of professionally qualified homeopaths and general information about homeopathy, contact:

North American Society of Homeopaths
P.O. Box 450039, Sunrise, FL 33345
Tel: 1-206-720-7000
Fax: 1-208-248-1942
Website: www.homeopathy.org
E-mail: NashInfo@homeopathy.org

National Center for Homeopathy
101 S Whiting Street, Suite 16,
Alexandria, VA 22304
Tel: 1-703-548-7790
Fax: 1-703-548-7792
Website: www.homeopathic.org
E-mail: info@nationalcenterforhomeopathy.org

HYPNOTHERAPY
By allowing external distractions to fade, hypnotherapy allows you to fully relax and understand the root cause of many of your problems, phobias, and addictions. To find your nearest practitioner, contact:

American Association of Professional Hypnotherapists
16055 SW Walker Road, #406,
Beaverton, OR 97006
Tel: 1-503-533-7106
Website: www.aaph.org

American Society of Clinical Hypnosis
140 N. Bloomingdale Rd., Bloomingdale, IL 60108
Tel: 1-630-980-4740
Fax: 1-630-351-8490
Website: www.asch.net
E-mail: info@asch.net

National Board for Certified Clinical Hypnotherapists
1110 Fidler Lane, Suite 1218,
Silver Spring, MD 20910
Tel: 1-800-449-8144 or 1-301-608-0123
Fax: 1-301-588-9535
Website: www.natboard.com
E-mail: admin@natboard.com

The Nutrition Source by The Department of Nutrition at Harvard University
Harvard University Nutrition Researchers put up the latest nutrition news along with recipes, resources, links to studies and other useful nutrition information.
Website:
www.hsph.harvard.edu/nutritionsource

IRIDOLOGY
Iridology is a method of analysis rather than treatment that is based on the theory that the whole body is reflected in the eyes. Using a magnifier, the practitioner examines the visible parts of the eyes to pinpoint physical and emotional weaknesses or potential areas that might be causing problems, either currently or in the years to come. For more information, contact:

International Iridology Practitioners Association
Tel: 1-888-682-2208
Website: www.iridologyassn.org
E-mail: iipacentraloffice@iridologyassn.org

The Guild of Naturopathic Iridologists (www.gni-international.org) recommends the following practitioners in the US:

David Pesek
375 Paradise Lane, Waynesville, NC 28786
Tel: 1-828-926-6100
Fax: 1-828-926-6084
Email: drpesek@juno.com

Farida Sharan
P.O. Box 7367 Boulder, Colorado 80306
Tel: 1-303-525-4502
Fax: 1-303-447-0881

KINESIOLOGY
Kinesiology is the science of testing muscle response to discover areas of impaired energy and function in the body. It is especially useful if you think you have a sensitivity or negative reaction to either a food or an external allergen. Kinesiology can also be used to test if the supplements you are taking suit your unique physiology. To find your nearest practitioner, contact:

American Kinesiology Association
P.O. Box 5076, Champaign, IL 61825
Fax: 1-217-351-1549
Website: www.americankinesiology.org

MANUAL LYMPHATIC DRAINAGE
Manual lymphatic drainage is a very gentle, pulsing massage that helps drain the lymph nodes, thereby reducing swelling and pain related to the lymph glands. This is a very useful treatment for ladies who have had breast and/or lymph surgery. It is also great for

reducing water retention anywhere in the body. To find your nearest practitioner, contact:

National Lymphedema Network
116 New Montgomery Street, Suite 235,
San Francisco, CA 94105
Tel: 1-800-541-3259 or 1-414-908-3681
Fax: 1-415-908-3813
Website:
www.lymphnet.org/resourceGuide/manualDraina
ge.htm
E-mail: nln@lymphnet.org

NATUROPATHY

Naturopaths treat the whole person, on a spiritual, physical, and emotional level, to discover any underlying dysfunctions in a patient's life. They then offer advice on dietary changes, supplements, and herbs to help improve or alleviate your condition. Many naturopaths are also qualified homeopaths and/or acupuncturists. They help provide the right tools for the body to heal itself naturally. Because naturopaths treat the person, not the ailment, any treatments are tailored to each individual. For more help contact:

American Association of Naturopathic Physicians
4435 Wisconsin Avenue, NW, Suite 403,
Washington, DC 20016
Tel: 1-866-538-2267 or 1-202-237-8150
Fax: 1-202-237-8152
Website: www.naturopathic.org
E-mail: member.services@naturopathic.org

American Naturopathic Medical Association
P.O. Box 96273, Las Vegas, NV 89193
Tel: 1-702-897-7053
Fax: 1-702-897-7140
Website: www.anma.org

In London, UK, I visit Bob Jacobs, who is a naturopath and homeopath—and a good friend.
Bob Jacobs
The Society of Complementary Medicine
3 Spanish Place, London, UK W1U 3HX
Tel: 011-44-20-7487-4334
Website: www.scmhealth.com
E-mail: admin@scmhealth.com

NEURO-LINGUISTIC PROGRAMMING

This is a profound, yet simple way to reprogram any negative thoughts or habits into more positive ones. It is great for phobias and panic attacks, as well as for attaining your goals in life. For further information on NLP, contact:

American Board of NLP
P.O. Box 531605, Henderson, NV 89053
Tel: 1-888-823-4823 or 1-702-456-3267
Fax: 1-702-436-3267
Website: www.abh-abnlp.com

You can also find an online database of practitioners at www.nlp-practitioners.com

NUTRITIONAL THERAPY
To find the nearest qualified nutritionist who can help you balance your diet and suggest the correct vitamins, minerals, and so on, contact:

Nutritional Therapy Association
P.O. Box 354, Olympia, WA 98507
Tel: 1-800-918-9798 or 1-360-493-0900
Fax: 1-360-528-2564
Website: www.nutritionaltherapy.com
E-mail: nta@nutritionaltherapy.com

ORGANIC PRODUCE

There are a number of organizations dedicated to helping you find places to buy organic, locally grown produce. Use the following websites to help find farmers' markets, family farms, and other sources of organic food in your area.

LocalHarvest
www.localharvest.org

Eat Well Guide
www.eatwellguide.org

Organic Consumers Association
www.organicconsumers.org

The Environmental Work Group also offers a Shopper's Guide to Pesticides that will help you reduce your exposure to pesticides and make better produce choices. Download the PDF version or the iPhone app at www.foodnews.org

OSTEOPATHY

Osteopathy is a system of healing that works on the physical structure of the body. Practitioners use manipulation, massage, and stretching techniques. If you suffer from chronic or sudden back, hip, neck, or shoulder displacement or injury, go to see an osteopath. To find your nearest practitioner, contact:

American Osteopathic Association
142 East Ontario Street, Chicago, IL 60611
Tel: 1-800-621-1773
Fax: 1-312-202-8200
Website: www.osteopathic.org

PILATES

This is a highly effective, low-impact, isometric form of exercise that you can practice even if you have suffered some kind of injury. It is very powerful but gentle. For more information, contact:

United States Pilates Association
1500 East Broward Blvd., Suite 250,
Ft. Lauderdale, FL 33301
Tel: 1-888-484-8772
Website:
www.unitedstatespilatesassociation.com
E-mail:
info@unitedstatespilatesassociation.com

QIGONG

Qigong is an extremely gentle form of exercise (like tai chi) that helps people with impaired mobility, such as severe arthritis. Anyone can practice qigong and no special clothes are needed. For further information, contact:

National Qigong Association
P.O. Box 270065, St. Paul, MN 55127
Tel: 1-888-815-1893
Fax: 1-888-359-9526
Website: http://nqa.org

Qigong Institute
617 Hawthorne Ave., Los Altos, CA 94024
Website: www.qigonginstitute.org
E-mail: qi@qigonginstitute.org

REFLEXOLOGY

Reflexology is the gentle stimulation of the reflex/nerve-ending points on the hands and feet that correspond to every part of the body. By working with pressure on these points, blockages in the energy pathways are released, which encourages the body to heal itself. This is a great way to boost circulation and is really relaxing. To find your nearest practitioner, contact:

Reflexology Association of America
P.O. Box 714, Chepachet, RI 02814
Tel: 1-980-234-0159
Fax: 1-401-568-6449
Website: www.reflexology-usa.org
E-mail: InfoARR@reflexology-usa.org

Also see also details of Advance Reflexology on page 422.

YOGA

The ancient principles of yoga are beneficial for staying healthy and supple well into your 80s and beyond. Yoga teaches relaxation and breathing techniques, together with gentle stretching exercises, which help keep the whole self fit for life. It is especially useful for keeping the spine strong. There is also a monthly YOGA magazine, especially for yoga enthusiasts. Visit www.yogamagazine.co.uk for more information or to subscribe.

To find your nearest class, contact:

American Yoga Association
P.O. Box 19986, Sarasota, FL 34276
Website: www.americanyogaassociation.org
E-mail: info@americanyogaassociation.org

Yoga Alliance
122 W. Lancaster Ave., Suite 204,
Reading, PA 19607
Tel: 1-877-964-2255
Website: www.yogaalliance.com

INDEX